THE PSYCHOLOGY OF RELIGION

Also Available

The Psychology of Prayer: A Scientific Approach
Bernard Spilka and Kevin L. Ladd

The Psychology of Religious Fundamentalism
Ralph W. Hood, Jr., Peter C. Hill, and W. Paul Williamson

The Psychology of Religion

AN EMPIRICAL APPROACH

FIFTH EDITION

Ralph W. Hood, Jr.
Peter C. Hill
Bernard Spilka

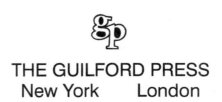

THE GUILFORD PRESS
New York   London

To Emery Grace Jorgensen
—Ralph

To Carol
—Peter

To Ellen, for 65 years of love,
support, and guidance.
My love for you continually grows.
—Bernie

Copyright © 2018 The Guilford Press
A Division of Guilford Publications, Inc.
370 Seventh Avenue, Suite 1200, New York, NY 10001
www.guilford.com

Printed in the United States of America

This book is printed on acid-free paper.

Last digit is print number: 9   8   7   6   5   4   3   2   1

Library of Congress Cataloging-in-Publication Data

Names: Hood, Ralph W., Jr., 1942- author. | Hill, Peter C., 1953- author. |
    Spilka, Bernard, 1926- author.
Title: The psychology of religion : an empirical approach / Ralph W. Hood,
    Jr., Peter C. Hill, Bernard Spilka.
Description: Fifth Edition. | New York, NY : Guilford Press, 2018. | Includes
    bibliographical references and index.
Identifiers: LCCN 2018031189 | ISBN 9781462535989 (hardcover : alk. paper)
Subjects: LCSH: Psychology, Religious.
Classification: LCC BL53 .P825 2018 | DDC 200.1/9—dc23
LC record available at *https://lccn.loc.gov/2018031189*

About the Authors

Ralph W. Hood, Jr., PhD, is Professor of Psychology and Leroy A. Martin Distinguished Professor of Religious Studies at the University of Tennessee at Chattanooga. He is past president of the Psychology of Religion division of the American Psychological Association and a recipient of its William James Award, Virginia Sexton Mentoring Award, and Distinguished Service Award. He is cofounder of *The International Journal for the Psychology of Religion*, for which he has served as coeditor and book review editor. Dr. Hood has also been editor of the *Journal for the Scientific Study of Religion* and is currently coeditor of *Research in the Social Scientific Study of Religion*.

Peter C. Hill, PhD, is Professor of Psychology at Biola University's Rosemead School of Psychology in La Mirada, California. He is past president of the Psychology of Religion division of the American Psychological Association and a recipient of its William C. Bier Award and Distinguished Service Award. He is editor of the *Journal of Psychology and Christianity*.

Bernard Spilka, PhD, is Professor Emeritus of Psychology at the University of Denver. He is past president of the Psychology of Religion division of the American Psychological Association and a recipient of its William James Award and Distinguished Service Award. Dr. Spilka has also been vice-president of the Society for the Scientific Study of Religion and president of the Colorado Psychological Association and the Rocky Mountain Psychological Association. Now retired, he continues to write on the psychology of prayer and on religion, evolution, and genetics.

Preface to the Fifth Edition

At the beginning of the 20th century, those who were to become highly esteemed figures in the history of psychology and its sister disciplines focused much of their interest and attention on religion. In academic psychology, scholars such as William James and G. Stanley Hall not only helped to found psychology, but manifested a great interest in the psychological study of religion. In psychoanalysis, a new field was created outside of academic psychology that nevertheless immensely influenced psychology. One cannot read Freud or Jung for long without encountering extensive discussions of religion.

The second quarter of the 20th century saw a rapid decline in the study of religion among psychologists. Behaviorism was indifferent to the topic, while psychoanalysts relegated it to the province of psychopathology. The net effect was that research in this area remained on the periphery of scientific respectability. The mid-1950s, however, saw a renaissance in the study of religion. Perhaps as psychology became more secure as a science, it could once again look with some interest into the serious investigation of religion. This time the study was less speculative, not as concerned with grand theory, and focused on issues other than the origin of religion. In a word, an *empirical* psychology of religion emerged. This was a more limited view, to be sure, but it demanded that statements about religion be formulated as hypotheses capable of empirical verification or falsification.

In rapid succession, journals devoted to the empirical study of religion emerged in the middle of the last century. Among these were the *Journal for the Scientific Study of Religion*, the *Journal of Religion and Health*, and the *Review of Religious Research*, as well as three journals with specific religious interests: the *Journal of Psychology and Theology*, the *Journal of Psychology and Christianity*, and the *Journal of Psychology and Judaism*. More recently, additional journals and annuals have appeared, including *The International Journal for the Psychology of Religion; Research in the Social Scientific Study of Religion; Mental Health, Religion and Culture;* and *Spirituality and Health International*. Since the fourth edition of this text was published, the American Psychological Association has introduced the journal *Psychology of Religion and Spirituality*.

Likewise, the *Archiv für Religionspsychologie* (*Archive for the Psychology of Religion*), once the yearbook of the Internationale Gesellschaft für Religionspsychologie (International Association for the Psychology of Religion), founded in 1914, has been revived and is now published as a journal; this indicates that the psychology of religion has proven to be a topic of truly international interest. The pertinent literature continues to grow at a rapid rate across the globe. Specialty journals such as the *Journal of Muslim Mental Health* address religious traditions other than Christianity, which has been long dominant in the work of American scholars of the psychology of religion. The domination of interpretative and conceptual discussions of religion in psychology is gradually yielding to data-based research and writing that are pulling the psychology of religion into the mainstream of academic psychology. Likewise, several general and specialty handbooks focusing largely on empirical studies of religion and spirituality have been published. The appearance of the fifth edition of this text is itself an indication of the vigor of our field. Finally, the psychology of religion is now a frequent topic in mainstream psychology journals, indicating the increased frequency of experimental studies in the field.

Our aim remains the same in the fifth edition as in the first four: to present a comprehensive evaluation of the psychology of religion from an empirical perspective. We are not concerned with purely conceptual or philosophical discussions of religion, or with theories that have little empirical support. Interesting as these approaches may be, they generate few, if any, hard data of relevance to their evaluation. We do not, however, ignore these theories when meaningful empirical predictions follow from their claims. When this occurs, they are considered, as are other hypotheses, tentative claims to be judged by the facts. We have not imposed a single theoretical perspective across all the chapters. However, we do see the issue of meaning and control as the single most general theme running through each of the chapters. We avoid siding unequivocally with any of the emerging grand theories, such as evolutionary psychology, that have been proposed to integrate the psychology of religion. Likewise, we do not give exclusive dominance to a single empirical approach, such as cognitive science; nor do we unequivocally endorse emerging areas of psychology, such as positive psychology. Instead, these theories, approaches, and areas are integrated where relevant throughout the text. We simply approach the field from an empirical perspective, broadly conceived to include any studies in which either quantitative or qualitative data are germane to establishing and/or resolving questions of fact. Although we are sensitive to the difficulties and limitations of a purely empirical approach, we have not abandoned the commitment to empiricism as the single most fruitful avenue to understanding the psychology of religion. However, as several of the chapters also reveal, the same empirical data can lend credence to radically different ontological claims. Since the work of William James, texts on the psychology of religion have suggested various metaphysical options under which the same empirical data can be viewed with radically different consequences. All we ask is that our readers not lose sight of the empirical data, so that various theoretical interpretations can be recognized and evaluated in terms of their relationship to these data.

While we retain the basic structure of the fourth edition, we have added much new material while trying to show the continuity of the field. However, as with the fourth edition, many chapters can be read independently, so instructors can reduce the range of material assigned on the basis of their own classes' needs. The rich variety of empirical research that continues to be published is itself a testimony to the vitality of the field.

We briefly acknowledge three major cultural influences that have affected our field. The first is the growth of spirituality outside of organized religion. A glance at the references for the fifth edition reveals numerous titles that reference spirituality, not simply religion. In some areas, such as health, few studies refer to religion alone, and many titles reference both religion and spirituality. How this growth of spirituality has occurred, and why, is addressed throughout the text.

The second is the role of the John Templeton Foundation in funding projects concerned with the psychology of religion and spirituality. Various splinter foundations established as offshoots have also heavily funded the scientific study of religion and spirituality. We simply acknowledge, although not without criticism, that the availability of such funding sources often guides the direction and prominence of research agendas.

Finally, September 11, 2001, remains a crucial date for psychologists who study religion. Fundamentalism in all its forms has become a major issue. Even those who thought that religion could be ignored as a topic of study have recognized that religion continues to have a powerful influence on the course of history.

Our hope is not only that this new edition fairly represents the research and scholarly literature, but also that it will encourage young psychologists to participate in the empirical study of religion, regardless of how they otherwise identify their own psychological expertise.

Acknowledgments

The fifth edition of a book represents a long history of searching for information, as well as support and direction, from others. We have relied strongly on guidance from scholars who convey to us points of view we might otherwise have overlooked. Despite our best efforts, we can never thank all who deserve recognition.

Ralph W. Hood, Jr.: I have benefited greatly from discussions with my colleagues and frequent coauthors Ron Morris, Paul Watson, and W. Paul Williamson on issues related to the psychology of religion. I am also very grateful for friendly and pertinent discussions with Jacob Belzen, Christopher Silver, Margaret Poloma, and David Wulff on the range and scope of psychology in general and of the psychology of religion in particular. I am especially grateful for cooperative research on projects of extended length, one with Heinz Streib and several with W. Paul Williamson. I am extremely thankful for a few days with Antoine Vergote that reminded me that scholarship and faith need not be antagonistic.

Peter C. Hill: It is again an honor to have my name associated with Ralph W. Hood and Bernie Spilka, who have been wonderful mentors and colleagues throughout the years. Much of my research has been funded by the John Templeton Foundation, for which I am exceedingly thankful. I am also grateful to Clark Campbell, Dean at the Rosemead School of Psychology, for his support. I appreciate the opportunity to learn much from my colleagues at Rosemead and at the Institute for Research in Psychology and Spirituality (IRPS), where ideas are discussed freely and openly. Finally, I express special thanks to Liz Laney and Shannon Maxwell, who helped greatly with research and the many details that go into a book like this.

Bernard Spilka: Special thanks to the editorial team at The Guilford Press. Editor-in-Chief Seymour Weingarten has always been highly supportive of our efforts. Senior Editor Jim Nageotte provided much needed guidance. Above all, we were blessed with a copy editor, Marie Sprayberry, whose proficiency and exactitude were truly exceptional. She has certainly taught all of us much about writing. I must also recognize the amazing ability and positive attitudes of the University of Denver, Anderson Academic Commons Library staff in finding essential information plus obtaining articles and books that were unknown to me. Specifically, I thank Christopher Brown, whose skill at finding the obscure and hidden is truly outstanding. Many thanks as well to the Pew Research Center's Forum on Religion and Public Life, for permission to include some of its exceptional survey material in my chapters. Last, the cooperation, helpfulness, and warmth of my colleagues in this venture made it a true labor of love.

Contents

Contents

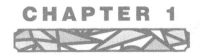

CHAPTER 1

The Psychological Nature and Functions of Religion

There is only one religion, though there are a hundred versions of it.

I assert that the cosmic religious experience is the strongest and the noblest driving force behind scientific research.

I am an atheist still, thank God.

The intractable mystery that was religion is now just another set of difficult but manageable problems.

Things have come to a pretty pass when religion is allowed to invade the sphere of private life.[1]

THE WHY, WHAT, AND HOW OF THE PSYCHOLOGY OF RELIGION

Why Should We Study Religion Psychologically?

There is a surprisingly simple answer to the question of why psychologists should study religion. Religion is of the utmost importance to many people, and many fascinating behaviors are performed in its name. Religion, especially in the "Abrahamic" traditions (i.e., Judaism, Christianity, and Islam—the three major traditions acknowledging Abraham as a prophet and founder), is an integral part of many aspects of our human existence. We surround ourselves with spiritual references, creating a context in which the sacred is invoked to convey the significance of major life events. Regardless of time or place, religion is omnipresent and affects people's lives. It is also true that religion has a dark side and may itself be viewed in negative terms. Some, such as Sam Harris (2004), may be right when they claim that more evil is done in the name of religion than in anything else. Indeed, newly emerging groups of atheists and nonbelievers are challenging the very basis of any and all religious thought as delusional (Dawkins, 2006). As we describe throughout this book, religion, including spirituality (we discuss the distinction between these two terms later in this chapter and throughout

---

[1]These quotations come, respectively, from the following sources: Shaw (1931, p. 378); Einstein (1931, p. 357); Luis Buñuel, quoted in Rogers (1983, p. 175); Boyer (2001, p. 2); Lord Melbourne, quoted in Cecil (1966, p. 181).

the text), has the capacity to bring out the best—and worst—in people. The highly respected personality and social psychologist Gordon Allport, who was also a leading scholar in the psychological study of religion, once said, "The role of religion is paradoxical. It makes prejudice and it unmakes prejudice" (1954, p. 444). Religion thus has both a bright and a dark side.

Is Religion in a Period of Decline?

There is a common perception that religion is losing its influence in society; 70% of Americans in one survey so indicated (The Gallup Poll, 2010a). The degree to which this is an accurate perception depends largely on how religion and spirituality are understood. Certainly there are cultural differences. Europe has already experienced a period where religion, especially institutional religion, has declined. There is evidence that the number of people who identify themselves as atheist or agnostic, as well as people who do not identify with any religion, has increased, but primarily in Europe and to a lesser extent in the United States and Canada (Pew Research Center, 2010). But this is not true everywhere. In fact, it is projected that by the year 2050, atheists and agnostics "will make up a *declining* share of the world's total population" (Pew Research Center, 2015a; emphasis added).

In the United States in particular, few human concerns are taken more seriously than religion. Research tells us that about 92% of U.S. residents believe in God (The Gallup Poll, 2011), and that about 90% pray (Gallup & Lindsay, 1999). Furthermore, 8 out of 10 Americans say that religion is very important (56%) or fairly important (24%), though these numbers have slightly declined in the past two decades (Newport, 2007b). Even among emerging adults, for whom religion is perceived to be losing its influence the most, 70% say that religion is important or very important in their lives (Harvard Institute of Politics [IOP], 2008), and spirituality remains important even in the context of college (Astin, Astin, & Lindholm, 2011; Hill, 2011). Simply put, most Americans see their religious faith as part and parcel of the larger picture of living their lives. Our role is to keep this larger picture before us as we attempt to understand the psychological role of faith in the individual personality. However, we are also cognizant that in many European countries, religion is of much less significance. Religion is more salient in some cultures than in others. Furthermore, religions outside the Abrahamic faiths, such as Hinduism and Buddhism, differ in substantial ways from the Abrahamic faiths and have been less studied by psychologists of religion—although, as we note, this is beginning to change.

The preceding discussion answers another fundamental question: "Why has religion attained such status?" This is a problem not only for both the social sciences and psychology; it is also one for religion, particularly for the theologians who justify and support each faith. Though we may not deal directly with theology, the topics and issues discussed in these pages are central to both psychology and religion, and therefore to religious people everywhere. Particularly in Western civilization, and especially in the North American milieu (for which psychologists have the most reliable empirical data), religion is an ever-present and extremely important aspect of our collective heritage.

What Is the Psychology of Religion?

Psychologists of religion want to know what religion is *psychologically*. However, just as scholars debate the definition of "religion," so do they debate the definition of "psychology." The discussions of psychology and methodology in most contemporary psychology textbooks lack a sophisticated philosophical treatment of various assumptions that are involved in a commitment to any given methodology (Belzen & Hood, 2006; Miles, 2007). This can be illustrated by the fact that the contemporary psychology of religion and spirituality is repeating the scenario that characterized the emergence of the discipline. Our acknowledgment of this will frame our exploration of the methodological options available for psychology of religion.

Even though our approach here examines the person in the sociocultural context, it focuses primarily on the individual; this distinguishes psychological analysis from sociology and anthropology, which examine religion in society and culture—though sometimes the distinction is difficult to make. Our commitment is to no single methodology or ontological perspective. Thus we cannot rest comfortably with any declaration presented as if it defined a discipline or required a priori ontological assumptions. Our discussion assumes "methodological pluralism" (Roth, 1987). That is, we believe that religion and spirituality are best illuminated by a variety of methods, each of which contributes something to our understanding. More controversially, we also assume the stance of "methodological agnosticism," in which transcendent realities remain as possible contributors to a full understanding of religion (Hood, 2012b; Newberg & Newberg, 2010; Porpora, 2006). Furthermore, we accept the call by Emmons and Paloutzian (2003, p. 395; emphasis in original) for "a new *multilevel interdisciplinary paradigm*" for the study of religion.

The perpetual issue for psychology has been to what extent, if any, it can include religious or spiritual constructs that explicitly involve transcendence. Many psychologists subscribe to what is known as the "methodological exclusion of the transcendent," arguing that an empirical psychology must remain within the limits of natural science and not admit any reference to transcendence as playing a causal role in psychology (Flournoy, 1903). In what remains a useful distinction, Dittes (1969) provided four possible options. Each has methodological implications—two that include the possibility of including transcendence, and two that necessarily exclude transcendence. The issue is relevant, insofar as some have argued that in order for psychology of religion to gain respectability, it must court mainstream psychological methods (Batson, 1977, 1979), while others have argued that mainstream psychology can be enhanced by adapting methods and topics unique to the psychology of religion (James, 1890/1950; Hood, 2012b).

Two of Dittes's options support methods that allow the psychology of religion to integrate with mainstream psychology. Dittes's first option is the claim that the only variables operating in religion are the same that operate in mainstream psychology. Therefore, the psychology of religion need have no unique methodologies, as its subject matter is not unique. The second option is that while the variables operating in religion are not unique, they may be more salient in religious contexts, and thus their effect is greater within religion than outside of it. However, they remain purely psychological variables. By definition, these two options adopt the principle of the exclusion of the transcendent first championed by Flournoy, as noted above.

Dittes's second two options allow for the possibility of the inclusion of the transcendent, especially in the study of spiritual experience. The least controversial of the first in this set of two options is that psychological variables uniquely interact in religious contexts, and thus the psychology of religion must acknowledge religion as a cultural phenomenon and study psychological processes that interact with religion (Hood, 2010, 2012b). The final option is that there are unique variables operating in religion that either do not operate in or are ignored by mainstream psychologists. This can include acknowledging the transcendent as an additional causal factor in spiritual experience (Hood, 2012b; Porpora, 2006). Obviously, Dittes's second set of options is more compatible with a nonreductive integrative paradigm for the psychology of religion and spirituality, which seeks to integrate theological and psychological constructs in meaningful research designs. It is also more compatible with the claim that at least some forms of science and some forms of spiritual experience are epistemologically similar (James, 1902/1985; Miles, 2007; Walach, Kohls, von Stillfried, Hinterberger, & Schmidt, 2009). We assume that a basic goal of the psychology of religion is to understand people within the context of their faith commitments. The psychology of religion is but one of many applications of this rather broad definition of psychology; in fact, over 50 specialties have been designated divisions of the American Psychological Association (APA). These divisions represent not only such basic psychological topics as personality, coping/adjustment, clinical psychology, psychological development, and social psychology, but also such specific domains as health psychology, psychology of women, gay and lesbian issues, and peace psychology. For us, the most pertinent one is Division 36, whose history can be briefly noted here as instructive of the diversity that characterizes researchers in the psychology of religion.

A Brief History of Division 36 of the APA

What eventually became Division 36 of the APA began when the Catholic Psychological Association began meeting as an interest group at the 1946 annual meeting of the APA. This interest group gradually morphed into a group named Psychologists Interested in Religious Issues (PIRI), a title formally adopted in 1970 with the intent of obtaining divisional status in the APA. After an initially failed attempt, PIRI obtained divisional status in 1974. In 1992, the division's name was changed to Psychology of Religion. The most recent change occurred in 2010, when Division 36 officially became the Association for the Psychology of Religion and Spirituality.

This brief history suggests tensions and commitments that continue both to unite and to divide psychologists of religion. Whether psychologists are "interested" in religious issues, want to explore psychology *and* religion, seek to identify a psychology *of* religion, or seek to be involved in an association of psychology and spirituality has implications that will become evident throughout this text. To cite but one example, recent handbooks reviewing our field tend to be titled with some variation of *Psychology of Religion and Spirituality*. Paloutzian and Park (2013a) initiated this trend, focusing upon Dittes's first two options. However, the official APA handbook in two volumes goes by the same name, with the first volume devoted to a review of the empirical literature (Pargament, Exline, & Jones, 2013) and the second devoted to clinical application that mesh nicely with Dittes's second two options (Pargament, Mahoney, & Shafranske, 2013). However, as Körver (2015, p. 252) has noted, many psychologists worry that the APA can be seen as promoting superstition and magic, especially among psychologists committed to Dittes's first two options and denying that there is a sacred or transcendent dimension. Finally, yet another handbook (Miller, 2012a; see Miller, 2012b, pp. 1–4) breaks fully with the restrictions of Dittes's reductionistic options and argues for a "postmaterialist" psychology of spirituality—one fully committed to the reality of a sacred transcendent dimension and questioning psychological science's fundamental core ontological assumptions. The diversity of these debates and of the methodologies they support is evident throughout this text.

Understanding Our Limits

We must always keep in mind that there is a major difference between religion per se and religious behavior, motivation, perception, and cognition. We study these human considerations, not religion as such. It is important, therefore, that psychologists of religion recognize their limits. The psychological study of religion cannot directly answer questions about the truth claims of any religion; attempting to do so is beyond its scope. A psychologist of religion may offer insights into why a person holds a specific belief or engages in a particular religious behavior, but this says nothing directly about the truth claim itself that may underlie the specific belief or behavior. However, having said this, we also acknowledge that psychology has implications affecting all of the domains just discussed—and, as we have noted above, psychologists vary widely in what ontological assumptions and methodological commitments they accept in the study of religion.

The Psychology of Religion in Context

By now, it should be clear that our approach emphasizes the empirical and scientific; we go where theory and data take us. But it should also be clear that we see value in different methods of collecting data (something discussed in Chapter 2). The fact that most psychological research has been conducted within the Judeo-Christian framework is reflected in this text. Wherever information is available outside the Judeo-Christian realm, however, we pursue it—and such information is increasing. Again, the essential psychological point here is that psychologists of religion do not study religion per se; they study people in relation to their faith, and examine how this faith may influence other facets of their lives. To do this thoroughly and accurately, however, a psychologist must respect the context of what a person believes to be true, whether it be a major religious tradition, a sect or cult outside the religious mainstream, a spirituality independent of a formal religious tradition, or an agnosticism or atheism (that also involves an orienting belief system)—and whether the psychologist agrees personally with that context or not.

Whereas sociologists and anthropologists look to the external setting in which religion exists, we psychologists focus on the individual. Ours is an internal perspective. Even while we adopt the psychological stance, we must never lose sight of the fact that people cannot really be separated from their personal and social histories, and that these exist in relation to group and institutional life. Families, schools, and work are part of the "big picture," and we cannot abstract a person from these influences. They constitute a large part of what we discuss in the following chapters, in light of the call noted earlier for a multilevel interdisciplinary paradigm.

How Should We Study Religion Psychologically?

We have already provided the short answer to the question of how to study religion psychologically: We advocate an empirical, scientific approach. Now we'll explain. From a scientific perspective, a psychologist desires to gather objective data—that is, information that is both public and capable of being reproduced. Even though there is contention in scientific circles about how to go about collecting such information, the problem for the empirical scientist is how to carry out research without letting his or her biases affect the outcome (Roth, 1987). The sociologist C. Wright Mills is reported to have declared, "I will make every effort to be objective, but I do not claim to be detached." As we will see, it is often not easy to remain either "detached" or "objective."

Perhaps the challenge of objectivity is even greater when the object of study is something about which people have strong opinions, such as religion. A fair question to ask is this: "Can a psychologist of religion who is also devoutly religious be objective?" From the standard scientific perspective, an individual who is both a believer and a scientist may experience a conflicting struggle for definitive answers, and thus may be less able or less qualified to be objective. We should note, however, that theological conviction is a problem not just for a religious psychologist, but for any psychologist who takes a stand regarding religion. The agnostic and the atheist likewise must constantly seek to avoid prejudices that may jeopardize objectivity.

Though it is certainly true that extreme positions exacerbate conflicts (Reich, 2000), "extreme" is in the eye of the beholder; that is, what is reasonable to either a committed believer or a committed scientist may seem unreasonable and extreme to the other. Examination of the "objective" realm may necessitate parallel examination of one's "subjective" commitments. Self-examination is a prerequisite to self-understanding and to the avoidance of short-sighted prejudices. At the very least, all researchers should acknowledge their own vulnerabilities to bias, and should resolve to prevent (as much as possible) those biases from driving their research and conclusions.

A scientific treatment of religion may be subject to the criticism that science is usurping religious prerogatives—something we have already stated we are trying to avoid. There are several ways to consider the relationship. First, in order to accomplish this goal, one might want to adopt an approach described by the late Stephen Jay Gould (1999). Gould argued that there is no inherent conflict between religion and science, insofar as science deals with facts and religion with values. Thus religion and science are nonoverlapping domains of teaching authority. This is a version of "giving to God that which is God's, and to Caesar that which is Caesar's." However, Gould's dichotomy is unsatisfactory to many faith traditions, which insist on the historical accuracy of what others see as myths, and which also accept as fact events (e.g., miracles) that are unacceptable to science. A second approach available to the religiously committed scholar is to consider science as an avenue to God. This implies that God primarily works through natural law and processes. Another religious judgment might claim that a religious psychologist gains insight into God's way in the world, and that humanity may possibly be endowed with a naturalistic awareness of God's existence. As interesting as these perspectives may be, if we are to be true psychologists of religion, we must wear the scientific mantle when we conduct our research and formulate our theories about faith in the life of the individual.

Let's Be Realistic

We have stated our hopes and ideals. The problem is the way people, including psychologists, tend to think and behave in real life. Professional psychologists are quite as subject to prejudices against religion (with a smaller number favorably prejudiced toward religion) as their religious peers have been to prejudices against (or for) psychology. Some clinicians perceive religion as inducing mental pathology and countering constructive thinking and behavior (Cortes, 1999). At times in this book, we will see that religion creates problems and can be "hazardous to one's health." We will also see that religion functions in a much more constructive manner for the majority of people. We further show that the kinds of religion being judged and the standards used to judge religion have an impact on any evaluation of the usefulness of personal faith. Indeed, anyone can selectively employ psychological research to make a case either for or against religion. The better quest is to understand religion in its manifold varieties.

It is obvious that a scientific, empirical approach is the one favored in this volume, but we do not take this in the narrow sense of focusing only upon laboratory-based experimental research. Any empirical method that helps us understand religion is accepted, including qualitative methods such as interviews and individual narratives. By taking this perspective, we intend to note the potential for biased views to enter the picture and to reduce such bias, even as we admit our own vulnerability to bias. Indeed, we three authors have varied faith commitments, and we hold varying values.

The Necessity of Theory

Knowledge has to be meaningfully ordered, and theories can provide that necessary order. Theory is therefore central to an empirical approach. The noted social psychologist Kurt Lewin is reported to have said that "there is nothing as practical as a good theory." Theories are the ways we have of organizing our thoughts and ideas, so that the data we collect make sense because all of the relevant variables have been studied. Without theories, we have little more than a random and confusing collection of research results. So we need to develop theories to tell us what factors or variables may or may not be pertinent when certain problems and issues are examined. Theories should first be formulated in interaction with any available data, and then should be used to guide research.

But where do these theories come from? The prime source for the psychology of religion has usually been mainstream psychology—primarily personality and social psychology, though clinical, developmental, and cognitive psychology have also provided theoretical foundations. Let us consider what Hill and Gibson (2008) have identified as three theories of continuing promise for the psychology of religion. First, attribution theory has been instrumental in guiding research in the psychology of religion and has been a central guiding theory in what is now the fifth edition of this book. Second, many issues in the study of personal faith involve personality, mental disorder, and adjustment; hence coping theory is of great importance. Third, there is much concern about how personal religion develops in early life and changes over the lifespan. As these examples suggest, psychology is a complex field with a large number of subdisciplines. All have the potential to provide theories for the psychology of religion.

Even though we usually look to the main body of psychological knowledge to guide us theoretically, there is no reason why the psychology of religion itself may not eventually provide us with new and constructive directions. Indeed, some of its findings do not fit well with other parts of psychology; this implies that these other subareas may be able to benefit from the psychological study of religion. For example, the recent positive psychology movement, particularly with its focus on human flourishing and the development of virtue, may draw many insights and ideas from the psychology of religion (Hill, 1999; Hill & Hall, 2018).

Clearly, we are not confined to psychology and its subdisciplines for theoretical guidance. Sociology, anthropology, and biology cannot be ignored. Indeed, because the significance of religion is of such breadth and magnitude, we cannot deny the possibility that fruitful ideas will come from other scientific and nonscientific sources. Even theologies themselves can serve as psychological theories (Spilka, 1970, 1976). But to say that we take ideas from such other areas does not mean that the ideas remain unchanged. They may be altered because the psychology of religion has somewhat different interests, or because modifications are necessary to enhance their fit with our data. The theories we hold are "open"; they are always amenable to new information. Closing our minds is the most impractical thing we can do. Our approach is therefore both theoretical and empirical, because neither aspect by itself is meaningful.

WHAT IS RELIGION?

To this point, we have tried to answer the "why," "what," and "how" questions about the psychology of religion. Before we go any further, maybe we need to step back and ask an even more fundamental question: The psychological study of religion requires that we understand what religion is in the first place. For thousands of years, scholars have been writing and talking about religion. Chances are that more books have been written on religion, or some aspect of religion, than any other topic in the history of humanity. With such impressive evidence of concern, who would have the temerity to ask, "Just what is it you are talking about?" Boldness notwithstanding, this is a very good question to pose to anyone.

There may be a tendency for some to disregard such questions as unnecessarily pedantic—one of those exercises that interest academics, but in which few others see value. "I know religion when I see it" is a common (but vague) response, and indeed there may be considerable agreement on some aspects of being religious, at least within a given culture. Such a response, however, not only fails to satisfy scientific and intellectual curiosity; it leaves any observation open to the phenomenon that social psychologists refer to as the "false-consensus effect" (Ross, Greene, & House, 1977)—the tendency to overestimate the extent to which others hold one's own opinions or views. There is no reason to think that religious perceptions and beliefs are uniquely immune from such cognitive bias. Hence what one person is sure to call religious may be far removed from another person's understanding, especially when we begin to analyze religion across traditions and cultures.

Is Defining Religion Even Possible?

Any attempt to define religion therefore immediately runs into trouble. We feel quite confident that we can come to a meeting of the minds if we deal with the Judeo-Christian heritage and the Islamic tradition, but once we go beyond these to the religions of eastern Asia, Africa, Polynesia, and a host of other localities that are not well known in North America and Europe—or even to the Native religious traditions of the United States and Canada—we find ourselves in great difficulty. Religion may encompass the supernatural, the non-natural, theism, deism, atheism, monotheism, polytheism, and both finite and infinite deities; it may also include practices, beliefs, and rituals that almost totally defy circumscription and definition.

The best efforts of anthropologists to define "religion" are frustrated at every turn. Guthrie (1996b) claims that "the term religion is a misleading reification, labeling a probabilistic aggregate of similar, but not identical ideas in individual heads" (p. 162; see also Guthrie, 1996a). In other words, we select a number of ideas and observations that we think belong together and call it "religion." The fact that we use one word to describe a complex of beliefs, behaviors, and experiences as "religious" is often enough for us to believe that religion is really one entity, and that we can expect to find the same or similar phenomena anywhere else in the world.

The assumption that the term "religion" really represents one entity leads to a second question: "On what basis do we group the components we now call 'religion'?" The evident answer is that we call upon our experiences, obviously in our own society and culture, and then uncritically generalize these to other peoples. For example, if idols are found, they are often considered representations of the Judeo-Christian God; rituals are frequently viewed as religious ceremonies; and trances are commonly termed "mystical religious states." We distinguish religion from other aspects of our culture, but such a distinction may be invalid elsewhere, and our interpretations can be very wrong. The noted anthropologist Murray Wax (1984) affirms "that in most non-Western societies the natives do not distinguish religion as we do" (p. 16).

The sociologist J. Milton Yinger (1967) maintained that "any definition of religion is likely to be satisfactory only to its author" (p. 18), and a noted early psychologist of religion, George Coe (1916), said that he would "purposely refrain from giving a formal definition of religion. . . . partly because definitions carry so little information as to facts" (p. 13). The situation has changed little in the past century. That said, it is important to recognize that there are important differences between religious traditions. Many of us in the West are familiar with Christianity but are less likely to know much about other major religions, so we now provide a brief review of the five major world religions. This is not a text on comparative religion, so we are not going into great detail; we focus primarily on the major substantive issues within each religious tradition that are particularly relevant to psychological functioning.

The Five Major World Religions

For people who identify with a religious tradition, religion often becomes an important source of cultural identity, especially when it is a minority religion. In fact, Cohen (2009) maintains that religion should be thought of as a cultural variable. Thus the ability to practice one's religious faith freely, without fear of repercussion or ostracism from the larger culture; to impart religious education to one's children; to mingle with other people of the same tradition; and to have access to places of worship are all important contributors to one's cultural identity (Tarakeshwar, 2013). To understand how religion and spirituality are formed and how they function within specific populations, it is crucial to understand their cultural manifestations in light of the specific claims made by the major religious traditions within which they are embedded.

Islam

Islam is a highly diverse religion, and only the most general Islamic beliefs and practices, common to most all Muslims, are reviewed here (for a more detailed description, see Esposito, 1998, or Gordon, 2002). Islam is a monotheistic religion that includes beliefs in divine judgment (heaven and hell) and predestination (though with allowance for free will that is granted by Allah) (Abu-Raiya, 2013). The Qur'an is Islam's holy book and is considered the direct word of Allah (God). All beliefs and ethical guidelines must be filtered through the Qur'an. Islamic practices include the "Five Pillars of Islam"—five required practices that reflect the human relationship with Allah, and that together constitute the Islamic ritual system and ceremonial duties (Gordon, 2002).

- *Shahada,* or the testimony of faith, is the oft-repeated act of stating with conviction that "There is no true god but Allah, and Muhammad is the messenger of Allah" during ritual duties.
- *Salah,* the ritual of prayer, is considered the single most important ritual, in that it alone is considered the supreme act of righteousness.
- *Zakah,* or alms giving, is the act of the annual distribution of material possessions to the less fortunate. The ritual has the spiritual significance of purification of one's soul, so that there will be no suffering in the next life.
- *Sawn,* or fasting during the month of Ramadan, involves a righteous intention of discipline whereby the Muslim cannot eat, drink, smoke, or have sexual intercourse from sunrise to sunset during Ramadan.
- *al-Hajj* is the once-in-a-lifetime required pilgrimage (for those who are healthy and can afford it) to Mecca.

There is no single Islamic document that provides explicit guidelines for ethical conduct. Rather, such guidelines must be understood through careful study of the Qur'an. Farah (1987, as summarized by Abu-Raiya, 2013) has identified 10 major Islamic ethical guidelines: (1) Acknowledge no other god but Allah, (2) respect and honor parents, (3) respect others' rights, (4) be generous, (5) avoid killing (except when totally justified), (6) commit no adultery, (7) protect the possessions of orphans, (8) deal equitably and justly in all relationships, (9) be pure, and (10) be humble and unpretentious.

Judaism

Jews, like members of every other religious grouping, tend to be diverse (e.g., Orthodox vs. Conservative vs. Reform Jews), and taking such differences into account is important in understanding Judaism's impact on psychological functioning. Nevertheless, certain characteristics of Judaism cut across such denominational differences and are both similar to and in contrast with the characteristics of other religious traditions. For example, compared to most other religious traditions, Judaism (as well as Hinduism) is a "religion of descent" (Morris, 1996); that is, one's religious identity is primarily determined by birth. One *is* a Jew; one does not *become* a Jew. In contrast, other religions might be considered "religions of assent," which emphasize the role of beliefs. Cohen and Hill (2007) have found, for example, that Protestant Christians are more likely than Jews (and, to a much lesser extent, than Catholics) to stress the importance of beliefs to one's religious identity. In contrast, Jews are more likely to stress the importance of practice. One important cultural implication is that Christians and Jews, for example, may use different criteria by which they make moral judgments (Cohen, Gorvine, & Gorvine, 2013). Jews may be less likely than Christians to consider thoughts morally diagnostic. It's the practice that counts, in other words.

Thus "Judaism is a religion concerned with ritual boundaries—kosher versus not kosher, Chosen versus Gentile, Sabbath versus not. Many aspects of the Jewish law first given in the Torah (the five books of Moses) have been extended to be more general so that one does not accidentally transgress a commandment" (Cohen et al., 2013, p. 667). As a result, it may be easier for a Jew to understand and even identify with the concept of "religious, but not spiritual" (a category with which a very small percentage of people in the United States self-identify), especially if the term "spiritual" is to be somehow dissociated from institutional religion (Sands, Marcus, & Danzig, 2008). This does not mean that theology, especially as it relates to beliefs, is unimportant in Judaism. It does suggest, however, that what one believes is less constraining in Judaism than it is in some other religious systems (e.g., Christianity); in contrast, what one does very much defines one's identity as a Jew. As Cohen et al. (2013) note, "Much Jewish practice is rooted in traditions that are hundreds and thousands of years old, and religious practice can for some Jews be less about expressing one's personal religious feelings than it is about participating in and continuing the arc of Jewish history, defined by the community's relationship with God" (p. 666).

Christianity

Roughly one-third of the world's population is Christian, with Roman Catholics constituting slightly more than half of the Christian population. Though Protestants are outnumbered by Catholics nearly 3:1 worldwide, they make up the majority of Christians in the United States. Beck and Haugen (2013) have used the statements found in the Apostles' Creed, a 4th-century statement of basic Christian belief, to arrange their discussion of the Christian religion. We provide a brief synopsis of that discussion.

Central to Christian belief is a Trinitarian God—the idea that God is composed of three divine "persons" who are unified into one "being": God the Father, God the Son, and God the Holy Spirit. Though cloaked in masculine terminology, the Trinity is not necessarily seen by Christians as a gendered being. Particularly distinctive is the role of Jesus Christ, the Son in the Godhead, whose life on earth (including his death and reported resurrection) is recounted in the four Gospels (the first four books of the New Testament). Christianity stresses that one can have a personal relationship with God, often described in the idiom of human relationships such as a parental or spousal relationship, through belief in Jesus's claims to be the Son of God. The legitimacy of Christ's claims is believed by Christians to be rooted in the Biblical recounting of his death (which sacrificially atoned for past, present, and future human sins) and resurrection (which demonstrated the power of life over death, such that believers will also experience their own resurrection for an eternal blissful life in the presence of God). The Holy Spirit is believed by many Christians to dwell within each believer in Christ to provide day-to-day guidance in the believer's spiritual journey.

The Bible is Christianity's sacred text. Though the Bible is revered by all Christians, there are different views on how to interact with the text. Some take a more conservative literalist approach to understanding the Bible, while others interpret the text more symbolically and moralistically.

Buddhism

More than the other major religious traditions, Buddhism is as much a philosophy and a psychology as it is a religion (Kristeller & Rapgay, 2013), and therefore has had perhaps a disproportionate connection with and influence upon psychology. The *dharma* is the communication and translation, in spirit and in content, of core Buddhist concepts into practice. The *dharma* originates from the teachings of the Buddha, which are supported by guidance from the *Sangha*, awakened beings who serve as spiritual leaders. The Buddha, who historically was the person of Siddhartha Gautama, is not a savior to be worshipped as much as it is simply the embodiment of teachings and principles; thus, to "take refuge in the Buddha means to commit to looking for the Buddha within" (Kristeller & Rapgay, 2013). Central to the dharma are the Four Noble Truths: (1) Life necessarily contains *dukkha*, or suffering, which is not to be avoided but understood; (2) the origin of *dukkha* is our desire to seek pleasure and to avoid discomfort; and (3) fully grasping and accepting the first two truths will provide the understanding for release from suffering through (4) following specific instructions known as the Noble Eightfold Path.

The Noble Eightfold Path consists of eight interrelated guidelines for pursuit of a better life, both spiritually and otherwise. The eight paths involve training that falls into three categories, all based upon the intellectual and experiential acceptance of Buddhist teachings: wisdom (two paths: right understanding and right intention); ethics (three paths: right speech, right conduct, and right livelihood); and meditation (two paths: right effort and right mindfulness). Spiritual and personal growth resulting from the intentional practice of these paths will diminish the hold of three life poisons: ignorance, craving, and aversion.

Hinduism

Branches of Hinduism vary considerably from each other, in that some are monotheistic and revere a personal God, while others are monistic and see divinity as pervading all reality. Thus any description of Hinduism in terms of common features is likely to be overly simplistic, and the best that can be done here is to represent a significant portion of the broad religious tradition. However, it is safe to say that common to virtually all religious Hindus is a belief "in a reality that transcends the mundane, empirical, or phenomenal world" (Puhakka, 1995, p. 123).

Most branches of Hinduism are pantheistic, though not in the way pantheism is commonly understood. There are an infinite number of gods who are only *avatars* (manifestations) of the three primary manifestations of the one true Godhead: the Vishnu (who are actually all one), the Trimutri (the three in one—sometimes called the "Hindu Trinity"), and the Brahman (the Supreme Being). The Brahman appears in many forms by emanation throughout the created order. As pointed out in the Vishnu Purana (one of the medieval collections of laws, stories, and philosophy that reflect the teachings of older scriptures):

> Just as light is diffused from a fire which is confined to one spot, so is the whole universe the diffused energy of the supreme Brahman. And as light shows a difference, greater or less, according to its nearness or distance from the fire, so there is a variation in the energy of the impersonal Brahman. Brahma, Vishnu, and Shiva are his chief energies. The deities are inferior to them; the yakshas, etc., to the deities; men, cattle, wild animals, birds, and reptiles to the yakshas, etc., and trees and plants are the lowest of all these energies . . . (Vishnu Purana 1.22)

Though such manifestations are phenomena of a world that is only temporary and partial and conceals total truth, they nevertheless reflect a certain divine immanence that places an emphasis, in positive psychology terms, on experiences of awe and appreciation (Haidt, 2003; Maltby & Hill, 2008).

The ultimate goal of the Hindu moral life is spiritual liberation, or the achievement of unity with the Brahman. To achieve this goal, one must initially also strive toward achieving the lower ideals of wealth, pleasure, and ethical merit. Ultimately, however, such goals must be transcended to achieve union with the Supreme Being, and this is accomplished through four spiritual paths: devotion (through such practices as prayer and rituals), ethical action (through deeds that bring pleasure to the Brahman rather than the self), knowledge (of spiritual bliss), and mental concentration (gaining mastery over one's mind). *Karma,* the teaching that suggests that people's past deeds have an impact on their present lives (as do present deeds for future living, including future lives), can offer a preliminary route to spiritual liberation (by the accumulation of good deeds)—just as it can create a barrier (by the accumulation of bad actions) to developing righteous tendencies and dispositions (Tarakeshwar, 2013).

There are, of course, other religious traditions, but these five are the largest, and their adherents together constitute the majority of the world's population. In addition, there are people who do not explicitly identify with these five (or any other) religious traditions, yet consider themselves as spiritual. This creates additional challenges for the psychology of religion. However, an early psychologist of religion (Dresser, 1929) suggested that "religion, like poetry and most other living things, cannot be defined. But some characteristic marks may be given" (p. 441). Following Dresser's advice, we avoid the pitfalls of unproductive, far-ranging, grandly theoretical definitions of religion. Quite simply, we are not ready for them, nor may we ever be. Many are available in the literature, but the highly general, vague, and abstract manner in which they are usually stated reduces their usefulness either for illuminating the concept of religion or for undertaking empirical research. Our purpose is to enable our readers to understand the variety of ways in which psychologists have defined religion by identifying, in Dresser's words, its "characteristic marks."

However, we admit that we are in a quandary. We deal largely in this book with the Western religious tradition (because that is where most research has been conducted), but we are saying that religion performs many functions for many different people. The extent to which research findings generalize to other religious traditions is still largely unexamined. Surely some of these functions may vary greatly in terms of their surface appearance; however, we feel that at their core they represent the same elemental human needs and roles, about which we will have more to say.

Spirituality and/or Religion?

"Spirit" and "spiritual" are words which are constantly used and easily taken for granted by all writers upon religion—more constantly and easily, perhaps, than any of the other terms in the mysterious currency of faith. (Underhill, 1933, p. 1)

This observation is perhaps even more applicable today than it was over 80 years ago. In the past few decades, "spirituality" has become a popular word. It is now common to refer to "spirituality" instead of "religion," but without drawing any clear distinction between them. Furthermore, much of Western society seems captivated by the notion of spirituality. It is not uncommon to see the topic as the cover story of popular newspapers such as *USA Today*, or news magazines such as *Time*. After reviewing the available literature on spirituality in the early 1990s, Spilka (1993), in his frustration, claimed that spirituality is so "fuzzy" that it has become "a word that embraces obscurity with passion" (p. 1). However, Hood (2003) has argued that "spirituality" is a fluid term often used in opposition to the clearly defined commitments of the religiously faithful. Though Daniel Helminiak (1987, 1996a, 1996b) has written a number of impressive scholarly psychological/philosophical treatises on spirituality, psychologists of religion have not taken his theoretical guidance and provided the kind of objective assessment we are stressing here. As a priest and a psychologist, Helminiak (2015) has completed his major work by arguing for an integration of neuroscience, psychology, spirituality, and theology. On the other hand, Gorsuch and Miller (1999) have suggested that the term "spirituality" can have meaning in the psychology of religion if clear operational definitions are made. As we will see throughout this text, progress is being made to allow clearer empirical distinctions between those who primarily define themselves as "both religious and spiritual" and those who define themselves as "more spiritual than religious" (Zinnbauer & Pargament, 2005).

The Spirituality–Religion Debate

The last few decades have witnessed a growing response to the question of spirituality that draws some distinctions between spirituality and religion. It is as if a "critical mass" of vague definitions has been reached. This has stimulated a new concern with the conceptualization of spirituality that directs our thinking toward its objective assessment and application through research (Hill et al., 2000; Hood, 2000b; W. R. Miller, 1999; Pargament, 1999; Pargament & Mahoney, 2002; Zinnbauer et al., 1997; Zinnbauer, Pargament, & Scott, 1999). Many current thinkers are therefore attempting to create theoretical and operational definitions of spirituality that either distinguish it from personal religiosity or show how the two concepts are related.

A traditional distinction exists between being "spiritual" and being "religious" that can be used to enhance our use of both terms (Gorsuch, 1993). The connotations of "spirituality" are more personal and psychological than institutional, whereas the connotations of "religion" are more institutional and sociological. In this usage, the two terms are not synonymous, but distinct: Spirituality involves a person's beliefs, values, and behavior, while religiousness denotes the person's involvement with a religious tradition and institution (Streib & Hood, 2016).

Psychologists seem to be embracing this distinction. It should be noted that only a minority of psychologists are religious in the classical sense of being affiliated with religious organizations, but that many more see themselves as spiritual (Shafranske & Malony, 1985). Despite the negative reaction the concept of "religion" engenders in most psychologists, aspects of it have become recognized as important for major areas of life. These include the benefits of meditation (Benson, 1975; Benson & Stark, 1996), as well as the evidence that religious people are less likely to use illegal substances, abuse alcohol, or be sexually promiscuous (Gorsuch, 1988, 1995; Gorsuch & Butler, 1976). As a result, religious persons possess better physical health than those engaging in these actions (e.g., Larson et al., 1989).

To some people, wanting only what is good from spirituality without the institutional baggage of religion is an "easy religion" or "cheap grace"; to others, it is "separating the valuable from the superstitious." Clearly, there is considerable debate regarding the potential separation of these concepts. Donahue (1998) forcefully claims in the title of a paper that "there is no true spirituality apart from religion." Pargament (1999) views the separatist trend with ambivalence, and offers guidance to prevent a polarization of these realms. Regardless of how the professionals debate this issue, the distinction may be sharpening on the popular level, with spirituality the favored notion (Roof, 1993). However, as Streib and Hood (2011) note, spirituality remains at best a form of privatized religion. This does not preclude the possibility that spirituality can occur both within and outside religious traditions: thus one can be "both spiritual and religious," or can be "spiritual but not religious."

It is still an open question whether the practice of spirituality outside religion can be adequately defined. Hood (2003) argues that it can be, and we discuss many empirical data supporting this claim throughout this text. If it can, will it then be found to relate to the same variables as religion? The proponents of Transcendental Meditation provide support that some effects of meditation are separate from those of religion (see Chapter 10), but this is a difficult area to research, for training people in a meditation style independent of a religion does not mean that they practice meditation apart from their faith. No one knows at this point whether spirituality will be a more viable psychological construct than religion once it is operationally distinguished from religion. However, the spirituality–religion distinction is gaining considerable empirical support. Distinctions are emerging that show religion to be associated with conservatism, while spirituality is associated with openness to change (Fontaine, Duriez, Luyten, Corveleyn, & Hutsebaut, 2005). Likewise, in a meta-analysis of several studies using the Schwartz Value Scale (Schwartz, 1992), Saroglou, Delpierre, and Dernelle (2004) found that religious persons scored higher on the Conformity and Tradition subscales. They also scored low on subscales assessing values associated with spirituality, such as Universalism. Thus religion may be an institutional expression of particular (but clearly not all) aspects of spirituality. Furthermore, as we discuss later in this text, spirituality is associated with many paranormal phenomena (see Chapters 10 and 11)—phenomena that both religion and science tend to reject.

Can We Distinguish Spirituality from Religion?

Defining "spirituality" in a manner distinct from "religion" can start from the past meanings of the ancient and complex term "spirituality." In Western thought, it has been a part of classical dualistic thinking that pits the material world against the spiritual world. Some things we can see, hear, smell, or touch, whereas elements that exist in the mental world can at best only be inferred from the material world. Non-Western thinkers have seen these two areas as more closely intertwined, but "spirit" still has the sense of being immaterial. For example, in Thailand, a house must be provided for the spirits of a parcel of land before it can be used (many Thai restaurants in the United States have such houses); although the spirits themselves dwell outside of ordinary experience by the human senses, they must still be appeased by a physical dwelling.

A contemporary illustration of setting spirituality apart can be seen in the way many Christian Protestant denominations and churches practice church governance. In these congregations, there are two governing bodies, often called the "deacons" and the "elders" (as they are defined in the New Testament). The deacons are concerned with the material aspects of congregational life, including maintaining a church's physical property and taking food to the needy. The elders are responsible for the spiritual welfare of the church. This includes taking the comforts of the faith to the sick and grieving, and encouraging activities that enhance the members' relationships to God. In other words, the elders are concerned with the inner being of the church members, and the deacons with the more physical aspects of the members' and the church's existence. Rarely do members have trouble defining the "physical" and "spiritual" matters of the congregation. But what these church members know, the psychology of religion (including the psychology of spirituality) needs to spell out—that is, to define operationally.

Another approach to defining spirituality from classical usage is to identify it with "spiritual disciplines." These have included not only such acts as prayer and meditation, but also fasting and doing penance for sins. For example, monks retire to a monastery to practice such disciplines, in order to lead a more spiritual life than is commonly possible outside the monastery. With the traditional Christian Protestant usage noted above and the set of spiritual disciplines, we could just divide the psychology of religion into personal practices (the spiritual) and communal practices (the religious). That is, we could employ both terms, but would not use them synonymously.

There are other ways of defining spirituality that shift the construct to new grounds, and so allow testing of whether "religion" and "spirituality" are just interchangeable terms. Here is one: "Spirituality is the quest for understanding ourselves in relationship to our view of ultimate reality, and to live in accordance with that understanding" (Gorsuch, 2002, p. 8). Streib and Hood (2016) note that if one accepts that for some transcendence can be vertical (Dittes's two nonreductive options) and for others it can be horizontal (Dittes's two reductive options), both religiously and spiritually committed persons can be identified in relation to transcendence. Some differences between this definition of spirituality and a definition of religion include the following:

- Spirituality is personal and subjective.
- Spirituality does not require an institutional framework. Its authenticity requires no consensus or "meeting of the minds."
- A spiritual person is deeply concerned about value commitments.
- A person can be spiritual without a deity (although some would say that the "view of ultimate reality" always includes what Alcoholics Anonymous refers to as a "higher power").
- Religiousness is a subset of spirituality, which means that religiousness invariably involves spirituality, but that there may be nonreligious spirituality as well.

There appears to be a growing consensus that these views are useful in distinguishing religion from spirituality; however, this consensus is still far from being unanimous. We do not intend to force any distinction on the profession—and, in fact, it is safe to say that even we three authors of this text do not fully agree with each other about the meaning of these terms. These are highly ambiguous terms, and the astute consumer of research needs to check carefully what is actually being measured, rather than to rely exclusively on any researcher's use of the term "religious" or "spiritual."

Defining Religion Operationally

From an empirical perspective, what is used to measure religion or spirituality in research is therefore the crucial element. "Operational definitions" literally focus on "operations"—the methods and procedures used to assess something. They are the experimental manipulations plus the measures and instruments employed. With respect to religion, what does it mean to be religious? How do we indicate religiousness? Operationally, we often identify people as religious if they are members of a church or other congregation, attend religious services, read the Bible or other sacred writings, contribute money to religious causes, observe religious holidays or days of fasting, pray frequently, say grace before meals, and accept religiously based diet restrictions, among other possibilities. Many psychologists also look to the beliefs that the devout express, as well as the experiences they report. Frequently, respondents fill out questionnaires about these expressions, and the questions they answer are the operational definitions for that study. There are a great many such operations that illustrate commitment to one's faith.

Basically, operational definitions tell us what a researcher means when religious language is used. For example, suppose we desire to evaluate the degree to which individuals believe in "fundamentalist" doctrines. We might then administer a questionnaire specifically designed to obtain agreement or disagreement with such principles. The Altemeyer and Hunsberger (2004) Religious Fundamentalism Scale might be selected, and we could report its scores for the sample tested. Fundamentalism is thus operationally defined by this measuring instrument. Of course, the scale itself is based on a conceptualization of fundamentalism that needs to be reasonable and testable. However, Williamson, Hood, Ahmad, Sadiq, and Hill (2010) have developed another measure of fundamentalism based on the theory of intratextuality developed by Hood, Hill, and Williamson (2005). Fulton, Gorsuch, and Maynard (1999) have used yet another scale that they call Fundamentalism. Finally, Streib (2008, pp. 58–59) and his colleagues have created a subscale of the Religious Schema Scale named Truth in Text and Teachings, which is also a measure of fundamentalism. This leaves us with at least four different operational measures of fundamentalism. It is important to examine the measures (as well as their underlying conceptual development) closely, to determine how similar and how different their items are. Throughout this volume, we emphasize operational definitions of different aspects or forms of faith. This is the only way we can understand religion from a scientific standpoint. Not all measures of religion are created equal; some are better than others, in that they conform more closely to certain standards of good measurement. We investigate those standards more thoroughly in Chapter 2.

THE NEED FOR MEANING AS A FRAMEWORK FOR THE PSYCHOLOGY OF RELIGION

The assumptions forming the fundamental framework for this book are that the search for meaning is of central importance to human functioning, and that religion is uniquely capable of helping in that search. Our framework suggests that the cognitive, motivational, and social aspects of finding meaning in life offer us the directions necessary for a rather "grand" psychological theory for understanding the role of religion in human life. When we look at cognition, we discover that people are active meaning-making creatures through whose efforts some sense of global meaning is achieved. The study of motivation in finding meaning focuses us on the need of people to exercise control over themselves and their environment. Social life, which we encapsulate in the concept of "sociality," recognizes that people necessarily exist within relationships. Not only must they relate to others to survive and prosper, but it is often through their relational selves that meaning is discovered. In short, people need people, and it is through others that a sense of meaning is often most fully experienced. We now turn our attention to each of these realms.

The Cognitive Search for Meaning

It is safe to assume that all mentally capable people, not just those who are religious, struggle at some point or another to comprehend what life is all about. People need to find their particular niche in the world. It is hardly surprising that pastor Rick Warren's (2002) book *The Purpose-Driven Life* is reported to be the best-selling book of all time, except for the Bible. Viktor Frankl, a survivor of the Auschwitz and Dachau concentration camps in World War II, wrote a book called *Man's Search for Meaning* (Frankl, 1962), which was identified in 1991 by *The New York Times* as among the 10 most influential books in the United States. The struggle with existential questions and the corresponding search for answers sometimes lead individuals to religion. Though there is a kind of scientific vagueness to the idea of "meaning"—and thus psychologists sometimes prefer to use other overlapping terms, such as "cognitive structure"—no other word seems to capture as well its inherent significance, and thus we employ the term without concern.

The first two editions of this book used attribution theory, a staple of social psychology for decades, as a framework for understanding the psychology of religion (see Spilka, Shaver, & Kirkpatrick, 1985, for a full explication of the application of this theory to religious experience). Attribution theory is concerned with explanations of behavior—primarily causal explanations about people, things, and events—and is therefore a theory of meaning making. Such explanations are expressed in ideas that assign roles and influences to various situational and dispositional factors. For instance, we might attribute a person's lung cancer to being exposed to the smoking of coworkers, to his or her own smoking, or to the view that "God works in mysterious ways." All of these are attributions. Research examining such meanings and their ramifications became the cornerstone of cognitive social psychology, and attributional approaches were soon extended to explain how people understand emotional states and much of what happens to them and to others (Fiske & Taylor, 1991). Among the factors that may be involved in understanding the kinds of attributions people make are situational and personal-dispositional influences; the nature of the event to be explained (whether it is positive, negative, or neutral); and the event domain (e.g., medical, social, economic). We will also want to know what cues are present in the situation. For example, does the event take place in a church, on a mountaintop, or in a business office? Similarly, when we turn to personal-dispositional concerns, we may need to get information on the attributor's background, personality, attitudes, language strengths and weaknesses, cognitive inclinations, and other biases. Research Box 1.1 presents a representative attributional study in the psychology of religion.

All of this is well and good. Attribution theory has been extremely useful to social psychology, and Hill and Gibson (2008) have suggested that it has been underutilized by researchers in the psychology of religion. As an effort to acquire new knowledge, the attribu-tional process appears to be a first step in making things meaningful (Kruglanski, Hasmel, Maides, & Schwartz, 1978). Making attributions, however, is only the first step and is there-fore only a small part of the total process. People (whether religious or not) do not talk about their attributions. They talk about what makes life meaningful. Rick Warren's book would hardly have sold if it had been titled *The Attribution-Driven Life*! In the third and fourth editions, and now (even more so) in the fifth edition of this text, we have therefore attempted to provide a more inclusive framework.

Scientists, of course, may not have the luxury of deriving and testing specific empirical hypotheses from such a broad construct as "meaning." For them, more specific theories such as attribution theory are better capable of providing the framework necessary for conducting empirical studies. Therefore, we return to attribution theory in Chapter 2 as a foundational component for the empirical study of religion. For now, though, it is helpful to consider this research in terms of the big picture of the need for meaning. In essence, people need to make sense out of the world in order to live and to adapt; it must be made meaningful. Heintzelman and King (2013, 2014) make the case that, given the adaptive value of meaning in life, people's ability to find meaning must be commonplace. Their review of the empirical data supports their contention. Several national surveys (e.g., House, 2008; Kobau, Sniezek, Zack, Lucas, & Burns, 2010; Oishi & Diener, 2014; Stroope, Draper, & Whitehead, 2013) consistently show that the vast majority of people (over 80% and sometimes about 90%) agree

RESEARCH BOX 1.1. General Attribution Theory for the Psychology of Religion: The Influence of Event Character on Attributions to God (Spilka & Schmidt, 1983a)

This research focused on the components of events that occur to people. When seeking explanations, is a person influenced by (1) whether the event happens to oneself or others; (2) how important it is; (3) whether it is positive or negative; and (4) what its domain is (economic, social, or medical)? Given these possible influences, the emphasis of this study was on the degree to which attributions are made to God.

A total of 135 youths from introductory psychology classes and from a church participated in the study. Twelve short stories were written to depict various social, economic, and medical occurrences. Of the four stories in each of these domains, two described incidents of minor to moderate significance, and two described important happenings. One of each pair was positive, and one was negative. In half of the stories, the referent person was the responder; the other half of the stories referred to someone else. The participants were thus dealing with variations in incident domain, plus the dimensions of how important the incident was, whether the occurrence was positive or negative, and whether it was personal or impersonal. In addition, each participant was able to make attributions to (1) the characteristics of the person in the story; (2) possible others, even if not present in the story; (3) the role of chance; (4) God; or (5) the personal faith of the individual in the story. Lastly, two experiments were constructed. In the first, all of the participants filled out the forms in a school setting; in the second study, half the participants were in a church and half in school. This was an attempt to determine situational influences.

No situational differences were found, but all of the other conditions yielded significance. Attributions to God were mostly made for occurrences that were medical, positive, and important. Many significant interactions among these factors occurred, and though the personal–impersonal factor per se was not statistically significant, it was in its relationships to the other effects. Other research on attributions to God has revealed similar influences (Gorsuch & Smith, 1983).

or strongly agree with such survey items as "My life has a real purpose." Of course, meaning can be found through a variety of sources, such as family and friends (Lambert, Stillman, et al., 2010), generativity to future generations (Erikson, 1964), or provision through occupation (Steger, Dik, & Duffy, 2012). Religion is only one source of meaning, but it is an important source (Park, Edmonson, & Hale-Smith, 2013; Stroope et al., 2013). For example, J. H. Jung (2015) has found that people who believe in direct divine involvement in life are more likely to see life as meaningful. When we turn to religion, we focus on higher-level cognitions and some understanding of ourselves and our relationship to others and the world. The result is meaning—the cognitive significance of sensory and perceptual stimulation and information to us.

Religion and the Search for Meaning

Contemporary forms of Aristotle's dictum "All men by nature desire to know" (McKeon, 1941, p. 689) include Argyle's (1959) claim that "a major mechanism behind religious beliefs is a purely cognitive desire to understand" (p. 57), or Budd's (1973) view that "religion as a form of knowledge . . . answers preexistent and eternal problems of meaning" (p. 79). Clark (1958) maintained that "religion more than any other human function satisfies the need for meaning in life" (p. 419). Why? What is it specifically about religion that entices so many people to look to it to find meaning? For some religious people, the answer is simple: It speaks truth, so they believe, and for some the truth it speaks is so exclusive that no other claims of truth can even compete. Others, of course, find such claims preposterous, even though they too may find meaning through religion. Religion fills in the blanks in our knowledge of life and the world, and offers us a sense of security. This is especially true when we are confronted with crisis and death. Religion is therefore a normal, natural, functional development whereby "persons are prepared intellectually and emotionally to meet the non-manipulable aspects of existence positively by means of a reinterpretation of the total situation" (Bernhardt, 1958, p. 157).

Park (2005) provides an important distinction between what she calls "global meaning," which refers to a general life meaning that involves beliefs, goals, and subjective feelings, and "meaning making," which occurs during times of crisis or difficult circumstances. The two concepts are not independent of each other, and religion is invoked in both senses of the term. "Meaning making" is "a *process* of working to restore global life meaning when it has been disrupted or violated, typically by some major or unpleasant life event" (Park, 2005, p. 299; emphasis in original), and we focus on this throughout many chapters in this book. In this introductory chapter, however, we wish to focus on global meaning, which in Park's model is important to everyday life.

Why Turn to Religion for Meaning?

Why is religion the framework to which so many people turn in their quest to find meaning? First, it must be acknowledged that not all people attempt to find the meaning of life through religion. For many, including those who have tried religion and found it unfulfilling, a subjective sense of meaning is often successfully found through means other than religion. We live, in the words of the social philosopher Charles Taylor (2007), in a "secular age," where the roles and functions of religion in society have changed. Taylor argues not so much that religion has been replaced, but that it has been transformed through an ever-continuing change of options. Each option becomes a new departure point through which new spiritual landscapes are explored; in some cases, people have traveled so far that the old religious mooring can no longer even be identified. So we have gone from a world where belief in God was a given to a world where even atheism is a legitimate option, as we discuss in Chapter 9. One set of continual changes described by Taylor has resulted in a redefined understanding of meaning or fullness from something that comes totally from "beyond" human life to something that can come from "within" human life. Thus, in our secular age, a sense of "transcendence" (something that goes beyond our usual limits) is no longer a necessary requirement for meaning; fullness or meaning in life may also be found in the "immanent" (the state of being within) order of nature, such as in our sense of human flourishing.

For many people, however, religion continues to serve well as a provider of meaning. Hood et al. (2005) have identified four criteria by which religion is *uniquely* capable of providing global meaning: "comprehensiveness," "accessibility," transcendence," and "direct claims." Let us consider each criterion. First, religion is the most comprehensive of all meaning systems in that it can subsume many other sources of meaning, such as work, family, achievement, personal relationships, and enduring values and ideals. Silberman (2005a) demonstrates religion's comprehensiveness by pointing out the extensive range of issues that religion addresses at both descriptive and prescriptive levels: beliefs about the world and self (e.g., about human nature, the social and natural environment, the afterlife); contingencies and expectations (e.g., rewards for righteousness and punishment for doing evil); goals (e.g., benevolence, altruism, supremacy); actions (e.g., compassion, charity, violence); and emotions (e.g., love, joy, peace). Religion's special meaning-making power is due in part to its comprehensive nature.

The second major reason for religion's success as a meaning maker is that it is so accessible (Hood et al., 2005). Many conservative religious groups often stress the importance of a religious "world view"—a religious belief that contributes to global meaning. The accessibility of such a view is often promoted through doctrinal teachings and creeds, religious education, and sometimes even rules of acceptable and unacceptable behavioral practices—often in the name of developing a system of values compatible with the religious tradition. Such people are what Robert Wuthnow (1998) refers to as "religious dwellers." Religious dwellers, as the term implies, are comfortable in establishing and living by the "rules of the house"; they find great comfort in a religion that is not only comprehensive, but also comprehensible. However, not all religious people are dwellers, and some may find religion useful as a different avenue of meaning making. Viktor Frankl (2000) maintained that "the more comprehensive the meaning, the less comprehensible it is" (p. 143), and indeed it is precisely religion's or spirituality's elusive character that makes it so attractive for many people. In contrast to the religious dwellers, Wuthnow (1998) calls these individuals "spiritual seekers"—people who are willing to explore "new spiritual vistas" and are comfortable negotiating "among complex and confusing meanings of spirituality" (p. 5). Such individuals may be more fascinated with the questions than the answers, and may enjoy the freedom from what are otherwise perceived to be the restraints of a religious community connection. Such individuals may still find meaning through their religion, but this meaning is often found more in the process of the search itself than in the answers uncovered or derived.

Religion, by its very nature for many, involves a sense of transcendence—the third reason identified by Hood et al. (2005) for religion's success as a meaning provider. S. M. Taylor (2007) persuasively argues that transcendence should not be insisted upon as a necessary criterion for a sense of significance and fullness. Nevertheless, a belief in a transcendent and authoritative being, especially when complete sovereignty is attributed to that being (as in the case of Western monotheistic religion), is the basis of the most convincing and fulfilling sense of meaning for many (Wong, 1998). Perhaps more than any other system of meaning, religion provides a focus on that which is "beyond me." Thus many people have "ultimate concerns" (Emmons, 1999) that require some belief in an ultimate authority, be it God or some other conception of transcendence in which higher meaning is found. Walter Houston Clark (1958) put it this way: "At the end of the road lies God, the Beyond, the final essence of the Cosmos, yet so secretly hidden with the soul that no man is able to persuade another that he has fulfilled the quest" (p. 419).

Finally, no other system of meaning is so bold in its proclaimed ability to provide a sense of significance. Meaning is embedded within religion's sacred character, so that it points to humanity's ultimate purpose—in the Judeo-Christian tradition, for example, to love and worship God. As S. M. Taylor (2007) notes, for the committed Christian, devotion to a loving or even judgmental God (as in the injunction "Thy will be done") is contingent on nothing else. Christ's sacrificial love for humans, a staple of Christian theology, caused the well-known 18th-century Christian hymn writer Isaac Watts (1707) to put it this way: "Love so amazing, so divine, demands my soul, my life, my all." For some, such bold and sometimes exclusive claims are perhaps reason enough for suspicion. Others find these claims so convincing that religion demands their "all."

The Motivational Search for Meaning: The Need for Control

Why is personal meaning so important in the first place? Philosophers and theologians have long debated the underlying causes of the search for meaning and significance. From the myriad of possibilities, one that is particularly intriguing and of heuristic value to psychologists of religion is that meaning helps meet perhaps an even greater underlying need for control—an idea that also has a long history in both philosophy and psychology. Control in the sense of power is central in the philosophies of Hobbes and Nietzsche. Reid (1969) spoke of power as one of the basic human desires. Adler termed it "an intrinsic 'necessity of life'" (quoted in Vyse, 1997, p. 131). Though the ideal in life is *actual* control, the need to perceive personal mastery is often so great that the *illusion* of control will suffice. Lefcourt (1973) even suggests that this illusion "may be the bedrock on which life flourishes" (p. 425). Baumeister (1991) believes the subjective sense of personal efficacy to be the essence of control.

The attribution process described earlier represents not just a need for meaning, but also for mastery and control. Especially when threatened with harm or pain, all higher organisms seek to predict and/or control the outcomes of the events that affect them (Seligman, 1975). This fact has been linked by attribution theorists and researchers with novelty, frustration/failure, lack of control, and restriction of personal freedom (Berlyne, 1960; Wong, 1979; Wong & Weiner, 1981; Wortman, 1976). It may be that people gain a sense of control by making sense out of what is happening and being able to predict what will occur, even if the result is undesirable. Hence we sometimes hear of people who, after being given a bad health prognosis, still feel relieved because they at least now know something and are no longer left wondering.

Early attribution research demonstrated individual-difference patterns in identifying causes of events: themselves, luck/chance, or powerful other individuals (Levenson, 1974; Rotter, 1966, 1990). Religious populations appear to downplay the role of luck or fate (Gabbard, Howard, & Tageson, 1986). Welton, Adkins, Ingle, and Dixon (1996) argued that God control represented an additional control construct to those observed by Levenson (1974). They found not only that God control was independent of belief in chance and powerful others, but that it was also positively related to well-being—benefits normally only associated with internal control (Myers & Diener, 1995). Thus much current research exploring the connections between religion and health (see Chapter 13) utilizes such newly created measures as the God Locus of Health Control Scale (Wallston et al., 1999).

Religion and the Need for Control

Religion's ability to offer meaning for virtually every life situation—particularly those that are most distressing, such as death and dying—also provides a measure of control over life's vast uncertainties. Various techniques strengthen a person's feeling of mastery, such as prayer and participation in religious rituals and ceremonies. An argument can be made that religious ritual and prayer are mechanisms for enhancing the sense of self-control and control of one's world. Gibbs (1994) claims that supernaturalism arises when secular control efforts fail. Vyse (1997) further shows how lack of control relates to the development of and belief in superstition and magic. Indeed, the historic interplay of magic and religion has often been viewed as a response to uncertainty and helplessness. When other attempts at control are limited (e.g., when a death is impending), religious faith alone may provide an illusory, subjective sense of control to help people regain the feeling that they are doing something that may work. This enhanced subjective feeling of control is often capable of offering people the strength they need to succeed.

Religion and Self-Control

Yet another important sense of control addressed by religion is self-control. "Self-control" can be defined as the active inhibition of unwanted responses that might interfere with desired achievement (Baumeister, Vohs, & Tice, 2007). Self-control, as an internal restraining mechanism, is a core psychological function underlying many of the virtues addressed by religion: compassion, justice, wisdom, humility, and so forth. Baumeister and Exline (1999) point out that a life of virtue frequently necessitates putting the collective interests of society and community above pure self-interest. In their estimation, the natural proclivity toward self-interest and personal gratification (the very definition in some religions of sin or personal evil), often at the expense of others, requires the necessity of self-regulation for the good of society. Self-control can thus be viewed as personality's "moral muscle," and therefore in some sense as a master virtue. Suggesting that "virtues seem based on the positive exercise of self-control, whereas sin and vice often revolve around failures of self-control" (p. 1175), Baumeister and Exline (1999) maintain that the seven deadly sins in traditional Christianity (gluttony, sloth, greed, lust, envy, anger, and pride) can best be thought of as the absence of self-regulation in overcoming excessive desire or striving toward inappropriate goals.

At the heart of the "self-control as a master virtue" argument is a view that human nature's general tendency is toward self-interest, and that the development of virtue must counteract this tendency. But this counteraction will require work. If indeed self-control is like a muscle, we should see evidence of both fatigue and eventual strengthening after continued use. Ironically, religion may be a contributor to both moral fatigue and moral fortitude. Consider, for example, both the person who feels defeated because of an inability to live according to the ideal expectations of the religious teachings, and the person who has developed healthy spiritual disciplines that provide a sense of meaning and joy.

The Social Embeddedness of Meaning: The Need for Relationships

Our emphasis on the cognitive and motivational aspects of the search for meaning should not be taken to mean that the search itself is conducted in isolation from others. Though it is perhaps true that the search for significance for those who profess to be "spiritual but not religious" does not, at first glance, require that the search receive validation and support from an identifiable group of people (Hill et al., 2000), the *need to belong* is a powerful human drive (Baumeister & Leary, 1995). A truly fundamental principle is that we humans cannot live without others. We are conceived and born in relationship and interdependence, and connections and interactions with others are indispensable throughout our entire lives.

Defining Sociality

"Sociality" refers to behaviors that relate organisms to one another, and that keep an individual identified with a group (Brewer, 1997). Included here are expressions of social support, cooperation, adherence to group standards, attachment to others, altruism, and many other actions that maintain effectively functioning groups. Faith systems accomplish these goals for many people, and in return the cultural order embraces religion.

Religion and Sociality

Religion connects individuals to each other and their groups; it socializes members into a community, and concurrently suppresses deviant behavior. As Lumsden and Wilson (1983) put it, religion is a "powerful device by which people are absorbed into a tribe and psychically strengthened" (p. 7). In this way, both religious bodies and the societies of which they are components strengthen themselves in numbers and importance.

There is a circular pattern in this linking of social life to faith. Religion fosters social group unity, which further strengthens religious sentiments. Current data show that church members possess larger social support networks than nonmembers do; in addition, there is more positive involvement in intrafamily relationships among the religiously committed than among their less religious peers (Pargament, 1997). Many of these observations have been attributed to enhanced feelings of social belonging and integration into a community of like-minded thinkers. This may mean that church members and those reared in churchgoing families also join more social groups than nonmembers do in later life. Data support this inference (Graves, Wang, Mead, Johnson, & Klag, 1998).

Moreover, the importance of marriage and reproduction is invariably stressed by religious traditions (Hoult, 1958). Expectations to marry and have children probably influence reproductive success in couples where both spouses attend the same church, as such couples generally show high birth rates (Moberg, 1962). There is a strong need for new research in this area, as there may be much variation across different religious bodies. It does seem to be true of some growing conservative groups, such as the Church of Jesus Christ of Latter-Day Saints (also known as the Mormons). This mutually reinforcing pattern is also likely to limit access to those whose religious beliefs differ, and could contribute to relatively high divorce rates plus low marital satisfaction when people of diverse religious affiliations marry (Lehrer & Chiswick, 1993; Levinger, 1979; Shortz & Worthington, 1994).

We may thus view religious faith as strengthening group bonds, welfare, and positive social evaluation. In addition, religion appears to eventuate in heightened reproductive and genetic potential. Obviously, religious affiliation opens important social channels for interpersonal approval and integration into society on many levels. We also note that the search for meaning is not one-sided, and that the psychology of religion is also focused upon the response to what may be perceived as ultimately real (Hick, 2010; Hood, 2012b).

OVERVIEW

In this introductory chapter, we have tried to present some broad contours of our field, and have done so in a rather condensed manner. We have proposed that the search for meaning provides a useful and integrating theoretical framework for investigating the psychology of religion. We have also stressed the importance of theory and objectivity. We seek knowledge that is both public and reproducible. Our aim is to achieve a scientific circumscription of the psychology of religion, and to convey the importance of such a framework. However, we caution the reader that although we attempt to cover a great deal of information in this text, psychologists and social scientists produce a massive literature, and hence our efforts have had to be selective. We have tried to choose and emphasize major points and issues, but such efforts can rapidly grow into volumes in themselves. It is worth noting that for almost every chapter in this text, there is at least one major handbook devoted to its topic. This is frustrating to all of us. We think, however, that even though we may not have covered the entire waterfront, we have treated a massive amount of information in the psychology of religion that remains indispensable for any overview of the field.

The next chapter describes this approach in further detail. When this effort has been completed, we show how religion relates to biology, as well as to individual development throughout the lifespan; describe the experiential expressions of religion; and finally discuss the significance of faith in social life, coping, adjustment, and mental disorder. Simply put, religion is a central feature of human existence, the psychological appreciation of which we try to communicate in these pages.

From a scientific point of view, the most important feature of our integrating framework is that it is testable. In brief, religious commitment should relate positively to measures tapping the cognitive, motivational, and social needs for meaning. Yet we must admit that such findings cannot prove that religion totally originates from the needs specified here. Religious and spiritual experiences are far too complex to be reduced to single sets of psychological principles, as compelling as they may be. However, many of the research findings reviewed in this book speak strongly to the idea that religion is a powerful factor in meeting human needs for meaning making, control, and sociality.

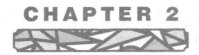

CHAPTER 2

Foundations for
an Empirical Psychology of Religion

Without knowledge of self there is no knowledge of God.

That's God's signature. God's signature is never a forgery.

. . . like most Americans, my faith consists in believing in every religion, including my own, but without ill-will toward anybody, no matter what he believes or disbelieves.

Religion is different from everything else; because in religion seeking is finding.

Man without religion is the creature of circumstances.[1]

THE EMPIRICAL STUDY OF RELIGION AND SPIRITUALITY

Psychology's status as a science is based largely on its methodology—that is, its use of scientific methods to study the phenomena of interest. The psychology of religion is no different from the psychological study of anything else. The problem is that religion and spirituality are exceedingly complex phenomena—so complex, as we have seen in Chapter 1, that they are difficult even to define. In this chapter, we demonstrate that they are also elusive to capture by standard scientific methods. On top of this, many people see religion and science as opposites that are in some type of conflict, and therefore see the use of one to help investigate the other as somehow problematic or at least inappropriate. Some religious people may even feel threatened by the scientific study of religion, for fear that it may somehow explain away something held as sacred. We attempt to dispel many of these concerns in this chapter. Still, the field is fraught with dangerous mines, and both the scientific investigator and student must be careful as they overturn each rock in their exploration.

These are serious and legitimate concerns that deserve special care. The psychologist of religion should not blindly enter the minefield without an understanding of the risks involved. But, as we shall see, there are useful tools to help us in our scientific study, and

---

[1]These quotations come, respectively, from the following sources: John Calvin, quoted in Kunkel, Cook, Meshel, Daughtry, and Hauenstein (1999, p. 193); Eddie Joe Lloyd, quoted in the online version of *The New York Times* (August 26, 2002); Saroyan (1937, p. 130); Cather (1926/1990, p. 94); and Julian Charles Hare and Augustus William Hare, quoted in *The Oxford Dictionary of Quotations* (1959, p. 237, No. 19).

so we need not be timid. In fact, since its earliest days, psychology has examined religion with confidence. In 1902, William James—a U.S. philosopher and one of the founders of our field—gave his famous Gifford Lectures at the University of Edinburgh. These were soon published in book form as *The Varieties of Religious Experience* (James, 1902/1985), a book continuously in print for well over 100 years—a rare feat indeed.

The success of *The Varieties* lies in several features that guide our discussions in this book. James explored questions about the nature of religion, already touched upon in Chapter 1, and compared religion to such concepts as psychic phenomena and superstition. James also asked whether religion is a help or a hindrance; that is, does the good it brings outweigh the harm that can be associated with it? In addition, he wanted to know the conditions under which religious conversion is likely to occur and the role that emotions play in religious experience. These questions are as much a part of the scientific study of religion today as they were in 1902, and we explore them throughout this book. Before we get to such substantive issues, however, we need to understand the empirical foundations of the psychological study of religion. Let us first do so by avoiding what is perhaps one of the most dangerous mines in the field—the temptation to reduce the richness and complexity of religious experience to a favorite psychological construct.

By beginning our discussion with the issue of reductionism, we are highlighting an important but sensitive philosophical shift in the psychology of religion—represented by Emmons and Paloutzian's (2003) call for a new multilevel interdisciplinary paradigm, which we have mentioned in Chapter 1. The new paradigm (the word "paradigm" means, for our purposes, a generally accepted perspective among a community of scholars in a given discipline) proposed is one that values multiple methods as legitimate and complementary in providing a more complete understanding of religious and spiritual phenomena. It also emphasizes interdisciplinary approaches, as the boundaries between such disciplines as sociology, psychology, and anthropology are becoming less rigid. As we shall see, in no way does this call for a paradigm shift lessen the discipline's resolve to be scientific. It does represent, however, an understanding of what constitutes legitimate science that may be somewhat different from the traditionally received view. In any case, part of the call for a new paradigm is to value nonreductive assumptions about the nature of religion and spirituality.

REDUCTIONISM IN CONCEPTUALIZING RELIGIOUS ISSUES

"Reductionism" is an attempt at explanation. It involves explaining a topic by variables independent of the topic itself, usually in the form of understanding the nature of complex things by *reducing* them to simpler, more fundamental phenomena. There are various types of reductionism (methodological, theoretical, ontological), and some may be more appropriate to understanding than others. We wish to avoid getting mired in the details of this philosophical debate, for the issues underlying reductionism are complex. Some defend reductionism as necessary to science, while others suggest that such a view involves a flawed understanding of science. It is safe to say, however, that as we attempt to scientifically explain broader and more complex issues (such as religious experience), we should greet reductionism with greater reservation. So, for example, when we utilize the need for meaning and purpose as a general framework for the study of religion, we should not assume that religion is *only* a useful device for finding meaning. Religion is much more than a meaning-making device. Reducing a complex concept may sometimes be appropriate, such as reducing a preschool child's church attendance to parental religiousness, and at times it may even be necessary for conceptualization purposes. In general, however, we caution against reductionistic tendencies in the psychology of religion.

Examples of Reductionism in the Psychology of Religion

Two traditions in the psychology of religion are selected here to illustrate reductionism: those of Sigmund Freud and William James. In both traditions, many of the reasons people give for being religious—primarily, beliefs—are ignored. The beliefs themselves are assumed only to reflect some psychological issue.

Freud assumed that religion is false, in the sense that its primary object (i.e., God) is not real. He was intrigued as to why people are religious when it is irrational to be so; since they believe in nothing that is real, there must be other foundations for these beliefs. In the introduction to *The Future of an Illusion*, Freud (1927/1961b) stated:

> . . . in past ages in spite of their incontrovertible lack of authenticity, religious ideas have exercised the strongest possible influence on mankind. This is a fresh psychological problem. We must ask where the inner force of those doctrines lies and to what they owe their efficacy, independent as it is, of the acknowledgement of reason. (p. 51)

Freud maintained that the inner force to which religion is reduced is infantile projection of the parental figure, a form of neuroticism. Other psychologists endorsed variants of this theme (e.g., Faber, 1972; Suttie, 1952; Symonds, 1946). In this view, the substance of religion—*what* a person believes, or the reasons behind certain religious behavior and practices—does not matter. If this is so, there can be nothing of importance to religious beliefs, so why measure them?

William James (1902/1985), a founder of the psychology of religion, treated religion with much greater respect than did Freud. Why people hold religious beliefs to be true was not an issue for James, since he approached religion pragmatically: Does it help people live? To this he resoundingly answered, "Yes." We will see throughout this text, particularly in Chapter 13, that James's answer has been supported by much contemporary research. James's form of reductionism is more subtle than Freud's, since James did not clearly take an atheistic position. In his view, nothing religionists claim in and of themselves as a basis for their religious faith needs to be examined; such beliefs are relevant only to the extent that they are functionally important—that they are of some benefit to the persons who hold them. For James, religious beliefs are reduced to their pragmatic functional value.

Religion as "Nothing but" Superstition

One common form of reductionism applied to religious experience is that such experience is "nothing but" some related concept. So, for example, one might believe that religion is nothing but superstition, and that if one can understand the basis of this superstition, then religious experience is explained. Let's consider this example in more detail.

A "superstition" has been defined as "any belief or attitude, based on fear or ignorance, that is inconsistent with the known laws of science or with what is generally considered in the particular society as true and rational; esp., such a belief in charms, omens, the supernatural, etc." (Guralnik, 1986, p. 1430). A superstitious person is one who acts on such beliefs. Examples of superstitious actions include walking under a ladder, avoiding the number 13, and tugging on one's cap before throwing a pitch in a baseball game.

These examples of superstition contain nothing that is called religious or spiritual. But can the "superstition" label be properly extended to religion as studied by psychology? *The Oxford Universal Dictionary on Historical Principles* (Onions, 1955) includes in its definition of superstition: "esp. in connection with religion" (p. 2084). This definition explicitly links the two concepts, but it also distinguishes between superstition and religion, since the two realms are not equated with each other.

One basis of superstition can be found in learning research. Though this type of research was originally conducted on animals by the noted psychologist B. F. Skinner (1948, 1969), superstition is obviously present in humans and may occur in one-trial learning, particularly with strong negative reinforcement (Morris & Maisto, 1998). Primarily when threat, pain, or much emotion is present, and is then resolved, irrelevant stimuli present in the situation become meaningful. For example, let us suppose that Joe, an athlete, was wearing a specific pair of socks when a problem with his athletic performance was alleviated; hence they become his "lucky socks," which he wears just in case they might make a difference in future similar circumstances. Joe knows full well that there is no rational basis for the lucky socks to affect the game, but he just feels better when wearing them. Of course, if success occurs, the incident will be cited as proof of the superstition's truth.

It is not surprising that some religious behaviors are also superstitious for a particular person. They meet the twin conditions of being nonrational and of avoiding a major negative outcome (i.e., being based in fear). We must, however, ask whether religion is *just* superstition.

Most religious beliefs and behavior do not meet the conditions of superstition. Religions usually have well-developed theologies that make religious behaviors rational, at least to those who hold them. The threat of avoiding a major negative outcome (e.g., going to hell) also seldom enters into daily religious behavior. Furthermore, the promise of hell is unlikely to take hold after one-trial learning, in that it involves complex social learning. Although religion includes conditioned responses, it is far more than just these responses (thus avoiding another form of reductionism); much social learning may be involved, and genetic and evolutionary factors may even play indirect roles. These factors are detailed in Chapter 3.

What do the data say? Can scientific investigation itself help answer whether religion is just superstition? If both religion and superstition involve the same psychological processes, then we should expect either (1) positive correlations between measures of religiousness and measures of superstition (i.e., those who are most superstitious are also the most religious), in that the two are functionally the same; or (2) negative correlations between religion and superstition, in that one serves as a substitute for the other. If they are independent of each other, we should expect little or no correlation between their measures.

Studies are few in this area, and further work is necessary. Using the statistical technique called "factor analysis," Johnston, de Groot, and Spanos (1995) found separate factors for beliefs involving the paranormal, superstition, extraordinary life forms, and religion; these results counter the "functionally the same" hypothesis. Sparks's (2001) review of work in this area confirms the distinctiveness noted by Johnston et al. (1995). Goode (2000), however, claims that there may be paranormal elements in certain religious concepts (e.g., creationism, angels, the Devil), and provides data to this effect. We discuss the empirical research relating to paranormal and religious experiences, including mysticism, in Chapters 10 and 11.

The limited data available suggest that religion and superstition should be treated as independent constructs. Thus we can tentatively say that a definition of either religion or superstition is more accurate if it does not include the other. To be sure, most psychologists of religion do not investigate superstition or psychic phenomena per se. Of course, superstition and psychic reports occur in almost all areas of life, and among religious people as well the nonreligious. They are, however, peripheral to the psychology of religion.

Reductionism: Conclusions

The empirical study of religiousness has many great challenges. The first of these challenges considered here is how to maintain the scientific standards of good empirical work—always the goal of science—without sacrificing the richness and depth of the object of study. We have gone to considerable lengths to make the case that religious experience should not be reduced to specific psychological processes. It is tempting to do so when one adopts the naturalistic perspective that underlies scientific investigation, and to ignore the meaning system of the people being studied. What is needed is some nonreductionistic accounting of the phenomena of interest, but without abandoning scientific methodology and thus failing to reap the benefits that it provides.

QUALITATIVE AND QUANTITATIVE RESEARCH METHODS

One way to avoid reductionism is to treat the individual as a holistic entity, instead of the typical psychological research approach of dividing the individual into traits, attitudes, beliefs, values, habits, responses, and underlying physiology. This holistic–atomistic distinction is not a sharp dichotomy, and many levels exist between these endpoints. The primary traditional scientific avenue to demonstrating valid knowledge is to obtain information that is empirical, public, reproducible, and reliable. This usually requires collecting data on a relatively large sample and is sometimes referred to as the "nomothetic" approach to research. However, some researchers maintain that by breaking the individual into such concepts as traits or attitudes and then abstracting these by a supposedly "objective" analysis, only a false and incomplete picture of the person is attained—a partial interpretation with a grain of truth to it. Instead, these researchers argue that a holistic, phenomenological, clinical approach is better. This approach often involves case studies and a greater reliance on various qualitative methods (as opposed to the quantitative methods of the nomothetic approach); it is sometimes called an "idiographic" or "idiothetic" research approach. The challenge, of course, is whether such an approach can meet standard scientific criteria.

The Complementary Nature of Qualitative and Quantitative Research

Qualitative data collection ranges from writing the biography of a religious person to chatting with several people about a religious topic, conducting interviews with open-ended questions, or having people tell a story about a picture they are given. Central to this process is how experience is interpreted. In short, it is "the interpretative study of a specified issue or problem in which the researcher is central to the sense that is made" (Banister, Burman, Parker, Taylor, & Tindall, 1994, p. 2), and is thus "(a) an attempt to capture the sense that lies within, and that structures what we say about what we do; (b) an exploration, elaboration and systematization of the significance of the identified phenomenon; and (c) the illuminative representation of the meaning of a delimited issue or problem" (Banister et al., 1994, p. 3).

The use of qualitative methods often allows researchers to "get behind" the quantitative data to uncover specific issues of meaning. People may have specific reasons—sometimes common and sometimes uncommon—for responding, for example, with a 4 on a 7-point scale as an indication of moderate agreement with a religious belief statement. Without qualitative methodologies to unpack what a 4 actually means, we have limited understanding of the phenomena of interest. At issue is the fact that many of our quantitative measures involve "arbitrary metrics" (Blanton & Jaccard, 2006), which do not tell us the absolute standing of an individual or group on an underlying psychological construct. For example, a score of 68 on a 100-point measure of depression does not tell us how depressed a person actually is. Such arbitrariness, of course, is not a death sentence for research, in that quantitative measures are used to test ideas and theories; therefore, the relative standing of scores is useful. We can say that a score of 68 on a measure of depression is more than a score of 38, and this difference, for example, may support or not support a hypothesis. However, what the score means in terms of the actual experience of depression is limited.

Therefore, several researchers in the psychology of religion have called for a greater role for qualitative methods (e.g., Belzen, 1997; Belzen & Hood, 2006). This call is especially relevant to an understanding of religion as a meaning system—the approach taken in this text. It also resonates well with the earlier-noted call by Emmons and Paloutzian (2003) for a new multilevel interdisciplinary paradigm that values multiple levels of analysis and nonreductive assumptions regarding the nature of religious and spiritual experience.

Qualitative methods are the methods of choice in idiothetic research, but many such methods are used in nomothetic research as well. Therefore, it is an error to equate qualitative methods with idiothetic research and quantitative methods with nomothetic research, as is frequently done. For example, determining what religious behaviors people perform in certain specific settings may call for a novel procedure. This could include observing missionary activity in a Third World village undergoing cultural change, or the behavior of congregants during a church service (Wolcott, 1994). In contrast, quantitative data collection techniques might ask people to rate how strongly they agree with a particular statement or to report how often they attend worship services. The major distinction is that quantitative measures give scores directly, but qualitative data must be processed by a rater or by a computer program for information.

A similar distinction can be made between qualitative and quantitative analyses of data. Qualitative treatment can involve a more or less subjective review that enables a scholar to make sense of the information and draw conclusions. A researcher employing quantitative analysis uses statistics such as means, standard deviations, significance levels, and correlations in order to draw conclusions.

Although quantitative methods have been typical of data collection and analysis in the sciences as well as in the psychology of religion, there is no doubt that they miss something. A description of a sunset in terms of physics is quantitative, but none would argue that a painting of that sunset is replaced by the physical description. Physics has never claimed to contain the whole of human experience regarding physical phenomena; nor does the psychology of religion claim to contain the whole of human experience regarding religion. Just as a personal experience with a sunset is meaningful in addition to the physics of a sunset, so a personal religious experience cannot be replaced by the psychology of that experience. Similarly, psychology does not directly cover the history of religions, the biographies of religious leaders, or the anthropology of religions, although they may be considered within the new paradigm insofar as interdisciplinary considerations provide a broader context within which to understand psychological findings (Hood & Williamson, 2008a, 2008b). The psychology of religion is an application of scientific methods to enhance our psychological understanding of religion.

Reliability and Validity

The acceptability of both quantitative and qualitative methods within the psychology of religion depends on whether they can be shown to meet the scientific criteria of "reliability" and "validity." For example, when Ponton and Gorsuch (1988) used an instrument called the Quest Scale in Venezuela, its reliability was low, so the authors were hesitant to draw any conclusions from it. Qualitative measures also need to demonstrate reliability. Do different raters or judges agree in their observations and/or interpretations? If they reach different conclusions as to whether a person feels God's presence during meditation, for example, then there is no reliability in their measure. Usually a minimal level of agreement is established before observations take place to determine whether or not there is sufficient reliability.

Once it has been shown that the qualitative or quantitative method is reliable, validity must then be established. Usually "content validity" is used. This means that psychologists examining the method agree that the items or interview or rating criteria are appropriate for whatever descriptive term is employed.

Since both qualitative and quantitative methods are acceptable if they meet the standards of being reliable and valid, why are quantitative methods so popular? One important problem is that reliable qualitative methods are rather expensive to use. Consider the question of how a victim becomes a forgiving person after major harm has been done to that person. Using an interview-based qualitative approach, a researcher might ask each of 100 people to describe a time when a person harmed them, and then, in their own words, to explain how they forgave that person and how their religious faith was a part of that process. The interviewing would take about 300 hours (including setting up the interviews, doing the interviews, finding new people to reduce the "no-shows," transcribing the interviews, etc.). Then the interviews would need to be rated by two people trained to use the same language to describe the processes that were reported, and differences would need to be reconciled with the help of a third rater (all this would take another 300 hours). At this point, a total of 600 hours would be needed for collecting and scoring the data.

By contrast, in quantitative measurement utilizing a questionnaire, a group of 100 people might take 2 hours to fill out the questionnaire. Scoring these responses would take another 4 hours. The quantitative approach would thus take an estimated 6 hours, versus 600 hours for the qualitative approach. Which procedure would you rather use in a research project?

In some cases, qualitative methods are the only ones we currently have to tap into the psychological processes being studied. It is, for example, difficult to understand children's concepts of God without using their drawings of God, which are then rated. And in models where a person makes a choice, it is also a problem to find out what options *spontaneously* occur to that person without utilizing at least somewhat qualitative methods. Throughout this text, we report many studies that use qualitative research methods, provided that those methods demonstrate sufficient reliability and validity. When they do meet adequate psychometric criteria, we can be just as confident in reporting the results of qualitative research as those of quantitative research.

An Example of a Qualitative Approach

There is no single qualitative method. Though a common element of virtually all qualitative methods is that they take an interpretive approach to their subject matter, the methods vary considerably in terms of their goals and aims. Some methods, such as discourse analysis or participant observation, may only produce descriptive information. Other techniques, such as interviewing and ethnography, may likewise be descriptive, but may also involve an explanatory interpretation by the coinvestigators (the researcher and the person being studied). Here we provide a single brief example of the use of qualitative techniques that is particularly relevant and applicable to the overall theoretical framework of religion as a meaning system used in this text.

"Narrative analysis" is a qualitative technique used to investigate the means by which individuals utilize the language of their culture to construct a story of their experience. Hood and Belzen (2005) suggest that this is a particularly useful technique to test ideas drawn from psychoanalytic theory. They recommend using archives of recorded interviews, and point to effective uses of this technique in studying a serpent-handling sect in Appalachia (Hood, 1998, 2005a) and the Word of Life congregation in Turku, Finland (Hovi, 2004). Let us consider the serpent-handling example. Williamson and Pollio (1999) analyzed the narrative form of serpent-handling sermons, while Hood (2005a) utilized an oral narrative of a handler. This team of researchers (Williamson, Pollio, & Hood, 2000) has also creatively used "phenomenological" methods to identify, from the snake handlers' perspective, the actual experience of handling a snake, especially in the context of religious commitment.

Sixteen open-ended interviews (Williamson, 2000) were then subjected to interpretations based upon a "hermeneutical methodology" developed by Pollio, Henley, and Thompson (1997) involving a group interaction by researchers trained in dialogical procedures (see Hood & Williamson, 2008a, for a more complete description). From this analysis, four fundamental beliefs of serpent handlers were identified: (1) Handling serpents is a Biblical mandate based on Mark 16:17–18; (2) handling serpents is a sign of enablement or power bestowed by God in response to obedience; (3) handling serpents is a sign of God's protection (handlers thereby acknowledge the danger of handling); and (4) the experience of handling serpents is a confirmation of God's power and blessing (Hood, Hill, & Williamson, 2005).

The point here is that what seems to outsiders a bizarre and pointless activity that is dangerous and even life-threatening (11 of the 16 interviewees had been bitten, and all knew of someone who had died from snake bite) carries great meaning for the serpent handlers through its Biblical justification. Understanding the richness of serpent handling as a religious meaning system could not have been attained through quantitative techniques only. Rather, what is necessary is the use of multiple techniques (including historical methodologies). Although qualitative techniques are fraught with potential bias and possible misuse and should therefore be used only according to strict guidelines, they serve as a useful complement that will greatly profit the psychology of religion.

Spirituality: From an Idiothetic to a Nomothetic Concept

In Chapter 1, we have pointed out the complexities of the term "spirituality." We have noted that it is not a word to be easily substituted for "religiosity"; nor is it really meaningful when those who have left an organized, formal religious body define themselves as "spiritual." We review the empirical distinctions between religion and spirituality more fully in Chapters 10 and 11. Here we confront the issue of how best to study spirituality in terms of the idiothetic–nomothetic distinction. We use it as an example to demonstrate why researchers so often gravitate to a nomothetic approach, even when it is better understood idiothetically.

Even though there are challenges in understanding precisely what spirituality is (Spilka, 1993), and there are controversies about the degree to which it is distinct from religiousness (Emmons & Crumpler, 1999; Hill et al., 2000; Hood, 2000b; Pargament, 1999; Zinnbauer et al., 1997), most commonly it is viewed holistically—that is, as a characteristic of a person *in toto*. Two overlapping systems have been proposed (Elkins, Hedstrom, Hughes, Leaf, & Saunders, 1988; LaPierre, 1994). Table 2.1 illustrates these two schemes. The criteria listed in the table suggest directions for the study of spirituality, but still possess an idyllic quality that remains unclear and ethereal. They also strongly suggest that it will be difficult if not impossible to assess spirituality in a holistic manner.

Hardy's (1979) approach, by stressing spiritual experience as the key element of spirituality, helped spur the movement from a holistic, phenomenological perspective to an objective, nomothetic analysis. By offering "a provisional classification" (p. 25) of reported experiential elements, Hardy grouped the elements into 12 major categories, each with further subdivisions until a total of 90 components were given. An exhaustive questionnaire treatment could undoubtedly result in many more items than this last number suggests.

As a result, today spirituality is largely measured nomothetically. The last few decades have witnessed a flurry of efforts to evaluate spirituality. Despite extensive lists

TABLE 2.1. Some Suggested Dimensions of Spirituality

	Elkins et al. (1988)
Transcendental dimension	"Experientially based belief [in] a transcendent dimension to life" (p. 10).
Meaning and purpose to life	Authentic sense that life has purpose and meaning.
Mission in life	Sense that one has a calling, a mission.
Sacredness of life	Belief that "all of life is holy" (p. 11).
Material values	Sense that material things do not satisfy spiritual needs.
Altruism	Belief that we are all part of humanity.
Idealism	Being committed to ideals and life's potential.
Awareness of the tragic	Awareness of and sensitivity to pain and tragedy in life.
Spiritual fruits	Sense that life is infused with spiritual benefits and experience.
	LaPierre (1994)
Journey	Belief that life has meaning and purpose.
Transcendent encounters	As above, belief in a higher level of reality.
Community	Belief that personal growth should occur within a loving community.
Religion	Beliefs and practices relating one to a supreme being.
Mystery of creation	Sense of connection to an environment, its creation and creator.
Transformation	Sense of personal change in relation to social involvement—of becoming.

of characteristics associated with spirituality, the holistic–atomistic problem remains unresolved. Gorsuch and Miller (1999) indicate the many qualifications researchers should consider in their assessment attempts, but few have been taken seriously. Still, there has been no dearth of efforts to measure spirituality, many since 2000 (Hill, 2013), as indicated later in this chapter in Table 2.3.

For now, we simply want to point out that the concept of spirituality and its operationalization demonstrate very clearly how a notion that was originally idiothetically conceived necessarily found nomothetic expression. As it was analyzed and measured, various beliefs and values of people entered the realm of scientific knowledge, and became useful both for research and for application to real-life problems.

THE MANY VARIETIES OF RELIGIOUS EXPERIENCE

In our effort to avoid a reductionistic approach to the study of religious and spiritual experience, we have cautioned against the "nothing but" argument—that religion is nothing but, for example, superstition. In so doing, we have made the claim that religious experience can and should be distinguished from other concepts, such as superstition. But there is another, perhaps more subtle message about the dangers of reductionism: One can easily fall prey to believing that all forms of religious experience reflect what one has directly and personally experienced. Thus, for example, one raised in a religious tradition that emphasizes the importance of what one believes, which is typical in much of Protestantism, may be surprised to learn that in some religious traditions what one believes is not as important as one's heritage or sense of social connectedness (Cohen & Hill, 2007). Morris (1996) has distinguished these two types as "religions of assent" versus "religions of descent." Indeed, religious and spiritual experience has many varieties, as William James (1902/1985) noted in the title of his classic book.

Dimensional Approaches to Religion

The human passion to be efficient—to summarize the complex, to wrap it all up in "25 words or less"—is often an enemy to real understanding. Words are symbols that place many things under one heading, and the term "religion" is an excellent example of this tendency. When psychologists first began research in this area, they simply constructed measures of religiousness or religiosity. Sophisticated thinkers, however, soon put aside notions that people simply vary along a single dimension with antireligious sentiments at one end and orthodox views at the other end. These proved unsatisfactory, and many new sets of dimensions—some covering a broad range, some narrower in their focus—began to appear in the research literature. Examples of these dimensions are listed in Table 2.2.

When we examine the many dimensional schemes that have been proposed, we see that some stress the purpose of faith, whereas others look to the possible personal and social origins of religion. Although some appear to mix psychology and religion, there are also those that take their cues exclusively from psychology and focus on motivation or cognition. However, two real problems exist: the presence of a "hidden" value agenda that implies "good" and "bad" religion, and a lack of conceptual and theoretical clarity. There is also great overlap among the various proposals, with essentially the same idea being phrased in different words—testimony to the excellent vocabularies of some social scientists. There is, however,

TABLE 2.2. Some Logically and Empirically Derived Dimensional Approaches to the Study of Individual Religion

Allen and Spilka (1967)

Committed religion — "Utilizes an abstract philosophical perspective: multiplex religious ideas are relatively clear in meaning and an open and flexible framework of commitment relates religious to daily activities" (p. 205).

Consensual religions — "Vague, nondifferentiated, ifurcated, neutralized" (p. 205). A cognitively simplified and personally convenient faith.

Batson and Ventis (1982)

Means religion — "Religion is a means to other self-serving ends than religion itself" (p. 151).

End religion — "Religion is an ultimate end in itself" (p. 151).

Clark (1958)

Primary religious behavior — "An authentic inner experience of the divine combined with whatever efforts the individual may make to harmonize his life with the divine" (p. 23).

Secondary religious behavior — "A very routine and uninspired carrying out ... of an obligation" (p. 24).

Tertiary religious behavior — "A matter of religious routine or convention accepted on the authority of someone else" (p. 25).

Fromm (1950)

Authoritarian religion — "The main virtue of this type of religion is obedience, its cardinal sin is disobedience" (p. 35).

Humanistic religion — "This type of religion is centered around man and his strength ... virtue is self-realization, not obedience" (p. 37).

Hunt (1972)

Literal religion — Taking "at face value any religious statement without in any way questioning it" (p. 43).

Antiliteral religion — A simple rejection of literalist religious statements.

Mythological religion — A reinterpretation of religious statements to seek their deeper symbolic meanings.

James (1902/1985)

Healthy-mindedness — An optimistic, happy, extroverted, social faith: "the tendency that looks on all things and sees that they are good" (p. 78).

Sick souls — "The way that takes all this experience of evil as something essential" (p. 36). A faith of pessimism, sorrow, suffering, and introverted reflection.

Lenski (1961)

Doctrinal orthodoxy — "Stresses intellectual assent [to] prescribed doctrines" (p. 23).

Devotionalism — "Emphasizes the importance of private, or personal communion with God" (p. 23).

McConahay and Hough (1973)

Guilt-oriented, extrapunitive — "Religious belief ... centered on the wrath of God as it is related to other people ... emphasizes punishment for wrong-doers" (p. 55).

Guilt-oriented intropunitive — "A sense of one's own unworthiness and badness ... a manifest need for punishment and a conviction that it will inevitably come" (p. 56).

Love-oriented, self-centered — "Oriented toward the forgiveness of one's own sins" (p. 56).

Love-oriented, other-centered — "Emphasizes the common humanity of all persons as creatures of God, and God's love ... related to the redemption of the whole world" (p. 56).

Culture-oriented, conventional — "Values ... are more culturally than theologically oriented" (p. 56).

one point on which all agree: Even though there is only one word for "religion," there may be a hundred possible ways of being "religious."

Logical Approaches

Some dimensional approaches to religiousness are logically derived; that is, they are based on concepts and ideas derived from induction. In other words, some theorists have observed and thought logically about religion, and from their many observations, they suggest what its multifaceted essence is. One particularly wide-ranging, comprehensive logical system of understanding religion is that proposed by Glock (1962), a well-known sociologist of religion. This system identifies and measures the following areas of religion (all quotes are from Glock, 1962, p. S99):

- *Experiential dimension:* "Religious people will . . . achieve direct knowledge of ultimate reality or will experience religious emotion."
- *Ideological dimension:* "The religious person will hold to certain beliefs."
- *Ritualistic dimension:* "Specifically religious practices [are] expected of religious adherents."
- *Intellectual dimension:* "The religious person will be informed and knowledgeable about the basic tenets of his faith and its sacred scriptures."
- *Consequential dimension:* This covers "what people ought to do and the attitudes they ought to hold as a consequence of their religion."

In addition to Glock's dimensions, it is possible to develop sets of logically derived psychological categories for understanding religion. One system for doing so would separate the personal from the interpersonal. This system is narrower in its focus than that of Glock, but it can be highly useful when detail on religious practices is desired. Because religion is at the same time unique to each person and yet part of a community, religion can be subdivided within each of these two areas. Here is one possible breakdown of religious practices:

- Personal
  - Prayer
  - Reading of scriptures
  - Meditation
- Interpersonal
  - Worshiping with others
  - Committee participation
  - Receiving and providing social support

Examining Logical Systems Empirically

Logical systems such as Glock's (1962) and our categories of religious practices help to organize our thinking and research. Although they are obviously useful, how they relate to each other is an empirical question. Proponents of a more empirical approach note that logical approaches to understanding religion may have poor psychometric properties. Glock's dimensions as described above are a good example. Although the *logic* distinguishing Experiential from Consequential is clear, *empirically* the two are strongly related (Faulkner & DeJong, 1966; Weigert & Thomas, 1969). This is true of all the categories: They correlate highly with each other. Statistically, then, one only needs to measure one or two, because the same conclusions will be reached regardless of which dimension is used. For instance, a person who has a religious experience is therefore likely to be concerned with the consequences of adhering to the faith.

Similar objections can be raised to the logically derived system of religious practices we have described. If a person engages in one personal category of religious behavior, it is quite likely that this person utilizes the other personal practices. And if the person engages in an interpersonal category of religious behavior, he or she probably also employs other interpersonal practices.

Logical approaches can evolve into systems that blend the logical and the empirical. This is what happened to a system proposed by Gordon Allport (1959, 1966). In attempting to understand prejudice, he noted that some Christians, in keeping with the Christian tenets of love toward all, are less prejudiced than non-Christians. He also noted, however, that some Christians are more prejudiced than other Christians and some non-Christians are, even though this is in violation of Christian doctrines of love. To explain this difference, Allport suggested that some are Christian for the sake of the faith itself, and thus are "intrinsically" committed; they try to live in accordance with Christian doctrines. Others are Christian for what they can personally get out of it; these "extrinsically" committed Christians pick what they need and ignore the rest, such as the teachings on loving others. Allport called these "religious orientations" and saw them as opposite ends of an Intrinsic–Extrinsic (abbreviated from here on in this chapter as I–E) continuum. Others developed similar constructs, including Allen and Spilka's (1967) Committed versus Consensual scales, and Batson's Internal versus External scales (Batson & Ventis, 1982).

It turns out that there are some problems with Allport's conception of I and E as opposites. For our purposes now, however, we should simply note that in the attempt to *measure* I and E, it was found that E items did not correlate strongly negatively with I items, which they should do if I and E are opposites. Allport and Ross (1967) then modified their stance from I versus E as the ends of a single dimension, to I and E as two distinct dimensions, each with its own separate set of items. Although there was (and generally continues to be) a low negative correlation between the I and E scales, I and E religious orientations are empirically distinct; thus some people are high (or low) on both. This is an example where empirical research helped modify a logically derived system. Our ideas need to be empirically tested, and the quality of empirical research depends greatly on our capability to measure the constructs of interest accurately.

MEASUREMENT IN THE PSYCHOLOGY OF RELIGION

To illustrate the importance of good measurement, we borrow an example from Hill, Kopp, and Bollinger (2007) involving Chicago's Lakeshore Marathon in 2005. This race was not one for the record books. In fact, the runners were perplexed by their unusually slow times and perhaps woke up the next morning to find themselves more sore than usual. The problem? It was discovered *afterward* that the course had been wrongly charted and they had actually run 27.2 miles—a full mile further than the usual grueling distance for a marathon. Indeed, accurate measurement is very much a relevant issue. Imagine that after you had already run 26.2 miles and your body was excruciatingly telling you that you should be finished, you had yet another full mile to run!

Without good measurement in research, the data that are collected in the process of doing a research study are of little if any value. Most measures in the psychology of religion are self-report scales. Participants completing such measures are asked to respond to multiple items designed to assess the many varieties of religious and spiritual experience. There are problems with self-report measures, and researchers do all they can to circumvent these problems. Fortunately, psychologists of religion have long recognized the importance of good measurement and have placed a high priority on it. As early as 1984, Gorsuch pronounced measurement to be the current paradigm (i.e., the dominant perspective or concern) of psychologists of religion. By the end of the 1990s, Hill and Hood (1999a) identified over 125 measurement scales available to psychologists of religion, and many more have been developed in the new century (Hill, 2013; Hill & Edwards, 2013). To be sure, there is a well-developed measurement literature in the psychology of religion. But what makes one scale better than another? Both theoretical and technical issues must be considered in determining the best measure.

Theoretical Considerations

Any attempt to measure a concept such as religiousness or spirituality requires that the concept be specified in measurable terms. Such an "operational definition" is especially important when applied to religiousness and spirituality, because, as we have seen in Chapter 1, there is considerable variety in how these terms are conceptualized. The importance of theoretical clarity extends beyond how the constructs are conceptualized; good theory is necessary in providing a framework for testable hypotheses as well. Furthermore, researchers must consider the various dimensions of religious and spiritual experience (a topic that we consider shortly) to help determine the appropriateness of potential measures.

We should also note that good measurement based on good theory will also keep the domains of cognition, affect, and behavior distinct. To these three, we perhaps should add habit, since there are important habitual components in religious experience. "Cognition" is primarily concerned with beliefs and how they are learned—in other words, how the ideological aspect of religion is conceptualized. The realm of "affect" emphasizes feelings and attitudes—the emotional, "like–dislike" facet of belief or behavior. The attitude concept is especially important to the psychology of religion, since attitudes are often important predictors of behavior. "Behavior," of course, consists of what people do and how they act. Finally, "habit" involves what people do regularly, consistently, and often automatically. The psychology of religion looks at individual religious differences within each of these areas.

Technical Considerations

The issues of reliability and validity, discussed earlier in the context of qualitative research, apply equally well to quantitative measures. The more reliable and valid a measure is, the more useful it is for conducting scientific research. Though brief scales (sometimes just one-item scales) may be appealing because they are time-saving and convenient, they also tend to be less reliable and perhaps less valid.

"Reliability" refers to the consistency of a measure and is usually assessed in terms of either (1) "consistency across time" or (2) "internal consistency." When one is assessing consistency of a measure over time, better known as "test–retest reliability," the reliability coefficient is a correlation between the test scores of a group of individuals who are administered the scale on two different occasions (usually at least 2 weeks apart). More common is the use of internal consistency as a reliability indicator. The better the fit among multiple scale items (as determined statistically), the higher the internal consistency. Internal consistency is most often measured by a statistic called Cronbach's alpha, which ranges from 0 to 1.00, with a higher value indicating greater consistency. Alpha levels of religious and spiritual constructs are preferably above .80, but frequently are acceptable at about .70.

Consideration of the scale's "validity," or the extent to which a test measures what it purports to measure, is also essential to good measurement. There are many different ways to think of and measure validity. For example, though it may be tempting to do so, we cannot rely simply on our subjective sense of whether or not the scale appears to measure what it is supposed to be measuring, referred to as "face validity." Face validity is subject to all sorts of human bias and is therefore not scientifically useful. "Content validity," as noted earlier, refers to whether or not a representative sample of the domain is being covered. For example, perhaps you are working with a measure of spiritual disciplines. If your measure inquires about prayer, fasting, and tithing, but does not address reading sacred texts or service, content validity is sacrificed—because the entire behavioral domain has not been included in your measure. "Construct validity" examines the agreement between a specific theoretical construct and a measurement device, and may rely heavily on what is already known about a construct. "Convergent validity" and "discriminant validity" are both subdomains of construct validity and can be considered together. Convergent validity asks, "How well does this measure correspond to similar measures of the same or similar constructs?"; discriminant validity asks, "How is this test unrelated to measures of different constructs?" Those who develop scales try to demonstrate as much reliability and validity as possible, though it is highly unlikely that any single measure will be perfectly reliable or score high on all types of validity just discussed.

Sample Representativeness

There are many measurement scales in the psychology of religion that adequately meet these technical criteria, but care must still be taken in their use. Why? Because these scales were developed on rather limited samples that may not represent the populations of interest in current investigations. The most common such limitation is that many of the scales were initially developed for a Christian population, but now many researchers wish to investigate religious and spiritual experience outside the confines of Christianity, or perhaps even outside the context of any formal religious tradition (Hill, 2013; Hill & Edwards, 2013). Even more problematic is that many of the scales were initially developed among white, young, middle-class, American (or, to a lesser extent, British) college students (Hill & Pargament, 2003). Four variables known to be strongly correlated with religious experience are age, socioeconomic status, race, and educational level (Hill, 2013); therefore, caution is necessary if one should choose to use such a scale for a population with a different demographic profile or outside the Judeo-Christian context.

Scales created on the basis of either unrepresentative samples or samples representing a narrow population (e.g., a single denomination) are usually insensitive or inapplicable to broader groups (Chatters, Taylor, & Lincoln, 2002). For example, Protestant African Americans—among the most religious of all ethnic groups in the United States—emphasize community service (Ellison & Taylor, 1996), as well as the notion of reciprocal blessings with God (Black, 1999). Both of these characteristics are ignored in virtually all measures of religiousness or spirituality, in favor of other issues that may be irrelevant to African Americans.

Hill and Dwiwardani (2010) provided a fascinating example of how difficult it is to transport the study of religious experience to other world religions when they attempted to apply Allport's I–E distinction to Indonesian Muslims. In order to make the scale that measures both I and E religious orientations applicable to the Muslim context, more than just the language of the scale needed to be changed (e.g., changing the word "church" to "mosque"). Because Islam is such a strong pillar of the overall collectivistic culture in Indonesia, the concept of the social basis of the E religious orientation as a form of immature religion is simply not as applicable to Muslims as it is to Christians. Fortunately, however, another group of researchers has provided the Muslim–Christian Religious Orientation Scale (Ghorbani, Watson, Ghramaleki, Morris, & Hood, 2002), which takes into account a social dimension in relation to the broader community and culture rather than to the mosque. It is important that we recognize the limits of our measures and seek to improve them for more diverse settings.

Measurement Domains

Because religiousness is a highly complex and varied human experience, good measurement must reflect this complexity. This does not mean that any single measure must reflect all of this complexity, since often the topic of interest is only a piece of the religion pie—for example, religious beliefs or specific religious behaviors. We have noted earlier that psychologists, especially social psychologists, frequently discuss the totality of human experience in three domains: "cognition," or how the ideological aspect of (in our case) religion is conceptualized; "affect," or the emotional facet of belief or behavior (which frequently includes attitudes and values); and "behavior," or what people do and how they act. To these, we have proposed adding "habit," or what people do regularly and often automatically. It is important that measures reflect these individual domains. Mixing these domains often leads to confusing research. So, for example, of about 125 measures identified by Hill and Hood (1999a), there was a cluster of measures stressing religious beliefs, another cluster emphasizing religious attitudes, and so forth. Sometimes it is desirable to have a single multidimensional measure, but even then there will usually be subscales (often determined by factor analysis) tapping more specific domains.

Table 2.3, based on Hill (2013), provides a summary of 13 common categories of measures that have been developed, with examples of measures from the literature that fit each category. One might be surprised by the number of measures available, especially since the measures and their respective categories in the table are not exhaustive. In fact, the table includes only a small percentage of measures, though Hill (2013) maintains that they represent some of the better measures in the psychology of religion. Notice that the first nine categories cover what Tsang and McCullough (2003) refer to as "Level I" measures, which represent "higher levels of organization reflecting broad individual differences among persons in highly abstracted, trait-like qualities" (p. 349). Level I measures may help assess how religious or spiritual a person is, and here we refer to this as "dispositional religiousness." The final four categories of measures represent "Level II" measures, which get at how religion or spirituality functions in a person's life, referred to here as "functional religiousness." For example, highly religious people may use their religion in different ways to help cope with life's stressful agents. In reality, the distinction between Level I and Level II measures is often blurred. Level I scales that assess, for example, religious social participation (Category 7) also include scales

TABLE 2.3. Specific Measures of Religion and Spirituality in 13 Common Domains

Level I: Measures of dispositional religiousness or spirituality

General religiousness or spirituality
    Mysticism Scale (Hood, 1975)
    Religiosity Measure (Rohrbaugh & Jessor, 1975)
    Spiritual Transcendence Scale (Piedmont, 1999)

Religious or spiritual well-being
    Spiritual Well-Being Scale (Paloutzian & Ellison, 1982)
    Functional Assessment of Chronic Illness Therapy—Spiritual Well-Being Scale
        (Peterman et al., 2002)

Religious or spiritual commitment
    Dimensions of Religious Commitment Scale (Glock & Stark, 1966)
    Religious Commitment Scale (Pfeifer & Waelty, 1995)
    Religious Commitment Inventory–10 (Worthington et al., 2003)
    Santa Clara Strength of Religious Faith Questionnaire (Plante, Vallaeys, Sherman, &
        Wallston, 2002)

Religious or spiritual beliefs
    Beliefs and Values Scale (King et al., 2006)
    Buddhist Beliefs and Practices Scale (Emavardhana & Tori, 1997)
    Christian Orthodoxy Scale (Fullerton & Hunsberger, 1982; Hunsberger, 1989)
    Love and Guilt Oriented Dimensions of Christian Belief (McConahay & Hough, 1973)
    Loving and Controlling God Scale (Benson & Spilka, 1973)
    Spiritual Belief Inventory (Holland et al., 1998)
    Spiritual Belief Scale (Schaler, 1996)
    Student Religiosity Questionnaire (Katz & Schmida, 1992)
    Views of Suffering Scale (Hale-Smith, Park, & Edmondson, 2012)

Religious or spiritual development
    Faith Development Interview Guide (Fowler, 1981)
    Faith Development Scale (Leak, Loucks, & Bowlin, 1999)
    Faith Maturity Scale (Benson, Donahue, & Erickson, 1993)
    Religious Maturity Scale (Leak & Fish, 1999)
    Spiritual Assessment Inventory (Hall & Edwards, 1996)

Religious attachment
    Attachment to God Inventory (Beck & McDonald, 2004)
    Attachment to God Scale (Kirkpatrick & Shaver, 1992)
    Attachment to God Scale (Rowatt & Kirkpatrick, 2002)

Religious social participation or religious/spiritual support
    Attitude Toward the Church Scale (Thurstone & Chave, 1929)
    Attitude Toward Church and Religious Practices (Dynes, 1955)
    Congregation Climate Scales (Pargament, Silverman, Johnson, Echemendia, &
        Snyder, 1983)
    Congregation Satisfaction Questionnaire (Silverman, Pargament, Johnson,
        Echemendia, & Snyder, 1983)
    Religious Involvement Inventory (Hilty & Morgan, 1985)
    Religious Support Scale (Krause, 1999)
    Religious Support Scale (Fiala, Bjorck, & Gorsuch, 2002)
    Spiritual Experience Index—Revised (Genia, 1997)

(continued)

TABLE 2.3. *(continued)*

Religious or spiritual private practices
  Buddhist Beliefs and Practices Scale (Emavardhana & Tori, 1997)
  Inward, Outward, Upward Prayer Scale (Ladd & Spilka, 2002, 2006)
  Religious Background and Behavior (Connors, Tonigan, & Miller, 1996)
  Types of Prayer Scale (Poloma & Pendleton, 1989)

Religious or spiritual history
  The SPIRITual History (Maugans, 1996)
  Spiritual History Scale (Hays, Meador, Branch, & George, 2001)

Level II: Measures of functional religiousness or spirituality

Religious or spiritual experiences
  Attitudes Toward God Scale (Wood, Froh, & Geraghty, 2010)
  Daily Spiritual Experiences Scale (Underwood, 1999)
  Index of Core Spiritual Experiences (Kass, Friedman, Leserman, Zuttermeister, & Benson, 1991)
  Religious Experience Episodes Measure (Hood, 1970)
  Religious Comfort and Strain Scale (Exline, Yali, & Sanderson, 2000)
  Spiritual Experience Index—Revised (Genia, 1997)
  Spiritual Orientation Inventory (Elkins, Hedstrom, Hughes, Leaf, & Saunders, 1988)

Religion or spirituality as motivating forces
  Duke Religion Index (Koenig et al., 1997)
  Intratextual Fundamentalism Scale (Williamson et al., 2010)
  Intrinsic–Extrinsic Scale—Revised (Gorsuch & McPherson, 1989)
  Quest Scale (Batson, Schoenrade, & Ventis, 1993)
  Religious Orientation Scale (Allport & Ross, 1967)
  Religious Internalization Scale (Ryan, Rigby, & King, 1993)
  Religious Fundamentalism Scale (Altemeyer & Hunsberger, 1992, 2004)

Religious or spiritual coping or struggle
  Attitudes Toward God Scale (Wood et al., 2010)
  Religious and Spiritual Struggle Scale (Exline, Pargament, Grubbs, & Yali, 2014)
  Religious Comfort and Strain Scale (Exline et al., 2000)
  Religious Coping Scale (RCOPE) (Pargament, Koenig, & Perez, 2000)
  Religious Coping Activities Scale (Pargament et al., 1990)
  Religious Pressures Scale (Altemeyer, 1988)
  Religious Problem-Solving Scale (Pargament et al., 1988)
  Spiritual Transformation Scale (Cole et al., 2008)

Religious or spiritual meaning and values
  Functional Assessment of Chronic Illness Therapy—Spiritual Well-Being Scale (Peterman et al., 2002)
  Meaning Scale (Krause, 2009)
  Purpose in Life Scale (Crumbaugh & Maholick, 1964)
  Seeking of Noetic Goals Scale (Crumbaugh, 1977)
  Sense of Coherence Scale (Antonovsky, 1987)

Note. Based on Hill (2013).

of religious or spiritual support, which is also a functional (Level II) benefit. More scales and more detailed discussions of scales can be found in a number of resources: Hill (2013), Hill and Edwards (2013), Hill and Hood (1999a), MacDonald (2000), and MacDonald, LeClair, Holland, Alter, and Friedman (1995).

Gorsuch's (1984) claim that the psychology of religion had been dominated by issues of measurement up to that time led him to conclude that measurement scales were "reasonably effective" and "available in sufficient varieties for most any task in the psychology of religion" (p. 234). Now, over 30 years later, we can say that Gorsuch was both correct and incorrect. Within the psychology of religion proper, and especially at Level I dispositional measurement, Gorsuch was correct. Researchers have a sufficient arsenal of measurement instruments at hand to adequately assess a person's level of religiousness or spirituality, even given the complexities of what it means to be religious or spiritual. The one caveat, however, is that measures within the psychology of religion will need to become increasingly pluralistic, to better represent (1) religious traditions other than Christianity and (2) those forms of spirituality that do not conform to any formal religious tradition.

However, Gorsuch (or anyone else, for that matter) was, quite understandably, unable in 1984 to envision the direction the field would take, particularly the move toward examining the many functional varieties of religiousness (Level II measurement) that would require further scale development. So, for example, in reviewing the significant association between religion and both mental and physical health (to be discussed in considerable detail in Chapter 13), Hill and Pargament (2003; see also Hill & Edwards, 2013, and Hill & Pargament, 2017) have highlighted ongoing advances in measurement (e.g., measuring perceived closeness to God, religious struggle) that help delineate *why* religiousness and spirituality seem to contribute (mostly positively, but sometimes negatively) to health and well-being. It is safe to say that measurement issues, particularly of the Level II functional variety, will continue to be of great interest and concern to psychologists of religion.

Implicit Measures

The final measurement issue we wish to discuss is an issue that plagues all of psychology—the field's overreliance on self-report measures. Every measure (including qualitative measures) discussed thus far in this section relies on self-reports, which of course may be biased for a number of reasons: intentional deception, impression management, personal bias, and many more. The accuracy of self-reports is especially suspect when the topic being investigated is personal and sensitive in nature (Dovidio & Fazio, 1992), which religion and spirituality often are. As a result, there has been an increasing interest in developing other measurement techniques (such as physiological measures, better behavioral measures, etc.), including the use of "implicit" measures, particularly as measures of attitudes (see Jong, Zahl, & Sharp, 2017, for a more complete discussion). Greenwald and colleagues (Greenwald & Banaji, 1995; Greenwald, McGhee, & Schwartz, 1998) have defined "implicit attitudes" as unconscious, automatic evaluations that influence thoughts, feelings, and behaviors. Probably the most common implicit measure is the Implicit Association Test (IAT; Greenwald et al., 1998), which uses response latency as a marker of one's unconscious and automatic attitudes. The IAT was first developed as an implicit measure of racial attitudes, whereby an associative strength between two concepts (e.g., objects and evaluative adjectives) is measured by the amount of time (measured in milliseconds) it takes to determine whether the concepts go together. Thus it may be easier for a racially prejudiced white person to categorize two objects that are congruent (and hence take less time to determine that the two concepts go together) in his or her thinking (e.g., white and good; black and bad) than objects that are incongruent (e.g., white and bad; black and good). Though there are many assumptions underlying the IAT (and the notion of implicit measurement in general), social-psychological research has shown it to be psychometrically adequate in terms of its internal consistency, temporal reliability, and validity (Rowatt & Franklin, 2004).

The utilization of implicit measures is not yet common in the literature on the psychology of religion. Some of these studies have investigated explicit (i.e., self-report) measures of religiousness or spirituality in relation to some implicit measure, such as race attitudes (Rowatt & Franklin, 2004), humility (Powers, Nam, Rowatt, & Hill, 2007; Rowatt, Powers, et al., 2006), attitudes toward homosexuals (Rowatt, Tsang, et al., 2006; Tsang & Rowatt, 2007), or attitudes toward other religious groups (Rowatt, Franklin, & Cotton, 2005). The results of much of this research are covered later in this book, particularly in Chapter 12. Others (e.g., Hill, 1994; Jong et al., 2017; Wenger, 2004), however, have made the case that religion itself may be a topic that can be implicitly measured, and several notable attempts have now been made (Bassett, Smith, et al., 2005; Cohen, Shariff, & Hill, 2008; Gibson, 2006; Jong, Halberstadt, & Bluemke, 2012; LaBouff, Rowatt, Johnson, Thedford, & Tsang, 2010; Wenger, 2004).

Here we describe two of these measures. LaBouff et al. (2010) have developed an implicit measure of religiousness/spirituality (abbreviated here as RS) in the IAT tradition by measuring the extent to which people consider themselves religious relative to others. In their RS-IAT measure, participants were asked to categorize words such as "I," "me," "my," "mine," "self," "they," "them," "their," "it," and "other" as applying to either "Self" or "Other." Similarly, they were asked to categorize such words as "religious," "spiritual," "faithful," "theistic," "believer," "nonreligious," "nonspiritual," "faithless," "atheistic," and "agnostic" as applying to either "Religious–Spiritual" or "Not Religious–Not Spiritual." People who were faster at categorizing Self/Religious–Spiritual and Other/Not Religious–Not Spiritual pairings than at categorizing Self/Not Religious–Not Spiritual and Other/Religious–Spiritual were considered (implicitly) more religious or spiritual. Scores on the RS-IAT were positively correlated with self-report measures of religiousness/spirituality. The measure was also able to predict people's attitudes toward gay men and lesbian women over and above self-reported measures.

Cohen et al. (2008) used reaction times to words as an implicit measure of religious beliefs. They presented participants with a series of words, along with the instructions to categorize these words as either "real" or "imaginary" and to do so as quickly as possible. Examples of words included words that were clearly real (e.g., "airplane," "George Bush"), clearly imaginary (e.g., "Captain Kirk," "tooth fairy"), objects of religious faith that are not directly observable (e.g., "Adam and Eve," "heaven"), and objects of secular "faith" that are not directly observable (e.g., "black hole," "molecules"). Indeed, religious people categorized religious items as real more than did nonreligious people. Furthermore (and of greater value for these reaction times as an implicit measure), the researchers found that people who reported themselves at the extremes (i.e., as either very religious or very nonreligious) were faster than people who self-reported as moderately religious in making the call of "real" or "imaginary." These differences were found only on the objects of religious faith and not on words that fit the other three categories, suggesting that this is an implicit measure of religiousness more than some other characteristic (such as make-believe).

This research is still in its earliest stages, with the implicit measures themselves needing more frequent testing before any judgment of their utility can be made. These attempts do represent, however, important efforts at getting beyond reliance on self-report measures.

ATTRIBUTION IN THE PSYCHOLOGY OF RELIGION

Considering the awe with which the power of God is regarded in the Judeo-Christian tradition, one might perceive a role for the deity only when events of the greatest significance are involved. A disaster takes place, and the insurance company defines it as an "act of God." A young person unexpectedly dies, and it is said to be an expression of "God's will." People who win millions of dollars in lotteries may attribute their success to the "hand of God." The unanticipated is often explained by such phrases as "God works in mysterious ways." Despite the fact that science has provided detailed naturalistic interpretations of birth and death, as well as reasons for good fortune and victory or for failure and defeat, for most people there still remains a sense of the miraculous about the rare and unique events that can greatly change their lives. From a personal perspective, science and common sense often do not satisfactorily answer such questions as "Why now?", "Why me?", or "Why here?" If someone is suffering from a severe illness or a terminal condition, pleas to God seem quite appropriate. Instances of remission when all appeared hopeless are frequently regarded as signs of God's mercy, compassion, favor, or forgiveness. Research confirms this view that God becomes part of the "big picture" for the significant things that happen (Spilka & Schmidt, 1983a). Defining what is important has a very individual quality: Sports teams may pray for extra achievement in the "big game," or gamblers may plead for divine intervention on a roll of the dice (Hoffman, 1992).

We have identified in Chapter 1 the search for meaning as the core theme in our framework for the psychology of religion. People are meaning-driven creatures, and religion is uniquely capable of providing meaning, even sometimes when applied to ordinary everyday events and experiences. There is, however, a problem with this framework for psychologists who empirically study religious experience: "Meaning" and "purpose" are broad and elusive concepts that are difficult to investigate empirically. What psychologists need are more specific theories capable of producing testable hypotheses within the larger framework of the search for meaning. In Chapter 1, we have described attribution theory as one such possibility. There are other approaches to studying religion as a meaning system, of course, and utilizing the search for meaning as an overall conceptual framework is but one of many ways in which the psychology of religion can be approached. Nevertheless, as we shall soon see, attribution processes are at work in how we find meaning in life (Kruglanski, Hasmel, Maides, & Schwartz, 1978), even though they are only part of the story, and we believe that attribution theory is indeed a useful framework for the empirical study of religious experience. We now look more specifically at how attribution processes are part of how people use religion.

We have noted in Chapter 1 that attributions involve creating causal explanations about people, things, and events. Such explanations are couched in ideas and statements that assign certain powers and positions to various situational and dispositional factors. By examining such meanings and their ramifications, attributional research became a major cornerstone of cognitive social psychology, and it was soon extended to explain how people understand their emotional states and many of the things that happen to them and to others (Fiske & Taylor, 1991; Hewstone, 1983a). It may also help explain much religious experience.

Motivational Bases of Attributions: Needs for Meaning, Control, and Esteem

The question of why people make attributions returns us to some basic motivational themes that underlie much religious thinking and behavior—namely, to needs for meaning, control, and esteem. Here we define "esteem" as a personal sense of capability and adequacy, which is a central part of sociality (as defined in Chapter 1) and is reflected in our relationships with others. Though other activating elements are important, depending on the topic and situation, we see meaning, control, and esteem as central concerns for the psychology of religion.

Forms of personal faith—for example, Allport's I, E, and Quest orientations—can be viewed as motivationally concerned with meaning, control, and esteem. Allport's (1966) idea of I faith as a sentiment flooding "the whole life with motivation and meaning" (p. 455), and as a search for truth, is explicitly directed toward the attainment of ultimate meaning. Garey, Siregar, Hood, Agustiani, and Setiono (2017) created a reliable scale to measure positive and negative attributions to Allah or God among disadvantaged adolescents in Indonesia. Although the majority of their participants were Muslim, among both Christians and Muslims positive attributions to God or Allah were related to both meaning and religiosity, indicating that even the important differences noted above on I and E for Muslims and Christians in Indonesia do not exclude similarities as well. It may be that regardless of faith tradition, positive attributions to ultimacy are related to meaning. Quest is a similar effort to attain answers to basic questions. Further analyses of these religious orientations easily yield connections with these motivations.

In addition to a "need to know," a "need for mastery and control" enters the picture, as Kelley (1967) and other central figures in attribution theory and research have noted. Bulman and Wortman (1977) suggested yet another motivational source of attributions, which has been buttressed by much research—namely, that "people assign causality in order to maintain or enhance their self-esteem" (p. 351). Self-esteem is also likely to be a consequence of the presence of meaning and a sense of control.

Our theoretical position asserts that attributions are triggered when meanings are unclear, control is in doubt, and self-esteem is challenged. There is, as suggested, much evidence that these three factors are interrelated.

Naturalistic and Religious Attributions

Given these three sources of motivations for attributions, an individual may attribute the causes of events to a wide variety of possible referents (oneself, others, chance, God, etc.). For the psychologist of religion, these referents may be classified into two broad categories: "naturalistic" and "supernaturalistic" (or "religious"). The task is to identify and comprehend those influences that contribute to the making of religious attributions. The evidence is that most people—even those who are highly religious—will in most circumstances initially employ naturalistic explanations and attributions, such as references to people, natural events, accidents, or chance (Lupfer, Brock, & DePaola, 1992; Ritzema & Young, 1983). For several reasons, however, this does not mean that naturalistic attributions necessarily discount the role of the supernatural. For example, people may still believe that multiple agents, some natural and some supernatural, are simultaneously at work (Legare, Evans, Rosengren, & Harris, 2012; Legare & Gelman, 2008), such as when God is perceived as working through a naturalistic cause (e.g., a person's altruistic act of kindness, a natural disaster). There is also a good likelihood for some people to shift to religious attributions when naturalistic ones do not satisfactorily meet the needs for meaning, control, and esteem (Hewstone, 1983b; Spilka, Shaver, & Kirkpatrick, 1985).

Extending Attribution Theory

Theories usually become more useful when they are combined with other theoretical speculations, and Wikstrom (1987) has added to an attributional framework with the role theory of religion first developed by the Swedish scholar Hjalmar Sundén. Sundén's theory proposes that religion, "psychologically speaking, seem[s] to provide models and roles for a certain kind of perceptual 'set'" (Wikstrom, 1987, p. 391). A frame of reference is established in which the person's actions and cognitions are now structured by a religious role. Wikstrom further tells us that "when the frame of reference is activated, stimuli which would otherwise be left unnoticed are not only observed but also combined and attributed to a living and acting 'other,' to God" (1987, p. 393). Moreover, "as a condition and as a result of the feedback from the role-taking experience . . . [the self-perception] . . . can be seen as something that provides meaning and a feeling of identity, and strengthens self-esteem" (1987, p. 396). Control is also brought into the picture, showing how role and attribution approaches seem to parallel each other. There is unexplored potential here: van der Lans (1987) shows how this kind of role theory predicts various aspects of religious experience. Unfortunately, this approach has not stimulated much research.

Our contention is that these two cornerstones of social psychology—the attributional process and role taking—are products of interactions between external situational factors and internal dispositional factors (Magnusson, 1981). In other words, all thinking and behavior take place in an interpersonal and sociocultural context in which situations are elements. We now identify some of these influences that contribute to the making of religious attributions.

Situational Influences

For many years, social psychology in general and attribution research in particular have emphasized the role of immediate environmental factors in the determination of thinking and behavior (Ross & Nisbett, 1991). This implies that much religious experience, belief, and behavior are subject to the vagaries of current circumstances. In other words, the information we researchers obtain may largely be a function of the settings in which people are studied and data collected. There is evidence to support this idea. Schachter (1964) claims that an individual "will label his feelings in terms of his knowledge of the immediate situation" (p. 54). Dienstbier (1979) has referred to this labeling as "emotion attribution theory," in order to explain how people define the causes of emotional states when ambiguity exists. Proudfoot and Shaver (1975) used the same basic idea to denote the bases of religious experience. Research suggests that up to three-quarters of intense religious experiences occur when individuals are engaged in religious activities or are in religious settings (Spilka & Schmidt, 1983a). Still, one must be cautious, for some studies have not shown the influence of religious situations on religious attributions (Lupfer et al., 1992). There is also reason to believe that personal factors need to be considered (Epstein & O'Brien, 1985).

Situational influences fall into two broad categories: "contextual factors" and "event character factors." The first category is concerned with the degree to which situations are religiously structured, while the latter stresses the nature of the event being explained.

Contextual Factors

Situations may be religiously structured by the locale in which activities or their evaluations take place (e.g., church surroundings; the presence of others who are known to be religious, such as clergy; or participation in religious activities, such as prayer or worship). The presence of such circumstances should elicit religious attributions, and, as noted above, this is obviously true when religious mystical or intense religious experiences occur. Certainly if other people are present and are religiously involved, their actions should aid in the selection of a religious interpretation. We might say that the likelihood of religious explanations is heightened by such factors. Work by Hood (1977) has further demonstrated the importance of situational influences in the creation of nature-related and spiritual experiences. Contextual elements apparently increase the chances that those affected will attribute what occurs to the intervention of God. The *salience* of religion seems to be the key influence here. That is, the more important, noticeable, or conspicuous religion is in a situation, the more probable it is that religious attributions will be offered. This suggests what has been called the "availability hypothesis" or "availability heuristic." Religious influences in situations increase the probability of making religious associations or arousing religious ideas (Fiske & Taylor, 1991), though simply being present in a religious institution may not be enough (Spilka & Schmidt, 1983a).

Event Character Factors

Religious attributions may also be affected by the nature or character of the event being explained. A possibility that introduces questions of meaning and control concerns the degree of ambiguity and threat that events convey. For example, medical problems may be least understood and have the greatest potential for threatening life. In contrast, as serious as economic disasters are, they seem to be understood more easily; they also leave an individual the possibility of starting over again. In other words, we hypothesize that situations involving high ambiguity and high threat may have the greatest likelihood of calling forth religious explanations.

Several possible aspects of the character of an event may have implications for religious attributions: (1) the importance of what takes place; (2) whether the event is positive or negative; (3) the domain of the event (social, political, economic, medical, etc.); and (4) whether the event occurs to the attributing person or to someone else. These factors have been shown to affect the intensity and frequency of religious attributions, and are likely to be influential to the extent that they enhance meaning, control, and esteem.

EVENT IMPORTANCE

At the start of this discussion of attribution theory in the psychology of religion, situations where people frequently invoke God as a causal agent—ones in which "acts of God" and

"God's will" are common expressions—have been identified. We are more likely to make such attributions to God when the events are important. Rarely do we think about the role of God for what is commonplace, such as a successful trip to a local grocery store. However, if that same trip involves a severe accident where we narrowly escape death, then we are more likely to see "God's hand" at work. Indeed, research shows that we are likely to attribute events to God when they are life-altering (Ray, Lockman, Jones, & Kelly, 2015), such as surviving a tsunami (Levy, Slade, & Ranasinghe, 2009).

EVENT VALENCE

An event's "valence" refers to how positive or negative the event is. For years, research suggested that attributions to God are overwhelmingly positive (Bulman & Wortman, 1977; Johnson & Spilka, 1991; Lupfer et al., 1992), and that people rarely blame God for the bad things that happen to them. Bulman and Wortman (1977) studied the reasons given by young people who became paraplegic because of serious accidents. They saw a benevolent divine purpose in what happened to them. As one such youth put it, "God's trying to put me in situations, help me learn about Him and myself and also how I can help other people" (quoted in Bulman & Wortman, 1977, p. 358). In another study, a patient with cancer told one of us, "God does not cause cancer . . . illness and grief do not come from God. God does give me the strength to cope with any and all problems" (quoted in Johnson & Spilka, 1991, p. 30). Rabbi Harold Kushner's (1981) well-known book *When Bad Things Happen to Good People* supports this idea that bad things should not be attributed to God. Much of the early empirical research on this topic was done with overtly religious samples.

Even though positive attributions to God prevail, some recent research suggests that people are willing to question God, especially under some circumstances such as human suffering (Gray & Wegner, 2010; Hale-Smith, Park, & Edmondson, 2012). Even then, however, they may not see God as causing the suffering as much as allowing it to occur (Miner & McKnight, 1999). When God is seen as causing something negative, people may respond with anger (Exline, Park, Smyth, & Cary, 2011), which could reflect ongoing spiritual struggle (Exline, 2013).

Furthermore, some people feel that they are being punished for their sins and may make negative attributions to God. This research suggests that this tendency reflects a negative coping style (Pargament, Koenig, & Perez, 2000). Clearly, the valence of events influences religious attributions, but we need to know more about why and under what circumstances positive or negative attributions are made to the deity.

EVENT DOMAIN

Certain domains appear "ready-made" for the application of secular understandings, while others seem more appropriate for invoking religious possibilities. We know that medical situations—especially those that are life-threatening—strongly elicit religious attributions, which may reduce death anxiety and provide a sense that God is in control (Kay, Gaucher, McGregor, & Nash, 2010; Kunst, Bjorck, & Tan, 2000). Social or economic circumstances, which may be more associated with naturalistic explanations over which we may have a greater sense of control, are less likely to elicit religious explanations unless they are highly unusual (Spilka & Schmidt, 1983a). In addition, religious institutions have been quite averse to glorifying money and wealth. References in the Bible to "filthy lucre" and the difficulty the rich will encounter in attempting to enter heaven leave little doubt that economic and spiritual matters are not regarded as harmonious.

Without question, when people are in dire straits in any domain, it is not uncommon to seek divine help. The issue may, however, revolve around the clarity of meanings and the sense of control a person has in various situations. Religion may best fill the void when the person cannot understand why things are as they are, and control is lacking—in other words, when ambiguity is great and threat is high.

EVENT PERSONAL RELEVANCE

There is little doubt that when events occur to us, they are much more personally important than when they happen to others. We can be deeply moved when we hear about a friend's or relative's serious illness, but when we suffer from such a condition ourselves, the question "Why me?" is suddenly of the greatest significance, and attributions to God are commonly made. If something particularly good happens to someone else, such as the winning of a great deal of money, we might say, "That's luck for you," and feel happy for that person. The one benefited is more likely to claim that "God was looking out for me." The idea that personal relevance may elicit more religious attributions has gained support, but not consistently. It does seem to be involved in interactions with other variables, so additional research is called for to resolve these ambiguities (Lupfer et al., 1992; Spilka & Schmidt, 1983a).

Personal relevance is one of those variables that overlaps the broad categories of situational and dispositional influences in that it is part of both realms. It is to the role of dispositions in the attribution process that we now turn.

Dispositional Influences

The Individual in Context

The strong emphasis on individualism in North American society causes us to look at people as if they act independently of their surroundings. Just as events take place in contexts, persons always exist in their individual life spaces, which vary with time and place. It may make a big difference if someone reacts in the morning before breakfast, or in the evening after supper. A religious experience that takes place in a church may have different repercussions than one that occurs when the individual is alone on a mountaintop does. Personal response is surprisingly situationally dependent. That does not mean, however, that there are no individual differences even when a person is in the grips of a powerful situation.

Personal Factors

Individual characteristics may be termed "dispositional," and these fall into three overlapping categories: "background," "cognitive," and "personality/attitudinal." Since we are not in a position to denote constitutional and genetic influences or their effects, these three realms imply that people pattern their attributions regarding the causes and nature of events so that some explanations are much more "available" or "better-fitting" than other possibilities. What is available or better-fitting for one person may not hold for another. This would hold true for the selection of naturalistic as opposed to religious referents. Specifically, it would be true for their decisions as to whether positive or negative event outcomes are a result of their own actions or those of others; are due to fate, luck, or chance; or are attributable to the involvement of God.

BACKGROUND FACTORS

It is a psychological truism to state that people are largely products of their environment as far as most behavior is concerned. The overwhelming majority of us are exposed early in life to religious teachings at home and by our peers and adults in schools, churches, and communities. These childhood lessons often follow us throughout life and are expressed by the use of religious concepts in a wide variety of circumstances. A common observation suggests that the stronger a person's spiritual background, the greater the chance that the person will report intense religious experiences and undergo conversion (Clark, 1929; Coe, 1900). Frequency of church attendance, knowledge of one's faith, importance of religious beliefs, and the persistence of religious ideas over many decades are correlates of early religious socialization (McGuire, 1992; Shand, 1990). In other words, the more conservatively religious or orthodox the home and family in which a person was reared, the greater the person's likelihood of using religious attributions later in life.

COGNITIVE FACTORS

One area of study that is drawing considerable attention is the cognitive science of religion. Barrett (2004) has suggested that the human mind possesses a "hyperactive agency detection device"—that is, a heightened tendency to detect intentional action by outside agents, both natural and supernatural, especially when it makes sense or is said to be "minimally counterintuitive" (Hornbeck & Barrett, 2013). So, it is natural for young children to believe in God (or other supernatural agents such as the devil, demons, angels, or ghosts). This may be especially true for adults under conditions that elicit awe (Valdesolo & Graham, 2013; Van Cappellen & Saroglou, 2012), such as a visit to Zion or Bryce National Park in Utah—or, conversely, in secluded and threatening situations (Barnes & Gibson, 2013). But this does not hold true for everyone. For example, cognitive style is a factor in that people who are more analytical (vs. intuitive) thinkers are less likely to use religious attributions (Pennycook, Cheyne, Seli, Kohler, & Fugelsang, 2012; Razmyar & Reeve, 2013; Shenhav, Rand, & Greene, 2012).

Attributions depend on having available a language that both permits and supports thinking along certain lines. Bernstein (1964) tells us that "Language marks out what is relevant, affectively, cognitively, and socially, and experience is transformed by what is made relevant" (quoted in Bourque & Back, 1971, p. 3). Such relevance is well demonstrated by studies showing that religious persons possess a religious language and use it to describe their experience. There is reason to believe that the presence of such a language designates an experience as religious instead of aesthetic or some other possibility (Bourque, 1969; Bourque & Back, 1971). Meaning to the experiencing individual appears in part to be a function of the language and vocabulary available to the person, and this clearly relates to the individual's background and interests. There is much in the idea that thought is a slave of language, and the thoughts that breed attributions are clearly influenced by the language the attributor is set to use (Carroll, 1956).

PERSONALITY/ATTITUDINAL FACTORS

The broad heading of "personality/attitudinal factors" includes a wide variety of dispositional factors that almost seem to defy classification. The language of personality is both difficult and complex, and different thinkers often employ different concepts to cover the same psychological territory. Schaefer and Gorsuch (1991) propose a "multivariate belief–motivation theory of religiousness" in an effort to integrate the often scattered ideas and research notions that associate traits and attitudes with religion. These scholars first recognize what they term a "superordinate domain" of religiousness, which comprises a number of subdomains. Their intention is to define the components of these latter spheres. The three they select for study are religious motivation, religious beliefs, and religious problem-solving style. Depending on the variables chosen to represent these subdomains, there may be room for argument as to whether one is looking at a cognitive or a motivational factor. Unhappily, most workers in the field have not been as rigorous as Gorsuch and his students where definition of variables is concerned. For example, many "personality" factors have been examined in relation to religiousness. Among these are self-esteem, locus of control, the concept of a just world, and form of personal faith. All four seem to possess a motivational quality, yet the last two strongly involve belief systems. The Schaefer–Gorsuch theory implies a need to distinguish motivational from belief components, or to identify a third, overlapping domain (Schaefer & Gorsuch, 1991). Obviously, this work is in its infancy, but it suggests a potentially fruitful way of organizing a mass of piecemeal findings into a coherent framework.

To illustrate the meanings of personality/attitudinal dispositions relative to the making of religious attributions, let us look briefly at what we know about two well-researched factors: self-esteem and locus of control.

Self-Esteem. Research on self-conceptions has been conducted for almost 60 years. For more than 30 years, many psychologists have focused on self-esteem—the regard people have for themselves (Wylie, 1979). The evidence suggests that this variable is quite basic to personality. One view is that attributions are often made to validate and enhance self-esteem; they perform a self-protective function (Hewstone, 1983b).

Needless to say, a fair number of researchers have examined self-esteem relative to religiosity. In general, high self-esteem relates to positive and loving images of God, and similarly to Allport's I religious orientation (Benson & Spilka, 1973; Hood, 1992b; Masters & Bergin, 1992). There may be a need here for consistency; this suggests that those who have negative self-views perceive God as unloving and punitive (Benson & Spilka, 1973). In other words, the person with a negative opinion of the self may think, "I am unlovable; hence God can't love me." Consistency further implies that favorable attributions to God ought to be associated with positive event outcomes as opposed to negative occurrences. This hypothesis has been supported (Lupfer et al., 1992; Spilka & Schmidt, 1983a).

Self-esteem does not stand by itself. It is enmeshed in a complex of overlapping personality traits and religious concepts and measures, such as sin and guilt, as well as the nature of the religious tradition with which one is identified (Hood, 1992b). This work indicates that different patterns of self-esteem and God attributions may be a function of one's religious heritage and its doctrines. If a prime role of attributions is to buttress self-esteem, we need to ask how religion performs such a function—especially in traditions such as fundamentalism, which may seem quite harsh on an individual's effort to express positive self-regard.

Locus of Control. "Locus of control" was initially conceptualized as a tendency to see events as either internally determined by the person or externally produced by factors beyond the control of the individual. This formulation has been extended and refined a number of times. External control factors were originally viewed as fate, luck, and chance until Levenson (1973) added control by powerful others, and Kopplin (1976) brought in control by God. Pargament et al. (1988) recognized the complexity of control relationships relative to the deity, and developed measures to assess what they termed a "deferring" mode (an active God and a passive person), a "collaborative" mode (both an active God and an active person), and a "self-directive" mode (an active person and a passive God). These notions illustrate different patterns of attribution for control to the self and God. In the deferring mode, individuals may pray and, having done that, attribute all the power to God: "It's in the hands of God." Those with a collaborative style are basically saying that both they and God have control: "God helps those who help themselves." Utilizing these coping styles relates to further attributions to the nature of God. Though the associations are stronger with the collaborative than with the deferring mode, the tendency for persons who adopt such control perspectives is to attribute generally positive qualities to the deity, along with their recognition of God's power (Schaefer & Gorsuch, 1991).

Although belief in supernaturalism affiliates with external control, Shrauger and Silverman (1971) found that "people who are more involved in religious activities perceive themselves as having more control over what happens to them" (p. 15; see also Randall & Desrosiers, 1980). This sounds like intrinsic religion, or at least orthodoxy, for this relationship is strongest among religious conservatives (Furnham, 1982; Silvestri, 1979; Tipton, Harrison, & Mahoney, 1980). Studying highly religious people, Hunsberger and Watson (1986) found that attributions of control and responsibility are made to God when outcomes are positive—a well-confirmed finding—but that when the result is negative, the tendency is to attribute the blame to Satan ("The Devil made me do it"). Issues of control, and questions of to whom or what control is attributed, have been extensively studied both within and outside the psychology of religion. These are concerns that should be kept in mind throughout this book.

Attribution Theory: Summary

In keeping with our theme that religion helps provide a sense of meaning, we have proposed attribution theory as a useful midlevel theoretical framework from which testable hypotheses about religion and religious experience are derived. How people attribute the causes of behavior both reflects and influences meaning systems, whether religious or otherwise. By drawing from mainstream social psychology, not only are we able to utilize theoretically well-grounded psychological notions that have stood the test of time; as we apply such theories as attribution to the psychology of religion, we may foster new insights into and understandings of the theories themselves, thus offering something back to the field (Hill, 1999; Hill & Gibson, 2008).

OVERVIEW

In this chapter, we have first attempted to distinguish what psychologists of religion study from similar concepts that have possible overlaps with religion but that are nevertheless different, such as superstition. We have then directed our attention toward the operationalization of religious concepts. To this end, we have examined various dimensions of religiousness, both logical and logical–empirical, in order to make our thinking clear about how we construct the instruments we employ.

Our long-term goal is to keep the psychology of religion integrated with the mainstream of psychology itself. Since the study of personal faith is largely regarded as part of social psychology, we have shown how various basic ideas in social psychology are realized in our work. We must clearly know the details and parameters of what we are talking about; hence our emphasis on cognition, affect, behavior, and habit, as well as on attribution theory.

Recognizing that the psychology of religion shares in (and is often plagued by) the same issues that the overall field of psychology continually confronts, we have also looked at questions concerning reductionism and the idiothetic–nomothetic controversy, which overlaps with the issue of holistic versus atomistic analysis. Maintaining our inclination toward the scientific, with its concern for making information public, reproducible, reliable, and valid, we have illustrated the idiothetic–nomothetic and holistic–atomistic issues by returning to the problem of spirituality, first discussed in Chapter 1. In the last few decades, this has become a "hot" topic. Psychologists have heretofore avoided spirituality, because it was (and still is) so much easier to assess religiosity in its various forms. We have shown how spirituality, which has usually been conceptualized as holistic, rapidly becomes multiform in both conceptual and psychometric analyses. We are thus forced to return to Meehl's (1954) conclusion that "the actuary will have the final word" (p. 138). We see no scientific alternative at the present time.

CHAPTER 3

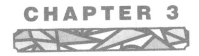

Evolution, Neuropsychology, and Other Biological Aspects of Religion

Probably in no other area has the encounter between Christianity and science generated so much misunderstanding or left such deep scars as in that of biological science.

The brain is the organ of the soul.

Biology has nothing directly to do with religion, and by no possibility can religion, such as we know, be based on biology.

Darwin was a most careful observer . . . there was great truth in the theory and there was nothing atheistic in it if properly understood.

Religion itself is one of the most striking possible examples of evolution.

If you are a Darwinist, I pity you, for it is impossible to be a Darwinist and a Christian at the same time.[1]

We have barely touched on relations between religion and science. Though Scott (1999) suggests four ways in which they are related, most attention has been afforded what she terms the "warfare model." This approach sets each domain against the other and implies, in their extreme form, that there can be no resolution of their conflict.

In contrast, the psychology of religion allows us to bring these broad realms together into a psychobiology of religion—a relationship that is rapidly growing in complexity and potential. Our task in this chapter is to explore psychobiological arguments and theory regarding the origins of religion plus a variety of its expressions. Ideas and information from neuroscience, evolutionary theory, and genetics, among other possibilities, are examined. In addition, their relevance to health is explored. Finally, some long-known relationships between specific religious groups and diseases are discussed.

When new ideas grip people's imaginations, enthusiasm often leaps ahead of the necessary sobering second thoughts. It is therefore important for us to step back and

---

[1]These quotations come, respectively, from the following sources: Hearn (1968, p. 199); Porter (1883, p. 38); Haldane (1931, p. 43); McCosh (1890, p. vii); Millikan (1935, p. 65); and Russell (1935, p. 76), quoting his boyhood tutor.

recognize the complexity of the field and the many cautions that should be observed (Azari, 2006; Kirkpatrick, 2006a; Vaas, 2009). Even though we must keep in mind the fact that our reference framework for the psychology of religion is science, it is not our intention to challenge theology or religious and spiritual frameworks. Theology may even serve as a source of theory and a guide for empirical research (Hood, 2012a; Spilka, 1976; Vaux, 1990).

UNDERSTANDING RELIGIOUS CONCEPTS

If there is one reality that must be confronted, it is that we can never actually find a provable origin for faith. We offer theories and hypotheses, and search for data that support or refute these ideas. Here we look primarily to biology for such information, and evolution immediately enters the picture.

It is quite easy for us to use the term "religion" and just move on in our presentation. We need, however, to appreciate its complexity, its multidimensionality. Given the almost unbelievable variety of religious and spiritual expressions in different cultures, this might seem an impossible undertaking. Still, social scientists have attempted such an endeavor. Vaas (2009) for example, suggests that religion covers seven main components—"transcendence," "myth," "morality," "mysticism," "rite," "ultimate relationships," and "ultimate purpose." The choice of different terms ("supernaturalism," "ceremonialism," "superhuman agency," etc.) by other scholars does not lighten the burden. Some practices may have different origins. Unfortunately, multiple usages further confound the problem. We therefore need to approach the problem of beginnings by appreciating the obvious fact that there may be a number of origins.

THEORIES OF THE ORIGINS OF RELIGION: HERITAGE AND DIRECTION

Early Development of Views on Religion in the West

In Western civilization, religion has been a source of interest and concern for millennia. Prior to the 17th century, it dominated virtually all aspects of social and cultural life. Religion was justified through ideas about the physical universe; the composition and nature of the human body and mind; human limitations; and the existence of suffering, disease, and death. Mythologies, especially nature myths, were often judged to be the antecedents of religion (Caird, 1893/1969; Hopkins, 1923; Muller, 1879, 1889; Tylor, 1896). The essential point is that for the West, the approved origins of religion resided in the Bible and the teachings of Judaism and Christianity.

The coming of the Enlightenment in the 17th century opened a door to science, yet religious institutional doctrines were still not to be questioned. A growing attention to consciousness and the human mind constituted the realm of mental philosophy. A "religious psychology" replaced this in the early to mid-19th century (Fay, 1939). Discussions of mental faculties such as intellect remained premised upon theology and institutionally established faith. By the late 19th century, however, science slowly came to predominate in psychology, with the establishment of research laboratories such as that founded by Wilhelm Wundt at Leipzig in 1879. Attention to mind and consciousness stimulated the development of questionnaires and interviews. A new emphasis on religious ideas in childhood and adolescence, and on the nature of religious experience and conversion, appeared (Hall, 1900, 1904; Starbuck, 1897). In 1902, William James produced his noted *The Varieties of Religious Experience*, which (as noted in Chapter 2) remains a "must-read" volume detailing religious functions in many aspects of life. It is worth of note that James's subtitle to this classic text was *A Study in Human Nature*. With these early developments, the psychology of religion became scientific in theory and research. Biology was present, but stayed in the background or psychology in general.

Introducing Biology

The science of biology "stuttered along" until the mid-19th century. The appearance of *The Origin of Species* (Darwin, 1972) revolutionized the field, and Darwin's theory was rapidly adopted by the early psychologists. Religionists were split, as some fought these new ideas while others embraced them. Quite independently of faith, evolutionary theory took center stage and has continued to grow, but still finds opposition and a public that is not sure of its truth. Currently, one-third of Americans either do not believe in evolution or interpret it erroneously. This number rises to 64% among white evangelical Protestants (Pew Research Center, 2013d).

Scholars have attempted to understand faith from many vantage points. Early psychologists such as Freud and Jung offered their theories, but as psychology identified with the rigorous perspectives of mainstream science, attention increasingly turned to observable and measurable behavior. The next step became the assessment of concepts such as perception, emotion, and cognition. Continuing this process, a very sophisticated emphasis on neuroscience is currently growing in importance.

Evolutionary and Genetic Possibilities: Modern Perspectives

The core principle of evolutionary theory is natural selection, meaning that evolution's ultimate expression is through reproduction, with those who live passing on their genes to the next generation. Natural selection sounds simple on the surface, but is far more complex than is usually understood. The main implication of evolution through natural selection is that whatever is passed on is adaptive. Not only is this not always true, but there is continual speculation and theory regarding what is adaptive (Bering, 2009). Boyer (2001) emphasizes the idea that natural selection structures the mind so that only certain religious ideas *can* be acquired. The ideas themselves are not the direct products of natural selection. Religious foundations are thus produced, not specific religious contents.

In contrast, another view posits that some physical and psychological factors are "by-products" (Gould, 2002). In the course of natural selection, various unrelated components may be attached to what is passed down through the generations. They are, in essence, genetic hitchhikers. Later these may become adaptive. The idea of God is considered by some scholars to be such a by-product (Kirkpatrick, 2005). The by-product approach, however, has recently been challenged. Though Boyer (2003) views adaptation as primary, he claims that religion itself is a brain by-product. The strong emphasis of Darwinian theory on adaptation via natural selection opposes the notion of evolutionary by-products that may have no present or past coping functions (Fetchenhauer, 2009; Kunz, 2009). Barrett (2007) offers an ingenious analysis of the by-product issue, particularly in relation to its usage against theism. This interesting paper constitutes a treatise against what Barrett perceives as antireligious biopsychological arguments in general.

Natural selection has been going on for over 3 billion years, and humans appeared approximately 5 million years ago. People as we know them have been changing for approximately 50,000 to 200,000 years, and signs of religion go back about 100,000 years (Burkert, 1996; Pfeiffer, 1982; Rice, 2007; Young, 1991). We thus need to ask why and how religion might have appeared in the course of evolution.

Since religion is essentially universal, for it to be genetically involved, relevant mutations must have occurred—probably in the distant human past. Crisler (1994) speaks in the abstract of a religious gene that resulted from a mutation very early in humanity's family tree. This probably occurred in Africa, before humans split into different groups and began populating Europe and Asia. Despite such speculation, no such gene has ever been identified.

There is more than a little vagueness when evolution is applied to religion and spirituality. The search is for something genetic, and theory and hypothesis abound in this endeavor. Along these lines, possibly relevant to Crisler's hypothesis of a religious gene is the research of Dean Hamer (2004), a geneticist. He feels that the title of one of his books, *The God Gene*, overstates what he has found. Still, he reports research identifying a specific gene that he argues relates to self-transcendence, a theorized component of spirituality. Reference is made to transcendence in the sense of going beyond oneself, of feeling as if one is part of the overall universe. This is an aspect of self-realization—a sense of involvement in other-worldly things, particularly of a spiritual nature.

The elements that constitute spirituality are in contention, but most of the writing on spirituality focuses on religious and mystical experience. Hamer (2004) feels that more than one gene is likely to be part of the religion–spirituality complex. The gene he identifies is involved in mood control and expression, a facet of the popular tie between religious experience and spirituality. Hamer further shows that this gene relates to an objective measure of self-transcendence. Even though his research suggests that this tendency is largely genetic, the gene he has studied actually makes a rather small contribution to an objective measure of self-transcendence. Hamer's work and writing have stirred up a storm of controversy and criticism, but he has opened another research door to a very complex area (Broadway, 2004; Langone, 2004; Mohler, 2004; Zimmer, 2004).

Instinct

A major key for biology and psychology was first seen in the concept of "instinct." Our early lack of biological knowledge permitted scholars to employ this undefined popular term. They spoke of "maternal instincts," "imitative instincts," "gregarious instincts," and hundreds of others (Bernard, 1924). Instincts were viewed as the basis of habits and traits. They were regarded as innate patterns of both motivation and behavior that made religion fully biological (Bristol, 1904). Of course, the phrase "religious instinct" was widespread. In other words, religion was seen as naturally built into humans, and once this view was offered, its proponents felt that nothing more need be said. Although this view had earlier been rejected by Muller (1879, 1889), who correctly argued that it did nothing more than substitute one unknown for another, many endorsed the idea of a religious instinct until Bernard (1924) sounded its death knell when he reported that there were 83 religious instincts in the literature.

The old treatment of instinct is essentially dead, but not the word, as demonstrated by recent books titled *The Faith Instinct* (Wade, 2009) and *The Belief Instinct* (Bering, 2011b). These works are radically different from their predecessors, in that their authors accept modern science, evolution, and genetics. They believe there is a behind-the-scenes religious influence factor that is the result of natural selection, and they attach the word "instinct" to this factor. Bering (2011b) views instinct as a composite of cognitive, motivational, and emotional elements that are accidental by-products of evolution and genetics. He treats these as independent of religion. He further sees the source of his belief instinct residing in the brain, and this is termed an "adaptive illusion" or a "cognitive illusion." Like Bering, Wade (2009) utilizes evolution and natural selection, but violates tradition by extending it to human groups instead of restricting it to individuals. In Wade's view, religion has become a sociocultural force for uniting people, thus enhancing social solidarity. Altruism may replace competition and self-interest. Religious supernatural agents, rituals, and doctrines are designed to bring people together, to help them support each other. The goal is to create and strengthen viable social bodies, and to counter individualism and ideas and actions that might disrupt cooperation and mutuality. Evolution thus implants morality and empathy into the brains and minds of individuals to create socially supportive frameworks. Wade (2009) stresses the fact that religion appears to be universal among all peoples and groups on our planet. Its harmonizing and socializing functions and principles also appear general. He further claims the existence of a "faith instinct" that shades into an inspiration for theology and religion. Still, it remains a product of evolution and natural selection, increasing the likelihood of survival and reproduction. The purposes of these instincts are very positive, but in the larger world picture they fall far short of the intentions, if not hopes, of those who posit their existence.

   Supporters of frameworks that suggest biological, built-in bases for religion often describe these bases as "wired" or "hardwired." The reference may be to genes and genetics (Clark & Grunstein, 2000) or to brain structure and organization (Begley, 2001b, 2009). Some researchers ask whether belief in immortality is hardwired (Emmons & Kelemen, 2014). Shermer (2000) speaks of a hypothetical "belief engine" that makes us seek meaningful patterns, implying that we are "hardwired to think magically" (p. 35). It is evident from this discussion that those who work on the biology of evolution in relation to religion are quite linguistically flexible. We briefly mention this so that individuals interested in the psychology of religion will be fully aware of the language they might encounter in this area.

   Even though we have offered a number of considerations regarding religion as a probable outcome of the operation of evolution and natural selection, two further approaches merit our attention. These are the more rigorous ideas of J. R. Feierman (2009) and the highly controversial views of E. O. Wilson on sociobiology.

Feierman on Religion and Evolution

Feierman (2009, 2016) examines behavior down to the activating level of DNA and genes. Formulating original views of what may be inherited, he stresses a biological foundation for submissive behavior, which he feels is associated with activities such as prayer and with how people act in religious institutional settings. In a somewhat radical manner, he refers to cultural evolution as parallel to biology. The idea of natural selection enters the picture with his suggestion that religious behaviors enhance the likelihood of survival and reproduction. Even beliefs and values are offered as evolutionary products. We need more analyses such as Feierman presents. His edited volume (Feierman, 2009) offers much to stimulate our thinking in this area.

Sociobiology

Entomologist E. O. Wilson first proposed his theory of "sociobiology" in 1971 (see Wilson, 1978). He felt that his experience with social insects could be validly applied to people. From the sociobiological perspective, religious belief becomes an evolutionary product shaped by natural selection and therefore conferring a genetic advantage on people. It is a universal human behavioral tendency that resides at the core of society and suppresses an individual's personal interests in favor of the groups with which people are affiliated. Survival and reproduction are enhanced via submission to the social body. This is largely accomplished by teaching various beliefs and having people participate in established rituals and ceremonies. The outcome is that genes contributing to conformity will increase in frequency, and those that counter acquiescence and obedience will slowly be eliminated. Wilson (1978) thus writes about a "cultural Darwinism" (p. 181). Especially in the past, failure to follow the rules not only threatened survival but made one less acceptable as a mate, reducing the likelihood of passing on certain genes to following generations. Sexual selection and reproduction among group members are reinforced, whereas unconventional and noncompliant behavior can lead to ostracism and in many societies to exile, imprisonment, or even death. In summarizing this perspective, Austin (1980) stated that "genes favoring readiness to be indoctrinated were selected for" (p. 197). He concluded that "religious beliefs are enabling mechanisms for survival" (p. 193). Sociobiology thus favors natural selection and adaptation, but leaves room for learning and environmental influence.

Sociobiology is considered controversial (Kirkpatrick, 2006a). Its advocates and opponents have established well-defined battle lines (Dawkins, 1976, 1986; Gould, 2002; Sober, 1984; Williams, 1966). Cloninger and Yokoyama (1981) further claim that "much of the theory is speculative and poorly documented" (p. 749). Caplan (1978) produced a volume on what he aptly termed *The Sociobiology Debate*. Although much in the theory is indeed debatable, this book is a fascinating read—as is the sociobiology literature in general.

ASSESSING GENETIC INFLUENCE

Since evolution and natural selection must work through genetics, we need to understand this topic in slightly greater depth. Because genetics is a highly complex area of study we can undertake only a limited exploration here of its nature and effects.

If one studies identical and fraternal twins, it is possible to determine the degree to which any characteristic is a result of heredity or environment. When data are available on twins who were separated early in life, the influence of shared and unshared environments can also be evaluated (Falconer, 1981).[2] Utilizing this approach, a fair amount of research has been conducted on the heritability of religion. Serious efforts to evaluate various religious measures for identical and fraternal twins reveal higher correlations for the former (Bouchard & McGue, 2003). A hereditary component in religiosity thus appears to be present, but no one has been able to identify what this might be. Bouchard (2004) presents data suggesting that the genetic effects found for adults are at least twice as strong as those for adolescents. Even though thousands of sets of twins have been studied, serious questions can be asked about the

---

[2]These analyses start with correlations between the twins. The correlation coefficient squared (r^2) indicates the proportion of the variance that is explained when predicting from one twin to the other. Since identical twins have the same genetics, the variance due to heredity (h^2) is 100% accounted for Fraternal twins, like regular siblings only share 50% of their genetic variance. In addition, twins (whether identical or fraternal) share the same environment (e^2) if reared together. Since $r^2 = h^2 + e^2$ for identical twins reared together and $r^2 = \frac{1}{2}h^2 + e^2$ for fraternal twins reared together, one can solve for the proportion of the total variance for heredity and environment for any measured characteristics.

RESEARCH BOX 3.1. Genetic and Environmental Influences on Religious Interests, Attitudes, and Values: A Study of Twins Reared Apart and Together (Waller, Kojetin, Bouchard, Lykken, & Tellegen, 1990)

Utilizing respondents from the famous Minnesota Twin Study, Waller and colleagues were able to obtain data on five measures of religious attitudes, interests, and values. These were well-known and highly regarded scales. The participants were 53 pairs of monozygotic (identical) twins and 31 pairs of dizygotic (fraternal) twins who had been reared apart. The measures were also given to 458 pairs of identical and 363 pairs of fraternal twins who had been raised together. Data analyses suggested that 49% of the variation in the scores on the religious measures was a function of genetic influences. In other words, in this study, genetic and environmental factors were almost equal in their effects regarding the origins of personal faith.

measures employed. Though these measures are often treated as if they are independent of each other, they may be highly intercorrelated. Research Box 3.1 contains an example of one of the better studies of this type (Waller, Kojetin, Bouchard, Lykken, & Tellegen, 1990). In this investigation, 49% of the variation in religious indicators was referred to heredity.

A more recent study (Bradshaw & Ellison, 2008) attempted to look at genetic and environmental influences in a broader range of eight religious and spiritual measures. Again, of course, all such indices are intercorrelated, but the authors did not provide this information. Still, their work and findings yield impressive coefficients of shared heredity, ranging from 19 to 65%. Similar data for environmental influences range from 13 to 53%. Summarizing data from different researchers prior to 1999, D'Onofrio, Eaves, Murrelle, Maes, and Spilka (1999) found a range for heredity from essentially 0 to about 50%.

WHAT HAS EVOLUTION ACCOMPLISHED?

Writing on the roles and effects of evolution has been rapidly growing. Theory dominates this literature. Often this leaves much room for speculation. In regard to the outcomes of evolution, scholars have emphasized two major aspects of contemporary psychology—namely, cognition and neuropsychology. We have previously stated that the psychology of religion is concerned with religious belief, behavior, and experience. Even though researchers have often focused mainly on belief, the data have overwhelmingly provided evidence for relationships among all three. For example, believers are likely to go to church and have religious experiences. Independence among these variables simply makes no sense. We therefore emphasize the products of religious evolution—namely, cognition and brain development. Relative to the former, Richert and Smith (2009) simply state that "religious concepts build on natural cognitive dispositions" (p. 181).

Cognition and Religion

A major feature of mainstream psychology during the last 100 years has been the relatively rigorous and even mathematical understanding of behaviorism and learning. The initial focus was on classical conditioning, associative learning, and reinforcement. Names such as Pavlov, Hull, and Skinner ruled the field. Exacting as such work was, attention slowly shifted away from white rats to people and higher mental processes. Center stage was now occupied by thinking and the acquisition of more elaborate forms of knowledge and thought, including reasoning, abstraction, synthesizing, inference, mental representation, and the like. The domain of cognition or cognitive science was born and has been developing in virtually all aspects of psychology, including the psychology of religion (Andresen, 2001; Barrett, 2011). Religious belief and experience are largely cognitive, although emotion is now viewed as part of how cognition functions. It frequently seems that there are no limits to cognition when the term is applied to thinking about religion. Hardy (1975), a marine biologist interested in religion, wondered whether a "capacity for belief" (p. 66) might be inherited, as well as the idea and experience of God. He struggled with what biological mechanisms might be involved, but offered none.

Religious beliefs and experiences may take place within or outside of formal religious systems, though for most people, the faith with which they are associated provides the backdrop for their spiritual perspectives. Lawson and McCauley (1990) refer to a generalized belief in a supernatural realm of superhuman agents. This and the knowledge of ritual practices constitute a person's cognitive system for religion. It is usually acquired and manifested from early childhood on; thus one learns about God or gods, with attendant figures such as spirits, angels, demons, saints, and so on. Definitions include a divine or holy realm or some other ethereal locality—a heaven, a hell, and the like. The complexity of such places and what they are said to be must be left to a system's theology. These ideas, however, build on a social-cognitive concept termed "agency." This refers to behavioral determination, or, more broadly, the initiation of action by beings, both natural and supernatural (McCauley & Lawson, 2002). Richert and Smith (2009) claim that most cognitive research on religion concerns "the human tendency toward agency attribution in concepts of supernatural agents" (p. 182)—in other words, belief in God/gods and other "superhuman agents."

At this point, let us simply recognize the obvious: Namely there is a biochemical basis for the neuropsychology of human thought and behavior. Many scholars implicitly accept an underlying physiological substrate for cognitive religious expressions. They simply assume it as fact and turn their attention to how it is demonstrated (Lawson & McCauley, 1990; McCauley & Lawson, 2002). Others focus extensively on this foundational level and may use it as a basis for their overall theory of religion (Atran, 2002; Boyer, 2001; d'Aquili, 1978; Feierman, 2009; Newberg, d'Aquili, & Rause, 2002). We will look at this further, but for now we focus on religious cognition, as first manifested in animism.

From Animism to Religious Cognition

The search for religious origins and expressions prompted early scholars to identify the concept of animism. By the mid- to late 1800s, this became a social-scientific truth. The Latin-derived term "animism" was introduced into anthropology by Edward Burnett Tylor in 1866. He defined it "as a minimum definition of Religion, the belief in spiritual beings." Animism is then said to be "the deep-lying doctrine of Spiritual Beings" (Tylor, 1873, pp. 72–73). It also includes the belief that inanimate things possess life or spirit, even intention and motive. Its origins were first assigned to prehistoric peoples once labeled "primitive savages" (Hopkins, 1923, p. 11), Modern psychology rejects such verbal chauvinism. The manifestations of mythological figures are commonly found in human cognitions. Tylor presented a massive exposition of such mythical beings, both philosophically and in the religious frameworks of a wide variety of peoples. Basically, the belief in such beings is "anthropomorphism," or the explicit assignment of human traits to that which is impersonal and often fanciful. A person might see divine anger in lightning and thunder. When a car breaks down, the driver sometimes responds as if it did it on purpose. When things go wrong, people often act as if a malign intelligence is behind what has happened. During World War II, if some equipment failed, a popular notion was to say in mock seriousness that "gremlins" (mythical beings) did it.

Although the word "animism" has more or less fallen out of favor cognition now serves the same purpose, and of course cognitive theory and research have developed extensively over the years (Von Eckardt, 1995). In modern parlance, the cognitions described above have now been termed "patternicity," which Shermer (2009, p. 1) simply defines as "the human tendency to find meaningful patterns in meaningless noise." We organize the stimuli that affect us so that they become meaningful to us. We make out faces in clouds, and random sounds may be perceived as muffled voices (Guthrie, 1993). Haldane (2006) cites an instance where "a 10-year-old grilled cheese sandwich" was said to look like "the Virgin Mary" (p. 8A). More recently, a young woman reported the image of Jesus in her chewing gum (Telegraph Media Group Limited, 2010). Bering (2011a) notes that God is seen in all sorts of events, such as earthquakes and tsunamis. This "predisposition" to see and believe that God or gods are ever-present has been studied in very young children and adults of all ages (Kelemen & Rosset, 2009). Barrett and Keil (1996) have examined the prevalence of anthropomorphism in God concepts. An interesting expression of these beliefs is a "sense of presence"—the feeling described by devout people that God is always nearby or "walks" with them. In like manner, the company they sense might be angelic or satanic (Shermer, 2010). The cognition that "God is watching you" increases prosocial behavior (Shariff & Norenzayan, 2007), in that one moves into line with a standard religious goal. Interestingly, a recent study reports that "children exposed to religion have a hard time differentiating between fact and fiction" (Ashtari, 2014).

Anthropologist Stewart Guthrie (1993) offers this principle as a way of explaining the origin of religion: Here is cognition—human thought and belief full-blown. Jane Goodall (1971) described what might be termed animistic behavior on the part of chimpanzees. This clearly implies a prehuman animistic beginning for religious thought and ritual, and certainly indicates a role for evolution. To sum up, we are saying that evolution has modified the brain, one result of which is that cognition has developed into a very complex pattern of understanding and expression. Many scientists now explain religion as primarily a cognitive product premised on an underlying neurological foundation (Barrett, 2000, 2007), and we discuss this foundation next.

Religion, Spirituality, and the Brain

The brain and nervous system are probably the most extremely complex structures in the human body. Needless to say, we cannot and do not want to delve deeply into the anatomy of the brain here; however, a few major areas should be identified, primarily the lobes of the brain. We mention research that involves the frontal, parietal, and temporal lobes and their potential roles relative to religion.

The barrier separating faith from the nervous system has been breached in a number of places. As stated above, the process began with redefining the relationship. Religion has invariably been placed in a cognitive context that emphasizes goal-directed thinking, and hence a search for meaning in which the individual struggles to make sense out of the world. The major stage of this search emphasizes religious beliefs and experiences. We know that churchgoers affirm a belief in God and the principles of their church. As a rule, about three-quarters of attendees further indicate that they have had religious experiences. The overlap is so great that belief and experience are not sharply distinguished here. At the same time, we should be sensitive to the way these terms are employed. Apparently various brain sectors are involved in a number of these expressions.

Neuropsychological research aims to identify neural circuits in the brain that underlie the cognitive-experiential responses described above. As noted earlier, contemporary popular language often suggests that we humans are "hardwired" for these expressions (Clark & Grunstein, 2000; Haldane, 2006; Hamer, 2004).

In order to understand how the brain functions, neuroimaging procedures are used. These are very briefly listed (along with the abbreviations commonly used to refer to them) and described in Table 3.1. Some research using these procedures has been offered in the neurobiological literature dealing with religion (Newberg, 2006b). They are also becoming increasingly popular in modern medicine and neuropsychology.

Religion and Epilepsy

The idea that initially implied an association between faith and the nervous system goes back almost three millennia. It involved epilepsy, which by the 5th century B.C. was known as "the sacred disease." The famous Greek physician Hippocrates rejected the religious identification, noting that "it is not, in my opinion, any more divine or more sacred than other diseases" (Jones, 1923, p. 139). He dealt with epilepsy solely as a medical condition (Simon, 1978). His next step was to explicitly deny the Aristotelian assertion that understanding and experience emanate from the heart. All such functions, including epilepsy, were now described as located in the brain (Adams & Kelly, 1939).

Although Hippocrates rejected a sacred origin for epilepsy, he and others recognized an association of epileptic seizures with religion. Medical recognition of such a connection

TABLE 3.1. The Main Neuroimaging Techniques Used to Assess Brain Functioning

Technique (abbreviation)	Description
Electroencephalography (EEG)	Use of brain waves to detect electrical currents in the brain
Magnetic resonance imaging (MRI)	Use of magnetic fields and radio waves to produce images of brain functions
Functional magnetic resonance imaging (fMRI)	Use of oxygen in hemoglobin to assess blood flow in the brain
Positron emission tomography (PET)	Use of radioactive tracers to measure glucose or oxygen metabolism and produce two- or three-dimensional images
Single-photon emission computed tomography (SPECT)	Use of radioactive tracers to determine active brain regions

was affirmed in the 19th century (Dewhurst & Beard, 1970; Wulff, 1997); however, the links with epilepsy in general were complex, unclear, and generally weak. A possible connection with temporal lobe epilepsy (TLE) in particular seemed more substantial, but even this had problems. There have been a fair number of papers published on TLE, the majority of which offer case histories of those who have these seizures. Most of these histories have little or nothing to do with religion. In the few cases where faith enters the picture, it is often with people who are religious to begin with. Many of these patients attribute their epilepsy to being cursed and punished by God for sins (Ismail, Wright, Rhodes, & Small, 2005; Khwaja, Singh, & Chaudry, 2007). Nevertheless, most papers indicate that a rather small percentage of persons with epilepsy manifest religious behavior. For example, Ogata and Miyakawa (1998) studied 234 such persons found that their sample contained only 3 cases, or 1.3%, who had religious experiences related to epileptic episodes. The highest percentage, 38%, was reported in a study by Dewhurst and Beard (1970). Other researchers who studied patients with TLE indicated no significant differences in religious beliefs, practices, or mystical experiences relative to respondents with other conditions or to people in general (Sensky, Wilson, Petty, Fenwick, & Rose, 1984; Tucker, Novelly, & Walker, 1987). An extensive review of this literature by Schachter (2006) resulted in the same conclusion.

In short, this research indicates that the combination of epilepsy with religious expressions may be quite striking when found, but that instances are not very common. Their dramatic nature may take precedence over their frequency. Still, some researchers indicate that those with TLE show either a relatively strong response to religious content or greater religious interest than is true of control subjects (McClenon & Nooney, 1999). Something that has been observed and commented on for almost 2,500 years deserves a more thorough explanation. Elements of personality and mental disorder may be hypothesized, but little if anything relative to these areas has been suggested. A more pertinent research direction has, however, been developing over the last few decades. This searches for direct neurological connections between the brain and religious expression.

Beyond Epilepsy

In the past few decades, research has opened a door to understanding how faith functions relative to the brain. Among the first to study such relationships were Michael Persinger and his associates (Makarec & Persinger, 1985; Persinger, 1987, 1993; Persinger & Makarec, 1987; Persinger, Bureau, Peredery, & Richards, 1994). Emphasizing the temporal lobe, they studied the religious ideation that accompanied the neuroelectrical activity termed "temporal lobe transients" (i.e., brief electrical discharges). These researchers felt that the left temporal lobe was most sensitive to electrical stimulation that resulted in religious content. Ramachandran and Blakeslee (1998) concurred with Persinger et al.'s findings, reporting God-associated mental content with TLE and limbic system involvement during epileptic episodes.[3] Virtually every religious possibility was reported (mystical experiences, conversions, strengthened religious beliefs, etc.). They further suggested the broader concept of a "temporal lobe personality," which they felt was "obsessively preoccupied with philosophical and theological issues" (p. 180). In keeping with Schachter's (2006) observation cited

---

[3]The limbic system consists of a number of the older and deeper brain structures, such as the amygdala, hippocampus, and limbic cortex. It has been viewed as the seat of the emotions and is involved in the expression and control of emotionally motivated behavior (Bear, Connors, & Paradiso, 1996).

above, however, these authors acknowledged that only a minority of patients display esoteric traits like religiosity" (p. 285). Researchers usually assert that the content of such seizures is learned by the affected individuals within their cultural context. The sociocultural shaping of religious content is well known (Poloma, 1995). Given the difficulty of conducting such research, it should come as no surprise that it has been challenged and sometimes not replicated (Granqvist et al., 2005).

Although Ogata and Miyakawa (1998) focused on the temporal lobes and the limbic system, they did not attempt to stimulate these brain structures as Persinger and colleagues did. Ogata and Miyakawa confirmed the earlier claims of Bear and Fedio (1977) that the seizures do not produce a specific psychological pattern.

Apparently not one to give up easily on the potential association of religious feelings with the temporal lobe, Persinger constructed a wired helmet called the "Koren Helmet" or more colloquially the God Helmet, which he believed stimulated religious experiences when it was worn (see Horgan, 2006). Comparing an experimental and a control group, he claimed that 80% "sensed a presence" when the helmet was activated. Only 15% of his control group reported such experiences. Since the participants in this research knew beforehand what effects they were expected to have, one may argue that expectations were induced and that a placebo effect resulted. A Swedish sample that had no such prior knowledge did not have the predicted experiences (Granqvist et al., 2005). This study was criticized by Persinger (Horgan, 2006). However, the "sensed presence" reported by Persinger could be any believed supernatural being, hence Persinger's research suggests such might be a "cerebral mistake" (p. 5). Furthermore, though Persinger claimed that his wired helmet resulted in 80% of 600 participant sensing that vague presence. No one else has yet reproduced anything close to these findings. These results could thus fall under Shermer's (2009) rubric of "patternicity"—namely, "the human tendency to find meaningful patterns in meaningless noise" (p. 1). In failing to replicate Persinger's research, Granqvist et al. (2005) claimed that when positive results did occur, they were due to suggestibility, not temporal lobe stimulation.

The indefinite nature of most of the writing on relationships between brain functioning and religion is further illustrated by the popularity of the phrase "God spot." This concept has been around for quite a number of years, but its location and definition remain unclear. Currently the term refers to a specific brain area that has been associated with religious and/or spiritual activity, usually meaning experience on the part of those taking part in psycho-religious-neurological research (Barber, 2012; Hamer, 2004).[4] Much of this writing tends to locate the "God spot" (or spots) in the temporal lobe. Epilepsy-related religiosity/spirituality and the work of Persinger are often cited. Biello (2007) asserts that Persinger is simply saying that religious experience and God belief are nothing more than the results of electrical activity in the brain.

The Neuropsychology of Religious Belief and Experience

We all believe in innumerable things that are simply self-evident: The sun will rise and set daily; objects when released will fall to the ground. Such expectations are fundamentally beliefs that our experiences reinforce. Supernatural beliefs in God, deities, spirits, angels,

---

[4]The terms "religious" and "spiritual" are often treated in an ambiguous way in the psychology-of-religion literature. Religiosity has achieved greater agreement than spirituality, though many researchers have focused on the latter concept in the last two decades.

and the like are found among all peoples. As natural as these notions are to believers, it has been inevitable for scientists to pen volumes on the biology of religious belief (Giovannoli, 2000; Newberg et al., 2001; Wolpert, 2006). These workers largely assume that religious beliefs are innate cognitions and genetically programmed (Bering, 2006).

Biology and Belief

Gazzaniga (1985) argues that "religious beliefs are inevitable" (p. 166). Furthermore, they are the product of a "brain process" (p. 167) that he locates on the left side of the brain and indefinitely terms "the left brain interpreter" (p. 166). Also with a measure of vagueness, he puts these ideas in an archeological context and offers "the assumption that something about the species (a property of our brains) inclines it to yield to a belief in a greater order than that perceived around it" (p. 169). Unfortunately, Gazzaniga does not offer us specific neural correlates of religious belief.

Similarly, d'Aquili (1978) has suggested that "belief in supernatural powers . . . like all universal human behaviors . . . derives its source from the functioning of neural structures" (p. 258). He terms these organized neural tissues "neurognostic structures" and "neural operators" (p. 258) in the brain. Six of these are posited, one of which he calls the "causal operator" (p. 259). d'Aquili and Newberg (1999) claim that the joint functioning of such operators creates the need to cognitively create powerful supernatural beings. These operators are theoretical, and though they seem potentially useful, they are not identified with observable referents in the brain. The present state of much brain research points to relatively broad but unfocused neural indicators, especially for religious beliefs and experiences.

More recently and in a more exacting manner, Kapogiannis and his associates (Kapogiannis, Barbey, Su, Krueger, & Grafman, 2009; Kapogiannis, Dehpande, Krueger, Thornburg, & Grafman, 2014) used fMRI (see Table 3.1) in two meticulous studies and identified some functional components of religiosity. The frontal lobes and cortex, along with the temporal lobe, were particularly involved in their rather detailed identification and causal analyses. In the neuropsychological realm, complexity is the rule.

Despite all such biological thinking, let us not lose sight of the fact that children are usually born into homes that are religious to some degree, and that these homes are in communities in which faith usually constitutes a strong value system. Obviously, the involvement of cultural learning cannot be discounted. d'Aquili and Newberg (1999) minimize such concerns and claim that "God or pure consciousness is generated by the machinery of the brain" (p. 18). There is, of course, disagreement with this view. Considering our present state of knowledge, we feel that brain activities apparently correlate with religious actions, beliefs, and experiences—but that we should not confuse correlation with causation.

God: Belief and Experience

A special problem concerns belief in God. Conjecture and theory range from the idea that the concept is learned to the view that it has roots in the evolution of how the brain develops and functions. A caution is in order here: The Abrahamic faiths (Christianity, Islam, and Judaism) stress the idea of God, but this is not true of certain Asian faiths, so what is discussed here may not be meaningful for all religions (Klass, 1995). Still, a number of social scientists consider the anthropomorphic tendency to see deities as taking human forms, or as acting and feeling like people is innate (Barrett & Keil, 1996; Guthrie, 1993). Hamer (2004) mentions Persinger's research on magnetic stimulation of the parietal and temporal lobes creating the experience of God, which he has called the "God spot" (see above). Another popular phrase in this literature is to speak of a "God module." In both these phrases, God is reduced to a location in the brain that deals exclusively with such beliefs. The notion of the God module has found some acceptance in neuropsychological quarters, but has also elicited criticism (Atran, 2002; Horgan, 1999; Richardson, 2000).

Regardless of terminology such as the "God spot" or "God module," we need to examine actual research and theory on brain correlates of religion. One of the first workers to address this issue was the late Eugene d'Aquili, a professor of psychiatry. He claimed that the parietal lobe (just above the ear) on the nondominant side of the brain is involved in deity perceptions (d'Aquili, 1978). More recently, Spinella and Wain (2006) have focused on the prefrontal cortex with regard to beliefs they consider religious and superstitious. Relying heavily on brain evolution, Persinger (1987) shifted attention from belief to the experience of God. As described above, he believes that this experience is localized in the temporal lobe and is associated with "temporal lobe transients" (p. 16), although he admits that these have not been shown to exist in all people. He further introduces the concept of "psychic seizures" (p. 17), which do not result in convulsions but are accompanied by a wide variety of visual, auditory, and olfactory experiences. Strong feelings and emotions may be present. All these findings have led Persinger to emphasize the temporal lobe, which he sees as the "biological basis of the God experience."[5] The God experience, however, is not distinguished from other mystical, cosmic, or religious/spiritual experiences

Some neuroimaging brain research has been conducted by Azari and her associates. Its results both overlap with and differ from those of d'Aquili and Newberg and of Persinger. Variations in research methodology, along with small samples, may account for some of these differences and disagreement among researchers. Azari (2006) summarizes much of her group's work relative to religious experiences among Protestant Christians and Buddhists. As we have done above, she warns against inferring causes from correlational findings. Rather, her research stresses changes in brain activity that accompany religious experience. This work suggests that the prefrontal and medial frontal cortex may play an especially important role in mediating religious experience. An example of her research on the biological underpinnings of religious experience is presented in Research Box 3.2.

Traditional psychologists may argue that the samples in Azari's study are too small to permit definitive conclusions. In addition, there are likely to have been motivational differences between the experimental and control groups in the different conditions. Research of this nature is extremely difficult to undertake and needs to be examined closely.

Spirituality

Much of what is generally considered religious belief or experience is not only part of traditional religion, but would today be considered features of spirituality. The current emphasis on mystical experience is usually identified this way. The classic problem of knowing where religion leaves off and spirituality begins may never be resolved, because the concepts overlap and disagreements exist regarding the definition and components of spirituality, as well as whether a wide variety of feelings (such as Hamer's [2004] concern with transcendence)

---

[5]The full title of the chapter in Persinger (1987) is "The Temporal Lobe: The Biological Basis of the God Experience."

RESEARCH BOX 3.2. Neural Correlates of Religious Experience
(Azari et al., 2001)

In pioneering research, Azari and her coworkers attempted to locate those areas in the brain that are active during religious experience. The researchers used positron emission tomography (PET) to image the brain during religious and other activities. Six different activation conditions (a religious state, a nonreligious emotion state, and appropriate control conditions) were constructed; in all conditions, the state achieved was self-induced and subjectively defined. Six religious and six nonreligious participants took part in the six religious and control conditions.

While reading the 23rd Psalm, the religious participants (all Christian Protestants) reportedly attained a religious experiential state. Of most importance, the PET scans for the religious respondents, when they reported being in a religious state, showed activation in the frontal and parietal lobes—areas that have been shown in independent studies to be central for complex cognitions. Limbic structures (specifically the amygdala) were not activated during the religious state, but were involved during the nonreligious emotional state. On the basis of these findings, Azari and her coworkers have proposed that religious experience is likely to be a cognitive process utilizing established neural connections between the frontal and parietal lobes.

should be considered spiritual. One also reads of "cosmic experiences," "other-worldly consciousness," "out-of-body experiences," "heightened enlightenment," and a host of other notions generally identified as anomalous experiences (see Chapter 10). Our emphasis in this chapter, however, is on their biological underpinnings

Hay and Socha (2005) analyze many of the issues underlying this work In doing so, they transform notions of traditional religious experience into the broader context of "spiritual awareness." A naturalistic biological state of "relational consciousness" (p. 597) is introduced. This appears similar to what Azari and colleagues infer from their brain research. Like Hardy and others, Hay and Socha believe that spiritual awareness is a naturally selected evolutionary product that was "useful in the preservation of the species" (p. 600). Why natural selection was operative with spirituality, if it really was, is still an open question. Hay and Socha, however, also adopt a radical stance by seeing natural selection as adaptive not only in nature but also in culture. This motif relative to culture has been around for some time. Its underlying mechanisms have yet to be demonstrated.

When the neurobiology of spirituality has been studied, it is usually reduced to some kind of religious experience, such as meditation (Begley, 2001a), but meditation exists in both religious and nonreligious forms. Newberg (2006a, 2006b) has extensively reviewed this research, with regard not only to the parts of the brain that show changes, but also to the neurochemistry of these changes. Because of the complexity of this work and the measurement problems it entails, Newberg mixes research findings with possibilities for future testing that imply the potential of neurobiological research for faith and spirituality. These findings are difficult to summarize because of differences in the experimental and analytic methods used. Research Box 3.3 presents one example of this research.

The literature on neurobiology and religion or spirituality is quite complex and badly needs coordination. For example, Newberg (2006a) reveals the wide variety of neurochemicals such as neurotransmitters that are part of the receptor-signaling and -activating processes present in religious experience and ritual. Suffice it to say that current work along these lines does not allow inferences about cause. They must be treated as fundamentally correlational in nature. No one has found God in the nervous system.

Meditation

Meditation is present in all five of the world's major religions—Buddhism, Christianity, Hinduism, Islam, and Judaism. The use of the term, however, varies in both meaning and practice. In fact, different words, concepts, and actions imply a variety of ideas and behaviors under this verbal umbrella. A terminology that is abstruse, imaginative, and often difficult to interpret is frequently employed.

A review of five meditation studies indicated that three showed some activation of the frontal lobes, often in conjunction with a variety of other neural structures (Ott, Hölzel, & Vaitl, 2011). Though MRI was employed in all of this work, other procedures were also used in a few studies. Most often observations suggest a thickening of the brain's grey matter, which relates to muscle control and sensory processes during meditation.

An early study of yoga meditation compared 11 meditators with a control group of nonmeditators (Elson, Hauei, & Cunis, 1977) reported differences in skin resistance and respiratory rate, among other changes differentiating the two groups. Definitive inferences are impossible to make, however, considering the small sample size and the often vague character of the observations. Unfortunately, these problems characterize much of the research in this area.

RESEARCH BOX 3.3. Religious Experience and Emotion:
Evidence for Distinctive Cognitive Neural Patterns
(Azari, Missimer, & Seitz, 2005)

The purpose of this study was to distinguish the neural networks involved in religious experience from those involved in a nonreligious emotional state.

Six religious individuals were compared with six who were not religious. The former were Christian Protestants who had conversion experiences. The groups were matched on a number of background, verbal ability, personality, and life satisfaction measures, as well as the capacity to visualize scenes. There were three conditions: (1) a religious state; (2) a nonreligious, happy emotional state; and (3) rest. Everyone underwent PET scans, and regional cerebral blood flow was studied. A self-assessment procedure was used to judge the degree to which participants attained the desired goal state for each task.

The groups were compared relative to task conditions. Specific neural patterns/networks were indicated. These revealed activity in prefrontal cortical areas that are involved in complex cognition, as opposed to activation of the limbic system, which is understood to mediate basic emotional responses. The religious participants described their "experiences in terms of cultivating an interpersonal relationship with God (in the person of Jesus Christ)" (Azari et al., 2005, p. 274). A concept of perceived "relational cognitivity" is thus proposed to explain the observations.

Using a small sample of Tibetan Buddhist meditators, and SPECT observations (see Table 3.1), Newberg et al. (2001) found that seven different brain areas were activated during meditation. Three of these involved the frontal lobes. There was a decrease of brain responsivity in the parietal lobe, which Newberg et al. (2001) felt might be associated with a sense of the body's unity with the external world. Such speculation needs more direct corroboration. Inferring cognitive and emotional meanings from brain activity is problematic. Using a small non-Buddhist sample, Moyer et al. (2011) trained 11 subjects in meditation training for 5 weeks and also found responsivity in the left frontal lobe. This pattern is said to be indicative of positive moods. The wide variety of meditational forms and purposes leads us to conclude that neuroanatomical expressions have, as yet, hardly been examined.

Ritual and Prayer

Religious ritual is an extremely complex realm that has been little studied in relation to possible neurobiological correlates. Volumes have been written on religious ritual, and any attempt to discuss this literature thoroughly from Tylor (1873) to d'Aquili, Laughlin, and McManus (1979) and McCauley and Lawson (2002) would take many tomes weightier than this one. d'Aquili et al. (1979) consider meditation a form of ritual. Since it also involves repetitive behavior, it is regarded as activating the brain's limbic system, which has been described earlier (see footnote 3). We are further informed that "religious ritual is always embedded in a cognitive matrix—a web of meaning" (p. 160). This calls into play the frontal lobe.

Like meditation, ritual is multidimensional. To study it adequately requires identifying and defining the cognitions and behaviors involved in the rites of an almost unlimited variety of religious groups. The initial step to effect such identification has yet to be taken, and, of course, definitions will undoubtedly vary with whatever form of faith is being studied plus possibly other factors. In less formal quarters, one humorous reference to *The Yearbook of American and Canadian Churches* stated that over the years 250 religious bodies plus or minus 10 are listed. Some have been with us a long time; others randomly appear and disappear. Each has its own rituals. d'Aquili et al. (1979) provide some insight into the theoretical and operational issues that must be confronted in this area.

This bleak situation unfortunately also affects research in the realm of prayer. To appreciate how elaborate and intricate prayer is, interested readers might consult the volume *The Psychology of Prayer: A Scientific Approach* (Spilka & Ladd, 2013). More than a century of research in the area merits critical assessment, and much of this literature is covered in that book.

To return here to the relevant research, Newberg, Pourdehnad, Alavi, and d'Aquili looked at meditative prayer and cerebral blood flow in a study of three Franciscan nuns and eight Tibetan Buddhists. Employing a rather complex procedure (which was not fully explained), plus a SPECT analysis, Newberg et al. found that the nuns showed increased blood flow in the prefrontal cortex and inferior frontal lobes. Previous work was confirmed that involved other brain structures and the temporal lobe. Despite these very small samples, very high and statistically significant correlations are given. At least the authors refer to these findings as "preliminary data" (p. 629).

Utilizing EEG in a study of six Protestants, Surwillo and Hobson (1978) observed a speeding up of brain waves in most of their participants. They further reported a confirmation of this finding in one participant. Again, small sample size makes inferences problematic

Considering prayer an interpersonal relationship between a praying person and God, Neubauer (2014) employed fMRI to study prayer in extremely conservative Christians (e.g., Pentecostals). After-scan questioning elicited responses including statements that respondents felt themselves to be in the presence of God. Brain areas supposedly activated in interpersonal relationships were claimed to be activated in this research.

In work somewhat similar to Neubauer's, Schjoedt, Stetkilde-Jorgensen, Geertz, and Roepstorff (2009) also used fMRI on 20 Danish Christians. These researchers placed interpersonal prayer in a social-cognitive framework, and considered it from both a formalized, structured, public perspective and a noninstitutionalized, private, personal perspective. This complex study had five conditions and allowed prayer both within the fMRI scanner and outside it. Though a number of neurological effects were found, emphasis was largely on activity in the prefrontal cortex. Variations in social cognition were noted in relation to the different conditions. There is much in this ingenious study to provide guidelines for other researchers dealing with neuroimaging and prayer.

Evaluating Neuroimaging Research

Before concluding this somewhat superficial discussion of the neuropsychology of brain–religion relationships, we must indicate that we have done little more than scratch the surface of a rapidly growing realm of research. Furthermore, we have left out efforts to develop theory and investigate the chemistry of religiosity (McNamara, Durso, Brown, & Harris, 2006). We might say that this is a "hot" area in the psychology of religion, but also one that leaves much to be desired.

The use of neuroimaging methods designed to show relationships between aspects of the brain and religious beliefs, behaviors, and experience has resulted in many interesting observations. Unfortunately, the combination of often quite small samples with the failure to replicate findings raises questions about the reliability and validity of these findings. In addition, there has been a general lack of confirmation because single-method neuroimaging approaches characterize studies in this area. Maybe somewhere in this literature, more than one technique has been employed; however, we have been unable to locate such work. In other words, for example, fMRI research has not been compared with research using PET or SPECT; PET research has not been compared with studies using other imaging methods; and so on. The issue of reproducing findings is rapidly gaining much support in psychology, and we cannot emphasize it enough (Novotney, 2014).

A very strong warning comes from the work of Cunningham and Yu (2014), which attempts to address the problem that "simply recording the neural activity does not automatically lead to a clearer understanding of how the brain works" (*Science Daily*, 2014). Challenges to and questions regarding the statistical analyses of neuroimaging studies are easy to find. In one analysis, the claim is made that researchers often select the highest, spurious correlations, thus giving readers the wrong impression about observed associations (Lindquist & Gelman, 2009; see also Vul, Harris, Winkielman, & Pashler, 2009). Horgan (2006) summarizes his evaluation by claiming, "The field suffers from vague terminology, disagreement about what exactly 'religion' is, and which of its aspects are most important" (p. 2). We add that if ever a biological domain needed replication and repeated confirmation, this is it.

Neurotheology

The concept of "neurotheology" was introduced by Aldous Huxley in his novel *Island*. He defined it as "what's happening in the brain when you're having a vision" (Huxley, 1962, p. 137). Unfortunately, the focus and extent of this popular concept have not always been clear. For many years, visions were elicited by drugs that produced transcendental, mystical, spiritual, and religious experiences (discussed in Chapter 10). Attention was soon directed at religious and spiritual activities such as meditation, yoga, and prayer, plus related psychological states such as sensory deprivation or heightened emotion. Religion further entered the picture via rituals and ceremonial practices that arouse intense feelings and trance states. All this became the substance of neurotheology. Whereas neuroimaging largely stresses the underlying brain biology, neurotheology shifted to the experiential side of this work. Ratcliffe (2008) has denoted this emphasis by suggesting the involvement of six kinds of experience—"interpretive," "quasi-sensory," "revelatory," "regenerative," "numinous," and "mystical." For further discussion, interested readers should consult Ratcliffe.

Neurotheology thus poses significant problems. Given its name, one would expect theology to be present, but there is no theology in sight. Still, Pigliucci (2006) points out that it leaves the door open to religious explanations when we encounter neuropsychological problems for which we lack answers. In other words, our desire to be rigorously scientific is subverted. Underwood (2001) concludes her popular analysis of neurotheology by asking "whether our brain wiring creates God or whether God created our brain wiring" (p. 57). This suggests that neurotheology may be an effort to keep one foot in religion and the other in science—a rather unstable stance.

HEALTH IN RELIGIOUS GROUPS

All humans develop genetic mutations that are either supported or eliminated by natural selection. When a group tends to be geographically isolated, or attempts to separate itself from other social bodies because of its culture and/or religion, the mutations created among its members are likely to persist because of within-group marital bonding. In other words, inbreeding is the rule. Some mutations may be positive, others negative. The latter are often more noticeable and seem to be more common. They certainly get more attention, as they largely involve deformity or disease. Inbreeding in small, isolated groups can become a particular problem with genetic conditions. This means that, in the simplest case, the likelihood that both parents will have the undesirable mutation may be high. When recessive, the genetic disorder will affect 25% of the children. Fifty percent will be carriers, and 25% will not evidence the problem. Such genetic disorders have been demonstrated among Anabaptist sects, such as the Amish and Hutterites—groups that came to North America largely between 1650 and 1750 to escape persecution in Europe. The Amish, Mennonite, and Hutterite Genetic Disorder Database has been established because of a lack of data and information for medical professionals who treat these groups (Payne, Rupar, Siu, & Siu, 2011). The Jews are another religious group that stands out with regard to both certain health conditions and cognitive qualities. All three of these faiths have histories of physical and/or social separation from others. We now examine some of the most pertinent research regarding these groups.

The Amish

In 2012, there were 251,000 Amish in the United States and Canada. This number is said to double every 21–22 years, as the average Amish family has seven children (Osborne, 2013). Although Amish communities are found in at least 21 states, most are in Pennsylvania, Ohio, and Indiana. These settlements are viewed as separate inbreeding subgroups. Hostetler (1980) states that the Amish and Hutterites are the "best defined inbred group(s)" in North America (p. 319). Because intermarriage across the distinct communities is relatively rare, each has its own pattern of genetic conditions.

Extensive genetic research has revealed a high incidence of certain inherited conditions among the Amish (McKusick, 1978). For example, one Pennsylvania community displays a form of hereditary dwarfism, the frequency of which is higher than that in the rest of the world. A different type of dwarfism is found in some other Amish populations. The Amish in Ohio evidence a high frequency of hemophilia (pathological bleeding), whereas in Indiana an unusual form of muscular dystrophy is present. In Pennsylvania, genetically based stillbirths have also been noted (Hostetler, 1980). Other problems observed include congenital deafness; neuromuscular disorders; types of anemia; thyroid defects; cardiac deficiencies; a genetic mutation that produces intellectual disability excessive numbers of fingers and toes; and dementias (McKusick, 1978; Osborne, 2013). The CBS *60 Minutes* show claimed several years ago that Amish children "have medical conditions so rare, doctors don't have names for them yet" (McKay, 2005).

The Hutterites

The Hutterites, another Anabaptist group that originated in the same general central European region as the Amish who came to North America for the same reason (i.e., to escape persecution), arrived in the middle to late 19th century and located themselves first in the Dakotas and then in western Canada. They maintain a strong ingroup communal society and actively resist outside educational influences.

For the Hutterites, as for the Amish, separation from outgroups and inbreeding have resulted in some negative genetic developments. An early general observation of their mental health suggested that neurotic manifestations are low, but that relatively high rates of certain major mental disorders are found (Eaton & Weil, 1955). Both schizophrenia and bipolar disorder (called "manic–depressive psychosis" at the time this work was done) possess substantial genetic components. The Hutterites have relatively low rates of schizophrenia, but a high rate of bipolar disorder. Since both disorders are also environmentally influenced, genetic factors do not tell the entire story. Overall, too, the prevalence of these disorders is low in relation to national data (Hostetler, 1974).

Research studies on genetically based illnesses among the Hutterites are older and fewer than those conducted with the Amish. Still, one sees many similarities (and a few differences) between the two groups. A Canadian Hutterite collective evidences a type of inherited muscular dystrophy similar to that found among the Amish (Frosk et al., 2005; Shokeir, Rozdilsky, Opitz, & Reynolds, 2005). A genetically based brain disorder associated with intellectual disability has also been reported by Schurig, Van Orman, Bowen, and Opitz (2005). In addition, some 38 genetic blood markers have been observed among Hutterites (Lewis et al., 2005). There is clearly a need for additional research with this religious group.

The Jews

Historical Background and Types of Genetic Disorders

Whereas the Amish and the Hutterites exist on the fringes of society, Jews have been a central group in Western civilization for millennia. To a considerable degree, Jewish history in the past 2,000 years has been a tale of anti-Semitic discrimination and of self- and other-imposed separation from Christian neighbors (the nadir of which was, of course, the Nazi Holocaust). Long before Jesus, however, the early Hebrews sharply distinguished themselves from others who resided near them in the Near and Middle East. This pattern continued into the Christian era, when the separation of Jews into their own communities was formalized in the Middle Ages by the creation of the ghetto. Contrary to general belief, the ghetto was often instituted by the Jews themselves, not by Christian authorities (Wirth, 1928). As Wirth (1928) noted, "To the Jews the geographically separated and socially isolated community seemed to offer the best opportunity for following their religious precepts" (p. 19). Administratively, the ghetto was an agency of social, political, and economic control that enforced the segregation of Jews from non-Jews. Considering the prevailing anti-Semitism of Christians, this separation also served their desires well.

This situation began changing rapidly in the 20th century. Prior to World War II, Jewish intermarriage rates were below 5%. By 1970, about 32% of Jews were intermarrying, and by the mid-1980s intermarriage rates of 40–60% were reported (Silberman, 1985). This is likely to change the genetic situation in the not too distant future. However, recent genetic marker analyses reveal that Jews from eastern and western Europe, north Africa, and the Near and Middle East are related despite over 2,000 years of the Diaspora (i.e., the Jews' dispersion from their roots in Palestine during Biblical times) (Ostrer, 2000).

Simply put, the physical isolation of the Jews for millennia offered an opportunity for mutations to appear; hence this group has been troubled by a fairly large number of genetically based disorders. Though Jews are prone to a wide variety of inherited illnesses, in many instances one can argue that lifestyle and other factors contribute to the expression of certain diseases (Koenig, McCullough, & Larson, 2001). We must also keep in mind that genetics is usually more probabilistic than deterministic (Barkow, 1982; Gould, 1978). Still, a number of heritable conditions evidence great discrepancies between Jews and non-Jews (Griffiths, Miller, Suzuki, Lewontin, & Gelbart, 2000; Post, 1973). For example, Gaucher syndrome—a metabolic disease that affects the liver, spleen, bones, blood, and possibly the nervous system—has a prevalence of 1 per 2,500 among Ashkenazi Jews (also known as Ashkenazim), but 1 per 75,000 among non-Jews.[6] Another condition occurring disproportionately in this group is Tay–Sachs disease, a degenerative disorder of the brain that results in blindness, deafness, paralysis, and death, usually by the age of 3 or 4. It is found in 1 of 3,500 Ashkenazic Jews, but only 1 per 35,000 non-Jews. Genetic testing for Tay–Sachs is a success story. Between 1970 and 2000, over 1 million Jews were tested for mutations for this condition, and the incidence of Tay–Sachs births dropped over 90% (Macmillan Science Library: Genetics, 2004).

A genetic predisposition to breast cancer has been identified in Jewish women (Egan et al., 1996). In a balanced manner, these authors also note the influence of lifestyle and

---

[6]Ashkenazim come primarily from central and eastern Europe and account for about 80% of all Jews. Sephardic Jews are found in southern Europe and the entire Mediterranean region, while a number of smaller groups may be found in Asia.

reproductive history on the development of breast cancer. Those who would like to peruse the medical literature on other genetic disorders among Jews might research essential pentosuria, familial dysautonomia, Niemann–Pick disease, and torsion dystonia, among other possibilities. Goodman's (1979) overview of genetic disorders listed some 22 conditions among the Ashkenazim.

Concern among Jews about these conditions resulted in a National Foundation for Jewish Genetic Diseases, which has since been absorbed into the Center for Jewish Genetic Diseases at the Icahn School of Medicine at Mount Sinai,[7] a voluntary, nonprofit health and research organization that gathers and provides information on research, care, and resources for those interested in and/or affected by any of the genetic diseases to which Jews are susceptible.

A Newer Theory: Genetic Diseases and Intelligence among Ashkenazi Jews

A more recent theory has associated the pattern of Jewish genetic diseases with the issue of above-average intelligence among Ashkenazim. Formulated by three non-Jewish scholars affiliated with the University of Utah, this theory has been termed "politically incorrect" by a number of evaluators (Wade, 2005), but that is a poor excuse for avoiding controversy. This is a radical perspective that ties biology to religion, specifically only to Ashkenazim (Cochran, Hardy, & Harpending, 2005). To put it mildly, it has stimulated much debate and disagreement. These scholars make the following points:

1. The genetic disorders described above have plagued Ashkenazi Jews for centuries.
2. From 50 to 80% of the variation in intelligence test scores has been attributed to genetics (Bouchard, 1996a, 1996b; Myers, 1998).
3. Observations indicate that Ashkenazi Jews, on the average, score 10–15 points higher on intelligence tests than the norm for such measures (Lynn & Longley, 2006).
4. A relationship involving neural development is hypothesized between high intelligence and the production of certain genetic diseases among Ashkenazi Jews.
5. This association is believed to be a function of the long-term effects of prejudice and bigotry on Ashkenazi Jews in central and eastern Europe from about 800 to 1800 A.D.
6. The inference is made that discriminatory treatment forced the Ashkenazim into occupations requiring intelligence, especially of a verbal and mathematical nature (but not spatial).
7. Such occupations (e.g., money lending, banking, business, etc.) selected over time for high intelligence.
8. These males were financially well off, married the daughters of similar Ashkenazim, and had large families.
9. The outcomes were high intelligence and high rates of certain neurological conditions.

Some of these points merit further elaboration. Research points to two clusters of genetic problems. The primary one is termed the "lysosomal" or "sphingolipid storage" cluster of disorders (e.g., Tay–Sachs disease, Niemann–Pick disease, mucolipidosis, and Gaucher syndrome). These disorders evoke disturbances in neural function that interfere with the speed of nervous signals, the insulation of nerve fibers, and the growth of connections among

---

[7]The center can be contacted via its website (*http://icahn.mssm.edu/research/jewish-genetics*).

nerve cells (Nuenke, 2005; Wade, 2005). The second group of disorders is labeled the "DNA repair" cluster and may be involved to a lesser degree in neural functioning. Still, sufferers from at least one of these defects, torsion dystonia, evidence uncommonly high intelligence (Cochran et al., 2005). Referring mainly to the first cluster, Cochran et al. (2005) claim that genetic neurological diseases with high rates among Ashkenazim "are known to elevate IQ" (p. 661).

With respect to the third point above, what may be of greater significance is not the average difference in IQ, but the probability that IQs above 140 may be six times more frequent among Ashkenazim than among non-Ashkenazim. This positive development was, however, accompanied by "an increased [rate] of hereditary disorders" (Cochran et al., 2005, p. 659). For example, studies of patients with Gaucher syndrome reveal high IQs and occupations requiring high intelligence.

Given the problems associated with rapid natural selection, particularly with genetically recessive disorders, those not disabled by their mutations—namely, carriers of the mutations—may well manifest high intelligence. They possess, however, the very undesirable likelihood of passing on their presently silent neurological defects to future generations. This implies a testable hypothesis: Compared to those without these mutations, Ashkenazi carriers of the mutations should reveal significantly higher intelligence (Cochran et al., 2005). One estimate suggests that 29% of Ashkenazi Jews may possess genetic mutations for these disorders (*Intermountain Jewish News*, 2006). These mutations may function in a manner similar to the one for sickle cell anemia, which, despite its very negative character, protects against malaria. Another consideration is that the mutations causing these diseases should be eliminated unless they are performing some adaptive evolutionary function.

High IQs would be meaningless if they were not manifested in concrete accomplishments in life. Stark (1998) has claimed that "The Jews rapidly became the most highly educated group in the United States . . . and have the highest family income of any racial, religious or ethnic group" (p. 298). Further evidence is found in regard to Nobel Prize winners: From the second half of the 20th century up to 2004, the Jewish population in the United States ranged from about 2 to 3%, but they accounted for 41% of those receiving Nobel Prizes. In addition, though approximately 0.33% of the world's population is Jewish, this group has produced over half of the world's chess champions (Cochran et al., 2005). Similar data may be cited for intellectual honors in a wide variety of fields.

As indicated earlier, the view of Cochran and his associates has been challenged. Metzenberg (2005) claims that the operative selective process is not Darwinian natural selection, but a system of self-selection more than two millennia old. He stresses a Jewish cultural emphasis on learning and study, with those who were most successful becoming highly valued in their communities. Actually, self-selection and natural selection would have been mutually supportive. Either way, the result was that community leaders chose these men for their daughters. The consequences were financial support for further study, plus large families. Despite some good arguments, Metzenberg's thesis has also come in for sharp criticism (Razib, 2005). Cochran et al. (2005) stress that their position is hypothetical, is capable of being tested, and provides an avenue for further research and evaluation. Though knowledgeable scientists and scholars have ranged themselves on both sides of the issue, this work shows the psychological complexities of religion in its historical–cultural context. Politically incorrect or not, it is likely to elicit polemics for some time to come.

OVERVIEW

In this chapter, we have briefly examined the main questions surrounding the relationship of religion to biology, with an emphasis on evolution/genetics and on neuropsychology. This is a realm about which volumes can be written. It is also one that rapidly becomes highly specialized and technical, as biochemistry and the neurosciences are part of the overall picture.

The relationship between religion and biology has been historically conditioned by the theory of evolution. Soon after Darwin presented his views, the religious community split—interestingly, with conservatives on both sides of the conflict. One group saw evolution as posing a dire threat to faith by doing away with the distinction between humans and other animals. The religious proponents of Darwinism saw evolutionary theory as testimony to the wondrous way God works through natural law. This battle is continuing into the 21st century, with science on one side and creationism and intelligent design on the other. As fascinating as this debate is, it is beyond the scope of the present volume, and much good writing on the various issues is available elsewhere (K. R. Miller, 1999; Ruse, 2006).

In current biological and social-scientific thinking, religion has become a popular topic. Grand, all-encompassing theories may be intellectually exciting, but unless they eventuate in fruitful research, they will essentially remain sterile.

Research on religion and the brain appears to be a "hot" research area today, but it is basically in its infancy. Work in this domain has, however, opened new avenues to understanding the biological correlates of religious belief, behavior, and experience. Much still needs to be done to unravel the issues of causes, effects, correlations, and relationships between religious expression and these physical processes. Looking into our indefinite future, we particularly recommend that readers examine the work of Feierman, briefly discussed in this chapter. His creative publications may be opening up new avenues for theory and research.

It is abundantly evident that religion, which seems so distant from biology, is actually intimately involved with it on many levels. The tip of this iceberg is now displayed, but more of its body is coming into view as science studies the various links between religion and biology.

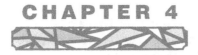

CHAPTER 4

Religion in Childhood

Dear God, instead of letting people die and having to make new ones, why don't you just keep the ones You have now?—Jane

Dear God, are You really invisible or is that a trick?—Lucy

King Solomon must have been fond of animals, because he had many wives and one thousand porcupines.

Mummy, in the Bible, there is a story about a flood and God promised that there would never be another flood. How come there was a flood in Texas then?

If Jesus is born every Christmas and crucified every Good Friday, how does he grow so quickly?[1]

RELIGIOUS AND SPIRITUAL DEVELOPMENT IN CHILDHOOD

With some exceptions, in this chapter we restrict our consideration of "religious development" to theory and investigations involving *children and young adolescents* (here taken to include persons through the midteen years). This purposely avoids many studies of college students and adults, unless such research has implications for child and young adolescent religious development. The research on religion and childhood can be divided into an earlier, largely theoretical period and a more recent empirical stage built on a newly emerging paradigm. Despite the facts that fewer than 1% of almost 150,000 studies identified in PsycINFO in 2005 included studies of religion in childhood, and that 45% of all dissertations addressing religion and childhood had been completed since 1990 (Boyatzis, 2005, p. 124), theories from mainstream psychology have dominated the study of religion, spirituality, and childhood. Largely identified as "stage theories," these theories conceptualize religious and spiritual development as involving subjective endorsement of beliefs and practices that gradually evolve as individuals mature (Mattis, Ahluwalia, Cowie, & Kirkland-Harris, 2006, p. 284). However, nearly three-quarters of all the research on religion and childhood has been published since 2000 (Boyatzis, 2013, p. 497). Much of this research is influenced by embedding attachment theory within the context of evolutionary psychology (Kirkpatrick, 2005).

---

[1] These quotations come, respectively, from the following sources: Paw Prints (n.d.); Paw Prints (n.d.); a child quoted in Goldman (1964, p. 1); Madge (1965, p. 14); and Madge (1965, p. 14).

However, even more of this research is influenced by a new multidisciplinary paradigm best identified as the "cognitive science of religion" (CSR). It is influenced by a multidisciplinary paradigm associated with and this paradigm also expands the psychology of religion to studies of children in other than Western countries (Barrett, 2013; Heiphetz, Lane, Waytz, & Young, 2016). The case of "more theory than data," long associated with stage theories, is beginning to be remedied. However, as we shall see, stage theories remain essential guides to religious development.

Stage Theories of Religious and Spiritual Development

The Influence of Piaget

As Hyde (1990) pointed out almost three decades ago, "The study of religion in childhood and adolescence has been dominated for thirty years by investigations of the process by which religious thinking develops" (p. 15), and this dominance has been largely attributable to the influence of Jean Piaget. Although Piaget is no longer held on a pedestal, his influence remains considerable. For many, it is hard to think of religious development in other than cognitive terms (Boyatzis, 2005, p. 126).

Piaget argued that "cognitive development" involves a series of stages. Beginning in the 1920s, he studied these stages in part by sitting on street corners and playing marbles and other games with his own and other children—asking about the "rules" of each game, posing problems for the children to solve, and so on (Piaget, 1932/1948, 1936/1952, 1937/1954). He was just as interested in the "errors" the children made as he was in "correct" answers to his questions, and noted that there were striking similarities among the ways in which children of the same age reasoned about things. Piaget concluded that there are four major identifiable stages of cognitive development, which reflect the general reasoning abilities of children of different ages:

1. *Sensorimotor stage* (birth to about 2 years). During this stage, children seem to understand things through their sensory and motor ("sensorimotor") interactions with the world around them (e.g., by touching and looking at things, and by putting them in their mouths). It is during this period that infants come to realize that objects continue to exist even though they are no longer immediately perceived ("object permanence"), and also that infants develop a fear of strangers ("stranger anxiety"). Both of these cognitive changes appear at about 8 months or soon thereafter.

2. *Preoperational stage* (about 2–7 years). During this second stage, children live in a very egocentric world, being unable to see things from others' perspectives. Preoperational children become quite at home in representing things with language and numbers, but lack sophisticated logical reasoning capability, and are unable to grasp more than one relationship at a time. Also, children at this stage are prone to errors, especially for concepts of conservation. That is, they have difficulty grasping the idea that such characteristics as volume, mass, or length of objects remain the same, in spite of changes in their outward appearance. For example, even when a child has seen the same amount of liquid poured back and forth between a short, fat beaker and a tall, thin beaker, the youngster may fail to understand that the amount of liquid in the two containers is the same. Rather, he or she may think that the tall, thin beaker holds more water because it "looks bigger."

3. *Concrete operational stage* (about 7–12 years). During this stage, children become capable of understanding the concepts of conservation that gave them so much trouble at the previous level. They are also able to reason quite logically about concrete events, to understand analogies, and to perform mathematical transformations such as those involving reversibility (i.e., 4 + 3 = 7; therefore, 7 − 3 = 4).

4. *Formal operational stage* (12 years and up). The last stage of cognitive development allows a move away from the concrete in thought processes. These older children are capable of complex abstract thinking involving the hypothetical—for example, by generating potential solutions to a problem, and then creating a plan to systematically test different possibilities in order to arrive at a "correct" solution.

Piaget's proposals have not escaped criticism (Boyatzis, 2005, pp. 125–126). One crucial assumption accepted by others influenced by Piaget is that cognitive growth proceeds sequentially, so that growing children can assimilate and deal with their environment, and can also alter their thinking in order to accommodate new information. In other words, it is assumed that each stage builds on the previous stages in order to further children's cognitive development. This assumption has important implications for religious and spiritual development. For example, it suggests that children are not cognitively capable of understanding the complex and abstract concepts involved in most religions of the adult world. Piaget did not write directly about the religious growth of children (Hyde, 1990), even though he wrote a book on moral development (Piaget, 1932/1948). It was left to others to relate Piaget's theories of cognitive stages to religion and spirituality.

Applications of Piaget's Stages to Religious and Spiritual Development

ELKIND'S APPROACH

David Elkind proposed that religion is a natural result of mental development, such that biological roots of intellectual growth interact with individuals' experiences. Specifically, Elkind suggested that four basic sequential components of intelligence (conservation, search for representation, search for relations, and search for comprehension) are critical in religious development, and that this sequence parallels the cognitive stages described by Piaget (Elkind, 1961, 1962, 1963, 1964, 1970, 1971). Three studies investigating Elkind's ideas about cognitive religious development are described in Research Box 4.1. Essentially, his research supported a Piagetian kind of progression as religious understanding emerges in children. A subsequent study (Long, Elkind, & Spilka, 1967) revealed a similar cognitive sequence for children's ideas about prayer.

Shifting from a child's sense of religious identity to children's religious experience, David and Sally Elkind (1970) studied the compositions of 149 ninth-grade U.S. students who were asked to respond to the questions "When do you feel closest to God?" and "Have you ever had a particular experience of feeling especially close to God?" (p. 104). The former question was assumed to tap recurrent religious experiences, and the latter acute religious experiences. The researchers concluded that the majority of respondents regarded personal religious experiences as a significant part of their lives, even though many resisted formal religious activities and participation. Across all respondents, 92% wrote compositions indicating recurrent experiences, and 76% wrote compositions indicating acute experiences (Elkind & Elkind, 1970, p. 104).

RESEARCH BOX 4.1. The Child's Concept of Religion (Elkind, 1961, 1962, 1963)

In three separate studies, Elkind posed a series of questions to Jewish, Catholic, and Protestant children, respectively, concerning their understanding of their religious identity and ideas. For example, in his 1961 study, Jewish children were asked questions such as these: "Are you Jewish?", "What makes you Jewish?", "Can a cat or a dog be Jewish? Why?", and "How do you become a Jew?" Elkind found considerable age-related cognitive similarity in children's responses to such questions across his three major religious groups. The development of religious ideas seemed to parallel Piaget's cognitive stages to some extent.

In the 5- to 7-year range (comparable to Piaget's late preoperational stage), children seemed to think that their denominational affiliation was absolute, having been ordained by God, and therefore it could not be changed. A few years later (ages 7–9, comparable to Piaget's early concrete operational stage), religious ideas were indeed very "concrete." Religious affiliation was seen to be determined by the family into which one was born, and if a Catholic family had a pet cat, it was thought to be a Catholic cat. At the next stage of religious development (ages 10–14, corresponding to Piaget's late concrete and early formal operational stages), children apparently began to understand some of the complexities of religious practices and rituals, and they could conceive of a person's changing his or her religion because they understood religion to come from within the person rather than being determined externally. Abstract and differentiated religious thinking was beginning to appear. In the end, Elkind concluded that children were not capable of an abstract "adult" understanding of religion before the age of 11 or 12 (i.e., the beginning of Piaget's formal operational period).

TAMMINEN'S RESEARCH

Kalevi Tamminen's (1976, 1994; Tamminen & Nurmi, 1995; Tamminen, Vianello, Jaspard, & Ratcliff, 1988) studies of the religious experiences of Finnish children and adolescents deserve attention in this chapter for several reasons. First, almost 3,000 young people have been studied. Second, this research program has produced limited but important longitudinal data. Third, and possibly most important, these studies have moved a step beyond the more traditional cognitive-stage approach by investigating the meaning and implications of religious *experiences* for children's lives, in addition to aspects of religious cognitive development.

Tamminen (1991) used the five religious dimensions of Glock and Stark (1965) to organize his longitudinal study of religious development in Scandinavian youths. Tamminen and his colleagues asked their participants, "Have you at times felt that God is particularly close to you?" They found a steady decline in the percentage of students reporting experiences of nearness to God by grade level. Tamminen's study is the only major longitudinal study to document the steady decline in the report of religious experience from childhood through adolescence in a highly secularized culture. It suggests that such experiences (or their report) are quite common in childhood, supporting the claims of Paffard (1973) and others as discussed later in this chapter.

Tamminen's research program is not without problems. It is difficult to know what to make of written questionnaire responses from relatively young children; probably the younger children were not able to express themselves well in writing, and it is not clear that their self-reported "religious experiences" are consonant with what adults would call "religious experiences." Also, questionnaires were administered in school classrooms, suggesting that peer pressure, contextual influences, and other such factors may have influenced responses. For example, children may have been reluctant to reveal personal religious experiences to an unknown adult, especially while sitting among their classmates. As Scarlett (1994) has pointed out, "These are surveys carried out in impersonal settings not conducive to tapping into what God and religious experience *mean* to adolescents" (p. 88; emphasis in original). Furthermore, the children and adolescents were fairly homogeneous in terms of their religious background (Lutheran), and it is not clear to what extent Tamminen's findings might generalize to children from other religious backgrounds or no religious background at all. For a better appreciation of differences in religious experience across religious traditions (though not specifically in childhood), the reader might consult the first six chapters of Hood's (1995b) *Handbook of Religious Experience*.

THE WORK OF GOLDMAN

Goldman (1964) applied Piaget's theory of cognitive development to religious thinking, claiming that "religious thinking is no different in mode and method from non-religious thinking" (p. 5). Working in England, he asked 5- to 15-year-old children questions about drawings with religious connotations (e.g., a child kneeling at a bed, apparently praying), as well as questions about Bible stories (e.g., Moses at the burning bush). He then analyzed responses to the questions by looking for evidence of Piagetian stages of development. He concluded, as did Elkind, that religious thinking does indeed proceed in a fashion similar to more general cognitive development.

A number of studies have confirmed these general conclusions about "cognitive stages," especially the implication that children are capable of more abstract religious thinking as they grow older (see, e.g., Degelman, Mullen, & Mullen, 1984; Peatling, 1974, 1977; Peatling & Laabs, 1975; Tamminen, 1976; Tamminen & Nurmi, 1995). There has also been some confirmatory cross-cultural work (see Hyde, 1990). Some studies have examined specific predictions of the Piagetian approach for religious development. For example, Zachry (1990) concluded that his data, obtained from high school and college students, were "consistent with the prediction of Piagetian theory that abstract thought in a specific content area such as religion depends on an underlying formal logic" (p. 405).

EVALUATING GOLDMAN'S FINDINGS

Some empirical work has not been entirely supportive of Goldman's conclusions about the development of religious thought. For example, Hoge and Petrillo (1978b) studied 451 high school sophomores in different Protestant and Catholic churches, and concluded that Goldman had overestimated the importance of cognitive capacity and underestimated the role of religious training in the development of religious thought. This conclusion, however, was apparently based primarily on differences between public and private school Catholics. Hoge and Petrillo attributed such differences to religious education at the private school, but there might well have been selection factors at work, such as socioeconomic status or parental religiosity. Hoge and Petrillo themselves acknowledged the bias in their sample, such that "the youth most alienated from the church refused [to participate] disproportionately often" (pp. 142–143).

Batson, Schoenrade, and Ventis (1993) reconsidered Hoge and Petrillo's (1978b) results and concluded that their conclusions were inappropriate. In fact, they suggested that Hoge and Petrillo's findings were "precisely what Goldman would have predicted" (1993, p. 62). The disagreement between these two groups of authors apparently hinges partly on a specific Goldman prediction concerning the level of religious *teachings* (e.g., "concrete thinking" about religious content) and adolescents' overall *capacity* for higher, more abstract ("formal operational") religious thinking. Hoge and Petrillo did not measure this "gap" directly, but assumed that higher absolute scores on a measure of abstract religious thinking meant that a smaller gap existed. Furthermore, their findings were not consistent across different measures of religious rejection or across different participant groupings, and the majority of reported correlations did not achieve statistical significance. It is not surprising that there was some disagreement as to the interpretation of these findings.

Some authors (e.g., Godin, 1968; Howkins, 1966; Kay, 1996; McCallister, 1995) have been quite critical of Goldman's general conclusions, especially the implications he drew for religious education. Apparently Elkind's research (see above) has escaped the severe criticism applied to Goldman's work, in part because Elkind avoided theological biases or assumptions (see Hyde, 1990), whereas Goldman "assumed a particular theological point of view" (Hyde, 1990, p. 35). For example, Greer (1983) has suggested that the cognitive tests of Goldman and those of Peatling, who developed a measure of religious cognitive development (Peatling, Laabs, & Newton, 1975), were biased in such a way that theologically conservative respondents would tend to endorse responses indicating concrete (rather than abstract) religious thinking.

In the end, although it has been argued that the religiosity of children is *not* dependent on cognitive development (Pierce & Cox, 1995), the works of Elkind, Goldman, and others have demonstrated the utility of a Piagetian framework for understanding the development of religious thinking. These researchers also set the stage for much subsequent work in related areas, such as faith development, moral development, and the emergence of the God concept and prayer.

Fowler's Stages of Faith Development

James Fowler (1981, 1991a, 1991b, 1994, 1996) has suggested that individual religious faith unfolds in a stage sequence similar to that described by Piaget for cognitive development, and by Kohlberg for moral growth (see below). He defines faith as "a dynamic and generic human experience . . . [that] includes, but is not limited to or identical with, religion" (Fowler, 1991a, p. 31). That is, although Fowler's use of the term "faith" does overlap with institutionalized religion, the two are also independent to some extent. Faith is seen as a deep core of the individual, the "center of values," "images and realities of power," and "master stories" (myths) involving both conscious and unconscious motivations. In other words, faith involves centers of values that vary from one individual to the next, but that are foci of primary life importance (such as religion, family, nation, power, money, and sexuality).

Furthermore, people tend to align themselves with power in this dangerous world—possibly religious power, but also sources of secular power, such as nations and economic systems. "Faith is trust in and loyalty to images and realities of power" (Fowler, 1991a, p. 32). Also, Fowler argues that faith involves stories or scripts that give meaning and direction to people's lives (e.g., what it means to be a good person or a part of a religious community).

Fowler and his colleagues have carried out extensive interviews with hundreds of people about these aspects of their faith. They have concluded that there are essentially seven stages in faith development, although some people never progress very far through these stages. Fowler's stages "aim to describe patterned operations of knowing and valuing that underlie our consciousness" (Fowler, 1996, p. 56). They are described in Table 4.1, with the approximate time of emergence of each stage shown in parentheses.

Fowler has concluded that it is extremely rare for people to reach the seventh and final stage in his sequence, but that people who have attained universalizing faith might include Mahatma Gandhi, Martin Luther King, Jr., and Mother Teresa. It is no coincidence that both Gandhi and King were assassinated. Fowler claims that people who achieve universalizing faith are in danger of premature death because of their confrontational involvement in solving serious problems in the world.

Fowler's analysis of stages of faith is rich in ideas, provides a framework for empirical work, and can potentially contribute to our understanding of what it means to be "religious." However, it has been pointed out that Fowler's conceptualization is complex and difficult to

---

TABLE 4.1. Fowler's Stages of Faith Development

1. *Primal faith* (infancy). This first stage involves the beginnings of emotional trust based on body contact, care, early play, and the like. Subsequent faith development is based on this foundation.

2. *Intuitive/projective faith* (early childhood). In the second stage, imagination combines with perception and feelings to create long-lasting faith images. The child becomes aware of the sacred, of prohibitions, of death, and of the existence of morality.

3. *Mythical/literal faith* (elementary school years). Next, the developing ability to think logically helps to order the world, corresponding to the Piagetian stage of concrete operations. The child can now discriminate between fantasy and the real world, and can appreciate others' perspectives. Religious beliefs and symbols are accepted quite literally.

4. *Synthetic/conventional faith* (early adolescence). During the fourth stage, there is a reliance on abstract ideas of formal operational thinking, which engenders a hunger for a more personal relationship with God. Reflections on past experiences, and concerns about the future and personal relationships, contribute to the development of mutual perspective taking and the shaping of a world view and its values.

5. *Individuative/reflective faith* (late adolescence or young adulthood). The fifth stage involves a critical examination and reconstitution of values and beliefs, including a change from reliance on external authorities to authority within the self. The capacity for "third-person perspective taking" contributes to the development of consciously chosen commitments and to the emergence of an "executive ego."

6. *Conjunctive faith* (midlife or beyond). In the sixth stage, there is integration of opposites (e.g., the realization that each individual is both young and old, masculine and feminine, constructive and destructive), generating a "hunger for a deeper relationship to the reality that symbols mediate" (Fowler, 1991a, p. 41) "Dialogical knowing" emerges, such that the individual is open to the multiple perspectives of a complex world. This enables the person to go beyond the faith boundaries developed in the previous individuative/reflective stage, and to appreciate that "truth" is both multidimensional and organically interdependent.

7. *Universalizing faith* (unspecified age). The relatively rare final stage involves a oneness with the power of being or God, as well as commitment to love, justice, and overcoming oppression and violence. People who have attained this stage of faith development "live as though a commonwealth of love and justice were already reality among us. They create zones of liberation for the rest of us, and we experience them as both liberating and as threatening. These people tend to confront others concerning their involvement in, and attachments to, dehumanizing structures which oppose 'the commonwealth of love and justice'" (Fowler, 1991a, p. 41).

comprehend, and it has failed to generate relatively rigorous empirical research. Also, Fowler has generally declined to analyze his own results statistically and has ignored related work in the psychology of religion (Hyde, 1990).

Streib (2001a) proposes that revisions to Fowler's faith development theory are needed—for example, to free the theory from "its almost unquestioned adoption of the structural-developmental 'logic of development' . . . in order to account for the rich and deep life-world- and life-history-related dimensions of religion" (pp. 144–145). Similarly, Day (2001) claims that "contemporary research challenges the fundamental assumptions of the cognitive developmental paradigm" (p. 173); therefore, we need to look elsewhere if we are to understand religious development. He has suggested that greater attention should be addressed to (religious) speech and narrative. McDargh (2001) focuses his critique of Fowler's theory more on its theological foundations, and claims that a more individually focused approach would be useful. McDargh (2001) and Rizzuto (2001) have both argued for more incorporation of psychoanalytic concepts and processes in analyzing faith development. However, Fowler (2001; Fowler & Dell, 2006) has defended his theory, arguing that it continues to serve after three decades of research as a useful framework for studying faith development at different levels (the individual, the family, and the social group).

One problem with Fowler's theory has been the difficulty in operationalizing the stages, and consequently there have been attempts to simplify the measurement of his proposed stages. For instance, Leak, Loucks, and Bowlin (1999) have developed an eight-item Faith Development Scale intended to measure Fowler's proposed stages. However, attempts to validate this scale have generated mixed results. Leak et al. (1999) have suggested either that this might be due to limitations of the scale, or that we should have "reservations on the beneficence of mature faith within a Fowlerian framework" (p. 122). More promising is the development of a Religious Schema Scale by Streib and his colleagues (see Streib, 2008, pp. 58–59; Streib & Hood, 2016).

Oser's Stages of Development of Religious Judgment

Fritz Oser, with Gmunder and other colleagues (Oser, 1991, 1994; Oser & Gmunder, 1991; Oser & Reich, 1990, 1996; Oser, Reich, & Bucher, 1994), has focused on a related aspect of religious development called "religious judgment." Apart from the work of Elkind, Fowler, and others, Oser (1991) has stated that

> there have been few investigations directed at building up a theory about the development of an individual's constructions and reconstructions of the religious experiences and beliefs. [Therefore we] are attempting to formulate a new paradigm of religious development, using a structural concept of discontinuous, stagelike development and the classical semiclinical interview method as our primary research strategy. (p. 6)

Oser's research has revealed five stages in the emergence of religious judgment, as qualitative changes occur in people's relationship to an "Ultimate Being" or God. Individuals move from a stage of believing that God intervenes unexpectedly in the world and that God's power guides human beings (Stage 1), through belief in a still external and all-powerful God who punishes or rewards, depending on good or bad deeds ("Give so that you may receive") (Stage 2). Individuals in Stage 3 begin to think of God as somewhat detached from their world and as wielding less influence, with people generally responsible for their own lives, since they can now distinguish between "transcendence" (God's existence outside the created world) and "immanence" (God's presence and action from within). In Stage 4 people come to realize both the necessity and the limits of autonomy, recognizing that freedom and life stem from an Ultimate Being, who is often perceived to have a "divine plan" that gives meaning to life. Finally, in Stage 5 the Ultimate Being is realized through human action via care and love. There is "universal and unconditional religiosity" (Oser, 1991, p. 10).

Oser and Reich (1996) have pointed to limited empirical support for this stage conceptualization of the development of religious judgment; some research (e.g., Bucher, 1991; Di Loreto & Oser, 1996, as cited in Oser & Reich, 1996; Roco & Ticu, 1996; Zondag & Belzen, 1999) has provided further support for Oser's proposals. Huber, Reich, and Schenker (2000) have argued that it is important to match the technique of measurement to the goals of an investigation in this area. Their findings suggest that combinations of methods may be appropriate.

Kohlberg's Stages of Moral Development

Lawrence Kohlberg's (1964, 1969, 1981, 1984) theory of moral development has served as a basis for the investigation of many issues related to morality. Building on Piaget's belief that the moral judgments of children derive from their cognitive development, Kohlberg attempted to identify cognitive stages that underlie the development of moral thinking. In a series of studies, he asked people what they thought about different "moral dilemmas."

Kohlberg's most famous dilemma involved a woman near death from cancer who could potentially be saved by a new drug developed by a nearby druggist. The druggist, however, wanted 10 times what the drug cost him to make—more than the sick woman's husband, Heinz, could afford—and refused to sell it for less. So Heinz considered breaking into the druggist's store to steal the drug for his wife. Respondents were asked to comment on the morality of Heinz's potential decision to steal the drug, and to indicate the reasoning behind their response. Based on such responses to such dilemmas, Kohlberg proposed that individuals pass through three broad levels of moral development, each with substages. As Sapp (1986) stated, "each stage is distinguished by moral reasoning that is more complex, more comprehensive, more integrated, and more differentiated than the reasoning of the earlier stages" (p. 273). Table 4.2 outlines the levels and stages of moral development proposed by Kohlberg.

Kohlberg's theory has been criticized (Darley & Shultz, 1990), and Bergling's (1981) extensive assessment of its validity suggests that the theory may have limited utility outside of Western industrialized countries. But there is some support for Kohlberg's conclusions that children do progress through moral stages, especially from the preconventional level to the conventional level of morality. Also, Snarey's (1985) review of the literature suggests that this progression *is* reasonably similar in different cultures.

One might expect that Kohlberg's conceptualization of moral development would be closely linked to religious growth, or that religious development would directly affect (and possibly determine) the emergence of morality. However, Kohlberg made it very clear that moral and religious development are quite separate, and that the two should not be confused. For example, he suggested that it is a fallacy to think that

> basic moral principles are dependent upon a particular religion, or any religion at all. We have found no important differences in development of moral thinking between Catholics, Protestants, Jews, Buddhists, Moslems, and atheists. . . . Both cultural values and religion

are important factors in selectively elaborating certain themes in the moral life but they are not unique causes of the development of basic moral values. (Kohlberg, 1980, pp. 33–34)

Research has confirmed Kohlberg's conclusion in this regard (Bruggeman & Hart, 1996; Cobb, Ong, & Tate, 2001; Gorsuch & McFarland, 1972; Selig & Teller, 1975), and other experts on moral development have taken a similar stance (e.g., Turiel & Neff, 2000). Moreover, Nucci and Turiel (1993) found that older children and adolescents were able to distinguish between moral and religious issues, and that they viewed moral rules as unalterable by religious authorities. However, this has not stopped many, many researchers from speculating about and investigating possible relationships between moral development and religiosity (e.g., Clouse, 1986; Fernhout & Boyd, 1985; Glover, 1997; Hanson, 1991; Kedem & Cohen, 1987; Mitchell, 1988). Such research has been facilitated by the development of a less subjective scoring system to evaluate stages of moral development.

TABLE 4.2. Kohlberg's Stages of Moral Development

Preconventional level (develops during early childhood)

Stage 1. Punishment and obedience orientation
The first stage is characterized by avoidance of punishment and unquestioning deference to power as values in themselves. Morality is seen as based on self-interest, and the goodness or badness of actions is determined by their physical consequences, regardless of any human meaning attached to these consequences.

Stage 2. Instrumental relativist orientation
This stage is defined by a focus on instrumental satisfaction of one's own needs as the determiner of "right." Reciprocity may be present, but is of the "you scratch my back and I'll scratch yours" variety.

Conventional level (develops during late childhood and early adolescence)

Generally, this level involves a move toward gaining approval or avoiding disapproval as the basis for morality; law and social rules are seen as valuable in their own right.

Stage 3. Interpersonal concordance or "good boy/nice girl" orientation
Early in the conventional level, the individual is driven by behavior that pleases or helps others and that receives their approval.

Stage 4. "Law and order" orientation
Subsequently, in the conventional level, the person focuses on the maintenance of the social order and the importance of authority and strict rules.

Postconventional level (may develop from late adolescence on)

People at this level tend to be concerned with morality as abstract principles. They are able to separate their own identification with groups from the principles and moral values associated with those groups.

Stage 5. Social-contract/legalistic orientation
The fifth stage involves recognition of the relative nature of personal values, and the importance of having procedural rules to reach consensus. The individual can separate the legal world from individual differences of opinion.

Stage 6. Universal ethical principle orientation
The last and highest stage of moral development, according to Kohlberg, involves defining "right" in one's own conscience, consistent with one's own abstract ethical principles, but with a sense of responsibility to others. There is a clear emphasis on universality, consistency, logic, and rationality.

Rest's (1979, 1983; Rest, Cooper, Coder, Masanz, & Anderson, 1974) Defining Issues Test (DIT) asks people to respond to a series of 12 statements concerning each of six moral dilemmas. The DIT was intended to be both simpler and more objective than Kohlberg's initial scoring of moral stages, and it has stimulated numerous studies on moral development and religion, though apparently few with children. These investigations have reported some relationships between level of moral judgment and religious orientation, though typically not strong ones (Clouse, 1991; Ernsberger & Manaster, 1981; Holley, 1991; Sapp, 1986). There have also been claims that people from fundamentalist denominations have lower DIT scores (Richards, 1991; Sapp, 1986). The validity of the DIT for conservative religious groups has been called into question, however, by Richards (1991; Richards & Davison, 1992). An improved measure of moral judgment, the DIT2, has since been published (Rest, Narvaez, Thoma, & Bebeau, 1999). It remains to be seen whether this revised measure will help to clarify the literature on moral development and religion.

Gilligan (1977) has criticized Kohlberg's theory and research for their failure to deal with unique aspects of women's moral development, especially the care and responsibility orientation of many women, as contrasted with the male justice orientation emphasized by Kohlberg. This could have implications for religious development—for example, in terms of gender differences in images of God, if God is seen as a person's anchor for morality. There is evidence that images of God diverge along gender lines, with women more likely to see God as supportive and men more likely to see God as instrumental (Nelsen, Cheek, & Au, 1985). Reich (1997) has pondered more generally whether such considerations might suggest the need for a theory specifically for women's religious development. However, he has concluded that there is no need to modify current theories of religious development, or to generate new ones in this regard. Others (DeNicola, 1997; Schweitzer, 1997) have been critical of Reich's stance; they have argued that, at a minimum, revisions to current theories are needed.

In general, Kohlberg's stages of moral development can at least stimulate our thinking about religious growth. For example, Scarlett and Perriello (1991) have suggested that Kohlberg's ideas could help in understanding aspects of the development of prayer. Furthermore, religion has much to say about morality, and understanding how moral development occurs is certainly relevant to the communication and understanding of moral issues at different ages. At the same time, we must take Kohlberg's warning to heart and not assume—as some researchers have—that moral and religious development are necessarily directly and causally related. (Other approaches to morality and religion are discussed in Chapter 12.)

Is a Unified Approach to Religious Development Possible?

Given the overlap among the various stage conceptualizations, it might be productive to attempt an integration and synthesis of Piaget's, Fowler's, Oser's, and others' stage theories of development, in order to delineate the common elements of these theories as they apply to the development of religious thought processes. Such an integration has been attempted by Helmut Reich (1993a, 1993b). He has attempted to summarize the "smorgasbord" of differing theoretical and empirical approaches to the study of religious development. In addition, he has attempted to distinguish between the degree of "hardness" and "softness" of stage theories. "Hard" stages describe organized systems of action (first-order problem solving), are qualitatively different from each other, and follow an unchanging sequence with a clear developmental logic: A later stage denotes greater complexity and improved problem-solving capacity. Each hard stage integrates the preceding stage and logically requires the elements of the prior stage (Reich, 1993a, p. 151).

The stage models of Piaget, Kohlberg, Elkind, and Goldman would be considered "hard." "Soft" stages, on the other hand, "explicitly include elements of affective or reflective characteristics (metatheoretical reflection) that . . . do not follow a unique developmental logic" (Reich, 1993a, p. 151). Oser's and Fowler's theories would fall into this "soft" category. The "hard–soft" distinction could be helpful in understanding and categorizing theories of religious development, as well as the circumstances under which one theory might be more appropriate than another. However, Fowler (1993) has criticized this approach, suggesting that the use of "hard" and "soft" categories is obsolete; that Reich's formulation does not incorporate the important work by Gilligan (1977) on the ethics of responsibility and care; and that Reich fails to acknowledge important differences between Oser's and Fowler's stage theories.

Reich's work does a considerable service by mapping common elements in different theories and empirical investigations, critically evaluating and integrating theories, and suggesting the need for clarification and some standardization in terminology and approaches. In reaction to Reich's proposed integration, Wulff (1993) has suggested that "in the long run . . . the psychology of religion and its practitioners will be best served if we not only recognize the limitations of these theories and their associated research techniques, but also strive to develop new ones more faithful to the traditions and life experience of the persons we seek to understand" (p. 185). Reich's beginning could stimulate further integrative conceptualizations. However, a single major integrative theory of religious development remains an elusive goal (see also Tamminen & Nurmi, 1995).

Critique of the Stage Approaches

Is a "stage" approach the best way to conceptualize religious growth and change? Certainly this approach has increased our understanding of the general processes involved in the emergence of adult religiousness. Furthermore, the numerous variations of stage theoretical approaches discussed above illustrate the dominance of such approaches prior to 2000. In their chapter devoted to religious and spiritual development in the authoritative sixth edition of the *Handbook of Child Psychology,* Oser, Scarlett, and Bucher (2006) have devoted considerable attention to the influence of stage theories and summarize their lasting contribution to our understanding of religious development with two empirical generalizations: (1) As children mature, they move from anthropological and mostly concrete conceptions of supernatural agents to more symbolic and abstract conceptualizations; and (2) children move from reliance on egocentric–imaginative thinking to more rational and decentered thinking as they mature (p. 972).

It is possible, however, that an obsession with stages may detract from our ability to understand the complexity and uniqueness of individual religious development. That is, the tendency to assume that such growth involves cognitive commonalities across all members of specific age groups can to some extent blind us to the idiosyncratic nature of religion in childhood and adolescence (see, e.g., Day, 1994, 2001; Streib, 2001a). Defenders of Piaget in particular have proposed methodological procedures by which Piagetian stages can retain their status as guides to cognitive development (Feldman, 2004). However, what Ferrer (2003, p. 39) has called a Western bias toward "cogniticentrism" remains a serious critique of stage theories indebted to Piaget. Furthermore, the stage approach implies a certain amount of discontinuity in religious development, whereas it may actually be a reasonably continuous process. Streib (2001a) suggests that we focus upon faith "styles" rather than "stages." Streib allows for religious schemas and faith styles to be continually available, and thus avoids the pitfalls of demanding invariant stages. Boyatzis (2005) has been vocal in noting the limitations of cognitive-developmental approaches to the study of religious and spiritual development in children. Others have argued that children and adults can employ similar thought processes, and that there is no necessity to postulate a sequence from magical to rational thought, such that children's thought processes are inevitably denigrated in comparison to "mature" adult thought (see Boyatzis, 2005, p. 126, for a discussion). These criticisms have suggested the limitations of an exclusive reliance upon stage theories and have contributed to a truly new paradigm in the study of religion—the CSR paradigm. Although this paradigm is still emerging, here we focus upon its assumptions and relevance to the study of religious development in childhood.

Cognitive Science of Religion

While evolutionary psychology has often been proposed as a paradigm within which psychological science should be embedded, it remains (as its name indicates) heavily psychological. For instance, Kirkpatrick (2005) has called for placing research on attachment (discussed below) within a comprehensive evolutionary psychology paradigm. However, though the CSR paradigm is heavily influenced by evolutionary theory, it is not simply psychological. CSR is unique in that "it was largely invented by nonpsychologists" (Barrett, 2013, p. 235). It is both multidisciplinary and methodologically pluralistic. Furthermore, many CSR studies use other than Western samples, avoiding the critique that North American psychology is primarily based upon the study of "WEIRD" people. WEIRD is an acronym for "Western, educated, industrialized, rich, democratic" cultures, which are the primary cultures studied in North American psychology, including the developmental psychology of childhood (Henrich, Heine, & Norenzayan, 2010, p. 17). If we can identify a single core assumption of CSR, it is that religious ideas are natural by-products of ordinary, universal human cognitive processes (Bering, 2006; McCauley, 2011; Xygalatas, 2016).

As noted by Oser et al. (2006) (who refer to CSR as "cognitive–cultural approaches"), CSR can be summarized as suggesting that (1) with age, children maintain conceptions of supernatural agents that are both anthropomorphic and nonanthropomorphic; and (2) beginning in childhood but persisting throughout the lifespan, humans sustain intuitive ontologies that can be perceived, which directly coexist with counterintuitive ontologies that cannot be directly perceived (p. 972). Perhaps CSR's unique position can be summed up with the suggestion that religion is a natural phenomenon, and thus humans are "intuitive theists" (Kelemen, 2004, p. 295)—or, as the title of a popular book puts it, *Born Believers* (Barrett, 2012).

A common assumption shared by many CSR researchers is that human cognition works on two levels. One is immediate, intuitive, and unreflective, and largely emotionally driven; the other is slower, deliberate, reflective, and relatively unemotional. Kahneman (2003) identifies the former as simply "System 1" and the latter as "System 2." Kahneman summarizes his elegantly simple theory, which is based on evolutionary theory, as follows: "Highly accessible impression produced by System 1 control judgments and preferences, unless modified or overridden by the deliberate operations of System 2" (2003, p. 716). Kahneman and other researchers committed to dual-process models of cognition have made important advances in understanding religion in childhood. However, while dual-process models vary, they all share the assumption that religion is a reflexive process that is constrained by a more intuitive process they seek to explain (Baumard & Boyer, 2013, p. 295). Children have natural propensities to believe, based upon System 1 processes, and these propensities can be expanded and expressed in explicit theological terms in System 2 processes. Thus a common folk psychology rooted in System 1 processes can be differentiated from a more reflective (and, for some, more theologically correct) understanding rooted in System 2 processes (H. C. Barrett, 2010; McCauley, 2011). Given that System 1 processes are intuitive, they often can best be identified by implicit measures, as discussed in Chapter 2 of this text.

The use of a dual-process model can correct "misguided" (Boyer & Walker, 2000, p. 140) studies that compare how children think with how adults ought to think, according to theological doctrine. Boyer and Walker have pointed out that we do not know whether adults' religious representations are indeed consistent with church doctrine (System 2 processing). Neither should we assume that children's religious development can be assessed by comparing it to adult religious thought. Possibly investigations of children's religion simply elicit "theologically correct" information. That is, children may say what their religious groups, parents, or cultures expect them to say, and this tells us little about, for example, religious concept development. In a similar vein, Harris (2000) has concluded that despite appearances to the contrary, the Piagetian legacy has actually led us to neglect the development of religious thinking—but, as noted above, this is not true of CSR. In fact, CSR has focused heavily upon the mentalization of children, using what has become noted as "theory of mind" (TOM).

Theory of Mind

TOM refers to processes associated with how children come to know about their own and other minds. TOM has been used by CSR theorists to make the remarkable claim that "Not believing in any sort of gods may prove to be a trait that is analogous to not being able to walk" (Barrett, 2012, p. 3). The reasons for this claim are rooted in three contributions CSR researchers using TOM have made to the study of religion, especially in childhood.

First, starting with the groundbreaking work of Guthrie (1993), CSR theorists have argued that humans have a natural tendency to anthropomorphize, or to see inanimate objects as if they were animate. This is an adaptive evolutionary trait, given that it is better to assume that a sound in the woods might be a threatening agent (e.g., a tiger) until it is proved otherwise. Thus the tendency to overdetect agents is an aid to survival, as a false positive is better for survival than a false negative! Barrett (2004) has gone so far (but with some regrets; see Barrett, 2013, p. 238) as to argue that humans have an "agency detection device" that for some may be "hyperactive."

Second, CSR theorists have argued that children have a natural tendency to reason about things teleologically (i.e., in terms of the purposes they serve). Kelemen (1999) goes so far as to refer to the tendency as "promiscuous teleology," in the sense that it is intuitively natural and need not be explicitly taught by parents. This tendency applies even to objects that upon adult reflection can have no purpose or agency (e.g., natural phenomena).

Third, CSR theorists have argued that children who naturally infer agency and purpose are thus also likely to think that things are created for a purpose. Kelemen (2016, p. 295) has noted how CSR has suggested the relevance of much of Piagetian theory. In particular, both children and adults have deep-rooted tendencies (System 1 processing) to use their own subjective experiences to assume that everything has, or is created for, a purpose. To cite but one example, creationism (as opposed to a naturalistic evolutionary explanation) need not be explicitly taught to children in order for it to be inferred as one possible explanation for not only their own, but the natural world's, existence (Evans, 2000). However, while the tendency to believe in gods may be innate and based upon TOM processes, the actual expression of the nature and number of gods believed to exist is dependent upon culture (Banerjee & Bloom, 2013).

EVOLUTIONARY PSYCHOLOGY AND ATTACHMENT THEORY

CSR is heavily indebted to evolutionary theory for the ultimate explanation of why the human mind is the way it is. However, there are wide disputes on precisely how to employ evolutionary theory as an explanation of religion, including whether or not evolution operates at the individual or group level and whether or not religion is an adaptation or not. These issues are hotly debated, and with respect to CSR (as with evolutionary theory in general), we should pay heed to Ruse's cautionary note that methodological naturalism need not lead to metaphysical naturalism (2013, p. 396).

With respect to attachment theory, the issues are less diverse. Most attachment research is done by psychologists, and hence attachment theory is almost exclusively psychological. Kirkpatrick, who began the close linkage between attachment theory and religion, now (in common with many attachment theorists) places this theory within an evolutionary theory seen as the master paradigm for modern psychology. Under this view, religion is not an adaptation, but rather emerged as a by-product of numerous adaptive psychological mechanisms (Kirkpatrick, 2005, p. 240). Thus attachment theory is seen as one adaptive mechanism of major relevance to religion. Religion itself is not seen as an adaptation.

Kirkpatrick (1992, 1994, 1995, 1997, 1998, 1999; Kirkpatrick & Shaver, 1990, 1992) has extended Bowlby's (1969, 1973, 1980) theory of parent–infant attachment to the realm of religion. In so doing, he has provided a unique approach for the study of links between early development and religion, and their implications for children's and adult's lives. As Kirkpatrick (1992) describes Bowlby's work, attachment theory "postulates a primary, biosocial behavioral system in the infant that was designed by evolution to maintain proximity of the infant to its primary caregiver, thereby protecting the infant from predation and other natural dangers" (p. 4). Attachment theory is not without its critics (e.g., Kagan, 1998), but Kirkpatrick has pointed out that this theoretical basis may help to explain individual differences in religiousness. For example, he has noted the extent to which the God of Christian traditions corresponds to the idea of a secure attachment figure. Similarly, religion more generally may serve as a comfort and a sense of security, especially during times of stress or other difficulties.

These observations led Kirkpatrick and Shaver (1990) to suggest that attachment and religion may be linked in important ways. They posited a "compensation hypothesis," which predicts that people who have not had secure relationships with their parents (or other primary caregivers) may be inclined to compensate for this absence by believing in a "loving, personal, available God." This was contrasted with a "mental model hypothesis," predicting that people's religiousness may be at least partially determined by early attachment relationships; that is, they may model their religious beliefs on the attachment relationships they experienced early in their lives.

In a study designed to test these ideas, Kirkpatrick and Shaver (1990; see Research Box 4.2) found some support for the compensation hypothesis, but only for people from relatively nonreligious homes. Findings generally contradicted the mental model hypothesis. Subsequent studies of adolescents (Granqvist, 2002b; Granqvist & Hagekull, 2001) and university students (Granqvist, 1998; Granqvist & Hagekull, 1999) in Sweden, and of adult women in the United States (Kirkpatrick, 1997), have also lent some support to the compensation hypothesis. Kirkpatrick's writings on attachment and religion have provided a rich source of ideas for empirical investigation and can be integrated with results from both CSR and object relations theory. For example, it has been suggested that attachment theory has relevance for understanding conceptualizations of God, religious behaviors such as prayer and glossolalia (speaking in tongues), and links between religious experience and romantic love (Kirkpatrick, 1992, 1994, 1997; Kirkpatrick & Shaver, 1992). However, it is also true that attachment theory has been criticized as a theory biased toward Western values and meaning (Rothbaum, Weisz, Pott, Miyake, & Morelli, 2000).

RESEARCH BOX 4.2. Attachment Theory and Religion
(Kirkpatrick & Shaver, 1990)

In this investigation, Kirkpatrick and Shaver tested the compensation and the mental model hypotheses (see text) with respect to links between childhood attachment to parents and adult religiousness. Data were collected from two surveys—one involving 670 respondents to a questionnaire in a Sunday newspaper, and the other including a subsample of 213 of these same people who agreed to participate in a further study. Various measures were used to tap aspects of religiousness, including the Allport and Ross (1967) scales for assessing Intrinsic and Extrinsic religious orientation (see Chapter 2). Child–parent attachment was measured in a standard way, which placed respondents into one of three categories (percentages in parentheses are from Kirkpatrick and Shaver's study): secure (51%), avoidant (8%), and anxious/ambivalent (41%).

Attachment did indeed serve as a predictor of religiousness, but in a somewhat complicated way. There was a tendency for those from avoidant parent–child attachment relationships to report higher levels of adult religiousness, and also for persons with secure attachments to report lower levels of religiousness, but only for respondents whose mothers were relatively nonreligious. The attachment classification apparently had a more direct relationship with reported sudden conversion experiences: Anxious/ambivalent respondents were much more likely to report such conversions at some time in their lives (44%) than were respondents from the other attachment groups (fewer than 10%). Home religiosity did not affect this relationship.

This study relied on adults' retrospective reports of earlier attachment and family religiousness, so memory and other biases may have affected responses. The authors pointed out that their investigation was very much an exploratory study of attachment–religion relationships. However, their initial findings are provocative and tend to support the compensation hypothesis (though only for people from relatively nonreligious homes in this study); they generally contradict the mental model hypothesis (i.e., that religiousness may be modeled after early attachment relationships). The reasons for this are not clear and call for further investigation.

Nevertheless, subsequent research has confirmed the utility of attachment theory for understanding the role of God or gods, at least within Western countries. These findings may be especially helpful when they are integrated with findings from other compatible orientations, such as object relations theory and CSR. For instance, Eshleman, Dickie, Merasco, Shepard, and Johnson (1999) interviewed 4- to 10-year-old children, and also surveyed their parents. Eshleman et al. concluded that their findings supported Kirkpatrick and Shaver's (1990) attachment theory model. For example, as children moved from early to middle childhood, their distance from parents increased as perceived closeness to God increased, just as attachment theory would predict. As a sidelight, these researchers also found that "perceiving God as male may distance God for girls and women" (p. 146). Dickie et al. (1997) also found evidence that seems to support attachment theory predictions; they concluded that "God becomes the 'perfect attachment substitute'" (p. 42) as children become more independent of parents.

Richert and Granqvist (2013, p. 167) have emphasized that God has a very special developmental standing, insofar that as a transitional object God is taken seriously by adults, and for the faithful is not an object to be abandoned. Rizzuto (1979), working from an object relations perspective, argues that by the end of early childhood most American children develop a God representation that is unlikely to be abandoned. This "living" God is associated with a safe haven. Research on children in other countries suggest that Finnish children report feeling close to God when lonely or in an emergency (Tamminen, 1994). Thus, as a safe haven, God is a readily available attachment figure. This fact has been supported by quasi-experimental research using symbolic God representations with not only American children (Eshleman et al., 1999), but also with Swedish (Granqvist, Ljungdahl, & Dickie, 2007) and Italian (Cassiba, Granqvist, & Constantini, 2013) children.

Granqvist and Hagekull (1999) found that retrospective accounts of attachment to parents suggested a positive association between security of attachment and socialization-based religiosity. Thus two major empirically supported hypotheses on attachment security and religiosity have emerged. One is Kirkpatrick and Shaver's (1990) "compensatory hypothesis," mentioned above, in which an insecure attachment history is linked to a greater need to establish compensatory relationships to regulate distress and obtain felt security. The other is the "correspondence hypothesis," in which a secure attachment history is linked to successful socialization. In a religious home, such successful socialization predicts an acceptance of a positively imaged God supported by specific religious beliefs (see Granqvist, Ljungdahl, & Dickie, 2007; Granqvist & Kirkpatrick, 2008).

In keeping with the new paradigm for the psychology of religion in general, dialogue between psychodynamic psychologies and mainstream psychology is desirable (Corveleyn & Luyten, 2005). Despite efforts to differentiate object relations theory clearly from attachment theory (Granqvist, 2006a, 2006b), their roots are intertwined (Rizzuto, 2006; Wulff, 2006). Luyten and Corveleyn (2007) have persuasively made the case for the reciprocal exploration of the findings of object relations and attachment theorists. Much of the distancing is due to philosophical differences in appropriate methodologies, which are no longer defensible. In the spirit of the new paradigm, multiple levels and interdisciplinary cooperation are required if our understanding of religion and spirituality is to be advanced. What attachment theory lacks in rich phenomenological description is balanced by its focus upon measurement. However, measurement must not trump description if we are to fully understand children's images and concepts of God. Roehlkepartain, Benson, King, and Wagener (2006) have argued that "the contrast between the call for deep, multidimensional theoretical frameworks and the 'shallow' measures often used in this domain represents one of the major challenges for the future of research in child and adolescent spiritual development" (p. 9).

SOCIALIZATION THEORY

Boyatzis (2005) has taken the lead in arguing for a clearer understanding of how socialization influences religious and spiritual development in children. Furthermore, he has noted the complexity of what actually is involved in the family mechanisms of socialization. Although generalizations such as "Religious families tend to produce religious children" remain true, they offer little insight as to *why* they are true. For instance, it is clear that even young children are not simply passive accepters of parental views. To take a secular example, Prentice, Manosevitz, and Hubbs (1978) showed that even among children whose parents taught them to believe in the Easter Bunny, almost one-fourth did not believe. Okagaki and Bevis (1999) have shown that parents' beliefs are not as important as children's perceptions of what their parents believe. Likewise, efforts to suggest that children naturally harbor anthropomorphic tendencies that can account for both their religious thinking and experience are balanced by studies showing that children recognize that God is *unique* and must be understood in *non*anthromorphic terms (Barrett & Richard, 2003). Boyatzis (2005, pp. 134–135) has provided effective critiques of studies in which children are asked to draw pictures of God, and then researchers interpret this as indicating anthropomorphic thinking! Heller (1986) has shown that Hindu children have complex views of God, attributing both personal and impersonal characteristics to God. Finally, Evans (2000) has shown that even children not raised with religious creationist beliefs tend to favor creationist views.

Thus, in contrast to anthropomorphic views derived from evolutionary models of general cognitive development (discussed in Chapters 3 and 10), socialization-oriented theorists favor a "preparedness" model in which children are assumed to have a natural tendency to be prepared to accept religious ideas. As noted above, this is consistent with many CSR studies. However, socialization theory notes that this natural tendency is enhanced when parents and others reinforce this with explicit religious instruction. Here religion, as an explicit system of beliefs, is grafted onto a spiritual awareness natural to children (Barrett, 2012; Nye, 1999). Quantitative longitudinal research has shown that as children mature, they tend to adopt the religious values of their parents (Wink, Ciciolla, Dillon, & Tracy, 2007). Qualitative research indicates that whether or not spirituality is religiously framed, children are naturally spiritual beings, insofar as they have a sense of interconnectedness with something larger than themselves (Coles, 1990; Hay & Nye, 1998; Reimer & Furrow, 2001). This has given rise to the "spiritual child" movement, largely spearheaded by Miller (2015). Boyatzis (2012, p. 153) summarizes several assumptions that undergird this movement: (1) Children are naturally spiritual beings; (2) children are socialized in ways that are supportive or not of their intuitive spirituality; and (3) spirituality is socially expressed in shared rituals and creeds associated with faith traditions. From these assumptions, it follows that attention not only to socialization practices, but also to parenting style, is essential.

Parenting Style

There is general agreement among developmental psychologists that parenting practices have important implications for child development (Darling & Steinberg, 1993). However, in spite of the likelihood that parental religious orientation influences parenting style (see Luft & Sorell, 1987), there has been little research relating parenting approaches, religion, and child development. A few early studies (e.g., Bateman & Jensen, 1958; Nunn, 1964) suggested the potential of such links. Subsequent theoretical and empirical work on parenting styles has provided new avenues for exploring the relationship between parenting and child religious development.

Baumrind (1967, 1991) has suggested that there exist four very different styles of parenting, based on parental responsiveness and demandingness: "authoritarian," "authoritative," "permissive," and "rejecting/neglecting." Authoritarian parents are high on demandingness but low on responsiveness, preferring to impose rules on their children and emphasize obedience. Authoritative parents tend to be both demanding and responsive, explaining why rules are necessary, and being open to their children's perspectives. Permissive parents make few demands, use little punishment, and are responsive to the point of submitting to their children's wishes. Rejecting/neglecting parents are neither demanding nor responsive, being generally disengaged from their children.

Correlational and longitudinal research has suggested that the authoritative style of parenting may have benefits for children's development, whereas the authoritarian and rejecting/neglecting styles may have some negative implications (Buri, Louiselle, Misukanis, & Mueller, 1988; Rohner, 1994). Other research suggests that parental emphasis on obedience is related to "cognitive accomplishment" (Holden & Edwards, 1989) and to personality development (e.g., right-wing authoritarianism; Altemeyer, 1988). There is also tentative evidence that permissive parenting is associated with an Extrinsic religious orientation, and that authoritative parenting may be related to an Intrinsic religious orientation among adolescent offspring (Giesbrecht, 1995) and to greater religiosity among parents (Linder Gunnoe, Hetherington, & Reiss, 1999). (See Chapter 2 for an explanation of the Intrinsic and Extrinsic orientations.)

The authoritarian parenting style bears some similarity to Biblical injunctions to emphasize obedience among children, and not to "spare the rod." Zern (1987) has argued that from a religious perspective, obedience is a preferred trait. In fact, research by Ellison and Sherkat (1993) has revealed that conservative Protestants (and, to a lesser extent, Catholics) tend to endorse an authoritarian parenting orientation, valuing obedience in children. Religion has also been linked with parental disciplinary practices (Kelley, Power, & Wimbush, 1992)—including a preference, among more conservative groups and those who subscribe to a literal belief in the Bible, for the use of corporal punishment (Ellison, Bartkowski, & Segal, 1996; Gershoff, Miller, & Holden, 1999; Grasmick, Morgan, & Kennedy, 1992; Mahoney, Pargament, Tarakeshwar, & Swank, 2001; Wiehe, 1990). Similarly, religiousness has been linked with emphasis on obedience to cultural norms generally (Zern, 1984).

As described in Research Box 4.3, Danso, Hunsberger, and Pratt (1997) found evidence that more fundamentalist university students (Study 1) and parents (Study 2) were more likely to condone the use of corporal punishment and to value obedience (rather than autonomy) in child rearing. However, mediation analyses suggested that the greater desire of fundamentalists to socialize their children to accept the (parental) religious faith was linked more closely to right-wing authoritarianism than to religious fundamentalism per se. One wonders, then, whether conservative religious groups (or religious fundamentalists more generally) might be inclined to use an authoritarian parenting style, with consequent implications for their children. Also, what role does right-wing authoritarianism as a parental personality trait play in such a relationship?

RESEARCH BOX 4.3. The Role of Parental Religious Fundamentalism and Right-Wing Authoritarianism in Child-Rearing Goals and Practices (Danso, Hunsberger, & Pratt, 1997)

These authors concluded that previous research had established links between stronger parental religiosity and a greater parental emphasis on obedience for their children, and also more positive attitudes toward corporal punishment (e.g., spanking) in child rearing. It was further hypothesized that parents' desire to raise their children to accept the family religion ("faith keeping") would have an influence on the goals that they set for their children. More fundamentalist parents were expected to place greater value on faith keeping, to emphasize obedience for children more strongly, and also to be more likely to condone the use of corporal punishment in child rearing. But beyond this, the authors explored how these factors were linked—suspecting, for example, that right-wing authoritarianism would mediate the relationship between religious orientation and child-rearing attitudes.

Two studies were carried out; the first involved 204 university students, and the second 154 mothers and fathers of university students. Measures included Faith Keeping, Attitudes toward Corporal Punishment, Autonomy, and Obedience scales developed for the research, as well as Religious Fundamentalism and Right-Wing Authoritarianism measures (the last scale was administered in Study 2 only). The university students were asked to respond to parenting items by imagining that they had children of their own. The parents were asked about their actual child-rearing attitudes when their (university student) children were between 7 and 12 years old.

The results of both studies indicated that religious fundamentalism was positively correlated with greater valuation of obedience, stronger endorsement of corporal punishment in child rearing, and the importance of socializing children to accept their parents' faith. Fundamentalism was also linked with weaker valuation of autonomy in one's children. In both studies, it appeared that faith keeping seemed to play a mediating role between fundamentalism and obedience attitudes. That is, more fundamentalist parents' child-rearing attitudes (e.g., increased emphasis on obedience, endorsement of corporal punishment) seemed to be a result of their stronger desire to have their children uphold the family's religious faith.

However, the addition of the Right-Wing Authoritarianism scale in Study 2 indicated that it was actually a more powerful mediating variable in these relationships than was faith keeping. That is, the fact that religious fundamentalism was strongly positively correlated with right-wing authoritarian attitudes "explained" the links between fundamentalism and child-rearing attitudes (e.g., the tendency to emphasize obedience, and condone the use of corporal punishment). The authors suggested that future researchers should consider the role of parental personality variables such as authoritarianism in studies of religion and child rearing.

The limitations of this research include the facts that university students were simply speculating about what their child-rearing attitudes would be *if* they had children (Study 1), and that parents had to reflect back 5–10 years to recall what their child-rearing attitudes had been at that time (Study 2). We do not know the extent to which such speculations and memories are accurate. Also, the authors do not discuss the "chicken and egg" problem of whether fundamentalism or authoritarianism comes first, or whether they may be causally related.

Darling and Steinberg (1993) have suggested that parenting *goals and values* should be distinguished from parenting *styles and practices*. In light of the discussion above, it seems apparent that religious orientation is likely to have some impact on parenting goals and values. Certainly, some conservative Christian books on child rearing emphasize the importance of authoritarian-like goals for parents—for example, by explicitly advising parents that raising obedient children is an important goal (Fugate, 1980; Meier, 1977). Such goals in turn are likely to influence both general parenting style as delineated by Baumrind, and specific parenting practices such as the use of corporal punishment to teach obedience (e.g., Danso et al., 1997). The role of religion in this process might even help to explain variations in the prevalence of different parenting styles in North American ethnic groups (Steinberg, Lamborn, Dornbusch, & Darling, 1992).

Parenting goals and practices can have important real-world implications beyond their direct effects for the children themselves. For example, in Aylmer, Ontario, Canada, seven children whose family belonged to a conservative religious group were taken from their parents by child welfare authorities (Saunders, 2001). The parents reportedly sometimes disciplined their children by hitting them with a rod or strap. When the authorities met with the parents, the parents justified their disciplinary methods by reference to their literal belief in the Bible, and they refused to assure the authorities that this practice would stop. The children were eventually returned to the family when the parents reportedly provided some assurance that they would not use certain types of physical punishment to discipline the children. However, the broader issues of the legality of such religiously based justification for corporal punishment, and of whether or not authorities should remove such children from their homes, have yet to be resolved.

It is important to note that the research and ideas discussed above involve conservative or fundamentalist religion groups and measures, and that the hypothesized relationships between conservative/fundamentalist religion and authoritarian parenting style may not hold for more general measures of religiousness. For example, Linder Gunnoe et al. (1999) did *not* find a positive link between authoritarian parenting style and a measure of the extent to which parents' religious beliefs played a role in their daily lives. Furthermore, Wilcox (1998) found that the strict discipline characteristic of conservative Protestant religious parents is tempered by the finding that conservative parents are also *more* likely to praise and hug their children. Wilcox has therefore argued that parents who hold theologically conservative beliefs may show aspects of *both* authoritarian and authoritative parenting styles. This possibility, as well as its implications for child and adolescent development, needs further investigation.

Other Aspects of Parenting

Religion may play more subtle roles in child rearing as well. Carlson, Taylor, and Levin (1998) found that the ways in which children use pretend play can differ across religious groups, even for different varieties of Mennonites. Ojha and Pramanick (1992) studied mothers in India and found that Hindu mothers began weaning and toilet-training their children earlier than did Christian mothers, on average, who in turn did so earlier than Muslim mothers. Of the three religious groups, Christian mothers were the most restrictive toward their children. The role of religion in these aspects of parenting and child rearing (and consequences for child development) has received little empirical attention to date.

Parenting techniques have been linked with religion in a somewhat different context. Nunn (1964) suggested that some parents invoke the image of a punishing God in an attempt to control their children's behavior. He hypothesized that relatively ineffective, powerless parents would be inclined to use God in an attempt to gain some semblance of power, telling their children such things as "God will punish you if you misbehave." Nunn's data supported this view of parents who formed a "coalition with God," and also suggested that this "God will punish you" approach had negative consequences for the children, who were reportedly more inclined to blame themselves for problems and to feel that they should be obedient.

Nelsen and Kroliczak (1984) have pointed out that there has been a general decline in people's belief in a punishing God, and that this decline is at least partly attributable "to parents being less likely to use coalitions with God. Hence, fewer children form this image" (p. 269). Nelsen and Kroliczak examined data from over 3,000 children in Minnesota elementary schools in an attempt to replicate Nunn's findings. They found a decreased tendency of parents to resort to the "God will punish you" approach (73% of respondents said that neither parent in a family employed this approach, compared to Nunn's 33%). But the children whose parents tended to use the "coalition" also tended to view God as malevolent, to have higher self-blame scores, and to feel a greater need to be obedient. Essentially, Nelsen and Kroliczak replicated Nunn's findings some 20 years later.

These studies have implications for the development of God images, but they also suggest that parents' approach to discipline may be important for children's religiosity, as well as for more general child development (e.g., tendencies toward self-blame and obedience). There may also be noteworthy ramifications for how parents deal with other child-rearing issues, such as illness. For example, research has indicated that parents who believe more strongly in divine influence are more likely to seek spiritual guidance in coping with (hypothetical) child illnesses (De Vellis, De Vellis, & Spilsbury, 1988). All of these findings are consistent with the suggestion that parenting goals, styles, and practices may have significant links with religious orientation.

Much of the research described above has assessed the extent to which parenting affects religion in one's children. We should not forget that religion can also affect parenting and parent–child relationships (e.g., Pearce & Axinn, 1998). There is also evidence that parenting can itself contribute to religious change in fathers (Palkovitz & Palm, 1998).

Child Abuse and Religion

Since the early 1990s, there has been increasing interest in possible links between religion and child abuse (e.g., Bottoms, Shaver, Goodman, & Qin, 1995; Capps, 1992; Greven, 1991). As we have noted earlier, evidence suggests that a conservative and fundamentalist religious orientation is linked with a tendency to condone the use of physical punishment in child rearing (e.g., Ellison et al., 1996). Greven (1991) has argued that the inclination of some religious groups and individuals to legitimize and promote the use of corporal punishment in child rearing can effectively condone child abuse. Whether or not this is true, abuse can apparently have implications for religiosity. Rossetti (1995) found, not surprisingly, that people who were sexually abused as children by Roman Catholic priests expressed less trust in the priesthood, in the Catholic Church, and in a relationship to God (see Chapter 12 regarding sexual abuse perpetrated by clergy). Similarly, others found that childhood sexual abuse more generally was associated with lower levels of religiosity (Doxey, Jensen, & Jensen, 1997; Hall, 1995; Stout-Miller, Miller, & Langenbrunner, 1997) or a more negative view of God (Kane, Cheston, & Greer, 1993).

However, some researchers have concluded that those who were sexually abused as children may turn to religion for support (Reinert & Smith, 1997), or at least may show some evidence of increased religious behavior, such as prayer (Lawson, Drebing, Berg, Vincellette, & Penk, 1998). Possibly such increased religiousness acts as a form of compensation, as discussed above in the context of attachment theory. Others (Gange-Fling, Veach, Kuang, & Hong, 2000) found that a group of individuals in psychotherapy for childhood sexual abuse did not differ in spiritual functioning from a group of people in psychotherapy for other reasons. However, both of these groups scored lower on spiritual well-being than people not in psychotherapy did.

In view of the apparently conflicting results of studies in this area, more research is needed. Possibly there are gender differences in response to abuse, and factors such as the religious environment before and after the abuse need to be taken into account, as well as the type, perpetrator, and context of the abuse.

Future Directions for Socialization Theory

Socialization theory is still in its infancy, insofar as psychologists seek to understand the actual dynamics of parent–child interaction. Heller (1986) has noted that parents are the primary interpreters of religious beliefs to their children. However, this is not a one-way street: Boyatzis and Janicki (2003) have focused on the bilateral and dynamic interaction between parents and children. The movement is clearly toward more specific empirical studies of the complex dynamics of religious and spiritual socialization, and away from stage-based theories (Boyatzis, 2006). Similar movement is evident in research focused on children's concepts and images of God.

CONCEPTS AND IMAGES OF GOD

When children think of God, what sort of an image forms in their minds? Many studies of religion in childhood have focused specifically on this issue. Some of this research was based on psychodynamic and object relations theories about the development of an image of God. For example, Freud (1913/1919, 1927/1961b) interpreted the God image as a father figure, a kind of projection of one's real father in the context of the resolution of the Oedipus complex. Jung (1948/1969) apparently agreed that there is some projection of one's earthly father into one's God image, but he felt that "archetypes" (images/symbols with biological roots, found in many cultures) also play a role in concepts of God. Although such analytic theories of the origins and development of a God image are difficult to test directly, they suggest that there should be a firm link between how children see their real fathers and their images of God. Object relations theorists have also explored the role of father figures in images of God (Rizzuto, 1982). What does the empirical research show?

Parent and Gender Issues

Empirical research has confirmed that God images are typically male-dominated in Western culture (Foster & Keating, 1992), possibly more so for girls than for boys (Ladd, McIntosh, & Spilka, 1998). But empirical support for the prediction that God images should be related to children's views of their own fathers has been mixed (Rizzuto, 1979, 1982; Spilka, Addison, &

Rosensohn, 1975). Vergote and Tamayo (1981) suggested that the God image may actually bear more similarity to the mother than to the father, and Roberts (1989) found a correspondence between images of God and images of self. There is also evidence that general qualitative aspects of relationships with parents may be related to positive (e.g., warm, loving) images of God (Godin & Hallez, 1964; Potvin, 1977).

Krejci's (1998) investigation of college students led him to conclude that God images were organized around three dimensions: "nurturing–judging," "controlling–saving," and "concrete–abstract." He found few gender differences, with the exception that control was more salient in men's God images. More gender differences appeared in another study (Dickie et al., 1997), which emphasized the importance of parents in affecting children's God images, both directly and indirectly. Dickie et al.'s results suggested that girls' God concepts were more closely related to attributes and discipline styles of parents than were boys' God concepts. Hertel and Donahue (1995) examined more than 3,400 mother–father–youth triads from data obtained through the Search Institute in the United States in 1982–1983. The young people in this study were in fifth through ninth grades. Results showed that although the relationships were not large, there were significant tendencies for parents' images of God to be reflected in young people's impressions of parenting styles. In particular, fathers' and mothers' loving God images both apparently affected children's images of their fathers and mothers as loving, respectively. In turn, parenting styles and parents' God images predicted youths' God images. These relationships remained even after social class, religious denomination, church attendance, and youths' ages were controlled for. Hertel and Donahue also concluded that there was a strong tendency for their participants to perceive God as love ("maternal") rather than as authority ("paternal"), and that mothers played a more important role in socializing their children's God images, especially for daughters.

At least one study has found evidence that teachers may be more important than parents in God concept development. De Roos, Miedema, and Iedema (2001) found that kindergarten children who evidenced a close relationship with their teachers also tended to display a loving God concept, whereas the mother–child relationship did not make a significant prediction in this regard.

In general, the literature on children's God images seems reasonably consistent in confirming the importance of parents in the development of these concepts. There is less agreement about gender differences in God images, the actual nature of those images (e.g., loving vs. authoritarian), and the relative impact of mothers and fathers in contributing to the development of God concepts (Rizzuto, 1982). However, what is clear is that insofar as teleological thought is integral to religion, its emergence is not simply a WEIRD phenomenon. For instance, Gelman, Mannheim, Escalante, and Tapia (2015) have documented that in a rural Quechua-speaking community in Peru, teleological talk between parents and children was found to be "surprisingly salient" (p. 372). A safe conclusion from a considerable body of emerging research is that teleological talk is an integral part of socialization and is not restricted to the modernized Western world.

Does a God Concept Develop in Stages?

Attempts to understand the developmental aspects of God concepts have typically focused on cognitive development. Some of these approaches are clearly Piagetian in orientation, whereas others have a more general cognitive focus. This area has benefited from research carried out in several different Western countries.

Harms (1944) suggested that previous investigations of children's images of God had erred by asking children to respond to fixed questions. Instead, he asked more than 4,800 U.S. children (ages 3–18) both to talk about and to draw their representations of religion, especially God. Their responses led Harms to conclude that there are three stages in the development of God concepts:

1. *Fairy-tale stage* (3–6 years). Children see little difference between God and fairy-tale characters.
2. *Realistic stage* (6–11 years). As children's cognitive capacities begin to expand, they see God as more concrete and more human. They are more comfortable using religious symbols.
3. *Individualistic stage* (adolescence). Adolescents no longer rely exclusively on religious symbols. They take a more individualized approach to God, resulting in very different conceptualizations from person to person.

Another major study of the development of God concepts was undertaken by Deconchy (1965) in France, though he did not include children under 7 years of age. He concluded that the development of God concepts occurs in three stages, revolving around themes of attribution, personalization and interiorization, respectively; these are described in Research Box 4.4.

There have been variations on these themes, but different authors describe similar stages in the development of God concepts (Ballard & Fleck, 1975; Fowler, 1981; Nye & Carlson, 1984; Williams, 1971), including some based on a Piagetian framework (Elkind, 1970; Goldman, 1964; Nye & Carlson, 1984). Others have simply noted the general change from fragmented, undifferentiated thinking through very simple, concrete God concepts to more abstract and complex images as children grow older (see, e.g., the review of European research on this topic by Tamminen et al., 1988). Attempts to further specify the parameters

---

RESEARCH BOX 4.4. The Idea of God: Its Emergence between 7 and 16 Years (Deconchy, 1965)

In this investigation, Catholic children and adolescents were asked to free-associate when they heard words such as "God." An analysis of their responses led Deconchy to conclude that these children exhibited three major stages in the development of God concepts. Those from about 7 or 8 to 11 years of age used predominantly "attributive" themes; that is, God was seen as a set of attributes, many anthropomorphic with overtones of animism. God concepts were relatively independent of other religious constructs, such as the historical events in the life of Jesus. The associations of children between 11 and 14 years of age emphasized "personalization" themes, such that God took on parental characteristics and was seen in more sophisticated anthropomorphic terms (e.g., "just," "strong," "good"). Finally, by approximately the age of 14 a further shift began to take place, focusing on "interiorization" themes. That is, in middle adolescence anthropomorphic characteristics of God disappeared, and God concepts became more abstract and tended to reflect relationships with God (e.g., involving love, trust) emanating from within the individual, rather than simply involving descriptive characteristics.

of such development, and the processes through which this unfolding occurs, have not been particularly successful (Ladd et al., 1998). For example, Janssen, de Hart, and Gerardts (1994) used open-ended questions about God in a study of Dutch secondary school students. They concluded that perceptions of God among their participants were complex and "can hardly be summarized" (p. 116). However, more recent research from the CSR perspective has shown that children's concept of God more resembles the implicit (intuitive, System 1) rather than the explicit (reflective, System 2) views of their parents (Heiphetz et al., 2016). Furthermore, the development of an omniscient God concept occurs only *after* children learn to distinguish the fallible minds they and their parents share from the radically different mind of God. In sum, considerable CSR research indicates that concepts shared with parents closely mirror each stage of development in children's mentalizing abilities (Heiphetz et al., 2016, pp. 129–131).

Variation in Concepts of God

Does the development of God concepts vary across cultures or different religious groups? Vergote and Tamayo (1981) found that although there are commonalities in God images across cultures, at least some cultural differences do emerge with respect to maternal and paternal symbolism. Ladd et al. (1998) found that God concepts developed similarly across Christian denominations, in a manner generally consistent with Piagetian theory, in their study of almost 1,000 children from eight Christian groups in the United States. These authors have suggested that more research is necessary to understand how and why very different religious education experiences do not lead to divergent concepts of God by adolescence.

Diversity of Method and Direction

Harms's (1944) call for less constraining measures of ideas about God has not been ignored. In addition to his own early attempt to allow participants greater freedom in description of their God concepts, other researchers have used diverse techniques: pictures or drawings (Bassett et al., 1990; Graebner, 1964; Ladd et al., 1998); word associations (Deconchy, 1965); adjective ratings (Roberts, 1989; Schaefer & Gorsuch, 1992); open-ended questions (Janssen et al., 1994); letters written to God (Ludwig, Weber, & Iben, 1974); semantic differentials[2] (Benson & Spilka, 1973); Q-sorts[3] (Benson & Spilka, 1973; Nelson, 1971; Spilka, Armatas, & Nussbaum, 1964); other card-sorting tasks (Krejci, 1998); standardized scales (Gorsuch, 1968); combination techniques such as "concept mapping" (Kunkel, Cook, Meshel, Daughtry, & Hauenstein, 1999); and sentence completions, essays, and "projective photographs" (Tamminen, 1991). There has been some interest in comparing the utility of the different approaches. One study (Hutsebaut & Verhoeven, 1995) concluded that closed-ended questions concerning God offered slight advantages over open-ended questions, but the participants in that research were university students. Comparative studies involving children are needed.

The measures used can apparently influence research findings. Tamminen's (1991) extensive research with Finnish children and adolescents (described earlier) involved both

---

[2]The semantic differential technique involves rating concepts on a series of bipolar adjective descriptors, such as "good ____:____:____:____:____:____:____ bad."

[3]The Q-sort technique involves having a person sort cards with words (e.g., "loving") on them into various piles according to how well they describe, for example, one's concept of God.

structured questions about God and unstructured methods, such as sentence completion and "projective photographs." His results were generally consistent with the stage approach outlined above. However, he noted that the images of God that emerged varied somewhat, depending on the measures used: "For example, God's effect on people, making them be good to each other, which was considered very important in the alternative answers chosen in the questionnaires, was not often mentioned in the fill-in sentences or essays" (Tamminen, 1991, p. 192).

The first edition of this book (Spilka, Hood, & Gorsuch, 1985) pointed out that despite the value of studies in this area, research has tended to be descriptive rather than carefully designed to test theories of cognitive development. This is less true today, as this research has become more interdisciplinary, with dialogues between advocates of classic Piagetian theory and proponents of CSR, and between attachment theorists and object relation theorists. Hyde's (1990) critique that research on children's ideas of God has been "occasional and sporadic, with no continuous theme" and "has tended to remain so, following the varied interests of those undertaking it" (p. 64) is no longer true. CSR and attachment theory have focused on the naturalness of religion, and the "spiritual child" theorists have documented the independent ontological validity of children's experience prior to explicit socialization with respect to religious creeds.

CHILDREN AND PRAYER

Children's concepts of prayer seem to develop in a manner consistent with Piaget's cognitive-developmental stages. For example, Long et al. (1967) interviewed 5- to 12-year-olds about prayer (see Research Box 4.5). The authors concluded that there was a clear tendency for these children's concepts of prayer to evolve in three stages: They moved from habits and memorized passages, through concrete personal requests, to more abstract petitions.

Other studies seem generally to be consistent with this Piagetian view of prayer development (see, e.g., the review by Finney & Malony, 1985a)—from relatively direct replication research by Worten and Dollinger (1986) to, for example, Brown's (1966) investigation of adolescents, which suggested less emphasis on the material consequences of prayer among older children. Scarlett and Perriello (1991) asked seventh- and ninth-grade Catholic school students, as well as college undergraduates, to write prayers for six hypothetical vignettes (e.g., a woman's best friend is dying of cancer). They found a shift from "using prayer to request changes in objective reality" (p. 72) among the younger students, toward prayer as a way to deal with feelings and become closer to God among the older participants. This shift is apparently consistent with the second and third stages of prayer outlined by Long et al. (1967), though at slightly older ages for the Scarlett and Perriello (1991) sample.

Tamminen (1991) also found some divergence from Long et al.'s (1967) stages in his Finnish young people. Personal conversation with God was important at younger ages (7–8 years) than Long et al. (1967) had found (9–12 years); moreover, petitionary prayer remained important up to age 20, whereas Long et al. reported decreasing importance of petitionary prayer as children grew older. Woolley (2000; Woolley & Phelps, 2001) also found that prayer and its connection to God developed years earlier (age 5) than Long et al. reported (9–10 years).

RESEARCH BOX 4.5. The Child's Conception of Prayer
(Long, Elkind, & Spilka, 1967)

In a Piagetian context, these researchers interviewed 80 girls and 80 boys ages 5–12 about prayer. They asked them open-ended questions, such as "What is a prayer?" and "Where do prayers go?", as well as giving them sentence completion tasks (e.g., "I usually pray when …"). Three judges independently analyzed the children's responses according to a scoring manual that outlined levels of differentiation and degree of concretization–abstraction. The results suggested three stages of prayer concept development:

1. At the younger ages (5–7), children responded to the questions with learned formulas based on memorized prayers.
2. Children ages 7–9 identified prayer as a set of concrete activities, with time and place defined; the purpose was also concrete, typically centered on personal requests.
3. For children between the ages of 9 and 12, prayer tended toward shared conversation rather than specific requests; prayer was also more focused on abstract goals than on material objects.

Thus, across the 5- to 12-year age range, prayer seemed to evolve from habits and memorized passages, through concrete personal requests, to more abstract petitions with humanitarian and altruistic sentiments. There was also an emotional shift noted: Praying was emotionally neutral for the younger children, but by the older ages prayer had important emotional implications (e.g., expression of empathy, as well as identification with others and the deity). All of this is quite consistent with the Piagetian conceptualization of cognitive development. The first two stages of prayer development parallel the preoperational (preconceptual substage) and concrete operational stages. Long et al.'s third stage is best characterized as transitional, giving evidence of the abstract thought characteristic of Piaget's stage of formal operations, which he felt did not begin until approximately 12 years of age.

Finally, Woolley and Phelps (2001) and Barrett, Richert, and Driesenga (2001) observed less tendency for children to anthropomorphize their concept of God than did Long et al. (1967). More research is necessary to determine the reasons for the differences across these studies. They could be attributable to culture, unique samples, method, time period of the research, and so on. For example, Woolley and Phelps (2001) pointed out that Woolley's sample came from religiously affiliated schools, compared to Long et al.'s private school sample. Also, her procedures involved new forced-choice questions and a variety of tasks, in addition to open-ended questions similar to those of Long et al.

Francis and Brown (1990, 1991) carried out investigations of influences on prayer, rather than cognitive stages in development of prayer. They found some denominational differences; for example, Church of England schools exerted a small "negative" influence on attitudes toward prayer, compared to the lack of influence in Roman Catholic schools. They also reported a shift in influence from parents (stronger among their 11-year-olds) to church (stronger among the 16-year-olds). They have interpreted their results as supporting a social learning or modeling interpretation of prayer, since prayer among children and adolescents seemed to result more from "explicit teaching or implicit example from their family and church community than as a spontaneous consequence of developmental dynamics or needs" (Francis & Brown, 1991, p. 120).

Some research has also attempted to relate prayer to (nonreligious) aspects of adjustment in children. For example, Francis and Gibbs (1996), in an investigation of 8- to 11-year-olds, found no evidence to suggest that prayer contributed to the children's self-esteem, or that low self-esteem led to prayer. Other studies have reported negative links between prayer and psychoticism scores on a personality test (Francis, 1997b; Francis & Wilcox, 1996; Smith, 1996).

Prayer has also been associated with identity status, such that private prayer was less frequent for college students with higher "moratorium" scores (an indication of searching for answers to religious and other questions, but without ideological commitment; McKinney & McKinney, 1999; see Chapter 5 for a discussion of identity status). McKinney and McKinney also found that the social identity reflected in the prayers of adolescents tended to be limited. Prayers involved family and friends, but usually did not involve the broader community.

It is surprising that more research attention has not been focused on prayer as it relates to religious development. Although there are problems in operationalizing and studying prayer (especially spontaneous personal prayer), prayer is an important religious ritual that could potentially serve as a "window" into more general religious development, as well as the meaning of faith to religious persons. Furthermore, there remain many questions about the nature and function of prayer in individual lives, as well as the nature of social and contextual factors in shaping prayer (Francis & Brown, 1991). Brown's (1994) book *The Human Side of Prayer* has initiated an exploration of some of these issues and provided an integrative review of the diverse research in this area.

Woolley (2000) has pointed out that there are "clear connections between magic and religion" (p. 118); in particular, prayer is conceptually similar to wishing, which in turn is related to magical thinking. Goldman (1964) also referred to magical thinking in the early stages of children's thought processes related to religious development. However, Woolley (2000) has also concluded that prayer is a more complicated process than wishing, since, for example, it involves an intermediary (God) between thinking and physical events. Research is needed to further explore connections between magical thinking in childhood and the emergence of religious faith and prayer.

Finally, efforts to socialize children to accept atheism as an ideology have met with only limited success (see Chapter 9). For instance, Zugger (2001) has noted that when the (then) Soviet Union occupied Poland, a heavily Catholic country, efforts were made to prove that God did not exist:

> Children were told to close their eyes and pray to God for candies and presents. When they opened their eyes nothing new was present in the room. Then they were told to close their eyes and ask the great Stalin for presents. Now when they opened their eyes, great heaps of goodies appeared on the teacher's desk. (p. 267)

However, most children saw through this deception, and the crude experimental effort to induce atheism in the children of a passionately Catholic country failed.

OTHER WORK ON RELIGION AND SPIRITUALITY IN CHILDHOOD

It is difficult to summarize the considerable literature on childhood religious development in a chapter such as this one. Up to this point, we have attempted to outline several major theoretical and empirical directions, and the resulting knowledge accumulated from many studies. We have given little attention to other theories (e.g., psychodynamic), and to the many articles that do not offer theoretical advances or that lack an empirical base (e.g., some in the religious education and pastoral counseling literatures). Furthermore, many empirical studies have not fallen neatly into the subcategories used in this chapter. Other authors (e.g., Benson, Masters, & Larson, 1997; Hyde, 1990) have summarized much of this other work. Here we offer a sampling of research directions not discussed above; broadly conceived, these fall under the rubric of the "spiritual child," in which the content and experience of children are taken seriously under the assumption that children are inherently spiritual beings (Miller, 2015; Boyatzis, 2012).

Paffard's Research

The focus on the spiritual child counters the old view that God becomes important only after childhood (Scarlett, 1994, p. 88). Certainly there is a rich description of the nature and content of children's and adolescents' self-reported "close to God" experiences in Tamminen's research (described above). His research should serve as a stimulus to other investigators to approach the topic of religious development from different perspectives—including CSR, which can be seen as not only compatible with, but also a revitalization of, a Piagetian focus on how children experience the world (Kelemen, 1999). A descriptively rich example is provided by the research of Paffard (1973), which deserves to be revisited in the light of CSR and the spiritual child movement.

Paffard was influenced by the research of Laski (1961), who identified mystical experiences among adolescents. Laski's research is discussed more fully in Chapter 11. In her interview sample, there were two girls ages 14 and 16, and one male age 10. This unwittingly opened the door to a series of studies identifying spiritual experiences among children and youths. Especially among those influenced by literary works, the poet William Wordsworth has given an implicit model of mystical experience relevant to children and adolescents. Laski (1961, p. 399) used two excerpts from Wordsworth's poetry in the literary texts she analyzed. In his autobiography, *Surprised by Joy*, C. S. Lewis (1956) extensively analyzed three boyhood experiences central to his religious development, noting that such descriptions had also been furnished by such poets as Wordsworth and could be "suffocatingly subjective" (p. viii). However, they gained ontological validity as they pointed to something "outer" and "other" (Lewis, 1956, p. 238). Paffard (1973) later titled a book that was partly based upon questionnaire responses from both British grammar school and university students *Inglorious Wordsworths*. Implicit in all these observations is a model purporting that children have an intense longing for transcendent experiences, which often are realized. Much of adult life is assumed to involve a longing for such experiences once again. Such a model can be contrasted with psychoanalytic and object relations theories, which assume mystical experiences to be regressive in a pathological sense. "Inglorious Wordsworths" have transcendent experiences that are valuable and healthy, and are capable of being recovered in adulthood.

As part of a questionnaire study, Paffard had both university students and sixth-form grammar school students in Great Britain respond to a literary description of an experience typical of Wordsworth's poetry—an experience that was specified as occurring in childhood, and one that involved consciousness of something more than a mere child's delight in nature (Paffard, 1973, p. 251). The actual text was from W. H. Hudson's (1939) autobiography *Far Away and Long Ago*. Participants were to describe in writing any experience of their own that they felt was is in any way similar to the one described in the passage. Paffard analyzed responses from 400 participants, half each from the university and grammar school samples; there were equal numbers of males and females in each sample. He found that 40% of the grammar school boys and 61% of the grammar school girls had had such experiences. In the university sample, the percentages were 56% for the men and 65% for the women (Paffard, 1973, p. 91).

Although Paffard's samples can be classified and analyzed in as many intuitive ways as Laski's, he did at least attempt some crude quantitative and statistical analyses. One quantitative effort was to have respondents check off, on a list of 14 words, those that applied to their experience. These results are presented in Table 4.3. It is interesting to note that whereas Paffard claimed, partly on the basis of his own transcendental experiences, that such experiences are part of the essence of what he termed "real" religion, his own respondents checked the two most religion-related words ("holy" and "sacred") quite infrequently. It is unlikely that the most frequently checked word ("awesome") was interpreted by the respondents in a religious sense.

Paffard found that transcendental experiences were most typical in the middle teens, under conditions of solitude. The experiences were positive, and most respondents wished to have such experiences again. However, they were less frequent in adulthood. One of the

TABLE 4.3. Endorsement of Words Characterizing Transcendental Experiences

Word	Frequency of endorsement	Percentage of subjects endorsing
Awesome	119	54
Serene	87	39
Lonely	81	37
Frightening	77	35
Mysterious	65	29
Exciting	64	29
Ecstatic	47	21
Melancholy	45	20
Sacred	39	18
Sad	33	25
Holy	28	15
Sensual	21	13
Irritating	7	3
Erotic	5	2

Note. Number of respondents = 222. Based on Paffard (1973, p. 262).

most common outcomes of the experience was some effort at creativity, although Paffard (influenced by Laski's work, as discussed in Chapter 11) specifically asked about creative acts following the experience, perhaps setting an expectation among respondents to list such activities.

Both Laski (1961) and Paffard (1973) found most mystical-type experiences discussed in Chapter 11 to be uncommon in childhood—Laski because she sampled so few children, and Paffard because his samples reported most such experiences in middle adolescence, even though the literary example he cited stated 8 years of age as the beginning of such experiences. Since in Paffard's sample sixth-form grammar school students would have tended to be age 18 and university students age 19 or above, his respondents may simply have reported their most recent experiences, hence minimizing reports of possible experiences in childhood. However, Miles (2007, pp. 16–18) reported a replication of Paffard's findings with sixth-form students, suggesting that transcendent experiences are indeed common in childhood. Likewise, Hay and Nye (1998) extensively studied small samples of children ages 6–7 years and 10–11 years. They suggest that children's spirituality is dominated by a relational consciousness that consists of "child–self," "child–God," and "child–world" consciousness.

Klingberg's Research

Klingberg (1959) sought to focus upon the study of religious experience in children, sampling only the age ranges from 9 to 13. Klingberg's study was done in Sweden in the mid-1940s, but was not published in English until 1959. Two sets of data were collected, intended to be "mutually supplementary" (Klingberg, 1959, p. 212); one of these consisted of adults' religious memories from childhood. Our concern is with compositions collected from 630 children (273 boys and 357 girls) in Sweden from 1944 to 1945. Most were 10–12 years of age. All children responded in writing to the statement "Once when I thought about God . . ." Of the 630 compositions received, 566 contained accounts of personal religious experiences (244 from boys and 322 from girls). An unspecified number of compositions contained accounts of more than one experience. Assessing the experiences for depth indicated "phenomena which call to mind the experiences of the mystic" (Klingberg, 1959, p. 213). These primarily included both apparitions of objects of religious faith, such as Jesus, God, and angels; more importantly for our interests, however, they also included a felt sense of an invisible presence. Although Klingberg recognized the facilitating role of a religious culture, school, and home in encouraging such reports among children, he claimed that the value of the study is that it shows that mystical experiences *can* take place during childhood. Klingberg argued that maturational mechanism cannot eliminate mystical experiences in children, and suggested their universality. Fahs (1950) has persuasively argued for the awakening of mystical awareness in children by avoiding narrow religious indoctrination, which might preclude a sense of wonder, curiosity, and awe. In sum, consistent with the spiritual child movement, the experience of children must be taken seriously. As Boyatzis (2012, p. 153) has noted, "during ontogenesis children's relational consciousness emerges *prior* to religious socialization."

If there is a valuable methodological lesson to be learned from the spiritual child movement, it is in the difficulty of getting children, especially at young ages, to understand and respond appropriately to questions about religion (e.g., Tamminen, 1994). This is likely an inappropriate commitment to classical Piagetian theory, in which it is assumed that children's views of religion are at a stage in which concreteness and anthropomorphism are prevalent, and that these views are at best seen as precursors to what will be theologically correct views in later stages of development. Francis and colleagues have noted tendencies for children's scores on attitudes toward religion to be positively related to "lie" scores on other scales (Francis, Pearson, & Kay, 1988), and also for children to bias their responses in a proreligious direction when a priest, as opposed to a layperson, is the test administrator (Francis, 1979). However, the methodological trick is not to confuse the language in which children try to express their experiences with the nature of the experience itself. The best conclusion seems to be that caution must be exercised in studies of children involving measurement of religion, and that appropriate checks should be included to assess possible biases or distortion of responses whenever possible.

Meaning and Implications of Religion in Childhood

We know relatively little about the meaning and implications of religion for children as they grow older, beyond the cognitive and experiential components discussed earlier in this chapter. We need to find novel ways of studying children's religious development without assuming that adult thought is the "gold standard" for comparison in this regard (see, e.g., Boyer & Walker, 2000). What impact, if any, does religion have on the day-to-day lives of children—including their physical and mental health, personal identity, and social relationships? How does childhood religion affect later religiosity, as well as nonreligious social attitudes? Does religious training affect a child's concept of death (see Florian & Kravetz, 1985; Stambrook & Parker, 1987)? What role, if any, does religion play in childhood psychopathology, and what role does (and should) religion play in the clinical treatment of children (see Wells, 1999)?

Findings suggest that a conservative or fundamentalist religious upbringing has implications for educational attainment and gender roles (see Sherkat, 2000; Sherkat & Darnell, 1999). A broad survey of children and young adolescents (fifth through ninth graders) led Forliti and Benson (1986) to conclude that religiosity was related to increased prosocial action, as well as to decreased rates of sexual intercourse, drug use, and antisocial behavior. They also concluded that a restrictive religious orientation was linked to antisocial behavior, alcohol use, racism, and sexism. These latter conclusions are not always consistent with those reached for older adolescents and adults (see Chapters 5 on socialization and 12 on morality). Also, given the moderately strong associations among right-wing authoritarianism, religious fundamentalism, and prejudice observed by Altemeyer (1988, 1996; Altemeyer & Hunsberger, 1992), it would seem appropriate to investigate the childhood antecedents of such relationships, as well as the developmental dynamics fostering such connections.

OVERVIEW

The area of religious development in childhood remains top-heavy in theory, especially stage theories of religious cognitive development and the more recent CSR. There has been a considerable amount of overlap in research that "tests" these theories, but integration remains elusive. Furthermore, there has been little or no empirical research on many issues related to childhood religious development, and some studies of religious development have little to say about *children*, having focused on older adolescents or young adults.

Theoretical conceptualizations of religious growth generally (Elkind, Goldman), and faith development in particular (Fowler, Streib), have apparently been stimulated by Piaget's formulations. And much other work on religious development (e.g., images of God, concepts of prayer) has also used the Piagetian framework as the basis for empirical studies. The results of numerous investigations have confirmed the utility of Piaget's cognitive stages for understanding various aspects of religious growth. CSR has revitalized interest in Piaget in terms of the naturalness of religion. As Bloom (2007, p. 151) notes, researchers have documented that children raised without a full-fledged language will naturally develop their own forms of expression—a phenomenon referred to by linguists as "creolization." These findings suggest that, indeed, perhaps children raised without religion will develop their own. This claim surely will guide future research, and it indicates that the spiritual child movement will frame much of the empirical research. It remains to be seen what paradigm will best illuminate religion from a developmental perspective. Currently a combination of stage theories associated with classical Piagetian thought, and cognitive–cultural approaches closely associated with evolutionary theory and CSR, seems to incorporate most of what we know about religious and spiritual development in childhood (Oser et al., 2006). Future research may be able to tease out socialized forms of religious thought from natural ones, after the manner of psycholinguistic research.

CHAPTER 5

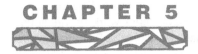

Religion in Adolescence and Young Adulthood

True love and religious experience are almost impossible before adolescence.

And further, contrary to the specific claim that Europe's secularity is exceptional, we will show that modernized societies outside Europe, such as Canada and even the US, are undergoing marked declines in religious beliefs and practices, especially among youth.

Adults appear to seriously underestimate the interest teens have in religion.

. . . doubt is not the opposite of faith; it is an element of faith.

When I was a boy of fourteen my father was so stupid I could scarcely stand to have the old man around, but by the time I got to be twenty-one I was astonished at how much he had learned in the last seven years.[1]

Early studies (Allport, Gillespie, & Young, 1948; Webster, Freedman, & Heist, 1962) of religion among college students found that the vast majority felt they needed religion in their own lives (e.g., 82% of the women and 68% of the men in the Allport et al. study), with only small percentages reporting little interest or no religious training. But these studies were carried out decades ago. Have times changed?

Some countries have apparently experienced broad-based and substantial decreases in church attendance and religious interest since about the middle of the 20th century. For example, Bibby (1987, 1993) has estimated that about 6 in 10 Canadians were weekly church attenders in the 1940s. However, this figure dropped steadily until the early 1990s, when the comparable figure was just over 2 in 10 people. This 20% rate continued to the year 2000 (Bibby, 2001) and was similar for Canada's teens and adults. Furthermore, the tendency toward decreased religious involvement has brought Canada more in line with Britain, France, Germany, the Netherlands, and the Scandinavian countries. Typically, in these European countries only about 10–15% of the population is involved in a religious group (Lippman & Keith, 2006), and regular attendance is correspondingly low (Campbell & Curtis, 1994). Francis (1989) noted a progressive trend in the 1970s and 1980s for British

---

[1]These quotes come, respectively, from the following sources: Kupky (1928, p. 70); Mason, Singleton, and Webber (2007, p. 58); Bergman (2001, p. 46); Tillich (1957, p. 116); Mark Twain (attributed).

adolescents to have less positive attitudes toward Christianity, and a general trend toward decreasing religious belief for British adults continued into the 1990s (Gill, Hadaway, & Marler, 1998). Also, religious involvement is much lower in Australia and Japan than in the United States (Campbell & Curtis, 1994).

However, religious involvement remains relatively high in the United States for both adults and adolescents, unlike the trends for many other Western countries. Though self-reported church attendance in the United States may be inflated (Chaves & Cavendish, 1994; Hadaway, Marler, & Chaves, 1993; Marcum, 1999), studies involving comparable data sources suggest that, relatively speaking, regular church attendance in the United States tends to be quite high, even when other factors are controlled for (see Campbell & Curtis, 1994). Overall, U.S. attendance rates for adults remained relatively stable up to the end of the 20th century (Chaves, 1989, 1991; Firebaugh & Harley, 1991; Inglehart & Baker, 2000). Similarly, belief in an afterlife was high (about 80%) and stable from 1973 to 1991, according to the General Social Survey data from the United States (Harley & Firebaugh, 1993).

Most research findings suggest that, in general, adolescents and young adults are less religious than middle and older adults in both North America and Europe (Dudley & Dudley, 1986; Hamberg, 1991). Moreover, religiousness is typically found to decrease during the 10- to 18-year-old period (Benson, Donahue, & Erickson, 1989), at least for adolescents in mainstream religious groups. However, such conclusions may reflect only certain measures of religiousness (e.g., involvement in institutional religion), and should not be construed to mean that adolescents are nonreligious or have little interest in spiritual matters.

In fact, a large nationwide survey of American college students conducted by the Higher Education Research Institute (HERI, 2005) at UCLA show that most college students report high levels of spirituality and espouse many spiritual and religious values (see also Astin, Astin, & Lindholm, 2011). To a considerable extent, students believe in the sacredness of life (83%), have an interest in spirituality (80%), search for meaning or purpose in life (76%), have discussions about the meaning of life with friends (74%), find spirituality as a source of joy (64%), and seek out opportunities to grow spiritually (47%). Also, they report believing in God (79%); pray (69%) and at least occasionally attend religious services (81%); discuss religious or spiritual matters with friends (80%) or family members (76%); and at least somewhat agree that their religious beliefs provide strength, support, and guidance (69%). Similar findings are reported by Smith and Denton (2005), based on data from the National Study of Youth and Religion: Adolescents in the United States believe in God (84%), believe that God is a personal being (65%), feel at least somewhat close to God (71%), and claim that their religious faith is at least somewhat important in shaping major decisions (80%).

The HERI has also conducted an annual survey of American college freshmen since the late 1960s. This survey found that in the 20 years from the early 1980s to the early 2000s, the percentage of those reporting no religious preference (vs. some other sort of religious identity) doubled from 8 to 16%, though during the same time period the percentage identifying themselves as born-again remained consistent at about 25% (as reported in Levenson, Aldwin, & D'Mello, 2005). Smith, Lundquist Denton, Faris, and Regnerus (2002) provided a broad picture of the religious participation of U.S. adolescents, based on data from three separate major national survey organizations. Longitudinal data indicate that between 1976 and 1996, weekly religious service attendance for 12th graders decreased by about 8% (from approximately 40% to 32%) and those "never" or "rarely" attending grew by about 4%. Just 44% of 12th graders reported being involved in religious youth group activities sometime during their 4 years in high school. Still, 85% of the 13- to 18-year-olds surveyed reported some kind of religious affiliation, with over two-thirds identifying themselves as Protestant (44%) or Catholic (25%). More females than males were religiously affiliated, and African American youths reported higher levels of church attendance than either European Americans or Hispanic Americans did.

The few studies to date of those who consider themselves "spiritual but not religious" have often been conducted by comparing them with those who self-identify as "spiritual and religious." Though much of the discussion has focused on critical antecedents of the "spiritual but not religious" development—most notably the "baby boomer" tendency to value individual conscience over institutional authority (Roof, 1993, 1999)—we are just beginning to get a handle on what these spiritual "seekers" are like (see Shahabi et al., 2002; Zinnbauer et al., 1997). Shahabi and her associates found that the seekers they studied were younger, better educated, less likely to be married, more likely to be white (vs. members of racial minority groups), and less likely to live in the South. Zhai, Ellison, Stokes, and Glenn (2008) found that the "spiritual but not religious" were more likely to be offspring of divorced parents (62%), possibly because divorce may interrupt the transmission of religious values from parents to children, may disrupt institutional religious practices (see Lawton & Bures, 2001), or may reduce the degree of supervision of children—all of which may contribute to the fact that children of divorced parents, compared to those raised in intact two-parent families, are less likely to adopt parental religious values and practices (Regnerus, Smith, & Smith, 2004).

It is not clear why adults and adolescents in the United States report much higher rates of interest and practice in religion and spirituality than do people in other countries. Perhaps it is the successful tendency for U.S. religious groups to "service the spiritual needs of Americans" (Bibby, 1993, p. 113), thus providing people with "social capital" that helps foster positive developmental outcomes through the religious context. Research by King, Furrow, and Roth (2002) on 413 high school students found that family and peers provide such capital. Perhaps in the United States disaffiliation is not simply indicative of a shift in religiousness; rather, disaffiliation is also symbolic in an important way, representing "a deep shift in outlook and lifestyles" (Hadaway & Roof, 1988, p. 31). Whatever the reason, it seems fair to conclude that "religious beliefs are an important aspect of adolescents' lives" (Cobb, 2001, p. 495) in the United States, and also that religion has a powerful impact on adolescents and their development (Benson et al., 1989).

INFLUENCES ON RELIGIOUSNESS AND SPIRITUALITY IN ADOLESCENCE

Many external influences have the potential to affect people's religiousness: parents, peers, schools, religious institutions, books, the mass media, and so on. Oman and Thoresen (2003, 2007) have argued that there has been no systematic framework for investigating how religiousness or spirituality is "caught" from the influence of others. They propose that Bandura's (1977, 1986) theory of social learning, with its emphasis on observation and vicarious learning, is capable of providing such a framework for the psychology of religion. Spiritual models, they suggest, whether they be major historical religious figures (e.g., Buddha, Muhammad, Jesus), contemporary spiritual leaders (e.g., Mother Teresa, Gandhi), or key individuals in a person's life (e.g., youth pastors, religious mentors), are overlooked influences on spiritual and religious development (see also Bandura, 2003, and Silberman, 2003).

External influences (parents, peers, etc.) affect individuals directly through, for example, explicit religious teachings or family practices. They can also affect people indirectly in many ways—for example, by influencing school, marital, and career choices, or through cultural assumptions, subtle modeling, or lack of exposure to alternative positions. People may be conscious of some religious socialization influences, but quite unaware of others. Cornwall (1988) has noted that the literature on religious socialization has traditionally focused on three "agents" of socialization: parents, peers, and church. We examine each of these in turn, along with a fourth factor that has been studied: education. Though we have already said much in Chapter 4 about the influence of parents, here we further consider their role as influence agents specifically in terms of adolescent religious and spiritual development, since there is general agreement that parents are the most important influence (e.g., Benson, Masters, & Larson, 1997; Brown, 1987; Cornwall, 1989). We consider church (or any other religious institution) simply as one of a number of "other factors" that have been suggested to affect the religious socialization process.

Our coverage of these potential influencing factors is largely restricted to the empirical work on religious socialization. There exists a rich body of literature in the psychodynamic and object relations traditions, especially with respect to the role of parents in the socialization process. The reader may wish to consult other sources for differing perspectives on these issues (see, e.g., Coles, 1990; Rizzuto, 1979, 2001).

The Influence of Parents

It is not a straightforward matter to tap parental influence in studies of religious socialization. Many highly religious parents sanctify their role as parents; that is, they see parenting as a sacred duty, with religious beliefs and values as among the most important things to be transmitted to their children (Mahoney, Pargament, Murray-Swank, & Murray-Swank, 2003). Some investigators simply focus on "keeping the faith"—the extent to which children identify with the family religion as they grow older. These investigations typically assume that keeping the family faith must result in large part from parental influence. Other researchers focus on parent–child attitudinal agreement regarding religious and other matters, assuming that greater agreement indicates more effective parental influence. Still others rely on direct self-reports of influence, asking children or adolescents about the extent to which parents influence their religiousness. Similarly, some investigators have asked older adolescents and adults to reflect back on their lives and consider to what extent parents (and other factors) influenced their religion. Collectively, these different approaches offer insight into parental religious socialization influence.

Studies of "Keeping the Faith"

A social-cognitive model of religious change in adolescence (Ozorak, 1989; see Research Box 5.1) predicts that both social factors (such as parental or peer influence) and cognitive variables (such as intellectual aptitude and existential questioning) influence adolescent religiousness. Ozorak's (1989) data supported the social-cognitive model, especially with respect to the positive link between parental and adolescent religiousness, and she concluded that parents are especially powerful influences in the religious socialization process. However, the influence of parents seemed more prominent for high school students than for college-age respondents, suggesting that parental influence may decrease as adolescents make the transition to adulthood.

RESEARCH BOX 5.1. Influences on Religious Beliefs and Commitment
in Adolescence (Ozorak, 1989)

Elizabeth Ozorak noted that various explanations exist for adolescent change in religious beliefs and practices. For example, it has been proposed that influence from parents, peers, or others may be powerful factors; that "existential anxiety" may be an initiating factor; or (as we have seen in Chapter 4) that cognitive development can serve as the stimulus for such change. Ozorak sought to test a variety of possible effects within a social-cognitive model of religious change. She proposed that social influences, especially parents, are the most powerful factors affecting adolescent religiousness; that there is a gradual polarization of religious beliefs in the direction established relatively early in people's lives; and that such cognitive factors as "existential questioning" are associated with decreased religious commitment.

After pilot-testing her materials on 9th and 11th graders, Ozorak studied 390 high school students and high school alumni from the Boston area. The subjects included 106 students in 9th grade, 150 students in 11th or 12th grade, and 134 alumni who had graduated 3 years earlier from two of the three high schools involved. Each participant completed a questionnaire including a wide variety of items and scales tapping religious affiliation, participation, beliefs, experiences, existential questioning, social "connectedness," family and peer influences, and religious change.

The data indicated that "middle adolescence is a period of [religious] readjustment for many individuals" (p. 455), with the average age of change being about 14.5 years. Social factors, especially parents, were powerful predictors of religiousness. For example, parents' religious affiliation and participation were positively related to children's religiousness. The influence of peers (discussed later in this chapter) was not so straightforward, though the data suggested that it too was related to adolescent religiosity. Cognitive factors also played a role; more existential questioning and higher intellectual aptitude were associated with religious change, but only for the oldest age group (high school alumni). In addition, there was support for a "polarization" interpretation of the data, such that the most religious participants tended to report greater change in a proreligious direction and the least religious participants reported decreasing religiosity over time.

Ozorak concluded that "parents' affiliation and their faith in that affiliation act as cognitive anchors from which the child's beliefs evolve over time. Family cohesion seems to limit modification of religious practices but exerts less pressure on beliefs, which become increasingly individual with maturation" (p. 460). This study is important because it reminds us of the powerful influence of *both* social and cognitive factors with respect to religious socialization. Furthermore, it emphasizes the critical role of parents in influencing religiousness and religious change in their offspring.

Other studies have also indicated that parental religiousness is a good predictor of adolescents' and even adult children's religiousness. Hunsberger (1976) found that a greater emphasis on religion in one's childhood home was associated with greater religiousness during college. A survey investigation of Catholic high school seniors led to the conclusion that the three main factors predicting adolescent religiousness were perceptions of the importance of religion for the parents, positive family environment, and home religious activity (Benson, Yeager, Wood, Guerra, & Manno, 1986). A national probability sample of more than 1,000 U.S. adolescents revealed that parental religiosity was a significant predictor of adolescent religious practice (Potvin & Sloane, 1985). The religious participation of Jewish parents was a powerful predictor of the religious beliefs and practices of their adolescent children (Parker & Gaier, 1980). Such influence may even extend into adulthood; a study of college teachers indicated that their parents' church attendance constituted the best predictor of their own religiousness (Hoge & Keeter, 1976).

Similarly, numerous studies have noted a strong tendency for children raised within a specific familial religious denomination to continue identifying with that denomination from childhood through adolescence and young adulthood (e.g., Altemeyer & Hunsberger, 1997; Bibby, 2001; Hadaway, 1980; Kluegel, 1980; see also Beit-Hallahmi & Argyle, 1997; Benson et al., 1989). In general, several different parental religion variables seem to be reasonable predictors of the extent to which adolescents and young adults maintain the family religion.

Parent–Child Agreement Studies

Is there what was popularly termed in the 1960s and 1970s a "generation gap"—"a kind of organized rebellion against parents by their teenagers, one component of which supposedly involves considerable discrepancy between teenagers' attitudes and those of their parents" (Hunsberger, 1985a, p. 314)? Some researchers (e.g., Friedenberg, 1969; Thomas, 1974) have concluded that there is such a gap, while others have contended that parent–adolescent attitudinal differences are relatively minor (Lerner & Spanier, 1980) or virtually nonexistent (Coopersmith, Regan, & Dick, 1975; Nelsen, 1981a). Also, parent–child attitudinal agreement may vary from one issue to another, and religious attitudes in particular may involve more parent–child agreement than some other domains (Bengtson & Troll, 1978). For example, Hunsberger (1985a) found stronger parent–child agreement on religious matters than on a number of other issues (e.g., self-rated happiness, personal adjustment, political radicalism).

Other investigations of mother–father–adolescent triads have led to similar conclusions, though relationships are sometimes weak. A study of triads from Catholic, Baptist, and Methodist homes showed weak to moderate correspondence between parents and their offspring on religious measures (higher for mothers than for fathers), with endorsement of a specific creed revealing stronger relationships (Hoge, Petrillo, & Smith, 1982). These relationships remained significant when the effects of denomination, family income, and father's occupation were partialed out, though Hoge et al. emphasized that extrafamilial influences (e.g., denomination) were also important in religious socialization. In a study of mother–father–child triads from Seventh-Day Adventist homes, modest agreement emerged across a series of religious and nonreligious values, with generally stronger relationships between offspring and mothers than between offspring and fathers (Dudley & Dudley, 1986). Glass, Bengtson, and Dunham (1986) carried out a study of three generations of family members, the youngest generation being between the ages of 16 and 26. They concluded that there was substantial agreement on religious and political issues for *both* child–parent and parent–grandparent dyads, suggesting that parental influence in these areas may persist into adulthood.

Such findings of weak to moderately strong parent–adolescent agreement on religious issues do not "prove" that parents are important influences in their children's religious lives, of course. However, the findings of these parent–adolescent agreement studies are generally consistent with recent conceptualizations of adolescence as a time of reasonably stable development and socialization, and a time when there is considerable similarity in values and attitudes between parents and their adolescent offspring. This is in contrast to earlier conceptualizations of adolescence as a time of turmoil and rebellion, resulting in a sizeable "generation gap." This shift in views of adolescence is reflected, for example, in Petersen's (1988) review of the adolescent development literature, and in some textbooks on adolescence (e.g., Cobb, 2001).

Self-Reports of Religious Influence

Studies involving a wide variety of age groups in North America and elsewhere have confirmed that individuals perceive their parents as the most important influence on their religiosity. Hunsberger and Brown (1984) asked 878 introductory psychology students at the University of New South Wales in Sydney, Australia to identify the three people who had the greatest influence on their religious beliefs. In this study, parents were listed as having the most important influence by 44% of all respondents (friends came next at 15%). In other studies, Hunsberger asked several hundred students at a Canadian university (Hunsberger, 1983b) and 85 older Canadians (ages 65–88 years; Hunsberger, 1985b) to rate the extent of religious influence that 10 possible sources of influence had exerted in their lives. Both the students and the older persons ranked their mothers and fathers first and third, respectively. Church received the second highest ranking.

One striking thing about these two studies (Hunsberger, 1983b, 1985b) was the extent to which the students and senior citizens agreed in their rankings. Also, the senior citizens generally reported stronger absolute proreligious influence in their lives than did the students; this was consistent with findings from other cross-sectional studies (Benson, 1992a; Hunsberger, 1985a) and a panel study of Swedes (Hamberg, 1991), which all showed a general increase in religiosity across the adult years. Furthermore, the rankings for the Canadian university students were quite similar to those given by the Australian university students (Hunsberger & Brown, 1984).

Francis and Gibson (1993) explored parental influence on religious attitudes and practices of 3,414 secondary school students in Scotland (ages 11–12 and 15–16). The authors concluded that parental influence was generally important with respect to church attendance, and that there was a tendency for this influence to *increase* from the younger to the older age groups. Consistent with some of Hunsberger's (1983b, 1985a) and Acock and Bengtson's (1978, 1980; see also Dudley & Dudley, 1986) findings, they also concluded that mothers had more influence than fathers on children's religion overall, but that there was some tendency toward stronger same-sex influence for both mothers and fathers. Also, parental influence was greater for overt religiosity (i.e., church attendance) than it was for more covert religiosity (i.e., attitudes toward Christianity).

In two studies of attitudinal predispositions to pray, described in Research Box 5.2, Francis and Brown (1990, 1991) concluded that parental influence was of primary importance with respect to church attendance for adolescents attending Roman Catholic, Anglican, and nondenominational schools in England. Church attendance in turn was positively related to attitudes toward prayer. Also, as in the Francis and Gibson (1993) study, they found that mothers seemed to exert more influence than fathers, although parental influence was stronger when both parents attended church.

As noted above, some findings suggest that mothers are more influential than fathers in the religious development of their offspring; however, not all studies confirm this generalization. Kieren and Munro (1987) concluded that fathers were more influential than mothers overall. And the findings of some other studies have been equivocal in this regard (Baker-Sperry, 2001; Benson, Williams, & Johnson, 1987; Hoge & Petrillo, 1978a; Nelsen,

RESEARCH BOX 5.2. Social Influences on the Predisposition to Pray
(Francis & Brown, 1990, 1991)

These two studies focused on predispositions to pray, as well as the practice of prayer, among two age levels of English adolescents. The first investigation involved almost 5,000 students age 11, and the second about 700 students age 16; all students attended Roman Catholic, Church of England, or nondenominational state-maintained schools. As well as self-reports of their own and their parents' religious behavior, participants completed a six-item scale assessing attitudes toward prayer (e.g., "Saying my prayers helps me a lot").

Results confirmed that the parents were powerful factors with respect to children's church attendance at both age levels, though mothers consistently exerted more influence than fathers. However, there were indications that parental impact on children's prayer had decreased somewhat, and that church influences (e.g., attendance) had increased, for the 16-year-olds. Attendance at Roman Catholic or Church of England schools did not seem to affect adolescent *practice* of prayer, after other factors had been controlled for; however, there was a slightly negative impact of Church of England schools on *attitudes* toward prayer.

The authors concluded their 1991 paper by stating that their findings "support the importance of taking seriously social learning or modeling interpretations of prayer. Children and adolescents who pray seem more likely to do so as a consequence of explicit teaching or implicit example from their family and church community than as a spontaneous consequence of developmental dynamics or needs" (p. 120).

1980). But the weight of the evidence suggests that mothers are more influential than fathers (e.g., Hertel & Donahue, 1995; see also Benson et al., 1997)—perhaps because they play a more nurturing role in child rearing; perhaps because they are more religious than men (e.g., Donelson, 1999; Francis & Wilcox, 1998); or perhaps because they tend to assume more child-rearing responsibilities (Smith & Mackie, 1995), which may include taking children to church or in teaching about religion.

However, it is quite possible that fathers also play an important role (see Dollahite, 2003; King, 2003). Fathers may serve as role models for continued religiousness or for rejection of religion after initial religious socialization. Thus mothers and fathers may play somewhat different roles, and have influence in different ways or at different periods, in their children's socialization. For example, a study of more than 400 families in rural areas of Iowa found that the roles of both mothers and fathers were important in religious transmission to their offspring (Bao, Whitbeck, Hoyt, & Conger, 1999). But when adolescents perceived that their parents were generally accepting of their adolescent children, mothers' influence was reportedly stronger, especially for sons. Such subtle nuances could well contribute to seemingly contradictory conclusions in the literature concerning the relative importance of mothers and fathers in religious socialization.

Other Aspects of Parenting

A number of studies have suggested that the *quality* of young people's relationships with parents can also affect religious socialization. For example, in a panel investigation spanning the years 1965–1982, children who reported while in high school that they had a warm, close relationship with their parents were less likely to rebel against religious teachings (Wilson & Sherkat, 1994). Furthermore, longitudinal data led Wilson and Sherkat to conclude that "Lack of closeness and contact have created a religious gap between parents and children rather than religious differences creating a distant relationship" (p. 155). Others have come to similar conclusions regarding the importance of the emotional relationship between parents and adolescents (e.g., Dudley, 1978; Herzbrun, 1993; Hoge, Petrillo, & Smith, 1982; Nelsen, 1980; Okagaki & Bevis, 1999). Myers (1996) interviewed parents and their adult offspring, and concluded that the main determinants of offspring religiosity were parental religiosity, the quality of the family relationship, and traditional family structure.

Cause and effect are not always clear, however. Most authors seem to assume that higher quality of family relationships "causes" increased religiousness in offspring. Of course, if the parents are themselves nonreligious, the higher quality of family relationships may then "cause" decreased religiosity in offspring. But Brody, Stoneman, and Flor (1996) concluded that degree of parental religiousness was the causal factor in their study of 9- to 12-year-old African Americans living in the rural southern United States. That is, they maintained that greater parental religiousness contributed to a closer, more cohesive family, as well as to less conflict between the parents. Additional research is needed to address the direction of cause-and-effect relationships in this area.

Are there any specific mechanisms that parents use to instill increased religiousness in their children? Dollahite and Marks (2005), utilizing a narrative approach based on 74 interviews from highly religious Muslim, Mormon, other Christian, and Jewish families, identified 10 central processes by which parents facilitate religious and spiritual development in their families. These include relying on God for guidance and support; living one's religious values at home (including religious traditions); resolving conflict with prayer, forgiveness, and repentance; loving and serving others; overcoming challenges through shared faith; abstaining from proscribed activities and substances; self-sacrifice of time, money, and comfort for spiritual reasons; nurturing growth in family members through teaching, discussion, and example; explicit obedience to God, prophets, parents, and/or commandments; and giving priority to faith and family over secular or personal interests.

Parental Influence: Summary

All of the different approaches to studying parental influence in the religious socialization process converge on a single conclusion: Parents play an extremely important role in the developing religious attitudes and practices of their offspring. In fact, few researchers would quarrel with the conclusion that parents are *the* most important influence in this regard, though such influence can sometimes be more indirect than direct (Erickson, 1992; Cornwall, 1988; Cornwall & Thomas, 1990). For example, parents to some extent are "managers" who control which "other influences" their children are exposed to (e.g., through church attendance, selection of religious vs. secular schooling, or control of what is viewed on television), and these in turn may have some influence on young people's religion.

The Influence of Peers

Some authors have concluded that peer groups play an important role in influencing adolescents generally (Allport, 1950; Balk, 1995; Sprinthall & Collins, 1995), but relatively few studies have investigated peer influence on religiousness. Those that have done so tend to report that peer group effects are weaker than parental influences. Such studies almost always rely on self-reports of peer influence, however, and the direction of the influence (positive or negative) is not always specified.

The impacts of parents and peers were compared in a study of 375 Australian youths ages 16–18 (de Vaus, 1983). Consistent with some previous research (Bengtson & Troll, 1978), it was concluded that parents were more influential for religious beliefs, and that peers tended to have more influence outside of the religious realm (e.g., with respect to self-concept); however, de Vaus found that peers also influenced religious practice to some extent (see also Hoge & Petrillo, 1978a). Erickson (1992) similarly found that peer influence was relatively unimportant in adolescent religiousness. But he pointed out that peer influence might be hidden because of the way in which effects were measured, and also because it was difficult to separate peer influence from religious education, which itself involved "a social/friendship setting" (p. 151) that might constitute a kind of peer influence. King et al. (2002) found that although parental influence tends to be the most significant, the influence of peers should not be overlooked. Whereas verbal communication tends to be the primary vehicle through which parents have an influence, peers tend to have an impact through both verbal discussion (surprisingly, they found the influence of discussion to be greater for boys than for girls) and shared religious activities. Similarly, Regnerus et al. (2004) found that though parents are the primary influence, the ecological contexts provided by friends and school matter as well in adolescent religious development, especially in self-rated importance of religion.

Similarly, Hunsberger's (1983b, 1985b) studies involving self-ratings of religious influences suggested that friends were well down the list of 10 potential influences for both university students (5th) and older Canadians (9th). Ozorak (1989) concluded that peers do influence adolescent religiousness, though this relationship is rather complex and is overshadowed by more important parental influences. Other researchers have confirmed the primary importance of parents in religious socialization, but have also found evidence that the religiosity of college students' current friends offers a kind of supplementary reinforcing effect (Roberts, Koch, & Johnson, 2001). In another investigation, both peer and family influences predicted adolescent religiousness (King et al., 2002).

Of course, peer influence may be stronger in some areas of religion than in others. For example, peers may have little influence on core religion measures such as frequency of church attendance, but may be more important with respect to youth group participation and enjoyment of that participation (Hoge & Petrillo, 1978a). Also, peer influence is probably complex, especially with respect to dating and heterosexual friendships. For example, particularly for adolescents of minority religions, religiously based attitudes toward interfaith dating may initiate a kind of filtering process in partner selection (Marshall & Markstrom-Adams, 1995). This filtering may in turn affect dating partners' interactions and reciprocal influence regarding religion (i.e., a type of peer influence).

In an exception to the usual self-report studies in this area, an unusual field experiment (Carey, 1971) involved randomly assigning 102 Catholic school students in seventh grade to one of three groups: proreligion, antireligion, or no influence (control group). Confederates (boys who were "leaders" in the same classes as the other participants) urged their classmates to comply or not to comply with a nun's talk on "Why a Catholic should go to daily mass." Actual attendance at mass was then monitored, and an effect did emerge for the position taken by the male confederates to influence their peers, but only for girls. Of course, the peer influence assessed in this study was very specific and short-term; we should be careful not to confuse such transitory impact with more general, long-term, and complex peer effects.

Finally, we should not assume that peer influence is relevant only to child and adolescent religion. Olson (1989) found that in five Baptist congregations, the number and quality of friendships were important predictors of adults' decisions to join or leave a denomination. And Putnam (2000) has pointed out that people who belong to religious groups tend to have more social commitments and contacts in their lives; this increased social interaction may allow for greater peer influence. Unfortunately, there has been little investigation of possible peer influence on religiousness in adulthood, beyond friendship networks.

Does Education Make a Difference?

The Impact of College

The extent to which education affects religious socialization has been a controversial topic. Early studies generally concluded that education, especially college, tends to "liberalize" the religious beliefs of students. For example, a review of more than 40 investigations led Feldman (1969) to conclude that these studies

> generally show mean changes indicating that seniors, compared with freshmen, are somewhat less orthodox, fundamentalistic, or conventional in religious orientation, somewhat more skeptical about the existence and influence of a Supreme Being, somewhat more likely to conceive of God in impersonal terms, and somewhat less favorable toward the church as an institution. Although the trend across studies does exist, the mean changes are not always large, and in about a third of the cases showing decreasing favorability toward religion, differences are not statistically significant. (p. 23)

Other reviewers (e.g., Parker, 1971) have similarly concluded that religious change may be considerable during the college years, especially in the first year. However, we should be cautious about such (average) trends toward decreased religiousness, because they may mask substantial change in the opposite direction for *some* students (Feldman & Newcomb, 1969). In addition, if change occurs, education itself is not necessarily the cause of the change. Shifts away from orthodox religion may be part of maturational or developmental change, or may result from the fact that some students are effectively away from parental control for the first time. Such shifts may also reflect either peer influence or a tendency for less religious (or more questioning) students to attend (and not to drop out of) college, or at least to avoid campus religious involvement. Madsen and Vernon (1983) found a (not surprising) tendency for more religious students to be more likely to participate in campus religious activities. More importantly, those students who participated in campus religious groups tended to increase in religious orthodoxy, but nonparticipants became less orthodox at college. It is also possible that apparent effects of college are actually due to other factors, such as religious background (Hoge & Keeter, 1976). For example, Sieben (2001) found in a Dutch study that the influence of education on a variety of variables, including orthodox religious belief and church attendance, was considerably overestimated when the impact of family background was not controlled for.

Furthermore, studies began to appear in the 1970s that were not always consistent with Feldman's conclusion that there is a general shift away from traditional religion. For example, Hunsberger (1978) reported a cross-sectional study of more than 450 Canadian university students, and a separate longitudinal investigation of more than 200 students from their first to their third university years, including an interim assessment of about half of this longitudinal sample during their second year. His data offered little support for the proposal that students generally become less religious over their university years. The only consistent finding across both studies was that third- and fourth-year students reported attending church less frequently than did first-year students. Thus there was limited support for a decrease in religious practices across the college years, but this change did not generalize to some other practices (e.g., frequency of prayer) or to scores on a series of religious belief measures. Finally, measures of "average change" did *not* mask frequent or dramatic individual religious change in different directions.

Hunsberger (1978) speculated that college-related religious change may have been more characteristic of the 1960s, since other subsequent studies (e.g., Hastings & Hoge, 1976; Pilkington, Poppleton, Gould, & McCourt, 1976) also found little or no change. In fact, Moberg and Hoge (1986) concluded that the decade 1961–1971 had seen considerable shifts toward liberalism in college students, but that the following decade (1971–1982) involved a slight change in the opposite direction (toward conservatism and traditional moral attitudes). Finally, Hunsberger (1978) suggested that religious change may be more likely to happen in the high school years, and may be relatively complete by the time students reach college—a suggestion supported by the research of others (Francis, 1982; Sutherland, 1988). However, some research has continued to show that higher education has at least indirect effects on young people's religiousness—by, for example, encouraging skepticism and a sense of religious and moral relativity (e.g., Bryant, Choi, & Yasuno, 2003; Hadaway & Roof, 1988; Reimer, 2010).

Studies in both Australia (Mason et al., 2007) and Great Britain (Savage, Collins-Mayo, Mayo, & Cray, 2006) of "Generation Y" young adults reveal a similar pattern of an emerging skepticism with respect to religious matters. For instance, in the two-stage Australian study, Mason et al. conducted intensive qualitative interviews with 91 persons born between 1981 and 1985, which made them 20–24 years old at the time of the study, followed by a national phone survey that resulted in 1,619 completed interviews. This wise use of mixed methods revealed that while 46% of interviewees identified themselves as traditionally Christian, such identification was associated with the belief that they could pick and choose among religious beliefs (Mason et al., 2007, p. 91). While some non-Christians identified with alternative religious views (19% identified with New Age beliefs, including beliefs in astrology and reincarnation), 28% were classified as secular. In Great Britain, Savage et al. (2006) found similar patterns. In both Australia and Great Britain, therefore, it appears that many Generation Y persons (defined for our purposes as those born between 1980 and 1990) have adopted what Mason et al. (2007) identify as "a liberal, secular individualism in its postmodern form" (pp. 331–332). This stands in opposition to a more classical acceptance of Christianity as a grand narrative providing a coherent and authoritative frame for life's meaning. Savage et al. (2006, pp. 38–89) provide an in-depth analysis of Generation Y persons' ability to utilize narratives centering on the here and now. Thus many in Generation Y in both Australia and Great Britain have framed a life of meaning and purpose without the necessity of resorting to grand narratives associated with religion or an appeal to the supernatural. They are satisfied with "happy midi-narratives" (Savage et al., 2006, p. 36). Similar studies in the United States suggest that as some adolescents advance through the college years, traditional religious beliefs and commitment to a single grand narrative may decrease.

Data from a national longitudinal research study (Astin et al., 2011; HERI, 2007) on college students from 2004 to 2007 in the United States provide limited support for the studies in Australia and Great Britain. In this study, students who were studied as freshmen in 2004 were administered the same set of questions as second-semester juniors in 2007 by the HERI at UCLA (mentioned at the beginning of this chapter). Results showed that religious engagement and charitable involvement decreased significantly over the course of the college years. For example, frequent attendance at religious services dropped from approximately 43% of the students to 25%. A similar decline was noted by the respondents in their friends' attendance at religious services. Students who reported frequent or occasional participation in such charitable services as volunteer work, community service, or participation in a clothing/food drive also significantly decreased during the 4 years of college. However, as we repeatedly argue throughout the text, attendance at religious services is not a good barometer of religious commitment; these other findings may be due to other issues (lack of transportation, scheduling conflicts, lack of resources and time, etc.). On the other hand, a number of religious or spiritual factors showed increases during the college years, including spiritual quest (e.g., developing a meaningful philosophy of life, attaining inner harmony, seeking beauty in life), equanimity (e.g., seeing each day as a gift, being thankful for all that has happened to one, finding meaning through hardship), spirituality (e.g., integrating spirituality into one's life, believing in the sacredness of life), an ethic of caring (e.g., helping others in difficulty, helping to promote racial harmony), and an ecumenical world view (e.g., improving one's understanding of other cultures, growing spiritually without being religious). Hill (2009, 2011), examining data from a nationally representative sample, concluded that some college students—such as those who attend conservative Protestant colleges, or who identify with religious organizations on secular campuses—may actually identify their years in college as providing a "moral community."

These results suggest that Feldman's (1969) conclusions (quoted above) are still partially true today. That is, as students progress through college, they do seem to become less conventionally religious, though the absence of church involvement may be uniquely associated with the college years. But the college years also appear to be a time of interest in spiritual matters, many of which are addressed by conventional religion (Astin et al., 2011; Hill, 2011).

Parochial School Attendance

Some investigations have compared public with parochial schools regarding the religiousness of their students. These investigations have generated rather muddy findings, possibly because of methodological shortcomings (Benson et al., 1989; Hyde, 1990). In the United States in recent decades, conservative Protestants (mostly evangelical or fundamentalist) have founded a growing number of "Christian schools" as an educational alternative to public or secular private schools. Also, some parents (again, especially conservative Protestants) are choosing to home-school their children, at least through some grades. Though there are many anecdotal accounts of the effects of such educational efforts, often used for promotional purposes, such programs have received little scientific scrutiny. Most of the research conducted to date has focused primarily on traditional mainline Protestant and Catholic schools.

Although some early researchers (e.g., Lenski, 1961; Greeley, 1967) concluded that parochial school attenders were more strongly religious in some ways than their public school counterparts, the relevant research sometimes failed to take background factors into account. Some investigators apparently assumed that differences between parochial and public school students were *caused* by the environments of the schools involved, and they ignored possible self-selection factors. More than 50 years ago, Mueller (1967) found that when he held religious background constant, he could find no differences in the religious orthodoxy and institutional involvement of college students. He concluded that "high orthodoxy is a direct function of a strong religious background rather than specifically of parochial school attendance" (p. 51).

Other research has supported this finding, including studies of fundamentalists (Erickson, 1964), Jews (Parker & Gaier, 1980), Lutherans (Johnstone, 1966), Mennonites (Kraybill, 1977), and Catholics and Church of England adherents (Francis & Brown, 1991). For example, Francis and Brown (1991) argued that a positive relationship between Roman Catholic school attendance and positive attitudes toward prayer was really a result of "the influence of home and church rather than that of the school itself" (p. 119). Furthermore, as indicated in Research Box 5.2, their investigation even detected a small *negative* influence of Church of England schools on attitudes toward prayer, after other factors were controlled for (gender, home, church, private practice of prayer). This finding is consistent with Francis's work (1980, 1993) with younger children and adolescents.

More recently, a study in the United Kingdom (Francis & Lankshear, 2001) similarly revealed very little impact of church-related primary schools on religiousness or religious activity in the local community. There was a tendency toward higher rates of religious confirmation in the preteen years (for voluntarily aided but not for controlled schools), but apparently no influence on older persons. However, such "minimal-impact" conclusions have been challenged by some authors (e.g., Greeley & Gockel, 1971; Greeley & Rossi, 1966), and Himmelfarb (1979) argued that church-related schools do indeed have a direct positive influence on the religiousness of their students.

In the end, there is probably variation across individual schools, different age groups (elementary, high school, and postsecondary students), and different religious denominations. Self-selection factors probably occur at many parochial schools, such that more religious students (or at least students with more religious parents) are likely to attend such schools. Findings may differ across studies, depending on whether they focus on religious beliefs or practices (Hunsberger, 1977). Effects may be unique to specific studies or may depend on combinations of factors. For example, Benson et al. (1986) found that Catholic high schools with a high proportion of students from low-income families tended to have a positive influence on religiousness *if* those schools stressed academics and religion, had high student morale, and also focused on the importance of religion and the development of a "community of faith." There may also be effects for some specific measures of religiousness, such as an increase in religious *knowledge* (Johnstone, 1966). It is often very difficult to separate the influence of parochial schools from the effects of parents and the family generally (Benson et al., 1989).

In light of the findings available, and their many qualifications, we are led to this conclusion: The bulk of the evidence suggests that church-related school attendance has little direct influence on adolescent religiousness, above and beyond the home influence per se. This is *not* to say that there is no influence, for influence can take many forms. It is likely that parochial school students come from more religious homes in the first place, and thus one role (among many) of such institutions may be the provision of a social and educational context where already existing religious values and beliefs are reinforced. The issue is not clear-cut and does not include the recent wave of Christian schooling in the United States, simply because research on such schooling that meets scientific criteria is not yet available. The reader may wish to consult more comprehensive reviews of the relevant literature (e.g., Hyde, 1990; Kanpol & Poplin, 2017).

Other Influences

Parents, peers, and education are not the only potential sources of influence on religiousness. Some studies have suggested that the particular church (or other religious institution) or denomination, as well as socioeconomic status, sibling configuration, city size, the mass media, reading, and so on, can also have some effect on the religious socialization process (see, e.g., Benson et al., 1989). For example, rural youths tend to be more religious than nonrural young people (King, Elder, & Whitbeck, 1997). However, self-reported ratings of influence (Hunsberger, 1983b, 1985b) and more indirect inferences (Erickson, 1992; Francis & Brown, 1991; Hoge, Hefferman, et al., 1982; Hoge & Thompson, 1982; Nelsen, 1982; Philibert & Hoge, 1982) suggest that factors related to the church (or to religious education, broadly defined) are the most important of various possible "other" influences on the religious socialization process. Francis and Brown (1991) have observed that church becomes a more important influence in middle adolescence, at roughly the time when young people are becoming less susceptible to parental influence with respect to religion.

In general, however, the various "other factors" discussed above have received scant empirical attention. There is a need for further investigation of attitudes toward the church; the role of the clergy; the influence of church-related peers compared to non-church-related friends, mass media effects, and so on; and the subtle interplay among these and other religious socialization factors.

The Polarization Hypothesis

Earlier in this chapter, we have discussed Ozorak's (1989) social-cognitive model of religious socialization processes, which allows for the possibility of a "polarization" effect in religious development. That is, Ozorak noted a tendency for more religious adolescents to report change in the direction of greater religiosity, whereas less religious adolescents reported a shift away from religion. As noted in Chapter 4, Tamminen (1991) found a similar religious polarization tendency among Finnish adolescents. This is consistent with the observation that more religious college students join campus religious groups, and also increase in religious orthodoxy while at college, but less religious students who do not join campus religious groups decrease in orthodoxy (Madsen & Vernon, 1983). In other words, the religious "distance" between these two groups increases at college. Similar self-reported polarization tendencies have been found among the most and least religious participants in a study of older Canadians (Hunsberger, 1985b). Reflecting back over their lives and "graphing" their religiosity across the decades, these senior citizens indicated that they had gradually become more religious across their lives since childhood if they were highly religious at the time of the study. However, senior citizens who were relatively less religious indicated that they had become progressively *less* religious across their lives, compared to their more religious counterparts.

These studies are limited by the retrospective, cross-sectional, and self-report nature of the data, as well as by the possibility that we are learning more about people's perceptions of reality than we are about reality itself. However, the findings are consistent with the possibility that general trends toward greater or lesser religiosity may be established quite early in life, and that these trends may continue long after early developmental and socialization influences have had their immediate effects.

Gender Issues

Social influences (especially the influence of parents) in the religious socialization process can help to explain some important gender differences in adolescent and adult religiosity. For example, women have typically been found to be "more religious" than men (see Donelson, 1999; Francis & Wilcox, 1998). That is, they attend worship services more often, pray more often, express stronger agreement with traditional beliefs, are more interested in religion, and report that religion is more important in their lives. Women's attitudes toward religion may also be developed at an earlier age (Tammimen & Nurmi, 1995). Such gender differences may be attributable to social influence processes in sex role training, either through sex differences that have implications for religiousness (e.g., women are taught to be more submissive and nurturing—traits associated with greater religiosity), or through direct expectations that women should be more religious than men. Similar "socialization" interpretations have come from others (e.g., Batson, Schoenrade, & Ventis, 1993; Nelsen & Potvin, 1981), though these are not the only possible interpretations of gender differences in religion (see Miller & Hoffman, 1995).

It is likely that religious socialization processes have important gender implications for other areas of people's lives, such as (nonreligious) attitudes, careers, and education. For example, national survey data from 19,000 U.S. women led to the conclusion that religious identification affects educational attainment more strongly than do other sociodemographic variables (Keysar & Kosmin, 1995). Women from more conservative, traditional, or fundamentalist backgrounds achieved less postsecondary education than did women from more liberal or modern religious backgrounds, on average. That is, "some gender inequality is indeed socially created by the influence of religion" (Keysar & Kosmin, 1995, p. 61). Although this was a correlational study, it does raise the possibility that religious socialization can ultimately affect "nonreligious" aspects of one's life.

There is also evidence that young men and women differ in their perceptions of God and in how they would react to a male versus a female God. Foster and Babcock (2001) asked university students to write a story about a fictional interaction with a male or female God. Men's stories involved more action, whereas women were more concerned with feelings. There was also more skepticism, criticality, and surprise in reaction to a female God than to a male God. Such gender differences may well develop during childhood as part of the socialization process—an issue ripe for future research.

Influences on Religiousness: Summary and Implications

We must be cautious in drawing conclusions about religious socialization influences, since it is often difficult to isolate parental, peer, educational, and other influences and their possible interactions. Many typical problems that face social-scientific researchers (e.g., self-report accuracy, sampling limitations) afflict this area of research as well. However, given the large numbers of relevant studies and the convergence of some findings, we are able to offer some general conclusions.

Parents are potentially the most powerful influences on child and adolescent religion, though their impact becomes weaker as adolescents grow into adulthood, and some of their influence may be indirect. Peers, education, parochial school environment, the mass media, and reading have been found to affect religious socialization to a lesser degree, though it is sometimes difficult to isolate the effects of specific causal factors. It has been suggested, however, that when parents and other potential influential agents (e.g., church, social network of friends) reinforce the same religious perspective, the resulting combined religious socialization effects may be especially strong (Hyde, 1990). Furthermore, trends established early in life for people to become more or less religious may continue into adulthood (as predicted by the polarization hypothesis).

Finally, it is important that we not lose sight of possible implications of religious socialization for other aspects of people's lives. We have seen that religious growth processes can have a potentially powerful impact on gender issues. No doubt the effects of religious socialization extend into many other aspects of people's lives as well, as discussed throughout this book.

DOES RELIGIOUS SOCIALIZATION INFLUENCE ADJUSTMENT AND NONRELIGIOUS BEHAVIOR IN ADOLESCENCE?

To what extent does religion affect other aspects of young people's lives? A review of the literature on adolescence and religion led Benson et al. (1989) to conclude that religion has a powerful impact on adolescents and their entire development. For example, adolescents who say that religion is important in their lives are more likely to do volunteer work in the community than are young people who say that religion is not important (Youniss, McLellan, Su, & Yates, 1999; Youniss, McLellan, & Yates, 1999). Also, it has been suggested that churches may serve a function of initiating youths into volunteer activity, and then sustaining this involvement (Pancer & Pratt, 1999). Some of this volunteering may result from church teachings about helping others and doing good. It is also possible that family religiousness is more generally linked to other group involvement, and that such effects may persist well into adulthood (see Putnam, 2000). For example, one study revealed that medical students' reports of family church involvement were positively associated with the number of group memberships they had some 39 years later (Graves, Wang, Mead, Johnson, & Klag, 1998).

Links have been found between stronger religiousness and decreased delinquent behavior for adolescents (e.g., Johnson, Jang, Larson, & Li, 2001), including lower rates of drug and alcohol use (e.g., Bahr, Maughan, Marcos, & Li, 1998; Corwyn & Benda, 2000; Francis, 1997a; Lee, Rice, & Gillespie, 1997; see also Donahue & Benson, 1995) and less deviant behavior in general (Litchfield, Thomas, & Li, 1997). Also, religiousness seems to be associated with both less sexual activity and delayed onset of sexual activity (e.g., Benda & Corwyn, 1999; Lammers, Ireland, Resnick, & Blum, 2000; Miller et al., 1997; Paul, Fitzjohn, Eberhart-Phillips, Herbison, & Dickson, 2000), but also with less condom use in adolescents (Zaleski & Schiaffino, 2000). Some of these links are explored in greater detail in Chapter 12 on morality. For our purposes here, however, it is important to note that such associations between religiousness and decreased substance use, deviant behavior, and sexuality are relatively common in studies of adolescents and young adults.

Other research has investigated possible links between religion and personal adjustment. For example, Blaine, Trivedi, and Eshleman (1998) concluded that "a large research literature . . . has established that measures of religious commitment, devotion, or belief strength are associated with a range of positive mental health indicators, such as decreased anxiety and depression, and increased self-esteem, tolerance, and self-control" (p. 1040). Others have come to similar conclusions (see Koenig & Larson, 2001; Maton & Wells, 1995; Seybold & Hill, 2001), including some studies that have focused on adolescents (e.g., Moore & Glei, 1995; Wright, Frost, & Wisecarver, 1993), although some authors have pointed out that religion may be associated with maladjustment as well (see Booth, 1991; Ellis, 1986; Shafranske, 1992). This literature is discussed in more detail in Chapter 13.

Some authors are inclined to conclude that in light of the relevant research, religion must *cause* improved mental health, decreased deviance, more prosocial behavior, and the like, especially during the adolescent years. This is indeed plausible, but one must also consider other causal possibilities. For example, young people who live more moral and mentally healthy lives may be more inclined to attend church, where they may find other like-minded persons who have similar behavioral inclinations. Causality is difficult to study in this area, and possibly as a consequence, few researchers have tackled the issue head-on.

Furthermore, if there are indeed connections between religion and adolescent behavior and adjustment, we might wonder about the processes that could explain such connections. There is no shortage of potential explanations, and many of them rely on the socialization literature. Religion may aid adjustment by providing social support, assisting in value and identity formation (King et al., 2002; Regnerus et al., 2004), and teaching social control (Wallace & Williams, 1997). Forliti and Benson (1986) have emphasized the importance of value development in early religious socialization. Religious socialization may also teach children and adolescents coping techniques such as praying when anxious, or may show them how to choose positive activities as alternatives to delinquency or substance use (see Hunsberger, Pratt, & Pancer, 2001b). Religious training may contribute to a more positive self-concept (Blaine et al., 1998), which in turn may have benefits for adjustment and behavior. These types of suggestions imply that the religious socialization process either directly or indirectly produces the desirable outcomes related to adjustment and behavior. However, two studies carried out by Hunsberger et al. (2001b), one with college students and one with high school students, found no differences on various adjustment measures between those raised in religious versus nonreligious homes.

There is a need for researchers to refocus their efforts in this area. There is no shortage of studies of adolescents and young adults that reveal correlations between religiousness variables and (decreased) destructive behaviors such as substance use, as well as improved personal adjustment. We now need investigations of the mechanisms and underlying causal patterns that generate such correlations.

RELIGIOUS THINKING AND REASONING IN ADOLESCENCE AND YOUNG ADULTHOOD

As we have seen in Chapter 4, a developmental shift in thinking about religious (and other) issues occurs as young people move from childhood to adolescence. In Piagetian terms, this shift is from concrete to formal operations, which (especially for religious concepts) involves a move away from the literal toward more abstract thinking. It has also been suggested that this trend toward abstract religious thought may be linked with decreased religiousness, and possibly with a tendency to reject religion in adolescence. Possibly adolescents' emerging abstract thinking capability "complicates" their religious thought, and may even stimulate new styles of thinking in order to deal with "difficult-to-explain" religious concepts and existential issues.

Reich's Notion of Complementarity Reasoning

Reich (1991) has pointed out that there are "many perceived contradictions and paradoxes that characterize religious life" (pp. 87–88; see also Reich, 1989, 1992, 1994). He has suggested that "complementarity reasoning" may develop in order to deal with such religious contradictions. That is, people may develop rational explanations for specific perceived contradictions, which make the contradictions seem more apparent than real. Reich gives the example of a 20-year-old who attempted to explain the seeming conflict between creationist and evolutionary explanations of humans' origins and development as a species: "The possibility of evolution was contained in God's 'kick-off' at the origin . . . but God probably did not interfere with evolution itself . . . and perhaps so far not all of the initial potential has yet come to fruition" (quoted in Reich, 1991, p. 78). Reich has suggested that complementarity reasoning is crucial to religious development, though it does not emerge in fully developed form until relatively late in life, and sometimes not at all.

Reich proposes that five different levels of complementarity reasoning appear in developmental sequence. Essentially, these levels evolve from a very simplified (true–false) resolution of different explanations, through careful consideration of various competing explanations, to possible links between competing explanations and possibly even the use of an overarching theory or synopsis to assess complex relationships among the different factors. This analysis bears some resemblance to the "integrative complexity" analysis of religious and other thinking (see below), and the complexity approach has the advantage of an established scoring system tapping different levels of thinking. Possible links between religious orientation and complexity of thinking processes have been investigated in several studies of university students.

Integrative Complexity of Thought

"Integrative complexity" is defined by two cognitive stylistic variables. "Differentiation" involves the acknowledgment and tolerance of different perspectives or dimensions of an issue, and "integration" deals with the extent to which differentiated perspectives or dimensions are linked. A manual for scoring integrative complexity (Baker-Brown et al., 1992) describes how such complexity is typically scored on a 1–7 scale. Lower scores indicate a person's tendency not to reveal (1) or to reveal (3) differentiation; higher scores (4–7) indicate the extent to which people integrate these differentiated concepts into broader structures. Research Box 5.3, which describes a study by Hunsberger and his colleagues on fundamentalism and religious doubt, gives examples of responses receiving different complexity scores.

Batson and Raynor-Prince (1983) found that a measure of religious orthodoxy was significantly negatively correlated (–.37) with the integrative complexity of sentence completions dealing with existential religious issues (e.g., "When I consider my own death . . ."). That is, people with a more orthodox religious orientation tended to think more simply about existential religious issues, as indicated by the sentence completion task. Also, scores on the Quest measure of religious orientation were significantly positively correlated (.43) with complexity scores for thinking about existential content. For both orthodoxy and quest, comparable correlations involving *non*religious sentence completions were not statistically significant. However, it should be noted that the integrative complexity scores were distributed primarily in the lower half (1–4) of the scale, suggesting that even those who differentiate well are not necessarily capable of integrating those differentiated concepts into broader structures. Furthermore, a series of investigations by Hunsberger and his colleagues (Hunsberger,

RESEARCH BOX 5.3. Religious Fundamentalism and Complexity of Religious Doubts (Hunsberger, Alisat, Pancer, & Pratt, 1996)

This interview study of university students provided examples of the integrative complexity anchor scores for content dealing with religious doubts. Students were asked questions about their religious doubts, and their responses were then scored for complexity of thought.

One question asked, "What would you say is the most serious doubt about religion or religious beliefs that you have had in the last few years?" The following response received a score of 1 (no differentiation), since it reveals just one dimension of religious doubt: "My only real doubt is why God could allow people to suffer so much in this world" (p. 207). Full differentiation (a score of 3) is illustrated by the following response, which outlines two different dimensions of doubt: "I have doubted why God allowed me to become seriously ill a few years ago. What was His purpose? Also, I could never understand why there is war and famine in the world if there is a God" (p. 207).

An example of a response showing integration of differentiated doubts (score of 5) is as follows:

> Over the years I have had various "little doubts." For example, I was bothered by the hypocrisy of some "religious" people, and the Bible seemed to not be very relevant to a lot of things happening today. After a while I sort of sat down and put all of these little things together and realized that in combination they made me doubt organized religion in general. (p. 207)

Scores of 7 are rare in this type of research, and no such score was found in this study. Scores of 2, 4, and 6 represent transition points between the odd-numbered anchor scores.

Results revealed a weak but significant correlation between the extent of one's religious doubts and the integrative complexity of thinking about those doubts. This finding is consistent with previous conclusions that complexity–religion relationships are restricted to domains involving existential religious content (Hunsberger, Pratt, & Pancer, 1994).

Pratt, & Pancer, 1994; Hunsberger, Alisat, Pancer, & Pratt, 1996; Hunsberger, Lea, Pancer, Pratt, & McKenzie, 1992; Hunsberger, McKenzie, Pratt, & Pancer, 1993; Pancer, Jackson, Hunsberger, Pratt, & Lea, 1995; Pratt, Hunsberger, Pancer, & Roth, 1992), using open-ended essay or interviews for a full expression of ideas, suggest that the complexity–religious orientation relationship may be restricted to issues involving existential content only (which, of course, are still clearly related to religious experience). In spite of these limitations, it is safe to conclude that not all people think about their religious faith with the same degree of complexity, and that one major predictor of integrative complexity is religious orientation.

RELIGIOUS DOUBTS

Of course, adolescents and young adults are not completely passive recipients of social influence when it comes to their religious beliefs. They think about religious issues, and they may not be willing to accept all that they are taught. Almost everyone has questions (e.g., "Does God really exist?", "Should I accept my parents' religious faith?") related to religious teachings at some time. Many people apparently resolve their questions to their own satisfaction, and their underlying religious beliefs are not substantially altered. Others, however, may have trouble resolving their questions, and this may lead to serious doubts and concerns about religious beliefs. These doubts may eventually lead them to abandon some or all of their beliefs. Let us examine this process in greater detail.

Questions and doubts about religion seem especially common in adolescence, though they may also occur among adults. Nipkow and Schweitzer (1991) analyzed 16- to 21-year-old German students' written reflections about God, and concluded that most of their respondents had "challenging questions" about God. These primarily involved unfulfilled expectations of God; whether or not the students continued to believe in God was determined by the extent to which their expectations were fulfilled. Similarly, Tamminen (1991, 1994) noted an increase in early adolescence in doubts about whether God exists, and whether prayers were answered, among his Finnish students.

However, research suggests that the mass media's depiction of young people as rebellious and questioning of parental values, implying that adolescents are boiling cauldrons of bubbling religious doubts, is exaggerated. Canadian studies of nearly 2,000 university students (Altemeyer & Hunsberger, 1997) and almost 1,000 high school students (Hunsberger, Pratt, & Pancer, 2002) revealed that average self-reported religious doubts were rated about 2 (a "mild amount" of doubt) on a 0–6 response scale. The greatest doubts in both studies were linked to (1) the perception that religion is associated with intolerance; (2) unappreciated pressure tactics of religions; and (3) other ways that religion seemed to be associated with negative human qualities, rather than making people "better." But even for these issues, the average doubt was rated less than 3 (a "moderate amount") on the 0–6 scale used. This mild to moderate level of doubt is not surprising, in light of evidence that adolescents' "reasoning is systematically biased to protect and promote their preexisting [religious] beliefs" (Klaczynski & Gordon, 1996, p. 317).

Correlates of Doubt

Is religious doubt unique to adolescents and young adults? One study did reveal a slight decline with age in scores on Batson's Quest measure ($r = -.19$), suggesting a decreased tendency among older adults to doubt, insofar as this measure taps doubting (Watson, Howard, Hood, & Morris, 1988). However, we should be careful not to conclude that doubt is virtually nonexistent among older adults, as mentioned previously. For example, Nielsen (1998) reported that about two-thirds of his adult sample provided written descriptions of "religious conflict" in their lives, although it is not clear how many of these descriptions would be classified as religious doubts.

Also, although absolute levels of doubting tend to be mild to moderate, religious doubting is apparently related to religious, personal, and social variables. Quite consistently, higher levels of doubt have been moderately to strongly associated with reduced religiousness, such as lower Christian orthodoxy (Altemeyer, 1988; Hunsberger et al., 1993, 1996); with lower religious fundamentalism and less religious emphasis in the family home, and less acceptance of religious teachings (Hunsberger et al., 1996); and with lower Intrinsic religion scores and an inclination toward apostasy (Hunsberger et al., 1993). Moreover, religious doubting has been linked with such personality characteristics as greater openness to experience (Shermer, 2000), lower right-wing authoritarianism (Altemeyer, 1988; Hunsberger et al., 1993), and less dogmatism (Hunsberger et al., 1996). Finally, it has been associated with some aspects of social activism (Begue, 2000), increased complexity of thought about religious issues (Hunsberger et al., 1993), and some aspects of ego identity development (Hunsberger, Pratt, & Pancer, 2001a), as discussed later in this chapter.

Doubt and Personal Adjustment

Research has also suggested that religious doubting is related to personal adjustment. As noted earlier, doubts were weakly but significantly positively related to perceived stress, depression, and self-reported life hassles for college students, and significantly negatively related to adjustment to college and relationships with parents, during students' first year in college (Hunsberger et al., 1996). Similarly, religious doubting has been associated with more psychological distress and decreased feelings of personal well-being in adult Presbyterians (Krause, Ingersoll-Dayton, Ellison, & Wulff, 1999). Krause et al. concluded that younger adults have greater difficulty with religious doubt than do older persons, since the association between doubt and depression scores was strongest at age 20 and decreased as age increased. These findings seem to support claims that religious doubt has negative implications for personal mental health, as suggested by earlier writers on the subject (e.g., Allport, 1950; Clark, 1958; Helfaer, 1972; Pratt, 1920), although supportive findings have not always been clear-cut (Kooistra & Pargament, 1999).

Why would religious doubting be associated with negative personal consequences? Several possibilities have been advanced (see Hunsberger et al., 2002; Krause et al., 1999). It has been claimed that various positive mental health and adjustment benefits are derived from religiousness, possibly through coping mechanisms that are associated with religion (e.g., prayer, religious social support; Pargament, 1997). Because doubt is associated with decreased religious faith, the resulting decreased religiousness may detract from one's coping ability, resulting in a less well-adjusted life. Also, doubt may be associated with feelings of shame or guilt, which in turn may adversely affect self-esteem (Krause et al., 1999). Doubt itself may be seen as a particular manifestation of Festinger's (1957) cognitive dissonance, and such dissonance is sometimes associated with psychological distress and negative affect (e.g., Burris, Harmon-Jones, & Tarpley, 1997).

Furthermore, Kooistra and Pargament (1999) found some (mixed) evidence that doubting may be linked to conflictual family patterns. They suggested that this might result from the general negative consequences that family difficulties seem to have for children's and adolescents' religiousness, such as negative God images, alienation from and negative feelings about religion, and decreased religiousness. However, Kooistra and Pargament studied only parochial high school students in the U.S. Midwest, and doubt was associated with conflictual families only for students at a Dutch Reformed school, not those at a Catholic school. Hunsberger et al. (2001a) were unable to replicate this difference between fundamentalist and Catholic students in Canada; rather, when they broke their findings down by major denominational groupings, relationships between doubt and poorer adjustment occurred only for mainstream Protestants.

Doubting may also have some positive associations. As noted earlier, religious doubting is an important component in the conceptualization of the Quest religious orientation (Batson et al., 1993), which has been linked with less prejudice, a tendency to help others in need, and some aspects of mental health (e.g., personal competence/control, self-acceptance, and open-mindedness/flexibility). Furthermore, Krause et al. (1999) have pointed out that doubt may be an important part of positive psychological development; this suggestion is consistent with research showing that doubt and uncertainty more generally might stimulate cognitive development (e.g., Acredolo & O'Connor, 1991).

Thus, strictly from a psychological perspective, we are hard pressed to say that religious doubting is either "good" or "bad." This is not to say that the predominant church attitude "that it is to be deplored as an obstacle to faith, at the worst a temptation of the Devil, at the best a sign of weakness" (Clark, 1958, p. 138) is necessarily wrong. It is to say, however, that judgments about religious doubts' being "good" or "bad" depend on how one defines these terms, and probably also on one's personal religious orientation.

Dealing with Doubt

Regardless of whether doubt is good or bad, most people who experience religious doubts are motivated to somehow resolve them. Hunsberger et al. (2002) investigated two ways in which young people attempt to deal with their religious questions and doubts. One way is to consult with people or reading materials that would likely push them in a proreligious direction. Scores on a self-report Belief-Confirming Consultation (BCC) scale were found to significantly predict increased religiousness 2 years later. A second approach is to consult resources that would be more likely to provide nonreligious or antireligious answers to questions (e.g., talking with friends with no religious beliefs, reading materials that go against one's religious beliefs). Scores on a self-report Belief-Threatening Consultation (BTC) scale significantly predicted reduced religiousness 2 years later. Of course, whom one consults may really be indicative of one's inclination to resolve religious doubts one way or the other in the first place.

Also, Hunsberger et al. (1996) found qualitative differences with respect to the nature of doubting, for respondents who were high and low in religious fundamentalism. "High fundamentalists" did not typically doubt God or religion per se; rather, their doubts were focused on others' failure to live up to religious ideals, or relatively minor adjustments that they felt should be made within the church (e.g., improving the role of women in the church). "Low fundamentalists," on the other hand, were more likely to be concerned about the underpinnings of religion, such as the existence of God, the lack of proof for religious claims, or the unbelievability of the creation account of human origins. Again, there was some evidence that people who reported more religious doubts tended to think more complexly about such doubts, and about existential material more generally.

APOSTASY

Broad-based survey studies suggest that disengagement from religion is most common for people in their late teens and early 20s. For example, it has been estimated that about two-thirds of all dropping out among Catholics occurs between the ages of 16 and 25 (Hoge with McGuire & Stratman, 1981)—essentially the same peak "dropping-out" years reported for Mormons (Albrecht, Cornwall, & Cunningham, 1988), Presbyterians (Hoge, Johnson, & Luidens, 1993), and broader religious groupings (Albrecht & Cornwall, 1989; Caplovitz & Sherrow, 1977; Hadaway & Roof, 1988; see also Schweitzer, 2000).

Furthermore, there seems to be a growing interest in atheism—as witnessed by the dizzying array of popular books on this topic (Dawkins, 2006; Dennett, 2006; Grayling, 2007;

Harris, 2004, 2007; Hitchens, 2007), often presented as the "thinking person's" alternative to the irrationality of religious belief. As already pointed out, the high rate of theistic belief in the United States seems to be an exception among postindustrial Western countries. In most European countries, the proportion of people claiming to have no religious affiliation increased steadily and sometimes dramatically in the 20th century. Even in the comparatively religious United States, the percentage of people saying that they had "no religion" jumped from 2% in 1967 to 11% in the 1990s (Putnam, 2000), and it is likely that a substantial part of this rise involved "apostates" (i.e., those who had abandoned faith).

Atheism is complex, and any single definition (of the many that have been offered), fails to capture the wide range of positions held by atheists. Philosophers have long debated whether atheism is a religion, or even whether it must involve belief. For example, a leading atheist philosopher, Michael Martin (2002), has argued that atheism must be defined entirely in terms of belief, though he distinguishes what he calls "positive atheism" (the explicit disbelief in God) from both "negative atheism" (simply the lack of theistic belief) and "agnosticism" (the lack of either belief or disbelief in God). It is beyond our purposes here to go into this debate. We note, however, that at least for the "positive atheist" as defined by Martin, as rational as atheism may appear to be, it does involve belief. Our focus here is on why people, some of whom were raised in religious homes, find either atheism or some other belief system more convincing. Of course, many of the same socialization processes that we have discussed in this chapter (influence of parents, peers, and other social factors) are likely to play a role in apostasy as well.

Problems in Definition and Measurement

Caution is necessary when one is comparing the results of different investigations of apostasy. The terminology used to describe disengagement from religion varies considerably from study to study, involving such terms as "dropping out," "exiting," "disidentification," "leave taking," "defecting," "apostasy," "disaffiliation," and "disengagement" (Bromley, 1988). Furthermore, operational definitions of these terms have varied from one study to the next. Some authors (e.g., Caplovitz & Sherrow, 1977; Hunsberger, 1980, 1983a) have studied people who say they grew up with a religious identification or family religious background, but who no longer identify with any religious group. Others have focused on cessation of church attendance for a specified period of time (e.g., Hoge, 1981, 1988); have incorporated elements of loss of faith, as well as disidentification (Altemeyer & Hunsberger, 1997); or have focused on aspects of the organizational structure of the religious group a person is leaving (Bromley, 1998).

Such differences could potentially lead to divergent findings. It is important in relevant investigations to be clear about the criteria used to define apostasy operationally, and also to be sensitive to how this definition will affect the findings. For example, it has been estimated that in the United States, about 46% of people discontinue church participation at some point in their lives (Roozen, 1980). Whether this estimate is accurate or not, there are many reasons for cessation of church attendance that do not necessarily involve loss of personal faith (Albrecht et al., 1988). Studying all nonattenders could seriously inflate the seeming number of apostates.

Yet another important issue to consider in defining and measuring apostasy is the degree to which it is a permanent abandonment of faith. Most of the research on apostasy has been conducted with college students, and there is some evidence of a tendency to return to religion (including institutional religion) soon after the college years, perhaps due to the influence of marriage and parenthood (Argue, Johnson, & White, 1999; Bibby, 1993; Chaves, 1991; Hoge et al., 1993).

An extensive longitudinal study of a U.S. national probability sample suggested that most religious dropping out probably occurs after age 16. Wilson and Sherkat (1994) followed the religious identification and other trends of 1965 high school seniors to 1973 and again to 1983. They managed to retain more than two-thirds of the original 1,562 participants. They focused their attention on those who reported a religious preference in 1965, but then reported no preference in 1973. For these dropouts, they found few differences between those who retained their apostate status in 1983 and those who had returned to religion. The returnees did report closer relationships with their parents in high school than did the continuing apostates. Furthermore, there was a tendency for early marriage and forming a family to be related to returning to religion, though this relationship was found only for men. Women were less likely to become apostates than were men, but women apostates were also less likely to return to the fold than were men. The researchers speculated that men are more likely to be religiously affected by transitions to marriage and parenthood.

Types of Apostasy

Some authors have attempted to define types of apostates, though the resulting groupings tend to focus on social and other characteristics of apostates (and some other disaffiliated individuals) rather than on the underlying apostasy process itself. For example, Hadaway (1989) used cluster analysis to derive five characteristic groups of apostates: (1) "successful swinging singles" (single young people who apparently were experiencing social and financial success); (2) "sidetracked singles" (single people who tended to be pessimistic and had not obtained the benefits of the "good life"); (3) "young settled liberals" (those who were dissatisfied with traditional values but who had a very positive outlook on life); (4) "young libertarians" (people who rejected religious labels more than religious beliefs); and (5) "irreligious traditionalists" (somewhat older, conservative, married people who maintained some religious moral traditions in spite of their nonattendance and nonaffiliation).

Others have offered different typologies (Bahr & Albrecht, 1989; Brinkerhoff & Burke, 1980; Condran & Tamney, 1985; Hadaway & Roof, 1988; Hoge et al., 1981; Perry, Davis, Doyle, & Dyble, 1980; Roozen, 1980). But no generally accepted categorization has appeared. These studies do indicate that we should not assume that apostates constitute a homogeneous group. The social characteristics of apostates may vary considerably, and the underlying processes of disengagement are not uniform.

Roots of Apostasy

A number of researchers (e.g., Caplovitz & Sherrow, 1977; Putney & Middleton, 1961; Wuthnow & Glock, 1973) have suggested that rebellion against parents and other aspects of society is at the root of apostasy. For example, Caplovitz and Sherrow (1977) proposed four factors that may contribute to the abandonment of faith: (1) poor parental relations, (2) symptoms of maladjustment or neurosis, (3) a radical or leftist political orientation, and (4) commitment to intellectualism. Underlying all of these processes is the apparent assumption that apostasy represents a deliberate rejection of previous identification, and a conscious acceptance of a new identification.

Early findings (e.g., Johnson, 1973; Hunsberger, 1976) had suggested that religious socialization tends to follow a "straight line," such that lower levels of religiousness are related to lower levels of emphasis on religion in the childhood home. That is, apostasy seems to represent *consistency* with a lack of parental emphasis on religion, rather than rebellion against parents and society. Three studies of university students were carried out to investigate this issue (Hunsberger, 1980, 1983a; Hunsberger & Brown, 1984). These investigations, from two different corners of the world, were consistent in finding that apostasy is most strongly associated with weak emphasis on religion in the home. Although this work involved Canadian and Australian university students, the essential findings have been replicated elsewhere in studies of Mormons (Albrecht et al., 1988; Bahr & Albrecht, 1989) and Roman Catholics (Kotre, 1971), as well as in studies of more representative U.S. samples (Nelsen, 1981b; Wuthnow & Mellinger, 1978).

In Hunsberger's studies, no support was found for two of Caplovitz and Sherrow's (1977) hypothesized predisposing factors—symptoms of maladjustment, and a radical or leftist political orientation. In a study of more than 600 U.S. and Canadian college students, Brinkerhoff and Mackie (1993) found that apostates reported being less happy in their lives than did "converts" (people who grew up with no religious affiliation but who now identified with a religious group), "religious stalwarts" (people who maintained the same denominational affiliation from childhood to young adulthood), and "denominational switchers" (people who had changed denominational affiliation since childhood). However, apostates typically did not differ significantly from these other groups on measures of self-esteem or life satisfaction. Although Brinkerhoff and Mackie (1993) concluded that apostates "are less satisfied in life, [are] less happy and have lower self-esteem" (p. 252), the statistical evidence supports this conclusion only for the general happiness item mentioned above. Apostates did report a more liberal world view, in the sense that they were "less traditional" than the religious stalwarts.

Also, Hunsberger found weak evidence that apostates have poorer relationships with their parents; he suggested that the poorer relationships could be *either* a cause or a result of apostasy. However, according to other researchers, their data suggest that poor relationships with parents are more likely to precede disengagement from religion (Burris, Jackson, Tarpley, & Smith, 1996; Wilson & Sherkat, 1994). Therefore, it may be that such poor relationships contribute to disengagement, rather than vice versa. In a similar vein, there is some evidence that parental divorce (and possibly the accompanying poor family relationships) may make offspring more inclined to change religious identity or to leave religion altogether (Lawton & Bures, 2001).

Going against the Flow: "Amazing Apostates" and "Amazing Believers"

Not everyone is equally influenced by the socialization processes of parents, peers, education, and church/other factors as described in this chapter. Though there is strong evidence that most people who become religious believers or apostates are behaving quite consistently with socialization theory predictions (i.e., most religious believers come from homes where religion was relatively strongly emphasized and modeling was readily available; most apostates come from homes where religion was only weakly emphasized and parental modeling of religion was not strong), there are rare exceptions to the rule. For example, just 2% of Canadian weekly church attenders in 1991 were going to church "seldom or never" as youngsters (Bibby, 1993), and just 10 of 631 Canadian and U.S. college students (1.6%) identified with a religious denomination after reporting that they grew up with no religion (Brinkerhoff & Mackie, 1993).

This is consistent with research on "amazing believers" and "amazing apostates"—people who seem to contradict socialization predictions. After screening several thousand students at their respective Canadian universities, Altemeyer and Hunsberger (1997) could find only 1.4% who met their established strict criteria for "amazing apostates" (those who were in the bottom 25% on a measure of orthodoxy but in the top 25% on a measure of religious emphasis in the home while growing up), and only 0.8% who met their equally strict criteria for "amazing believers" (top 25% on orthodoxy, but bottom 25% on religious emphasis).

The 46 amazing apostates who were interviewed confirmed that they had generally rejected family religious teachings, in spite of strong socialization pressures to accept religious beliefs. They were unique people whose "search for truth" had led them to question many things, especially religious teachings, often from an early age. Many of these people reported initial guilt and fear about dropping their religious beliefs (consistent with the findings of Etxebarria, 1992), but in retrospect they believed that the benefits of leaving their religion far outweighed any costs involved. The 24 amazing believers interviewed were more likely to have had *some* religious training early in their lives (in spite of a general lack of religiousness in the home), to be influenced by friends or significant others, and to have "found religion" in an attempt to deal with crises in their lives. Emotional issues such as fear, loneliness, and depression seemed to drive many of the amazing believers' conversions. For example, some were attempting to escape from a dependence on drugs, alcohol, or sex; others were grappling with serious illness or tragedy in their lives.

In spite of the relatively small samples in this study, the findings are fairly clear and intriguing. A small percentage of people do seem to "go against the flow" and reject religion in spite of strong childhood religious emphasis and training; a smaller percentage of others become strongly religious in spite of having mostly nonreligious backgrounds. In the end, as rare as these amazing apostates and believers are, such "exceptions to the rule" can potentially help our general understanding of the religious socialization process. (A further discussion of nonbelievers is provided in Chapter 9.)

RELIGION AND IDENTITY DEVELOPMENT IN ADOLESCENCE

Some promising research has linked adolescent identity development with religion. Identity development has roots in Erikson's (1968, 1969) theory of psychosocial development, especially the importance of the appearance of a secure identity in adolescence (vs. the danger of role confusion). In theory, religion can be an important contributor to the process of establishing a secure identity (e.g., Erikson, 1964, 1965)—for example, by helping to explain existential issues, by providing a sense of belonging, and by offering an institutionalized opportunity for individuals to commit to a (religious) world view ("fidelity"). Four identity statuses have been proposed by Marcia (1966; Marcia, Waterman, Matteson, Archer, & Orlofsky, 1993), based on the extent to which crisis (exploring alternatives) and commitment (investment in a particular identity) are apparent in adolescent lives (see Table 5.1).

Evidence confirms that the emergence of identity is a progressive developmental process, with "foreclosed" and "diffused" statuses the least developed, and relatively immature. The most advanced or mature status is "achieved," with "moratorium" being intermediate (e.g., Waterman, 1985). That is, a "diffused" young person (who has done little or no exploring

TABLE 5.1. Marcia's Classification of Identity Status Based on Crisis and Commitment

Crisis	Commitment	
	Present	Not present
Present	Achieved	Moratorium
Not present	Foreclosed	Diffused

in the religious realm, and who has not made any firm religious commitments) would be considered to be relatively immature in terms of religious identity development. But someone who has done a lot of thinking about (exploring) religious issues and conflicts, and as a result has decided to accept (commit to) a particular religious ideology, would be accorded the more mature "achieved" identity status.

Several studies have indicated that more religious commitment tends to be linked with more general identity achievement and foreclosure—the identity statuses that involve ideological commitment (Markstrom-Adams, Hofstra, & Dougher, 1994; Tzuriel, 1984). But these findings have not always been clear-cut, possibly because many studies have relied on self-reported church attendance, which is not necessarily a good measure of religious ideological commitment (see, e.g., Markstrom, 1999). Also, since women are more likely than men to make a commitment in the religious realm (Pastorino, Dunham, Kidwell, Bacho, & Lamborn, 1997), failure to control for gender could contaminate results (see also Alberts, 2000). In spite of such gender differences in commitment, however, some evidence indicates that both genders use the identity process similarly in the religious domain (e.g., Archer, 1989).

Some studies have examined links between religious orientation measures and identity status. Markstrom-Adams and Smith (1996) found that the Intrinsic religious orientation was associated with achievement status (apparently because of the greater religious commitment of intrinsically oriented persons), and that the Extrinsic orientation was linked with diffused identity status (apparently because of the lack of religious commitment and the lack of crisis or exploration for extrinsically oriented people). However, measurement of religious commitment and crisis was limited to the Intrinsic and Extrinsic religious orientation scales (Allport & Ross, 1967), and these might not be good measures of the extent of religious commitment and (especially) crisis.

In a study of college students, Fulton (1997) also found that Intrinsic orientation scores were linked with identity achievement (and Extrinsic orientation scores with foreclosure), as expected. In addition, Quest scores (see Batson et al., 1993) were associated with moratorium status, apparently because of the doubt exploration inherent in the Quest measure. However, a more recent investigation found no link between identity status and Quest scores (Klassen & McDonald, 2002).

Hunsberger et al. (2001a) attempted to improve on previous studies' limited measures of religious commitment, and especially of religious exploration/crisis. They carried out two studies, one of high school students before and after they finished high school, and another of university students. Their results generally confirmed the expected links between identity status and religion. For example, religious commitment was stronger for students with more achieved and foreclosed identities, and commitment was weaker for students with more diffused and moratorium identities. Also, religious crisis was positively correlated with moratorium (but not achievement) scores, and negatively related to foreclosure and diffusion scores. Finally, this research indicated that specific styles of religious crisis (belief-confirming vs. belief-threatening consultation for religious doubts) were also usually linked with identity status, as predicted (see Research Box 5.4).

In summary, recent findings suggest that ego identity status is relevant to the study of religion and could help us to understand religious development, especially during adolescence. It is possible that variables such as right-wing authoritarianism affect both religious development and more general identity development in this regard, since high right-wing authoritarianism is linked with both greater religiousness (e.g., Altemeyer, 1996) and foreclosed identity status (Peterson & Lane, 2001); however, the exploration of such relationships is left to future studies. Also, because the resolution of religious doubt is potentially an important task in the development of a secure identity in adolescence and young adulthood,

---

RESEARCH BOX 5.4. Adolescent Identity Formation: Religious Exploration and Commitment (Hunsberger, Pratt, & Pancer, 2001a)

These researchers used a Religious Doubts scale (Altemeyer, 1988) in order to tap religious "crisis" (see McAdams, Booth, & Selvik, 1981) more directly than had been done in previous studies. They also included several ways of looking at religious commitment (e.g., self-reported current religiousness, church attendance), to ensure that any relationships found were not unique to a specific measure of commitment. Using the Objective Measure of Ego Identity Status (Adams, Bennion, & Huh, 1989) in two studies, they found that high school and university students revealed links between broadly defined identity status, and religious crisis and exploration generally, as expected. People with more achieved and foreclosed identities did score higher, and people with more diffused and moratorium identities did score lower, on measures of religious commitment. Also, moratorium status was related to more religious doubting, as expected, but achievement status was (surprisingly) not linked with doubting. The authors speculated that religious doubting may have occurred earlier in more achieved people's lives, and therefore may not have been adequately detected by the measures used. Finally, lower levels of doubting ("religious crisis") should be evident among more foreclosed and diffused people, but this was true only for foreclosed identity status. To summarize, these two studies then offer general (but not complete) support for hypothesized links between religion and identity status.

These same studies also investigated the ways in which people dealt with religious doubts by means of the BCC and BTC scales, discussed earlier in this chapter. The authors suggested that BCC and BTC scores would be related to identity status, based on Berzonsky and Kuk's (2000) finding that identity status is related to the ways in which people process information. The evidence generally supported their hypotheses. For example, higher achievement scores were linked with both higher BCC and higher BTC scores, and diffusion was associated with both lower BCC and lower BTC scores. Finally, longitudinal data in the second study allowed Hunsberger et al. to assess relationships over time. Again, relationships were generally (though not always) as expected. For example, foreclosure scores significantly predicted reduced BTC scores and less overall religious doubting 2 years later. These findings have been interpreted as partially supporting Berzonsky and Kuk's (2000) suggestion that identity status is linked with social-cognitive information-processing styles within the religious realm.

it is possible that information-processing styles contribute to young people's approaches to religious doubts, and ultimately to the ways in which such doubts are resolved.

Another issue that needs to be addressed is the extent to which identity status measures are "contaminated" by content that asks explicitly about religion, since one-third of the content of some identity status measures (e.g., Adams, Bennion, & Huh, 1989) is in the religious domain. That is, to what extent are the links reported between identity status and religion a result of common religious content in measures of these two supposedly different concepts? In this regard, it may be inappropriate to think in terms of overall identity status, since there is some indication that identity development can be quite uneven in different content domains. For example, De Haan and Schulenberg (1997) concluded that covariation between religious and political identity was low and inconsistent. Skorikov and Vondracek (1998) found that religious identity development lagged behind vocational identity development. Possibly researchers should focus on *religious* identity development, with purer (religious identity) measures that are not complicated by content from other domains (e.g., politics, career).

OVERVIEW

In this chapter, we have focused on a socialization approach to the development of adolescent and young adult religiousness. There are certainly other ways of conceptualizing religious development as children move into adolescence; as we have seen, however, much evidence is consistent with a socialization perspective, especially one based on social learning theory. Empirical work confirms that parents are the strongest influences on adolescent religiousness, though their influence seems to decrease as young people grow older. Other religious socialization agents have sometimes been presumed to be active, such as peer groups, education, and the church.

Generational effects occur, such that adolescents and young adults are "less religious" than older adults. However, although religiosity has apparently decreased substantially in many parts of the world, religion itself is hardly on the verge of disappearing. The United States seems to be an exception to the "decreasing religiousness" rule, since rates of regular church attendance have been relatively stable, with about 30–40% of high school seniors reportedly attending weekly. Furthermore, there appears to be considerable interest in topics of religion and spirituality among college students.

Some evidence suggests that the religious socialization process may affect the ways in which people think about existential religious issues. Research on integrative complexity has indicated that more orthodox and fundamentalist persons think less complexly about such issues. Possibly these stylistic thought differences are related to the ways in which people resolve conflicts, questions, and doubts concerning religious teachings. The evidence suggests that questions and doubts about religion are common (though certainly not intense, on average) during adolescence and early adulthood, and that those with more doubts tend to think in more complex terms about religious doubts and conflicts. Work on apostasy has suggested that leaving the family religion is generally consistent with socialization explanations of religious development. People who abandon the family faith tend to come from homes where religion was either ignored or only weakly emphasized. Thus apostates often simply "drift" a bit further away from a religion that was not important to their family members in the first place. Apostates tend to have poorer relationships with their parents, and cognitive factors are probably involved in apostasy to some extent, since apostates are more likely to question, doubt, and debate religious issues earlier in their lives than are nonapostates.

Other research has linked ego identity status with religious exploration/crisis and commitment in predicted ways. Apparently religious development is associated with Erikson's hypothesized establishment of a secure identity, as opposed to role confusion, in adolescence. Moreover, evidence suggests that identity status can be moderately successful in predicting religious doubt levels and ways of dealing with doubts 2 years later; this is consistent with the suggestion that unique information-processing styles may characterize different identity statuses.

The research reviewed in this chapter constitutes a considerable body of knowledge concerning religious socialization processes. We continue to learn more about how young people become religious, how they think about religion, and why they sometimes leave a religious background. However, research has tended to focus on description rather than explanation. It *is* important to understand the integral role of parents (and the relative unimportance of some other factors) in the religious socialization process. It *is* valuable to gain insight into the thought processes and correlates of religious doubt and apostasy. It *is* worthwhile to devise typologies of apostates. And so on. But it is also important that we generate testable explanations concerning *why* these processes occur as they do, and what the causative factors are with respect to religious development. Too much attention has been devoted to the social correlates of religious socialization and religious change, and not enough attention has been focused on factors within individuals (e.g., styles of thinking, ways in which people approach and resolve information that challenges their beliefs). Correlational studies, which are the norm in this area, can help us to understand the processes involved, but do little to clarify cause-and-effect relationships. The issues discussed in this chapter therefore have considerable potential for future research.

CHAPTER 6

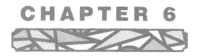

Adult Religious Issues

I consider myself a Hindu, Christian, Moslem, Jew, Buddhist, and Confucian.

Anyone who thinks sitting in church can make you a Christian must also think sitting in a garage can make you a car.

Among all my patients in the second half of life—that is to say, over thirty-five—there has not been one whose problem in the last resort was not that of finding a religious outlook on life. . . . none of them has really been healed who did not regain his religious outlook.

Religion reveals itself in struggling to reveal the meaning of the world.[1]

Culture and habit have set the start of adulthood at 18 or 21 years. Such ages are little more than widely accepted practical cues that are often used in our society and culture. They frequently provide definitions in the law, such as when someone may obtain a driver's license or vote in an election. Similarly, society has a history of designating age 65 as a transition point into the "elderly" category. In the United States, this might legally define when someone gets Social Security or various kinds of medical care. For simplicity's sake, we accept adulthood as extending roughly from 18 to 65 years of age.

Given these labeling issues, we normally think of certain behaviors as representative of adulthood. Here we find love, sex, and marriage; concern with work and economic matters; and involvement in politics and major social issues. In addition, religious thinking and activity probably attain their greatest complexity in adulthood.

THE FAITH OF AMERICAN ADULTS

Questioning People: Surveys

When we need information about people, we ask them questions. Commonly, we conduct surveys that very often deal with thousands of people. Kosmin, Mayer, and Keysar (2001) questioned over 50,000 persons in the American Religious Identification Survey (ARIS),

---

[1]These quotations come, respectively, from the following sources: Gandhi, quoted in Peter (1977, p. 450); Garrison Keillor (available at *www.goodreads.com/quotes* 5979); Jung (1933, p. 229); S. H. Miller, quoted in Simpson (1964, p. 204).

which replicated and extended the National Survey on Religious Identification (NSRI) of 1990. The most recent large-sample effort by the Pew Research Center's Forum on Religion and Public Life, the Religious Landscape Survey, did a phone sampling of 35,071 people in 2014 (Pew Research Center, 2015b). The 2012 General Social Survey (GSS) assessed 4,820 people on 1,030 variables. Efforts like these are tributes to the scholars and organizations involved in religious research (General Social Survey, 2016).

Surveys such as the ARIS and the NSRI are conducted by university centers, public service groups, and businesses (e.g., the famous Gallup Poll organization). This is a complex research area, and diverse findings may simply be functions of slight differences in the wording of questions that survey researchers employ. Variation in samples could be present, for example, in terms of the sections of the country where people live, rural versus urban residency, educational level attained, economic status, gender, or age. A Gallup Poll recently looked at adults who stated that they had no religious preference and found, instead of ARIS's 14%, only 10% in this category. Since the Gallup Poll's data go back to 1968, the pollsters found a trend for those taking this stance to have increased from 3 to 10% over a 37-year period (Winseman, 2005).

Religious Identifications

Defining the parameters of religion in the American cultural milieu is not as simple as one might think. For example, we may talk about Judaism and Christianity without recognizing that each has its formal denominations and subgroups (sects and even cults). In the United States, these major designations are expressed in over 200 classifications. Membership has been determined in different ways, which result in different numbers.[2]

The Association of Statisticians of American Religious Bodies (ASARB, 2014) used two different approaches in its 2010 U.S. Religion Census. Focusing on congregations by counties, the ASARB found that one procedure resulted in 344,894 congregations, and the other in 335,397. Respectively, the member counts were 150,596,792 and 105,460,999. Obviously, a considerable proportion of the American population is formally affiliated with religious bodies. Although, again, differences in methodology raise questions about assessment accuracy, such numbers clearly suggest the potential power and importance of religion in both U.S. society and Americans' individual lives. As we will shortly see, some of the differences between percentages may be small, but when researchers are questioning thousands of people, a little variation when generalized to a large population may be very meaningful.

Before going further, let us look at the state of religion in America today. Tables 6.1 and 6.2 offer us recent selected data that we discuss further.

Is Mainline Religion Weakening?

In 1956, the Gallup organization defined a possible maximum religiosity score of 1,000. At that time, the American score was 746; by 2004, however, it was down to 648 (Lyons, 2005). The Pew Forum's Religious Landscape Survey found that 28% of American adults left the faith in which they were reared to affiliate with another religious body or none at all (Pew

---

[2]We have not commented on non-Western faiths (Islam, Buddhism, Hinduism, etc.), the numbers of which in the United States are changing rapidly due to immigration.

TABLE 6.1. A Selective View of the State of American Religion in 2014, Compared with the 2007 Survey

Groups	2014	2007	Change
Christian groups	70.6	78.4	−7.8
Catholic	20.8	23.9	−3.1
Protestant mainline	14.7	18.1	−3.4
Evangelical	25.4	26.3	−0.9
Non-Christian groups	5.9	4.7	+1.2
Jewish	1.9	1.7	+0.2
Muslim	0.9	0.4	+0.5
All other faiths	3.2	2.6	+0.6
Unaffiliated	22.8	16.1	+6.1
Atheist	3.1	1.6	+1.5
Agnostic	4.0	2.4	+1.6
Nothing	15.8	12.1	+3.7

Note. Data are population percentages. Survey sample = 35,071 adults. Data from Pew Research Center (2015b).

TABLE 6.2. Gallup Polls: Some Feelings over Time about Religion in the United States

Issue	2013–2015[a]	2007	2000–2001[b]
Religious preference			
Protestant	37	51	52
Catholic	23	23	25
Jewish	2	3	2
None	16	11	8
Confidence in religious institutions			
Great deal/quite a lot	42	53	56
Satisfaction with organized religion			
Very/somewhat satisfied	53	56	64
Importance of religion in personal life			
Very/fairly important	78	82	88
Religion is increasing its influence	21	33	36
Member of church/synagogue	59	61	68
Attended church/synagogue last 7 days	39	41	44
Religion can answer all/most problems	56	59	65
Belief in God	86	92 (1967)[c]	98 (1954)[c]
Bible is the actual/inspired word of God	75	82	76

Note. Data are percentages. Data from *www.gallup.com/poll/1690/religion.aspx.*
[a]The dates for various items range from 2013 to 2015.
[b]The dates for various items range from 2000 to 2001.
[c]This question was last previously given at these dates.

Research Center, 2013a). Christian groups lost 7.8% of their members between 2007 and 2014 (Pew Research Center, 2015b). Similar indications have been reported by the Gallup Poll. In 2000–2001, 88% of Gallup's respondents felt that religion was personally fairly or very important. By 2013–2015, this percentage was down to 78%. In regard to American life in general, 63% believed in 2000–2001 that religion was losing its influence. By 2013, this number had actually increased by 13%, to 76%. During this same period, church and synagogue membership dropped by 11%, from 70 to 59% (The Gallup Poll, 2014). Atheists and agnostics increased from 4.0 to 7.1%, almost doubling their numbers. Given the multiple thousands of persons polled, numbers like these are quite meaningful. Apparently these data suggest that measured "religiousness" is decreasing. Finally, relative to persons without any religious identification, "nones" Pew Research tells us that in 2007 16% of adult Americans fell into this category; by 2015, 23% did so (Lipka, 2015).

This overall trend may be due to many factors; however, three stand out. The first is a reduction of confidence in religious institutions, leading some to identify themselves as "spiritual but not religious," as noted in earlier chapters. Another possible influence may be inferred from questions about the ethical standards of clergy; these are thought to result primarily from the sex abuse scandals of a small percentage of Roman Catholic priests. A third intriguing reason advanced by Wulff (2011) is that church membership is declining because pastors' sermons have become increasingly irrelevant to modern life. Current preaching seems to have little or no applicability to a contemporary high-powered electronic world where one sees virtually unbelievable developments (in modern medicine, robotics, astrophysical investigations of other worlds, drones, etc.). These may be affecting personal faith, primarily among younger adults. Research into such a possibility is worth pursuing.

There are indications that the percentage of those identifying themselves as Christians has also been decreasing. In 1990, it was 87%, 10% higher than a decade later (U.S. Bureau of the Census, 2008). The Pew Research Center (2015) claimed that such identification dropped 7.8% between 2007 and 2014. In the same period, Protestants and Catholics no longer religiously affiliated went from 16.1% to 22.8%. Unfortunately, little research has been directed toward the reasons for either the declines or the increases just noted. The Gallup Poll reported an investigation of the latter, albeit rather superficially (Newport, 2007b). This study found that 23% of churchgoers claim they attend for "spiritual growth and guidance," and another 20% feel that church attendance "keeps them rounded/inspired" (p. 2). Some are there simply because it is their faith (15%); others attend because they desire to worship God (15%) or just believe in God or religion (12%). We cannot dismiss the influence of habit, which probably accounts for this last statistic. Clearly, more detailed interview questioning is necessary if we are to understand what is actually taking place.

In 1990, the NSRI reported that 86% of the population was Christian; 11 years later, in the ARIS of 2001, 77% of respondents stated that they were Christians (Kosmin et al., 2001). The 2008 Pew work suggests a flattening out of this decline, with 78% designating themselves as Christians. This dropped to 70.6% by 2013–2014. Still, there seem to be noteworthy shifts in the numbers claiming to be unaffiliated with Christianity or any other type of religion. In the 1990 NSRI, 8% fell into this category; however, by 2001, the corresponding percentage in the ARIS was 14%, and the 2014 Pew data place it at 22.8%. Without question, this appears to be an important trend that calls for further research and explanation—especially since we might hypothesize that adults claiming to be atheistic or agnostic would be responding in a socially undesirable manner. Certainly in the realm of politics, to deny or even qualify a religious stance would be unacceptable in the contemporary United States.

Even though those directly involved with churches make much of relatively small changes in attendance, little work has been undertaken to identify and comprehend a wide range of factors that influence attendance, including mobility of attendees, income modifications, lifestyle changes, variation in beliefs, and personal importance of religion. Gallup (News Gallup, 2018) offers data regarding this last possibility. Reporting in 2-year intervals from 1993 to 2017, we see increases and decreases from no change to 5%. Over the total 24-year period, a reduction of 7% was found. This is an area requiring much further study.

Classifying Adult "Generations"

A popular way of understanding adult religious identifications and expressions adopts the notion that people fall into various age cohorts or generational classifications. Three groups currently existing in the United States have been popularly referred to as the "baby boomers," "Generation X," and the "millennials." The first cohort is defined as those born in the post-World War years, between 1946 and 1964; the second is roughly identified as those coming into the world from 1964 to about 1980; and their successors are the millennials, born between about 1980 and 1995. Labeling these cohorts in this way implies that each possesses a distinctive character, which, of course, is untrue. General propensities with much overlap are more realistic.

Religion and the Baby Boomer Generation

The "baby boomers" stand out because of their radical stance in the 1960s and 1970s against authority per se, the Vietnam War, and long-accepted traditions in many areas (ranging from education and politics to personal appearance). Their involvement in drugs, social communes, and "hippie" subcultures also distinguished them. Actually, those who engaged in these activities constituted a rather small minority of the population in their age brackets, albeit a very noticeable one. At this writing, the baby boomers are entering the ranks of the elderly, since the oldest of them are now in their early 70s. Certainly, they have demonstrated the struggles adults can go through in establishing a satisfactory religious stance. Many baby boomers pursued spirituality outside the religious mainstream through alternative religions, Transcendental Meditation, Scientology, and many other New Age possibilities. With respect to faith, the noted sociologist of religion Wade Clark Roof (1993) has called them *A Generation of Seekers*. In the first stage of his major study of boomer religion, Roof (1993) employed a sample of 1,599 people in four states spanning the nation. A second phase utilized 536 people who were in the initial sample. He distinguished three groups: "loyalists," "returnees," and "dropouts." Loyalists, as the word implies, stayed within America's customary religious mold; the returnees often deviated considerably in their personal experiments with faith before rejoining the religious establishment; the dropouts either moved away from or were never affiliated with mainstream religious institutions. These data indicate that conservative Protestants and Catholics, particularly the most orthodox religious subgroups, were more successful in keeping their members as active religionists than were mainline Protestants. In addition, about twice as many of the latter shifted to different faiths. These effects may be an expression of the power of conservative religious bodies. Still, Roof (1993) found that over 60% of all the young adults with conventional religious backgrounds had dropped out of their churches. When they did come back, 13% moved toward fundamentalism, and 21% were denoted as conservative (technically, "evangelical moderates"). Anderson (2008) labels returnees "baby boomerangs," and, like Roof, he views them as seekers of spirituality. He further claims that the role of raising their own children helped bring the "boomerangs" back to established churches. One should not underestimate the significance of family life in connecting people to religious organizations.

We see some possible contradictions when we look at attitudes toward churchgoing and actual weekly attendance among Roof's participants. For example, when asked whether a good Christian must attend church, a strong majority indicated "no." Agreement percentages ranged up to 94%, however. Churchgoing became an issue of personal determination and choice. Roof (1993) described this as the "new voluntarism" (p. 110).

Perkins (1991) studied a subset of the baby boomers, called "yuppies" ("young, upwardly mobile, urban professionals"). On the average, though religious commitment conflicted with yuppie values, many yuppies identified with traditional faiths. In addition, a religious stance was positively associated with a sense of happiness. Greater insight into the religious perspectives and needs of the yuppies would have nicely supplemented Roof's research.

In allied work, Roof (1990) compared older and younger boomers. The younger group revealed a more conservative Christian stance, although it included fewer loyalists, fewer returnees, and more religious dropouts.

Continuing his research in the mid-1990s, Roof (1999) administered a third round of questions to 409 of the 536 respondents who had participated in the second stage. Now he identified five subcultures: "dogmatists," "born-again believers," "mainstream believers," "metaphysical believers," and "seekers and secularists." The complexity of the religious scene for the baby boomers was evident. Even though such tendencies were probably always present among American religionists, they became most obvious in the boomer generation. Religion was extended well beyond immediate church experience to such issues as love, justice, the environment, and a host of similar concerns. Boomers now became active and involved in politics and government, and it is easy to perceive their influence today. Still, their search for spiritual meaning was troubled. They manifested strong inclinations to move on, as only 43% of returnees were still actively religious after 7 years. Of the 86% of strong believers in 1989, only one-third held such a position in 1996 (Johnson, 2001).

Using poll data, Waxman (1994) studied a sample of 801 Jewish baby boomers. Unfortunately, very few questions were employed. On the surface, this group seemed quite different from those studied by Roof. If, however, we assume some correspondence between Roof's category of "loyalists" (Protestants and Catholics identifying with their traditional faith) and Waxman's "personal importance" distinction, Jewish identification among Waxman's respondents appeared greater than that of traditional Catholics or Protestants among Roof's Christians. From 31 to 39% of Roof's groups were classified as loyalists, whereas Waxman found that 85% of his sample regarded being Jewish as important to some degree.

Sometimes one hears the term "cultural Jew," which may be valid here. Christianity is rather strongly tied to religion, whereas Judaism often refers to both a faith and a culture, especially in the United States. One rarely if ever hears of "Christian Americans," but "Jewish Americans" is a common referent (Goldstein & Goldscheider, 1968). Though being Jewish was considered important by Waxman's baby boomers, half of them (49.8%) were not married to Jews; by contrast, almost 80% of an older comparison sample of 46- to 64-year-olds had Jewish spouses. This favors the "cultural Jew" argument, rather than one based on conformity to Jewish religious principles.

Neither the work of Perkins (1991) nor that of Waxman (1994) approaches the depth of Roof's (1993) effort, yet we can easily ask for more. Interview data are excellent for the development of hypotheses that can be quantitatively assessed. As poignant as the struggles of individuals are, they point to subgroups that need further delineation and exploration. Studies of background motivational and experiential factors are largely lacking. Among Jews, distinctions among Reform, Conservative, and Orthodox affiliations need to be examined. Whether Jewish or Christian groups are studied, there are seekers, rejecters, and those who are simply apathetic about religion. There is much more to be learned about the life histories of such persons.

Generation X Religion

Though the baby boomers represented a rather sharp break from their pre-World War II forebears, they largely aged back into a cultural quietude that accepted traditional values. Rarely, however, do people totally leave behind the hopes of their younger years; hence Roof (1993) and others have stressed boomers' desires for self-improvement, plus their continuing search for life's basic meanings. Their temporal followers, "Generation X" or, more popularly, "Gen X"—seem to be employing a similar adaptive process by putting forth both conservative and liberal feelers for a future that is not easy to define. We are probably observing here a general tendency to seek self-understanding, regardless of age.

Overall, the Gallup Poll index of leading religious indicators showed a considerable decline from 1956 to 2004 (Lyons, 2005). Except for minor shifts since the late 1990s in attitudes toward the Bible and the existence of God, the boomers and Gen X look alike (Newport, 2006a, 2007b). More boomers than their Gen X successors see religion as very important (44% vs. 34%), and more boomers describe themselves as religious (35% vs 27%). The Gen X respondents appear comparable in their aspirations to the boomers when they were younger.

Additional detailed questioning is necessary, as potential disagreements keep surfacing in the polls. Beaudoin (1998) stresses that Gen X focuses on personal experience and feels that this experience should be spiritually expressed. This generation is, however, described as challenging Christianity or more broadly institutionalized faith, according to The Barna Group (2007). This organization conducted a study of 16- to 29-year-olds. Eighty-four percent expressed some degree of negativism toward Christianity, with only 3% being favorable toward evangelicals. "Half of young churchgoers said they perceive Christianity to be judgmental, hypocritical and too political" (The Barna Group, 2007, p. 2). Whereas approximately 75% of boomers identified themselves as Christians, only about 60% of Gen X'ers did.

Miller and Miller (2000), in attempting to define Gen X religion, emphasize that it is not expressed in any simple manner. Basically, they recognize that a so-called "generation" includes people who evidence their faith in many different ways. Because of this, Flory (2000) has moved to a higher level in order to characterize religionists in the Gen X age range. Like the boomers, Gen X'ers are viewed by Flory as a deeply spiritual generation searching for the fundamental meanings and purposes on which they feel their existence is premised. Although they are disinclined to accept the view that traditional religious avenues can satisfy their needs—Miller and Miller (2000) have described them as "bruised by their parents and disappointed by their society" (p. 10)—Gen X'ers do appeal to organized religion for structure and authority. This fits well with Flory's (2000) characterization of this group as rootless, yet one that seeks an authentic religious identity via a personal anchoring of the self in the community via their church connections. Though variety and diversity are endemic among Gen X'ers, they appear to avoid traditional religious orientations in favor of newer churches that employ current music and media to aid the search for personal spiritual experience. Much of this sounds similar to what the young boomers wanted in order to validate their own individuality away from community existence. In contrast, Generation X builds on a community base—but, rather than that of their elders, one that represents contemporary styles of living. Implied in much of this work is the suggestion that religious conservatism positively relates to age.

Much was discussed earlier regarding those who are unaffiliated. If we look at this group from the Silent Generation (born 1928–1945) through the baby boomers, Generation X and the millennials, there is an obvious major and orderly increase from 2007 to 2014. The Unaffiliated increase from 11% (Silent Generation) to 36% (Younger Millennials). Clearly data such as this indicates a great need to find the cause for a growing tendency toward unaffiliation (Pew Research Center, 2015).

Basically, we have been observing the foundations and effects of sociocultural change over the last 70 or so years. The psychology of religion must be direct its efforts in order to understand the plight of people in our time.

RELIGIOUS BELIEFS AND BEHAVIORS

In essence, we have been examining how religion has been collectively structured. Beliefs range from the almost universal to specifics associated with denominations, sects, and cults within sociocultural units of every magnitude. However, very little research has done more than simply determine the numbers of people who accept such notions as miracles, heaven, hell, and the Devil. Surveys often yield quite different estimates, as if respondents are not sure what they should believe. For example, in 2007 the Baylor Religious Survey (BRS) reported that only 32% of its sample felt that miracles occur. Neither the Gallup organization (Newport, 2007b) nor the GSS asked this question. As for belief in the devil, the BRS number was 53.6% in 2007, but Gallup that same year found 70.0%. Respectively these same organizations claimed 62.3% and 81.0% for heaven. Variation this great raises all sorts of doubts and possibilities about concepts' meanings, samples, and questions' reliability. Rather than speculate about these and other similar observations, let us begin with a focus on the most well-researched domain—namely, belief in God.

Belief in God

The concept of God is without question the most central consideration in Western religion and has been studied by anthropologists and historians back to possible prehistoric origins. Probably the most recent scholarly effort has been made by Sheridan (2014), a professor emeritus in engineering and psychology at the Massachusetts Institute of Technology. His approach is fully scientific, as he interprets the idea of God in a totally nonreligious manner. His goal is to be so exact that no room is allowed for theological, counter theological, or emotionally based arguments. Sheridan is, however, not at war with religion or religionists. The psychological approach we pursue here simply attempts to be as objective as possible. In both realms, the referent "God" is conceptually highly variable.

Granted that problems of sampling over the years produce slight variations in percentages, one wonders whether belief in God may be decreasing in the United States. A few decades ago, the polls regularly provided estimates of 95–98%. Gallup and Lindsay (1999) found 95% averring such a belief. In 2004, a Gallup Poll observed 90%, and in 2007 belief in God was down to 86% (Newport, 2007b). This was still true in 2014–2015. The BRS reported in 2007 that only 63.4% of its sample had "no doubts that God exists." Another 13.6% was simply unsure. If God is associated with alternative language ("universal spirit," etc.), we are back to 86% (The Gallup Poll, 2014)

If we look at belief in God in other parts of the world, Greeley's (2002) landmark study of European nations indicates that Poland (with 94%) and Ireland (with 95%) are comparable to the United States. This contrasts sharply with the findings of Burkimsher (2014), whose data are much more recent. Most countries examined by Burkimsher reported numbers in the 50–70% range in response to these items.

The Significance of God Belief

Table 6.2 has shown that more adults believe in God than in any other religious referent. We must first recognize that people hold many different notions and ideas about the deity (Gorsuch, 1968; Spilka, Armatas, & Nussbaum, 1964). These references are only the initial two in an extensive literature on how people perceive and define God. The Spilka et al. (1964) work found that an Old Testament view of a vindictive and punishing God was quite widely held. Closely following was an image of a less punishing deity, but one who evaluates behavior along an unyielding–permissive continuum. A third view stresses the "omni" quality of the deity—omnipresent, omniscient, and omnipotent. These were succeeded by numerous other possibilities, which emphasized "patient," "eternal," "sovereign," "holy," "divine," and other widely held views. Building on this initial work, Gorsuch (1968) found alternative overlapping definitions that focused on two sets of traditional Christian views, plus three others (see Research Box 6.1). Given that this research conducted over 50 years ago demonstrated the complexity of God beliefs, it is surprising that extremely little research has since been carried out on correlates of specific understandings of God concepts. Hill and Edwards (2013) have undertaken the most recent analyses of work in this area among adults.

Apparently our images and ideas of God are sensitive to conceptual analyses ranging from the psychological to the anthropological. In a sense, they show such distinctions to be somewhat arbitrary. For example, one recent study reveals that people in harsh living environments are likely to believe in moralizing gods (Botero et al., 2014). In other words, history, ecology, and social conditions may be involved in religious interpretations. The "how" and "why" of such involvement have yet to be determined. Since psychologists often fail to comprehend the complexity of environments, the psychology of religion may suffer as a result. We must keep in mind that religion reaches far beyond the individual.

Shifting to a more traditional psychological approach, we may first note that those who believe that their undesirable desires and behavior are biologically determined are more likely to be angry with God: He "did it." Motives viewed as environmentally created correlate with a more favorable attitude toward God (Grubbs & Exline, 2014b). Still, people are more likely to associate the deity with positive outcomes and Satan or the Devil with negative occurrences (Ray, Lockman, Jones, & Kelly, 2015). A recent illustration was provided by a Georgia school principal who made racist remarks and blamed the Devil for them (Holley,

---

RESEARCH BOX 6.1. The Conceptualization of God as Seen in Adjective Ratings (Gorsuch, 1968)

Refining the earlier work of Spilka, Armatas, and Nussbaum (1964), Richard Gorsuch selected 28 of their 63 adjectives and added 28 more to provide a broader basis for conceptualizing God. He had these evaluated for three degrees of descriptiveness of God by 585 respondents from eight Protestant denominations, as well as by Catholics, Jews, and a small number of respondents from other religious groups. Their ratings were then subjected to the multivariate statistical procedure known as "factor analysis." This provides a way of taking a large number of stimuli (here, the descriptive words) and grouping them into much smaller units of possible reliable tests or scales. This analysis further organized the data into several levels or orders of meaning. The final results were these meaningful concepts:

    I. Traditional Christian conceptions
      A. Companionable deity
        1. Evaluation
        2. Kindliness
        3. Relevancy
      B. Benevolent deity
        1. Lack of deistic-ness
        2. Eternality
        3. Kindliness
   II. Wrathfulness
  III. Omni-ness
  IV. Potently passive deity

These findings were compared to previous work, and a number of research possibilities were proposed. Unfortunately, these interesting and sophisticated findings have not resulted in further study.

2015). In some quarters, this attribution might have been seen as excusing her, but she lost her job.

A number of researchers have looked at the significant issue of God beliefs relative to life satisfaction (Granqvist & Kirkpatrick, 2008). This work found that God beliefs are positively affiliated with church attendance, among other possibilities. The latter is rarely statistically removed or controlled for, though one can see why it too is a favorable correlate of life satisfaction. This brings up the fact that the variety of religious beliefs and behaviors has not been exactingly studied, so that virtually any characteristic (e.g., prayer) is confounded with other aspects of faith plus the issue of test reliability.

A more general psychological approach stresses attachment theory (Kirkpatrick, 2005). Created by John Bowlby (1969), this framework has loosely been perceived as primarily appropriate to children. Though also discussed elsewhere in the present volume (see Chapters 3 and 4), it is best understood as a product of natural selection with lifelong significance. Kirkpatrick, an outstanding scholar, has applied it to religion and more specifically argued that "God 'really' is an attachment figure" (Kirkpatrick, 2005, p. 55). Though we cannot detail the thinking that justifies this simple statement, we strongly recommend that psychologists of religion read Kirkpatrick's very meaningful volume *Attachment, Evolution, and the Psychology of Religion.* Needless to say, it is cited a number of times in the present text. Let us look at a few recent examples of work stimulated by this approach.

Using a national sample of Presbyterians, Bradshaw, Ellison, and Marcum (2010) studied attachment to God and psychological distress. Distinguishing secure and anxious forms of attachment, they found that distress was negatively associated with the former and positively affiliated with the latter. A more focused study of alcohol usage, which may be viewed as an expression of distress, observed that an insecure attachment to God resulted in turning inward and away from traditional religion and God (Hernandez, Salerno & Bottoms, 2010). Such self-direction was tied to insecurity and alcohol usage; in contrast, those with secure God attachments drank less alcohol.

Kirkpatrick (2005) has also noted that Christian belief increases as risk-taking behavior lessens. This is supported by Ellison and McFarland (2011) with regard to gambling. Still more recent work argues that "thinking about God makes people bigger risk-takers" (Kupor, Laurin, & Levav, 2015, p. 374). Obviously, more work to resolve these questions needs to be undertaken. Attachment theory has yet to be explored in depth; however, these few examples show that it may have a rich potential.

The Acceptance and Rejection of Institutional Religion

Becoming Involved with Religious Institutions

There are many reasons for people to affiliate themselves with religious institutions. These range from an automatic, habitual continuation of family tradition to deep personal struggles with understanding one's place in life and society. A fine example of work in this area was carried out by Roberts and Davidson (1984), who recognized the importance of psychosocial factors in church involvement (see Research Box 6.2). These researchers utilized two major approaches to the problem: (1) the importance of religious meaning to the individual, and (2) religion as a social phenomenon (e.g., the significance of belonging to a church and relating to its members).

Choosing to become involved with a church is often quite complex. Meaning systems and social relationships are important and probably not independent of each other. For example, both may relate to socioeconomic status and to the nature of the church under consideration (Roberts & Davidson, 1984). Surprisingly, in this research, religious beliefs were the least important of a complex array of motivations. Because this effort was basically correlational, low variability worked against obtaining the kinds of data (correlation coefficients) that might better reveal the significance of religious beliefs. In addition, keep in mind that correlation does not imply causation. We also need researchers to replicate their findings, and assess the power of their tests not just offer us an uncorroborated result.

Utilizing a slightly different theoretical approach, Cornwall (1987) asked two basic questions: "How do adults come to their religious perspectives?" and "What maintains these outlooks?" Her answer to the first query was religious socialization by family and friends. Once this framework is established, a connection to a "personal community" of like-minded believers supports and strengthens one's attachment to a specific religious system.

O'Hara (1980) suggests some differences between Protestants and Catholics in why church participation persists from childhood to adult life. For Protestants, the dominant

RESEARCH BOX 6.2. The Nature and Sources of Religious Involvement
(Roberts & Davidson, 1984)

Seeking to answer the basic question of why people become involved in their church, Roberts and Davidson studied 577 members of two Methodist and two Baptist churches in relation to four sets of possible predictors of involvement. These were (1) one's personal meaning system, (2) social ties to church members, (3) sociodemographic factors, and (4) religious beliefs. Specifically, these variables were assessed as follows:

Meaning: How one makes sense out of the world—theism, science, nonreligious materialism, social humanism.
Social relations: Connections to other church members, a sense of belonging to the church community.
Demographic factors: Age, gender, socioeconomic status (education, occupation, income), denominational affiliation.
Religious beliefs: Beliefs in existence of God, divinity of Jesus, miracles, virgin birth, and life after death.

Using the statistical methods of correlation and path analysis, Roberts and Davidson observed a complex set of associations among the measures. Meaning and social relations were positively correlated, which suggested that others confirmed and supported one's personal meaning system. These two factors directly contributed most to church involvement. Religious beliefs were weakly and indirectly influential. Sociodemographic variables were also indirectly effective, largely through their influence on one's meaning system. Older church members and women tended to be most involved, but most important was membership in the liberal (Methodist) or conservative (Baptist) denomination being studied. Overall, meaning and social ties were the big determiners of church involvement. More research of this nature would help us understand further the connections among the predictor variables—in particular, the role of religious and social beliefs.

influence is "accommodation," or how one deals with the social pressures exerted by significant others. Second is meaning via cognition—namely, the degree to which the faith that is embraced resolves basic questions about life, death, God, and the supernatural. Third is socialization, or being part of a religious group that has established norms for religious belief and behavior. The order of these factors for Catholics is cognition, accommodation, and lastly socialization. These differences between Catholics and Protestants are probably functions of historically conditioned practices.

The processes of becoming and remaining involved in religion are similarly complex. Sociocultural influences operate on a large scale. Psychologically, we contend that religious behavior, belief, and experience are gratifying to the individual. Religion simply makes people feel good: It helps them resolve conflicts, answers fundamental questions, enhances their sense of control in life, and brings like-minded people together. One meta-analysis of 28 studies concluded that among adults, subjective well-being and religion are positively associated (Witter, Stock, Okun, & Haring, 1985). Apparently religious activity is more important than belief, but both contribute to the sense of self-satisfaction generated by religious participation. These positive feelings probably result from social integration, which, according to Durkheim (1915), makes life more meaningful.

Beliefs That Distinguish between Two Broad Patterns of Faith

Peter Benson (1988a, 1988b), a scholar known for studying the big problems in the psychology of religion, undertook extensive research on what he termed "mature faith." His approach employed the Intrinsic–Extrinsic distinction as formulated by Allport and Ross in 1967 (see Chapter 2). Mature faith has much in common with Allport's Intrinsic religious orientation— namely, a deep religious commitment that includes social sensitivity and "life-affirming values" (Benson, 1988a, p. 16). The latter constitute Saint Thomas Aquinas's classical duties to oneself, others, and God (Spilka, 1970). In mature faith, then, a healthy lifestyle is combined with an appreciation of human welfare, equality, personal responsibility, and what sounds like the role of faith in everyday life.

Utilizing thousands of respondents, Benson found religious maturity to be an outgrowth of literally being steeped in one's faith through family, early religious education, and affiliations throughout life with others who possess similar outlooks. Maternal and spousal influences (which may be translated into support and reinforcement) also appear to be central in maintaining strong attachments to religious principles and church doctrines (Benson, 1988b).

We can see that becoming truly involved with religious institutions has many facets, among which are the need for personal meaning, identification with a like-minded community, and (probably most important of all) a family background with ties that stress the pertinence of religious faith to the way life is lived. Undoubtedly, there is room for utilitarian attachments to religion, as Allport's concept of Extrinsic religious orientation conveys.

We've looked at a number of psychological factors that connect people to their faith— beliefs, cognitions, familial connections, and even personality inclinations. Let us, however, also recognize the broader social-scientific context. People prefer to associate with others who are like themselves ethnically (Pew Research Center, 2013a). Similarities such as ethnic identity, educational level achieved, age, and well-being (Barkan & Greenwood, 2003), as well as similar attitudes (pro- or anti-science, etc.; Evans, 2013), cannot be ignored. Political conservatism has also been examined. Without question, institutional religion cannot be arbitrarily separated from the complexities not only of psychology, but of the social order in which people exist.

Some Meanings and Correlates of Church Attendance

As we shift from examining belief to looking at behavior, the most obvious action suggesting religious attachment and commitment is church attendance. Many if not most people probably attend religious services because the practice was a regular family function (Green, 2014). In other words, churchgoing for such persons is an expected habitual practice, probably with little deep meaning. For other churchgoers it represents a true religious commitment. Their faith is intrinsic. For still others it is largely utilitarian and hence extrinsic, serving possibly social, economic, or other societal ends. In-depth research into the motives and correlates of attendance at services has yet to be done, though the relatively few efforts now available are tantalizing.

Studying almost 6,000 youths, Petts (2014) found that attending religious services with parents was positively associated with a personal sense of well-being. Other work has confirmed that attendance also relates favorably to physical health among both Christian and Jewish adults (Levin & Markides, 1986; Levin, 2015). A Baylor University Institute for Studies of Religion project found that over 5,000 Jewish adults who attended synagogue reported better health than nonattenders (Levin, 2015).

In addition, well-being and happiness have been examined in this research. Central in much of this work is the idea that church attendance is positively associated with social cohesion among those going to services. In other words, one becomes attached to companion attenders. This has been shown a number of times, especially among older attendees (Barkan & Greenwood, 2003; Childs, 2010). Childs (2010), however, suggests another factor in such satisfaction, namely, how positive people perceive relationships with God to be. The more favorable this appears to be, the stronger the attendance–happiness association.

We have briefly looked at the most obvious aspects of how people relate to their faith. Throughout history, religion has often been formalized and controlled by clergy and political authorities, in part to maintain power and control over the general population. Behavior has most often been defined by adherence to religious rules largely conveyed through attendance at services. This activity is supported by religious and spiritual beliefs and experiences that usually involve the messages of sermons. Central among such concerns is the idea of God plus Godly requirements and expectations about human behavior.

Deviation from the Traditional

Deviating individuals are often classified as atheists, agnostics, and apostates. Here let us focus on the last group, namely those who may still hold some feeling for religion or spirituality. Atheists and agnostics are usually viewed as rejecting such orientations (Streib & Klein, 2013). Simply put, "apostasy" denotes leaving the faith with which one has been associated. In other words, it largely refers to disaffiliation, as we have noted in Chapter 5. One may convert to a different religion, just drop out of a church, or simply reject religion *in toto*, embracing either agnosticism or atheism. Between 2008 and 2014, The Barna Group Frames project (2014) surveyed over 23,000 self-denoted Christians who were "unchurched" or "churchless," meaning that they had not attended a regular church service in the preceding 6 months. Utilizing this research, Barna and Kinnaman (2015) estimated that 114 million people fit this description. This does not mean that these people rejected religion. Throughout their lives, only 23% had never gone to a church except for some special occasion such as a marriage or funeral. The remaining 77% had been associated with one or more churches. Three-quarters owned a Bible, and about 60% had prayed during the week prior to responding to the poll (The Barna Group, 2014). Of these, 34% identified themselves as "deeply spiritual." Fifty-one percent claimed to be "actively seeking something better spiritually" (p. 3). Many if not most might best be described as "spiritual but not religious." Oppenheimer (2014) suggests that this characterization "isn't necessarily vague or wishy-washy. It's not nothing, although it may risk being everything" (p. A14). In other words, it is psychologically significant yet rather poorly defined. In many places throughout this volume, spirituality is discussed. It may be treated by some favoring this term as an avenue to apostasy, while others may still value much that traditional faith offers.

In studying this area, we need to direct our attention toward both the past and the future. Specifically, we need to ask *why* people put aside their previous religious identifications or commitments and select new alternatives. One study identified three kinds of "unchurched" Protestants (Perry, Davis, Doyle, & Dyble, 1980). Those regarded as "estranged" and "indifferent" held similar traditional beliefs, but differed in commitment: The latter just became inactive, whereas for the former, religion was no longer salient in their lives. This was also true for "nominal" Protestants, for whom traditional beliefs were irrelevant.

After interviewing respondents in six counties across the United States, Hale (1977) offered a scheme that demonstrates how complex the realm of unchurched individuals is. Table 6.3 details this framework. A system such as Hale's begs for rigorous, objective study, because there is a high likelihood that such categories might reflect personal and social dispositions for which religion is a convenient scapegoat or expression.

TABLE 6.3. A Taxonomy of Unchurched Individuals

Unchurched type	Description
Anti-institutionalists	See themselves as truly religious, "better Christians" (Hale, 1977, p. 40).
The boxed-in	Church was too restrictive.
The constrained	Feel limited by doctrinal rules.
The thwarted	Feel suppressed from growing by church insistence on conformity and dependence.
The independents	Independent, nonconformists.
The burned-out	Feel exhausted, drained, emptied.
The used	Feel exploited, worked over.
Light travelers	Feel no need to continue a deep commitment, just "take it easy."
The cop-outs	Never really committed, involved.
The apathetic	Can "take it or leave it."
The drifters	Establish no real attachments.
Happy hedonists	Either utilitarian or leisure-oriented; seek gratification.
The locked-out	Feel rejected or victimized.
The rejected	Claim that the church has not accepted them.
The neglected	Assert that the church ignores them.
The discriminated	Argue that the church is biased against them.
The nomads	Religious vagrants, expect to move on and up; casually attached.
The pilgrims	Seekers and searchers who believe.
The publicans	Self-righteous; feel "better than others." Can't find their "true faith" in church.
The scandalized	See power seekers, factions, and divisiveness in church.
True believers	Hold alternative or antichurch position.
Agnostics/atheists	Don't know if God exists, or fully reject the idea.
Deists/rationalists	Rely on reason, not revelation.
Humanists/secularists	Committed to human ideals outside of the church.
The uncertain	No reason for nonaffiliation.

Note. Data from Hale (1977).

Some of these characteristics are also present in a classificatory scheme proposed by Hoge (1988) for Catholic dropouts. Though there is overlap with Hale's (1977) framework, new, more personal and familial factors are described by Hoge, who further noted that dropout in his study was a function of both age and an orientation toward life. Those under 23 were mostly in the "family tension" group, where adolescent rebellion was expressed. In contrast, "weary" and "lifestyle" dropouts were commonly found among those older than 23. Obviously, problems with faith may evidence personal and social needs with which one struggles in early and middle adulthood.

The situation with Jews is noteworthy. The Pew Research Center's large Religious Landscape Survey surveyed 3,475 self-identified Jews and revealed considerable change in their religious commitment over the years (Pew Research Center, 2013c). From 1914 to 1927, 7% of Jews left Judaism. After 1980, this number increased to 32%. In other words, Jews who identified as such went from 93% down to 68%. When child rearing was examined, if both parents were Jewish, 96% of their children were raised Jewish, but with a non-Jewish spouse, the percentage dropped by 76% down to 20%. Before 1970, 17% of Jews married non-Jews; this number increased by 2013 to 58%. These data reveal a truly major reduction in Jewish identification, with an increase of those claiming to be atheist and agnostic. If these trends continue, this faith, which currently accounts for about 1.7% of the American population, may account for only 1% in a surprisingly short period of time.

Finding a New Faith: Switching Religions

Even though most people remain with the religion in which they were reared, there is a fair amount of movement across the major religious bodies. Some disagreement exists among the pollsters as to the level of switching. When examining movement from one major religion to another, the Pew Research Center (2009) reported that 28% shifted from the faith in which they were reared; when denominational switching within Protestantism was included, the number increased to 44%. Approximately 7% claimed that they were raised in unaffiliated homes, yet adults accounted for 16% of this group. Overall, the greatest shift occurred in the Catholic Church, which experienced a net loss of 7.5% of its members. The traditions that managed to hold on best to their childhood members were the Jews (76%), various Eastern Orthodox bodies (73%), and Mormons (70%). Catholics, with 68% remaining, came in fourth. Younger people were more likely to leave their faith altogether, while the oldest members usually sought another denomination within their general identification (e.g., Protestant). Unfortunately, there does not seem to have been any major study of the motives for switching. A number of smaller, focused investigations have been undertaken, however.

Research on religious switching is a troubled area. According to Flanagan (2015), the Pew Research Center claims that "about half of all Americans change their religious affiliation at least once in their lives" (p. 1). Confounding all of these estimates is the fact that faith is part of a much broader context that involves ethnicity, socioeconomic status, and geographic region.

For example, Albrecht and Bahr (1983) described some unexpected findings about those who either left Mormonism or abandoned their original churches to become Mormons. Most ex-Mormons simply became nonreligious. The next largest group of "leavers" turned to Catholicism, implying that they remained religiously conservative. Ex-Mormons may experience severe identity crises when they find that previous moral views may not be supported in their new socioreligious environment (McAlexander, Dufault, Martin, & Schouten, 2014). By contrast, most converts to Mormonism come from mainline Protestant bodies, and possess rather orthodox outlooks that the Mormon faith can effectively satisfy.

An interesting hypothesis is offered by Albrecht and Bahr (1983) in regard to either dropping out altogether or switching to a new faith. Switching may be seen as more deviant than dropping out. It means going public with a rejection of the previous identification (in this case, Mormonism). A switcher considers another group to be "better." A person who just drops out can, however, be viewed as a "lost soul" who has not found any real alternative. The first action can stimulate hostility; the second, pity from former coreligionists. The dropout may be considered potentially salvageable; the switcher may not be. One wonders whether pity might turn to rage and ostracism if a dropout publicly denies the existence of God. This could add even more insult to injury than switching. The major reason identified by Albrecht and Bahr for switching or leaving the church seemed to be disagreement with its teachings (40%). Another 38% of their respondents claimed to have found a more fulfilling faith. Nineteen percent of young adults fell into this last category, while only 9% of those between ages 50 and 64 acted similarly. Age thus appears as a possible stabilizing factor.

Hadaway (1980), using Gallup Poll data from national samples, also notes that switchers are mostly conservative religious seekers. The motivation to change is frequently associated with a religious experience, particularly among evangelicals. Apparently a period for integration of the meaning of the experience takes place during the process of reaffiliation into a group that values such encounters.

Institutional Disaffiliation

Simple institutional disaffiliation may occur for a number of reasons, not the least of which is the prevailing influence of secularization in modern society (Nelson, 1988). We have noted that some of these are suggested in the labels ("dropouts" and "unchurched") that researchers now normally apply to those who leave a church. These people often remain personally religious, but churches, temples, and synagogues no longer seem relevant to their lives in the modern world. Causes for this strain between individuals and religious institutions also reflect the degree of physical, social, and economic mobility that prevails in much of early and middle adulthood. People are often "too busy" to consider questions of ultimate meaning or even to feel a need to relate to a specific religious community. With respect to a wide variety of attitudes and beliefs, those who are religiously disengaged tend to be more liberal than churchgoers on many social, moral, and political issues (Nelson, 1988).

Regardless of the reasons for leaving formal religion behind, the tendency has increased in recent years, as already noted. Younger people do not see this as bad, while their older cohorts do. A third of U.S. adults under the age of 30 and a fifth of the overall public had no religious affiliation in 2012. Eleven percent saw this as good for American society, while 48% felt it was bad (Pew Research Center, 2013b). Unfortunately, we know very little of what this means from either personal or social perspectives.

Extreme Rejection: Atheism and Agnosticism

Atheism and agnosticism are indeed end points in the rejection of religion. A possible movement in this direction has recently been getting much recognition. A 2012 survey by the Pew Research Center (2013b) examined the "growth of the nonreligious." This work reported that "about one-fifth of the public overall—and a third of adults under age 30—are religiously unaffiliated" (p. 1). We have, however, noted that such lack of affiliation does not mean denial of the existence of a deity or, more vaguely, of a universal spiritual force or power. In addition, about a third of American adults do not consider themselves religious. As yet, though, the percentages of those openly identifying themselves as atheists or agnostics are much smaller: "Survey data from 2014 suggests that 3.1% of 'religious nones' claim to be atheists and 4.0% accept the agnostic label" (Lipka, 2015). Both these groups have been growing very slowly.

The prime reason for becoming an atheist appears to be the conflict between religion and science. Next comes the issue of "theodicy" (namely, trying to understand why evil exists). In third place, the phenomenal worldwide variety of faiths and their expressions stimulate atheistic rejection. Many other personal reasons exist (Blackford & Schüklenk, 2009).

Negativism toward atheists is widespread in the United States. According to Jacobs (2015), it is due to two factors: (1) Atheists are distrusted and believed to be low in morality, and (2) they challenge the personally gratifying idea of an afterlife. Though the second theme needs further corroboration, the idea of distrust and threat has gained considerable support (Gervais, Shariff, & Norenzayen, 2011). Distrust here is not a narrow concept, but rather encompasses a broad range of personal and cultural values with which people in our society strongly identify. Since atheists and agnostics deviate religiously from the societal norm, they are literally considered bad people.

Many famous scientists (e.g., Richard Dawkins, Niels Bohr, Richard Feynman, and Stephen Hawking) have publicly accepted atheism; hence the hypothesis has been advanced that atheists are more intelligent than nonscientists (see Chapter 9 for further discussion). A number of studies have shown that atheists score 3–4 points higher on intelligence than Christians. This difference is actually trivial and of no consequence (Lindgren, 2014). Of greater significance is the question of how atheistic scientific parents deal with religion in their family settings. Research Box 6.3 presents work on this important issue.

RESEARCH BOX 6.3. Atheists and Agnostics Negotiate Religion and Family
(Ecklund & Lee, 2011)

Searching for atheists and agnostics at elite academic institutions, Ecklund and Lee focused on scientists. Beginning with 2,198 faculty members in the natural and social sciences, they finally selected 79 atheists and 87 agnostics. They then conducted 275 interviews, ranging in length from 20 minutes to 2½ hours.

Though the term "religious identity" was actually undefined, the idea of spirituality rather than a formal religious identity was emphasized. Still, the involvement of children in religious communities and organizations was largely decided "jointly by spouses rather than unilaterally" (p. 737). The scientist–atheist parents justified exposing their children to religion as a way of seeing that they learned positive social and moral values. Though they tried to avoid God language, they also saw constructive ritualistic experiences as a means of enhancing child and family group identification. These parents further stressed a "schema of 'free thinking'" (p. 740). In sum, the scientist–atheist parents justified family involvement in religion as an avenue to positively socializing the family unit with constructive community values.

Even though this study offered new information, surprisingly there were no comparisons of atheists and agnostics on any variable. Throughout the discussion reference was made to "atheists and agnostics," except for a brief interlude which cited only atheists. Still, even this is not offered as distinct from agnostics. A search was undertaken to determine if either of the authors might have followed up with additional work and no further research was found.

RELIGION IN LOVE, SEX, AND MARRIAGE

If anything defines a person as an adult, it is concern with love, sex, and marital commitment—topics that place the individual in a matrix of biological, historical, sociocultural, and psychological forces. Alfred Adler (1935) termed love one of the three great tasks of life. The biology of love, translated into sex and procreation, has been analyzed in relation to evolution (Ackerman, 1994; Fisher, 1983). The historical, cultural, and psychological aspects of love and intimate relationships have also been widely discussed and researched (Brehm, 1992; Fincham & Beach, 2013; Hunt, 1959).

Even though the modern world has seen a considerable liberalization of religion, there remains a fair degree of tension, ambivalence, and discomfort in the religious context with regard to love, sex, and marriage. Historically, much of this is associated with institutional religion's sexist treatment of women (O'Faolain & Martines, 1973; Ruether, 1975). Furthermore, in recent years homosexuality has also "come out of the closet," and same-sex marriage must now be understood as an integral part of contemporary life. The world openly confronts established faiths with many love- and sex-related problems that in earlier times were suppressed or ignored. In addition to the ones already noted, we may think immediately of premarital sex, extramarital sex, and divorce—all of which involve religion.

Religion and Heterosexuality

History and Context

The relationship between religion and sexual behavior has a long and troubled history, as just noted. This is particularly true for homosexual behavior, which is treated in a later section; our present discussion is confined to heterosexuality. Conflict, ambivalence, and outright insensitivity have characterized the way organized religion has often dealt with sexual needs and expressions. To borrow a term from one book title, religion and sexuality have often been "intimate enemies" (Bach & Wyden, 1969). Indeed, at best, they have often been poor bedfellows.

Historically, religion has always attempted to control sexuality (Burkert, 1996). The Judeo-Christian perspective, in part, reflects an earlier Greek view that placed pleasures of the mind above those of the body. This was sometimes equated with the notion that the body is corrupting, whereas the exercise of mind through reason reaches toward enlightenment. Early Christian ascetics often claimed that the body interferes with the attainment of a mystical union with the divine. In certain quarters, this translated into the association of the body with sexual activity (Bottomley, 1979). This kind of thinking was a step toward the justification of celibacy for those dedicating their lives to the church.

Another step in this process was to identify sexuality with women and to associate the two with evil, as in Tertullian's reference to woman as "the Devil's gateway" (O'Faolain & Martines, 1973). Although one can selectively view scripture as emphasizing the mandate to "be fruitful and multiply," implying a positive and constructive purpose to sex, stress was often placed on the role of Eve in the fall of humanity, in order to generalize wrongdoing to all females. By the 3rd century A.D., elements of Manicheism filtered into Christianity (Mathews & Smith, 1923). This movement emphasized the conflict between good and evil, and even regarded marital sex negatively. Such views probably influenced Saint Augustine and other early church fathers to relegate sensuality, sexual relations, and women to a lower and more sinful realm (Ruether, 1972, 1974).

Annette Mahoney (2010) argues that religion and spirituality may influence relationships on three levels: the individual, the family unit per se, and the wider religious community. Further investigation reveals that faith may be involved in various aspects of family planning, procreation, child rearing, marital stability, and divorce, among other aspects of marriage. There is also evidence that "the family that prays together, stays together." Though love in this context is supposed to be associated with marriage, the sexual aspect begins with adolescence via puberty. We thus start our discussion with premarital sex, which in our time is definitely out in the open.

Premarital Sexual Behavior among the Religious

In regard to premarital sex among people in general and religious people in particular, the data are often challengeable. We do not know about excessive denial or admission of such experience. Gender may be a factor, with men trying to appear very experienced and women desirous of presenting images of chastity and purity. According to *The Janus Report on Sexual Behavior* (Janus & Janus, 1993), 67% of the married men and 46% of the married women who were surveyed had engaged in premarital sex. Janus and Janus also noted that the more religious people were, the less likely they were to be sexually active before marriage, or at least to admit it. Nevertheless, they reported figures of 52% for "very religious" men and 37% for such women. Obviously, these findings are far from the religious ideal of abstinence prior to marriage.

A large-sample study of approximately 2,000 Christians revealed the lowest rates of premarital sex among Pentecostals, Mormons, and Jehovah's Witnesses (Beck, Cole, & Hammond, 1991). These groups were denoted "institutional sects," as opposed to other conservative groups (e.g., Baptists). Since all of the mainline Protestant, Catholic, and conservative Protestant bodies included in the study held the same negative religious views of premarital involvement, the authors claimed that the lowest rates for institutional sects were a function of the "level of commitment and social integration" (p. 179) of young people in these groups.

Looking at data from 418,000 people worldwide, Hartnett (2013) observed that Muslims reported least involvement in premarital sex, with a probability of slightly more than .60; Christians were just under .80, while Jews were above .80.

Even though religious commitment reduces the probability of premarital sexual behavior, evidence of such activity is abundantly evident (Uecker, 2008a). Reynolds (1994) notes signs of a potentially serious error in such research—namely, a failure to identify and control for forced intercourse or rape. She suggests that 20–30% of premarital involvement by young people, particularly teenagers, may involve coercion. If this is true, and if such instances are statistically removed from the data, religious effects should become much more strongly negative.

Though the rate of intercourse is lower among religiously active, single evangelical Christians than it is in the general population, some are sexually active, contrary to their faith. In a study by Wulf, Prentice, Hansum, Ferrar, and Spilka (1984), 59% of such individuals reported no such involvement, while 18% were active once a month or more. These data were gathered on 365 respondents, and the prediction of who was engaged in these behaviors proved to be fairly reliable. Older men and women who had previously been married and currently had a close friend of the opposite sex were likely to be sexually intimate. Though the relationships were not strong, high scores on Allport's Intrinsic scale of religious motivation opposed sexual involvement, while high Extrinsic scores were positively related to sexual activity.

Studying a large sample of never-married adults, Barkan (2006) found that religiosity supported involvement with one or a small number of premarital sexual partners. Low religiosity was strongly associated with having many partners. Otherwise, there seemed to be no evidence that being religious reduced premarital sexual involvement per se.

It has often been asked whether premarital sexuality has later repercussions. The most recent large-sample work on over 6,500 women indicates high marital dissolution rates for women who were premaritally involved with men other than their future husbands (Teachman, 2003). Teachman claims that "premarital sex and cohabitation have become part of the normal courtship pattern in the United States" (2003, p. 453). This is further implied in the "2014 State of Dating in America" report, in which 61% of Christians "said they would have sex before marriage" (O'Neil, 2014).

Religion, Sex, and Pleasure after Marriage

Three nationwide studies have attempted to examine factors affecting sexual activity and associated attitudes after marriage. The faith with which one is identified appears to have little if any relationship to frequency of sexual activity (Michael, Gagnon, & Laumann, 1994; Laumann, Gagnon, Michael, & Michaels, 1994). These researchers explain the weak association they found for Roman Catholics as possibly due to Catholicism's definition of intercourse as solely for reproduction.

Another issue that has been examined is the extent of sexual pleasure reported by religious people. The famous mid-20th-century sex researchers Masters and Johnson (1970) claimed that religion adversely affects sexual pleasure. Among the difficulties discussed, it is suggested that orgasm may be inhibited and sexual satisfaction diminished. These views have not been borne out by research. Indeed, reported sexual activity levels are higher for very religious people than for those who are irreligious. In addition, the frequency of such activity appears to have increased in the 3 years preceding the Janus and Janus (1993) study, and more so for those who were "very religious" than for their nonreligious counterparts. Tavris and Sadd (1977) found no difference in frequency of orgasm between religious and nonreligious women. Mathews (1994) studied the sexuality of conservative, evangelical, submissive wives and found that "accountability to God for a wife's happiness and sexual satisfaction is part of exercising headship in the home" (p. 12). Fifty-seven percent of the men and 49% of the women in these marriages gave themselves a 10 or 10+ on a scale of sexual fulfillment. Religion thus appears to be no impediment to sexually gratifying relations.

Some social scientists are reluctant to accept the positive testimony of religious women. Suggestions have been made that they probably "don't know what they are missing," or are responding to researchers in a socially desirable way. No evidence to support these interpretations has been forthcoming. Although Tavris and Sadd (1977) believed that such women may have lower sexual expectations and are less willing to believe widely purveyed popular fantasies about ecstatic sexual gratification, again no data backing such assertions have been produced. In short, efforts to cast religion in repressive or suppressive roles relative to sexual expression have not gained research support.

Sexual activity and pleasure obviously have their place in marriage, but this overlaps with the issue of contraception and family planning. Church attendance links to more negativity about contraception and attitudes toward family planning seem to point toward disapproval. One problem with this research concerns significant but low correlations, which might imply a need for more complex, even multivariate analyses. Replication should also be taken into consideration (Barrett, DaVanzo, Ellison, & Grammich, 2014).

Religion and Gender Traditions in Marriage

In classic Christianity, the man is the head of the household. One survey of evangelicals (both males and females) indicated that approximately 90% affirmed the Biblical injunction of male domination in the family, and that about 40% would deny women any positions of power in the church (Kosmin & Lachman, 1993). Tradition has it that women should be subject to male control, and the more orthodox a religious body is, the more such a doctrinal view prevails.

Carolyn Pevey's (1994) study of a fundamentalist Southern Baptist church shows that theory may be one thing and practice another. Pevey found that wives were sometimes forced to submit, but when necessary, these religiously conservative women subverted masculine claims to authority. Usually, however, husband–wife relationships seemed to be mutually supportive and cooperative rather than combative (albeit within an authoritarian framework).

The employment of wives when spouses are members of a conservative religious body also raises conventional arguments about "woman's place." Tradition has the man going to work while the wife stays home and cares for children. No longer is that simple formula a rule; cultural reality, social progress, and economic necessity currently and commonly take precedence over such ideas. What about when wives go to work? See what Research Box 6.4 says about this.

Religion and Marital Adjustment

Dating precedes marriage, and singles are more willing to date than to marry someone outside of their religious group. Furthermore, the characteristics that are appealing in dating are often different from those desired in a marriage partner (Udry, 1971). The choice of a potential mate entails a shift to more stable, lasting behaviors that also support the creation of a successful marriage and home life. This includes a heightened emphasis on religion.

RESEARCH BOX 6.4. Wives' Employment Status and Marital Happiness of Religious Couples (Johnson, Eberly, Duke, & Sartain, 1988)

Mixed results have plagued research on satisfaction in marriage and the employment of wives. Theory has it that religiosity should correlate positively with the happiness of wives. Researching Mormons, Johnson and colleagues primarily selected wives for study. Even though Mormon women are members of a conservative religious group, they are as likely to work outside the home as members of any other denomination in the United States. Data were, however, gathered for both husbands and wives on religiosity, education, age of children, and the full- or part-time nature of wifely employment outside the home.

Greatest marital happiness and religious commitment was observed for both husbands and wives when the latter worked full-time outside the home. Least satisfaction was evident for those working part-time. Husbands responded similarly in relation to wives' employment. Husbands of traditional homemaker wives (i.e., wives who did not work outside their homes) were next. Among the wives, traditional homemakers were most pleased with their situation. The least wifely satisfaction among those working part-time may have been due to such factors as stress from remaining full-time homemakers as well. In addition, part-time jobs might not provide enough income.

As might be expected, Dudley and Kosinski (1990) found that the more similar husbands and wives are in religious behavior and attitudes, the greater their marital satisfaction. In particular, marital fidelity is enhanced by religion in a number of ways. Couples claim that their faith sanctifies their devotion to each other; joint religious activity enhances marital commitment, strengthens moral values, and improves their relationship to God and to each other (Dollahite & Lambert, 2007). In related work, religious couples described a variety of ways that God was involved in their marriage, all to the benefit of their union (Goodman & Dollahite, 2006).

When both spouses are religiously committed, they are also likely to be involved in a moral community. This helps explain many of the findings reported on religion and morality. In one study, marital happiness was positively correlated not only with agreement on religious matters, but also with the belief that love had continued to grow since the spouses married. These findings parallel increasing satisfaction with both oneself and one's mate (Hunt & King, 1978). Extrinsic religion is also operative here, suggesting that faith performs a utilitarian function—one that is beneficial both to the marital union and to its members as individuals.

Evans, McIntosh, and Spilka (1986) found that spouses with equivalent religious orientations/motivations expressed greater marital satisfaction. Since this work was correlational, those with high scores on the Intrinsic and Extrinsic religious measures either acquired mates with similar perspectives or increasingly grew to share the same religious outlook, thereby enhancing the success of their marriages along with their personal happiness. Regardless of the process, the outcome was beneficial.

There is more to personal faith than attitudes and public observance, both of which were concerns of the two studies just described. Recognizing the lack of attention to private devotional practices, Gruner (1985) looked at the frequency of prayer and Bible reading, and found that both were associated with marital adjustment. With respect to religious affiliation, the relationship between Bible reading and marital satisfaction was strongest for members of sects, somewhat less strong for evangelicals, and weakest for Catholics and members of liberal Protestant denominations. Of interest would be information on the degree to which members of such groups perceive prayer and Bible reading as pertinent to their marital state. Certainly sects and evangelical bodies do emphasize Bible reading more than other groups, but we know very little about the effects of private devotional practice on other aspects of an individual's life. The probability is that Bible reading may be more of a joint spousal activity in conservative than in liberal faiths. In sum, regardless of the measures used, religiosity and marital happiness go together (Filsinger & Wilson, 1984).

What about the other side of the coin—namely, those who describe themselves as having "no religion," or who conceive of their religion as outside of established faiths? The data suggest what the studies above imply: Religious independents are more likely to be unmarried, separated, divorced, or remarried than those who are affiliated. In addition, they reveal lower levels of satisfaction, personal fulfillment, and social integration (Bock & Radelet, 1988).

The evidence is strong that marital adjustment and longevity are functions of the "sanctification of family relationships" (Mahoney, Pargament, Murray-Swank, & Murray-Swank, 2003). This means that spouses who consider their marriage a sacred covenant are happier with their union and are more devoted to each other than are those who do not view their partnership in religious terms. Regarding a marriage as "made in heaven" is a powerful force in producing a happy family.

Intermarriage

INTERMARRIAGE AND RELIGIOUS SWITCHING/DROPPING OUT

McCutcheon (1988) indicates a rather orderly increase in the number of "intermarriages" or "exogamous marriages" (i.e., marriages outside the religious group in which each partner was reared) among Protestants, Catholics, and Jews throughout the 20th century. The more conservative the faith in which people were raised, the less often switching occurs (Hadaway & Marler, 1993). Over 80% of conservative Protestants and Catholics maintain their original church affiliation. If a person is brought up within a specific religious tradition, and marries someone of the same persuasion, the probability that either spouse will change affiliation is extremely low (Hadaway & Marler, 1993). The Pew Research Center's 2014 Religious Landscape Survey shows a continuation of these trends: Between 2010 and 2014, 39% of marriages were religiously mixed; this translates into a loss of 7.8% or 5.3 million Christians (Murphy, 2015).

Claiming that 45% of marriages in the first decade of this century involved interfaith unions, Naomi Riley (2013a), a member of such a union, sponsored a study of 2,450 couples. In keeping with the results of similar research, she found a greater likelihood of unhappiness and divorce than in withinfaith marriages. Jews were most likely to marry outside their faith and Mormons least likely. She further noted that the older such persons were, the greater the probability of participating in these matches. This is an area of increasing importance in U.S. society, and those interested in understanding its complexity might well benefit from reading Riley's (2013b) book, *'Til Faith Do Us Part: How Interfaith Marriage Is Transforming America.*

INTERMARRIAGE AND DIVORCE

The data are clear and consistent in showing that interfaith marriages have a much higher likelihood of ending in divorce than within-faith unions (Lehrer & Chiswick, 1993; Levinger, 1979; Mahoney, Pargament, Tarakeshwar, & Swank, 2001). The problem is not only that intermarried spouses often have different backgrounds and expectations, but that they also may vary in degree of religiousness. When the "honeymoon is over," and the spouses face the realities of married life, religious issues can take on a new importance. This frequently occurs after children are born and the new parents clash over needs for religious identification and education. One estimate suggests that religious differences are mitigated through conversion, which takes place in about 50% of these marriages (McCutcheon, 1988).

The evidence suggests heightened levels of conflict in intermarriage. This is more likely to occur when there is a greater religious distance between the spouses (e.g., one is low in religiosity while the other is strongly attached to a religious group, or each spouse is firmly committed to his or her own faith). Interreligious distance appears to have deleterious effects upon the children of such unions. The latter are more likely to become involved with drugs and alcohol (Petts & Knoester, 2007). It should come as no surprise that divorce adversely affects the spiritual growth of children (Blomquist, 1985). Lawton and Bures (2001) have shown that the experience of parental divorce among those who intermarry commonly eventuates in religious switching on the part of their children.

Interfaith marriage has been steadily increasing for over 50 years (Murphy, 2015). In the 1960s, 22% of marriages were between individuals from different religious bodies. As already note, this percentage has steadily increased, reaching 39% between 2010 and 2014.

Most of these unions are between Christian spouses who are religiously unaffiliated. Prior to 1960, these affiliations accounted for 5% of marriages; this percentage increased to 18% by 2010. Forty-nine percent of currently unmarried couples consist of persons of different faiths. Members of religious bodies that are not in the Christian mainstream show much lower intermarriage rates. Staying within their own group are 91% of Hindus, 82% of Mormons, 79% of Mormons, and 65% of Jews (Murphy, 2015).

Again, there are a number of possible reasons for switching. First, religion may be unimportant to two people from different religious backgrounds. If they marry, religion may never be a problem. In many other instances, the initial unimportance of faith changes for one or both spouses when children enter the family. Individually or together, the new parents may become seekers, as many baby boomers were. Community and family social pressures frequently enter the picture. American society, with its high level of religiosity, makes separation from a religious or spiritual framework increasingly difficult with the passing years.

WHO SWITCHES?

About 20% of switchers do so because of intermarriage; one spouse usually takes the faith of the other. Using national data on approximately 8,000 respondents, Musick and Wilson (1995) found; the least switching for marital reasons among Jews (3.4%), Baptists, Mormons, and Catholics (each about 5%). The highest switching rates for intermarriage occurred among Disciples of Christ, Lutherans, Presbyterians, and members of the United Church of Christ. Still, intermarriage is the main route to religious change for Jews, Catholics, and Lutherans. With regard to the details of switching for marital purposes, Musick and Wilson suggest that liberal religionists tend to affiliate with conservative religious bodies, while conservatives move toward the liberal end of the spectrum. Interestingly, Catholics shift to the no-religion category when marriage is an issue. The need for greater in-depth analyses of factors that relate to marital switching is abundantly evident.

SWITCHING AMONG JEWS

There is a real problem in determining the actual percentages of people who marry outside their religious groups. This is most evident in Jewish intermarriages.[3] Between 1900 and 1920, only 2% of Jews reportedly intermarried; between 1966 and 1972, 31.7% reportedly did so (Reiss, 1976). By the 1980s, Silberman (1985) suggested a rate of 24%, but noted that others put the rate as high as 60%. The 3.4% rate given by Musick and Wilson (1995; see above) is suspect, but considering their use of national data, their findings must be noted. To suggest that the actual numbers range between 3 and 30% is not very informative. Some of this variation might be explained by where and how samples are gathered; in areas where there are few Jews, the rate of intermarriage is high. A distinction also needs to be made between first and second marriages, as the latter have an intermarriage rate about 50% higher than that for first marriages. This also means that older Jews are more likely to intermarry than their younger cohorts (Mayer, 1985). Despite these numbers, one study reported that in 1990, 94% of those who were born Jews maintained their religious identification as Jews (Fishman, 2000).

---

[3] Religious change in general among Jews has been discussed earlier. Here we are concerned with change related to intermarriage.

Interestingly, 39% of intermarried Jews have spouses who are Catholics (Goff, 2008). Though not specifically studied, theory suggests that this selection probably occurs because both groups largely live in the northeast United States in urban areas, attend the same schools, and share faiths that emphasize formal holidays with standard rituals.

Intermarriage usually occasions considerable unhappiness on the part of parents and religious officials (Petsonk & Remsen, 1988; Stark & Bainbridge, 1985). A 1965 survey of Jews in Boston found that almost 70% felt that the Jewish community had "an obligation to urge Jews to marry Jews" (Geffen, 2001, p. 7); according to Geffen, a more recent survey still indicated that about 40% of Jews would be greatly distressed if their children married outside the faith.

Changing one's religious affiliation may involve a formal conversion; however, such switching does not always involve serious commitment. A convert for whom faith doesn't mean much may simply take on the affiliation of the more devoted spouse to please him or her. Unfortunately, long-term discrepancies between spouses in terms of religious observance commonly result in conflict and divorce (Gordon, 1967).

There is another effect that merits study: What about the religious identification of the children of intermarried couples? A study of Jewish intermarriages in New York City showed that if the wife is Jewish, the children are raised as Jewish in three out of four families; if the husband is Jewish, the ratio is one out of four (Silberman, 1985). This issue has been studied with Catholic, Protestant, and unaffiliated parents (Nelsen, 1990).

Religion and Heterosexual Sex, Marriage, and Family: Directions for a Summary

We have only sampled some of the main work on religion and heterosexual sex, marriage, and the family. An immense amount of additional theory and research may be found in this literature. Happily, some scholars have produced outstanding coordinating and summarizing papers (Mahoney et al., 2001; Weaver et al., 2002).

Religion and Homosexuality[4]

When the third edition of this book was being written, only 3 U.S. states had made same-sex marriages legal. By 2014, this number had risen to 36. On June 26, 2015, the Supreme Court extended such legality to all 50 states.

Historically, Western religion has been hostile toward homosexuality, citing scripture as the basis for its negative outlook. Many contemporary religious groups, especially liberal ones, have challenged the traditional Judeo-Christian stance. Among others, Daniel Helminiak (2000), a Catholic priest and a noted psychologist of religion, has examined in depth the Biblical bases for antipathy and fear of homosexuals. He raises serious questions about the unfavorable scriptural heritage that has pervaded Western religious thought on this topic.

Placing homosexuality in a broader, anthropological light, Carlsson (1997) explains the great variation in the way homosexuals are regarded across cultures. He feels that one reason for this is variation in the relative frequency of homosexuality. In societies where it is

---

[4]Though we have titled and emphasized in this section, homosexuality, the current literature goes far beyond this concept with the identifying abbreviation LBGT. Respectively this stands for Lesbian, Gay, Bisexual, and Transgender. We have thus selected and treated a limited literature.

common, it seems to be treated in a positive manner; where it is rare, strong efforts to suppress it are present. Without question, the valuation of homosexuality is culturally defined. In one study of 76 societies, 49 did not treat homosexuality as undesirable or deviant (Farb, 1978). Furthermore, whether it is viewed as culturally normal or not, in many of these societies homosexuality is defined in supernatural and religious terms (Hoebel, 1966; Katchadourian, 1989). Attitude change toward same-sex marriage in the United States over the last 20 years has been extensive, with acceptance going from 27 to 51% and still continuing to increase (Dillon, 2014). Though considerable opposition still exists, it is obviously decreasing at a surprising rate. Between 2001 and 2017, support for gay marriages increased by 22% among white Evangelical Protestants. The positive change for the same period among Mainline Protestants was 30%. Respectively for these two groups the percentages approving same-sex marriage in 2017 was 35 and 68%. 67% of Catholics also approved these unions. Those unaffiliated showed 85% approval (Pew Research Forum, 2017).

The Judeo-Christian Tradition: An Extreme View

Pargament (1997) describes a harsh religious view advanced by one Christian critic, who perceived AIDS as God's punishment for homosexual activity. As for those innocents who contract AIDS, "they, too, must pay the price for the moral depravity of a society that tolerates such abominations" (quoted in Pargament, 1997, p. 326). Stances like this can be exceedingly dangerous. Being homosexual and part of an orthodox religious community can eventuate in such a degree of shame and fear that a person not only remains "in the closet," but may even deny being infected with AIDS, seriously jeopardizing life (Bieser, 1995).

Clerical Perspectives

Just as attitudes toward homosexuality have demonstrated a slow but orderly movement toward its acceptability, extreme differences among individual clergy and religious groups exist.

One approach has us reading in the popular media about pastors who refuse to preside at the funerals of lesbians (Mitchell, 2015; Paul, 2015). In like manner, baptism was initially denied to the son of a gay father, although this decision was later reversed (Blumberg, 2015). General calls to clergy to avoid participation in civil ceremonies when gay persons are involved are common (Oppenheimer, 2015). Conflict relative to same-sex marriages has, however, been noted among evangelicals (Graham, 2015), even though a majority (70%) oppose such unions.

Approving stances are increasingly common. *The Wichita Eagle* recently reported that a United Methodist conference of 1,000 Kansas and Nebraska pastors passed and sent a petition acknowledging "diverse beliefs regarding homosexuality" to the Methodist General Conference (Riedl, 2015). In a parallel action, the Presbyterian Church (U.S.A.) endorsed same-sex marriage (Goodstein, 2015).

Following the legalization of gay marriage in Ireland, *The New York Times* headlined a column "On Same-Sex Marriage, Catholics Are Leading the Way" (Bruni, 2015b, p. A19). The author noted that nine other nations in which Catholicism is the dominant faith had previously taken action similar to Ireland's.

Among religions in the United States, the highest support for same-sex marriages comes from Buddhists, with an 84% favorable response. Jews follow, with a 77% positive response (Jewish Telegraphic Agency, 2015).

Hochstein (1986) examined the stance of pastoral counselors, overwhelmingly clergy, in regard to lesbian and gay clients. Though no distinction was made with regard to mental health between homosexuals and heterosexuals, 30% of the counselors scored high on a measure of homophobia. The main finding was that sex stereotyping was present. Interestingly, heterosexual males were seen as less masculine than heterosexual females, gays, or lesbians. Unfortunately, Hochstein provided no data that would distinguish the outlooks of male and female counselors. In addition, the data for his study were gathered over three decades ago.

The problem of homophobia in Western religion is both individual and institutional. Even relatively liberal churches officially maintain the biases of their more conservative peers. Recent years have, however, witnessed counterresponses by pastors and backtracking by church officials. In 2001, the United Methodist Church "ruled that practicing gays cannot be in the ministry" (Culver, 2001, p. 11A). By 2005, gay and lesbian ministers were being approved by Methodist ruling bodies. Apparently, Lutheran churches now accept lesbian and gay pastors if they remain celibate (*The Denver Post*, 2001). Even though a recent overview of 1,331 Christian churches showed an overall increase in acceptance of gays and lesbians, there was still a broad range of positions that may or may not be rigidly adhered to in practice (Masci, 2014). Homophobia often remains official doctrine, but it is clearly in retreat.

The Issue of Conversion Therapy

Regardless of the reasons for homosexuality, many conservative religionists believe in what has come to be known as "conversion therapy" (Haldeman, 1991, 1994, 1996). The intention is to convert homosexuals into heterosexuals (celibacy seems acceptable to the proponents of this therapy). In orthodox circles, the notion of therapy implies that homosexuality is at best, an illness. Neither the American Psychiatric Association nor the American Psychological Association currently holds such a view

In an impressive effort to get past isolated anecdotal statements regarding the effectiveness of conversion therapy, Shidlo and Schroeder (2002), using rigorous selection criteria, were able to interview 202 recipients of conversion methods administered by a total of 308 therapists. The majority of these therapists (66%) were licensed mental health practitioners, and 14% of these were explicitly identified with a particular religion. Of the unlicensed therapists, 55% were religious counselors. Two-thirds of the clients were religious. Eighty-seven percent of the respondents regarded their therapy as a failure; only 13% felt that it was successful to some degree. Moreover, approximately half of the "successes" experienced relapses or participated in alternative practices that implied continuing adjustment difficulties. There was also evidence that such therapy could eventuate in considerable psychological harm.

The landmark research of Shidlo and Schroeder is much more complex than this brief summary indicates. It spanned some 5 years, and provides very little support for those who consider conversion or reparative therapy a productive alternative to homosexuality. Strong emotional biases cloud any serious attempts to evaluate all of the issues involved in changing homosexual behavior (Winfield, 2002). Shidlo and Schroeder offer the kind of solid scholarship that this troubled realm needs. In previous work, Haldeman (1991, 1994) simply concluded that there is no evidence that conversion therapy changes sexual orientation.

As of mid-2015, although 18 states had introduced legislation to ban conversion therapy, only 3 states had adopted such laws. In April 2015, President Barack Obama condemned it as lacking scientific support plus having the potential of harming clients (*Monitor on Psychology*, 2015).

Before we leave the issue of conversion or reparative therapy, let us recognize that homosexuals are subject to the same psychosocial pressures that confront their straight associates. They thus share the therapy needs of heterosexuals in our society. There is, however, a significant difference: Being homosexual means also having to deal with the stresses and potential rejections of all who possess minority status. Social work, clinical psychology, and psychiatry are increasingly becoming aware of these difficulties (Bowland, Foster, & Vosler, 2013; Levy & Reeves, 2011). Again, the issue of life's growing complexity challenges all of us.

Right-Wing Authoritarianism and Anti-Homosexual Sentiment

The antipathy of fundamentalists and other religious conservatives toward gays and lesbians has been well documented (Altemeyer & Hunsberger, 1992; Hunsberger, 1996). Even though scripture serves as its justification, one may ask whether an antihomosexual stance is simply another form of prejudice. Laythe, Finkel, and Kirkpatrick (2001) looked at this question with respect to personality/attitude characteristics that might foster bias. Distinguishing religious fundamentalism (RF) from right-wing authoritarianism (RWA), which is also part of fundamentalist ideology, they observed that even though RWA and RF were positively correlated, RF was associated with antihomosexual feelings, but not with racism when RWA was statistically controlled for. RWA was tied positively to both forms of prejudice. After obtaining some contradictory findings in two additional studies, these researchers concluded that RF is at best weakly related to antihomosexual feelings. The culprit really seems to be RWA.

Hunsberger (1996) extended the relationship among RF, religious RWA, and anti-homosexual sentiment to Hindus, Muslims, and Jews. Even though the non-Christian samples tended to be small, the correlations showed that the same association between RF and a similar stance was found across all of the groups. Even when we restrict ourselves to the large Christian samples in four different studies, the connection is clear. These data show that RWA is indeed the problem, as four of the five partial correlations become nonsignificant when RWA is removed from the RF–RWA relationships. Some coefficients are only of borderline strength. Still, when RF is removed, all of the coefficients are statistically meaningful, further indicating that the RWA component causes the difficulty.

The complexity of this realm prompted Tsang and Rowatt (2007) to look more closely at questions this research has raised. Examining different religious orientations, they observed that, contrary to expectations, Intrinsic faith and an Extrinsic perspective were both tied fairly strongly to negative attitudes toward gays and lesbians. Even with controls, the Intrinsic influence persisted. RWA remains in the picture as above, but we must ask: Why the Intrinsic involvement? In such work, one can always point to the nature of the sample or the measures employed. We know that measures of orthodoxy relate highly to Intrinsic faith, and some research implies that this includes a "narrow orthodoxy" that supports bigotry (McIntosh & Spilka, 1990). Such orthodoxy may be a factor here. More research is called for.

Alternative Religious Organizations and Approaches for Gays, Lesbians, and Bisexuals

The rejection homosexuals encounter in mainline churches often causes them to respond in kind to those who spurn them. A common development is for lesbians, gays, and bisexuals to search for accepting religious groups or to establish their own churches and religious/spiritual organizations. A representative group is Dignity, an association for Catholic gays and lesbians (Wagner, Serafini, Rabkin, Remien, & Williams, 1994). Sometimes these bodies take unusual forms. Stark and Bainbridge (1985) describe a militant lesbian commune that organized as Wiccans, peaceful practitioners of contemporary witchcraft who pray to a "Great Goddess." One can view such actions as a struggle to obtain a sense of power.

Helminiak (1995) speaks of a nontheist spirituality, particularly among gays with HIV. He also notes that there are ministers who go beyond the traditional limits of their religious bodies to care for the spiritual needs of gay men and lesbians. Marshall (1996) details the problems of women who are in the process of developing lesbian identities. She specifies procedures and other considerations that pastoral caregivers can employ in their work with such women.

Since HIV/AIDS continues to be a major problem among homosexuals, it will come as no surprise that those suffering from this disease complex search for religious meanings to deal with their dilemma. One creative interview study revealed four major approaches involving religion (Jacobson, Luckhaupt, Delaney, & Tsevat, 2006). These are detailed in Table 6.4.

Effects of Religion-Based Hostility on Homosexuals

There is no reason to believe that the religious needs and desires of homosexuals are any different from those of heterosexuals (Goodwill, 2000; Haldeman, 1996; Lynch, 1996). The hostility of traditional religionists can therefore have serious deleterious effects on lesbians and gay men (Clark, Brown, & Hochstein, 1989; Grant & Epp, 1998; Haldeman, 1996; Lynch, 1996). But what are these effects? Quite often, homosexuals reject traditional religion (Clark et al., 1989; Goodwill, 2000). One study suggested that up to 50% of Catholic homosexuals may leave the church. This is commonly associated with confused and contradictory images of God, as well as with negative self-concepts (Marcellino, 1996). The latter tendency may be one adverse effect of damaged identity development (Grant & Epp, 1998). Homophobia can also be internalized as part of a pattern of self-hatred (Wagner et al., 1994).

TABLE 6.4. Religion-Related Meaning Patterns among Patients with HIV/AIDS

Group	Meaning pattern
1. Deferring believers	Deference to a God who will make the decisions.
2. Collaborative believers	Belief that God and the patients will work together.
3. Spiritual/religious seekers	Unsuccessful search for spiritual/religious meanings that will help them cope.
4. Self-directed believers	Belief that the patients must find their own spirituality to deal with their problem.

Note. Deferring, collaborative, and self-directed believers relate to the coping styles of Pargament (1988).

Influence of Religious Orientation
in Heterosexuals' Views of Homosexuals

The influence of religious motivation or orientation in heterosexuals' views of homosexuals has also been studied (Batson, Floyd, Meyer, & Winner, 1999; Fulton, Gorsuch, & Maynard, 1999). The results have been confusing.

Batson et al. (1999) undertook an experiment in which heterosexual participants could monetarily help a same-sex peer who disclosed homosexual inclinations or gave no such information. In the case of the former, the respondent self-identifying as homosexual indicated that the money donated would go either to a cause that promoted homosexuality or to one that did not. Heterosexuals with an Intrinsic orientation gave less to the discloser, regardless of where the money would go. This was seen as reflecting a bias against homosexuality. In order to resolve some of these difficulties with religious orientation, let us examine Research Box 6.5, which presents the work of Fulton et al. (1999). That this is a troubled topic goes without saying. One can argue that social change in recent years has entered this realm, and that prejudice against alternative sexual styles is clearly under attack. The psychology of religion needs a continuing research program to understand what is taking place both sociologically and psychologically.

RESEARCH BOX 6.5. Religious Orientation, Antihomosexual Sentiment, and Fundamentalism among Christians (Fulton, Gorsuch, & Maynard, 1999)

This study attempted a systematic evaluation of the role of the major forms of religious motivation in fostering antihomosexual sentiment. Measures of Intrinsic (personal) and Extrinsic (social) religious orientation plus their total, as well as scales assessing a Quest orientation and Fundamentalism, were employed. In addition, indices of antihomosexual sentiment and prejudice against African Americans and other groups were used. A measure of social distance was also administered to evaluate attitudes toward practicing and celibate Christian and non-Christian homosexuals. Because Intrinsic faith has been confounded with religious orthodoxy, the Fundamentalism scores were partialed out to obtain a purer measure of Intrinsic motivation.

Intrinsic faith was associated with rejection of prejudice against blacks and antihomosexual sentiment. Even though homosexuals were not the object of Intrinsic bias, homosexual behavior was still regarded as a moral problem. Extrinsic motives correlated positively with antiblack and antigay indices. There were few significant correlations with the Quest scale; where present, these were weaker than, but similar to, those of Intrinsic religion with attitudes toward homosexuality. The Fundamentalism scale was independent of antiblack measures, but those with high Fundamentalism scores were strongly negative toward homosexuals. Distinctions were not made between active and celibate homosexuals.

Clearly, different religious motivations need evaluation when feelings about homosexuality are studied. The authors concluded that "not all negative sentiment toward homosexuals by Christians should be interpreted as prejudice, while not all committed Christians are bound to express negative sentiment toward homosexuals" (p. 21).

Research from Gay and Lesbian Perspectives

When we evaluate the foregoing research, we must note that virtually none of it has been conducted from the perspectives of lesbians or gays themselves. Kirk Foster and his colleagues have attempted to correct this bias. They identified three aspects of the homosexuality–religion complex—namely, the integration of sexual orientation and religion, the ways in which theological meaning becomes understood, and finally the need to locate a supportive congregation. Resolving these issues relates to the development of lesbian and gay resilience (Foster, Bowland, & Vosler, 2015). These workers have opened a door. Let us now see more such work.

THE TRADITIONAL IMPORTANCE OF RELIGION AMONG WOMEN

Possible Explanations

Though historically and contemporaneously, men have overwhelmingly dominated the Judeo-Christian tradition, with few exceptions, women appear to be more religious than men. The question of why one finds more women at religious services cannot be easily answered. The complexity of this issue has been discussed at length by J. Francis (1997). He suggests that five theoretical explanatory positions have been advanced, and that these may be subsumed under two headings: sociocultural and psychological. Adherents of the former group claim that women are not more religious than men, but are simply socialized to accept religious and spiritual values and attachments more thoroughly than males, and hence manifest greater involvement in religious institutions. Adherents of the second group look to personality theories, ranging from Freudian theory to trait and response tendencies in which women are viewed as more sensitive than men. Francis (1997) also introduces some interesting research possibilities that can contribute to further understanding of this male–female issue relative to religiosity.

Looking more empirically at gender, a Gallup Poll indicates that in the adult age range chosen here, women feel more strongly than men that religion is very important to daily life (2006c). The percentage differences range from 13 to 16%.

On the level of culture, anthropologists and sociologists suggest that males are socialized to be dominant, and females to be dependent and submissive; as a result, lower status is commonly accorded to women, and this has repercussions in terms of the division of labor. In many societies, women are defined solely as homemakers and caretakers of children. Not being in the work force, they are regarded as having more time for religion and as demonstrating greater church attendance and stronger religious beliefs and commitments than are true for men. Religious participation is then treated as natural to the traditional female role (Miller & Hoffman, 1995).

Psychologically, Miller and Hoffman (1995) interpret the female social position in terms of risk taking. Being in a weaker cultural position than men, women should be less willing to take risks and more likely to adopt psychosocially safe positions such as religion. In other words, women are expected to confront life stresses and ambiguities conservatively. A case can also be made that males are reared to be independent, and hence to become risk takers. This may explain gender differences in many aspects of life in which females are more risk-adverse than males. As expected, the research shows that risk aversion is positively associated both with religiosity and with being female (Miller & Hoffman, 1995).

The lower status and power of women (McGuire, 1992; Pargament, 1997) have been analogized by Hinde (1999) to the "religion of the oppressed"—namely, the need of the powerless to turn to their faith when all other avenues fail. He further proposes that femininity is biologically affiliated with a greater propensity for social connections and relationships with others. Both of these inclinations may be gratified through institutional faith. As has so often been said, however, the times are changing. The secondary situation of women relative to salaries has recently been decried by Pope Francis, who has called it a "scandal" and criticized how men "want to dominate women" (*The Denver Post,* 2015, p. 14A). Bruni (2015a), however, considers Francis's statement trivial, noting that "pay isn't the primary issue when the symbolism, rituals and vocabulary of an institution exalt men over women" (p. A23). This is further detailed relative to male domination in the Catholic Church.

This greater attachment to religion on the part of women has some interesting implications. One is that religion is likely to possess more utility for women than for men, and the evidence suggests that this is true (Pargament, 1997). The more personally important religion is, the more helpful it becomes in coping with life's problems.

Another fascinating possibility that may partially explain the religion–women connection involves biology. Whitney (1976), citing data from many mammalian species, shows greater social cohesiveness and cooperation among females than among males. That religion and in-group social cohesion go together has been suggested by Durkheim and others (McGuire, 1992). Arguments in favor of women's religion and spirituality stress cooperation and cohesion (Conn, 1986). Could there be a genetic component in the propensities of women for religion and social unity? Hypotheses like this must be very carefully examined, as they may be perceived as "politically incorrect" and in fact may be used against women to buttress male control and female subjugation.

A further argument may be derived from the theory that in most instances, women seem to be the "religious culture carriers." A fascinating demonstration of this role across the centuries is illustrated by the work of Janet Jacobs (1996, 2002) on the function of women in the survival of "crypto-Jewish culture."

Crypto-Jewish culture is a result of the 15th- and 16th-century persecution of Jews by the Spanish Inquisition. Facing death or conversion to Catholicism, many Spanish Jews either left Spain or "converted." This frequently meant that their Judaism "went underground" but persisted until the present day in concealed form. Currently, crypto-Jews live primarily in the southwestern United States and Mexico, though some are also found in the eastern United States among Hispanic émigrés from the Caribbean.

Jacobs (1996) attributes the survival of crypto-Jewish culture to the women in these families. This framework of beliefs and behavior, both historically and contemporaneously, has been kept secret from outsiders, often beneath a veneer of Catholicism. Support for crypto-Judaism is associated with the maintenance of classical Jewish rituals, primarily by the women in the home. Among these, Jacobs has observed the lighting of Sabbath candles; enforcement of dietary laws; and the celebration of Jewish holiday ceremonies for Passover, Purim, and Chanukah. Since the families are often overtly Catholic, the Jewish festival of Purim may be practiced as the Festival of St. Esther, and Chanukah may be masked as the festival of Las Posadas (a celebratory representation of the journey of Joseph and Mary). Often central to this Catholic–Jewish syncretic activity is the preparation of food, which in these families is strictly a female duty. The importance of secrecy plus the maintenance of classic Jewish rituals and practices endows the women in these crypto-Jewish families with both power and responsibility. The mothers must protect the family's religious integrity in each generation, and pass on to their daughters the heritage they have received from their forebears. Jacobs does not deny that the men in such religious settings may play some role in preserving the old religious traditions; however, the women are the dominant force in teaching their faith to the children.

Women's Changing Roles in Life and Religion

Across the centuries, a few exceptional women in every generation have broken the psychosocial bonds that essentially held them captive. Major changes in women's position and status were initiated in the 20th century, as women began rebelling against male control in virtually all aspects of their lives. The classical roles of women in relation to religion also started to change radically by the 1960s. Subservience was often replaced by self-direction. Instead of following the paths set by males, many women developed new ways of realizing their capabilities and achieving their own directions.

These possibilities took several forms. First, women spoke openly of their religious/spiritual struggles and aspirations (Meadow & Rayburn, 1985; Ware, 1985). Next were attempts to realize these hopes by critiquing traditional religious-institutional structures and their theological justifications (Christ & Plaskow, 1979; Plaskow & Romero, 1974; Ruether, 1974). Rejecting their second-class citizenship, women now took long-overdue leadership positions in churches and synagogues (Conn, 1986; Ruether & McLaughlin, 1979). Chaves (1997) argues that pressures for gender equality were a major force in spurring the ordination of women—a trend that has increased rapidly since the 1970s.

It is hard to believe that broad-based concern with the religion of women only started in the 1960s with the rise of the women's movement. Former President Jimmy Carter claims that religion is "one of the 'basic causes of the violation of women's rights'" (quoted in Kristof, 2010, p. WK11). Mary Robinson, "former president of Ireland and United Nations high commissioner for human rights[,] asserts if there's one overarching issue for women it's the way that religion can be manipulated to subjugate women" (Kristof, 2010, p. WK11). There is no comparable enlightenment on the religion of men, as it was taken for granted that men should naturally dominate both women and religion. Historically, clergy were males, and scripture was used to validate the controlling role of men in both the family and the Judeo-Christian heritage. Even when women such as Catholic nuns serve the church, the real power still resides in the hands of a masculine hierarchy.

Cultural change is often slow and troubled. This is evidenced in recent work on the conflicted attitudes of women in conservative Christian and Jewish groups. While arguing for equality in self-expression and opportunity outside of their conservative faiths, they appear ambivalent regarding the liberalization of their roles in church and home. There is also a tendency to oppose feminism explicitly, while implicitly accepting its ideas when these are framed in conservative terminology (Manning, 1999). One can argue that such inclinations to control females have increasingly gone underground in a social-psychological sense. Women also appear more willing to utilize legal and political avenues to realize their aspirations.

Studying the feminist identity of Jewish women, Dufour (2000) encountered a situation similar to that found by Manning. Dufour perceives the process of coping as one of "sifting." Judaism is examined, and doctrinal selection takes place in order to resolve the conflict between spiritual and religious identities. Beliefs and actions that do not satisfy feminist spiritual needs are thus "sifted" out.

RELIGION, WORK, AND OCCUPATION

> Waste of time is thus the first and deadliest of sins. . . . Loss of time through sociability, idle talk, luxury, even more sleep than is necessary for health . . . is worthy of absolute moral condemnation. . . . it is at the expense of one's daily work. (Weber, 1904/1930, pp. 157–158)

This statement from Weber's *The Protestant Ethic and the Spirit of Capitalism* situates work at the heart of the Judeo-Christian tradition. The association of religion with work and labor is said to go back 1,500 years within Catholicism. It was considered a divine principle dictated by God and reinforced by the papacy (Carroll, 2013). During the Protestant Reformation in the 16th century, God was replaced by individual responsibility. Salvation, however, became evidenced by financial success, and this line of thought was used to justify capitalism. These views became central ideas in Protestantism; hence the adoption of the "Protestant work ethic" (PWE) as a central moral theme in Judeo-Christian economics. This Calvinist idea of the value of work and labor may seem a bit extreme by today's standards, but the notion is clearly well embedded in Western civilization. Though infrequently verbalized, these views lie at the sociocultural core of personal faith and success, as well as the capitalist economic order (Rotenberg, 1978; Tawney, 1926).

Mueller (1978) has suggested a contrasting, anticompetitive Roman Catholic ethic that values "a steady state economy and society . . . cooperation, security, and authority" (p. 143), and hence support for the status quo. This may in part explain the relatively low achievement of Catholics in North America (Riccio, 1979; Stark, 1998). Some scholars argue that this condition has been changing over the past 50 years, however (Porterfield, 2001; Roof & McKinney, 1987). A precursor to this change was offered by Greeley (1963), who found that Catholics and Protestants had similar economic aspirations.

Achievement Motivation and Occupational Success in Different Religious Groups

Underlying work and labor, in the perspective of the PWE, is the motivation to achieve. This has three components: activism, individualism, and a futuristic orientation (Riccio, 1979). As just noted, Catholicism has been theorized to counter activism and individualism (Rosen, 1950; Tawney, 1926).

Judaism has no source of central control, and certainly no direct PWE influence. The need for freedom from bigotry and oppression stimulated Jewish immigration from Europe to North America. The United States in particular offered many opportunities, including education. Jews often gravitated toward security-enhancing professions such as medicine and law (Gorelick, 1981). New chances to succeed in business were rapidly adopted. Jewish families now saw learning and higher education as avenues to honor and economic success, and strongly inculcated achievement values in their children (McClelland, 1961).

Training children in the home for later independence is a positive correlate of achievement motivation, and Rosen (1950) has shown earlier independence training among Protestants and Jews than among Catholics. He also found that independence training and achievement motivation go together, further supporting the underpinnings of the PWE. This is also realized in the vocational aspirations of Jewish and Protestant mothers for their children. The occupational goals selected by both groups have tended to be higher than those chosen by Catholics. In other words, until the late 20th century, Catholic mothers were more satisfied with lower-status occupations that offered stability and job security for their children than were their Jewish and Protestant counterparts (McClelland, 1961).

Lenski (1961) and Mayer and Sharp (1962) took the next step and compared religious groups in terms of socioeconomic status, primarily using measures of income, self-employment, occupational positions, and education. The patterns they observed were in harmony with the findings of Rosen (1950): Jews and Protestants exceeded Roman Catholics in all of these indicators. Bronson and Meadow (1968) reported a similar finding when Catholic and Protestant Mexican Americans were studied; the latter also revealed higher achievement needs than the former. A review of such studies by Riccio (1979) showed that the majority of American adults supported the PWE by that time; however, its acceptance was higher among Protestants and Jews than among Catholics.

When Is Work Considered a "Calling"?

A basic empirical question regarding the relationship of religion to work has been asked by Davidson and Caddell (1994). One assumption of the PWE is that work is not simply a career, but possesses religious significance and is therefore a "calling." Studying 1,869 respondents from 31 Catholic and Protestant congregations, these scholars found that about 15% of their sample did consider work a "calling." Secular cost and benefit factors dominated how respondents viewed their own labor and occupations. Davidson and Caddell (1994) concluded that interpreting work religiously is most likely to occur when people are intrinsically committed. As might be expected, such a perspective infuses all aspects of life with religious and spiritual significance, including work.

The Phenomenon of Jewish Achievement

As noted above, Jews found that many new opportunities were open to them when they left Europe and came to North America. The result is well stated by Stark (1998): "The Jews rapidly became the most highly educated group in North America . . . and have the highest average family income of any racial, religious or ethnic group" (p. 298). Stark further claims that male Jews are overrepresented in the professions and among managers and proprietors, and underrepresented in blue-collar occupations. This message, along with information on the economic achievement of Jews and other religious groups, has likewise been provided by Lehrer (2004) in a key paper.

Explaining the continuing level of Jewish achievement in a number of areas requires more than the bare-bones theory presented above. A number of theoretical possibilities have been advanced (Stark, 1998). Readers are referred to the theory and citations provided by Cochran, Hardy, and Harpending (2005), which are discussed in Chapter 3.

Integrating Religion and Work

Religion and Vocational Choice

Koltko (1993) has proposed a theory about the influence of religious values on vocational choice. He sees four dimensions of religion as crucial in this process. These are belief structures (theology); the history of the religious group studied; its social structure and socialization (religious practices, organization); and lifespan milestones (standardized practices relative to life events).

Unfortunately, these rather interesting directions for research do not appear to have been taken up by psychologists of religion. Wuthnow (1994) points out that we really know very little about how people in the United States integrate religious beliefs with economic motivations. His impressive survey reveals that even though religion's role in U.S. economic life is muted, it exerts a subtle pressure as a background variable. For example, Calvinistic/ Puritan ideas counsel morality in business dealings. Likewise, appeals to thrift and economic advantage probably find responsive minds when purveyed in advertisements by banks, investment firms, stockbrokers, insurance agencies, and other financial "movers and shakers."

When asked directly about the role of religion in choosing a job, about 22% of Wuthnow's (1994) sample felt that their faith might have been operative in their decision. A comparison of churchgoers with the total labor force on a wide variety of characteristics revealed none that really distinguished these two groups. With regard to their sense of personal worth, the former valued their relation to God much more than was found in the overall labor force. Slight differences showed churchgoers favoring familial, social, moral, and community values over personal pleasure and gain. These tendencies are in line with research revealing that leanings toward Intrinsic/committed faith are associated positively with social, altruistic, and proreligious values. As Wuthnow (1994) theorized, those who subscribe to a utilitarian/ Extrinsic faith orientation are more concerned with status, materialism, achievement, income, and security (see also Spilka, 1977). The classical Calvinistic idea that hard labor is pleasing to God still prevails. Wuthnow (1994) claimed that 53% of the total work force and 68% of weekly churchgoers affirmed this view.

Given the foregoing findings, one might reasonably ask about ties between religiosity and job satisfaction. Validating earlier research, Wuthnow found that religiosity was correlated positively with job satisfaction. He has also suggested that religious beliefs and activities might reduce job stress. His data as a whole imply that faith endows work with meaning, and that it constructively helps integrate work into one's life.

Religion and Ethics in the Workplace

Continuing his examination of the potential influence of religion in work settings, Wuthnow (1994) examined the possible role of ethics and found a number of factors related to faith commitments. In defining what work ethics entail, weekly churchgoers were more likely than the work force in general to stress honesty and fairness. Regarding major work decisions, moral absolutism was again present, along with a theistically premised moralism and altruism. These inclinations countered an individualistic/opportunistic utilitarianism. In other words, Wuthnow's respondents felt that personal desires and benefits should give way to religious and humanitarian considerations. They also felt that moral concerns should take precedence over personal ones; hence those who subscribed to absolutist moral and theistic perspectives were likely to adhere to ethical rules and regulations in the workplace. These positions were held most strongly by those affiliated with religious fellowship groups, again revealing the behind-the-scenes role of religious involvements.

In summary, even though Wuthnow's (1994) work is generally in line with Koltko's (1993) recommendations, data on the specifics of the four dimensions identified by Koltko are still lacking.

Religion and Spirituality in the Workplace

The 20th century ended with an essentially new perspective relating spirituality, religion, and workplace values (Mitroff & Denton, 1999). Possibly because of the potential for conflict, this perspective appeared to shift rapidly to spirituality, with religion taking a back seat. Stress was now placed on one's inner life and sense of meaning and purpose, plus the idea that those working together could be joined in a community that would increase personal satisfaction in the workplace (Hill, Jurkiewicz, Giacolone, & Fry, 2013). Research and writing on these ideas has burgeoned in recent years and does not appear to be slowing. A recent overview of 15 studies encompassing 38 variables (commitment, job satisfaction, work unit performance, etc.) showed 34 positive outcomes and only 4 that were negative (Benefiel, Fry, & Geigle, 2014).

Social Change and New Considerations

The 20th century witnessed almost unbelievable events and developments in all aspects of life, and religion did not escape these changes. In order to assess contemporary religious and spiritual views in relation to work, the impressive studies of Roof (1993) and Wuthnow (1993, 1994) may be considered models that require follow-up. Similar work detailing the beliefs of scientists is again necessary. We must keep in mind that beliefs in God and an afterlife can take many forms, so simplistic assumptions and generalizations about what intelligent and intellectually sophisticated people believe cannot be made lightly.

Much has been made of the importance of socioeconomic status for understanding how vocation relates to religion (Roberts, 1984). Findings from the 1980s and later place Episcopalians, Congregationalists, Presbyterians, and Jews at the top of the economic ladder, and Baptists, other Protestants, and sectarian groups at the bottom. Catholics have slowly been moving up ladder (Porterfield, 2001; Roberts, 1984; Roof & McKinney, 1987).

As noted earlier, Koltko's (1993) interesting theory has not been very thoroughly investigated to date. We have largely noted what might be termed broad social-structural variables, but possible psychological ties between vocation and religion have yet to be studied.

OVERVIEW

The complexity of adult religion has barely been touched upon in this chapter. Still, when we talk about religion, it is generally in terms of adult use and understanding. Without question, we can look at any aspect of adult religious belief, behavior, and experience individually and collectively in relation to any aspect of behavioral and social science. In all likelihood, we would find some work exploring a relationship. Needless to say, this chapter in its entirety, or any of its individual sections, could be expanded into a distinct and separate volume.

CHAPTER 7

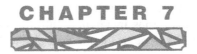

Religion, Aging, and Death

If the rich could hire the poor to die for them, the poor
would make a very good living.

Every man knows he will die, but no man wants to believe it.

You've heard of the three ages of man: youth, middle age,
and "you're looking wonderful!"

It is impossible to experience one's death objectively, and
still carry a tune.[1]

SOME BASIC CONSIDERATIONS

In 1929, noted author and world-famous anthropologist Ruth Underhill interviewed a
92-year-old Papago woman who put a number of life's truths together in her statement: "It's
not good to be old; it's not beautiful. When you come again, I will not be here" (quoted in
Underhill, 1936, p. 64). This may be the basic story of the last stage of our lives, but faith
has much to say about how this time can be lived and what it may mean for all of us. The
significance of death in all theologies cannot be overestimated; this is a worldwide religious
concern (Reynolds & Waugh, 1977). The treatment of age in Western society has, however,
ranged from negative to positive.

Life expectancy is continually increasing. In 1900, at birth the average American could
expect to live 47.3 years U.S Census Bureau, 1999, Table 1421). In 2008, life expectancy
reached 77.8 years; an estimate for 2015 was 79.5 years (U.S. Census Bureau, 2012, Table
104). This trend will probably continue, and along with it an expanding elderly population
whose voices are loudly heard—and must be heard—in religious circles. When we speak of
"the elderly" or those euphemistically called "seniors," habit and even the law have tended
to identify age 65 as the legal time to retire or be forced out of one's work situation. The Age
Discrimination in Employment Act of 1967 ended such discrimination in the United States.
In the popular mind, however, 65 remains the age at which a person tends to be considered
"old."

---

[1]These quotations come, respectively, from the following sources: Rosten (1972, p. 177); Rosten (1972,
p. 172); Cardinal Spellman, quoted in Peter (1977, p. 366); Woody Allen, quoted in Peter (1977, p. 134).

When a person is referred to as "old," a number of largely undesirable stereotypes are imagined. Chief among these are a fairly well-defined pattern of physical and mental infirmities, as well as reduced capabilities in virtually all areas of life. Declining health is a correlate of age, along with reductions in mental and physical skills and strength. Still, we should not lose sight of the tremendous variability among older persons. Many can surpass their younger associates in a wide variety of activities, and their many years of experience can be a valuable personal commodity. Research on religion and aging overwhelmingly focuses on what religion does for the elderly, and not as much on how the elderly may contribute to their church and the well-being of themselves and others. Largely due to the work of Krause (2013), research on church involvement is increasing at a rapid rate.

THE FAITH OF THE ELDERLY

In recent work, Smith (2012) examined belief in God for samples from 30 countries. Over time, God belief declined for 27 nations but not the United States, where 80.8% claimed that "I believe in God now and I always have." Only Chile and the Philippines scored higher. Table 7.1, using data collected from 1972 to 2014 by the General Social Survey (GSS, 2015) of the University of California, shows that such belief in God tends to be highest among the elderly.

Unfortunately, Smith offers no explanation for his observations, but it is possible that religious teachings may have been more prevalent, respected, and influential in previous generations. Krause (2013) basically states that this could be a function of being close to death, and that faith may reduce the anxiety activated by death ideas. Similar inclinations were reported in a Gallup Poll (Newport, 2006c), which found that religion steadily increased in importance with age: Whereas 47% of 19- to 29-year-olds claimed that religion is very important in their lives, 72% of those over age 65 felt similarly. Within the latter group, 78% of women and 63% of men took this position.

The greater religious inclinations observed among the elderly go beyond seriousness of God belief. Krause (2013) cites older persons' rates of church attendance, which are confirmed

TABLE 7.1. Certainty That God Exists (Affirming Percentages) among Americans of Different Ages

Age group	%
Under 28	53.8
28–37	59.4
38–47	55.0
48–57	63.8
58–67	69.0
68+	66.0

Note. Data for 1972–2014, from General Social Survey (2015).

by the GSS data: Whereas 23–36% of those ages 18–60 go to church, 52.6% of seniors in the 70–80 age range are steady attenders. A 4% drop in those ages 80–90 may well reflect the physical limitations of these people. We also note that these oldsters engage in more praying and Bible reading at home, plus seeking forgiveness, than younger persons. Table 7.2, again using GSS (2015) data, offers two further items that more deeply assess feelings about God. For both of these questions, once again the oldest respondents indicate the strongest commitment to their faith. Krause (2013), however, notes a lack of theory development and the widespread use of cross-sectional methodology, both of which raise serious questions about the validity and meaning of research findings. If we take some other data at face value, doubt enters the picture. One Gallup Poll (Gallup & Lindsay, 1999) examined church attendance and found that 67% of 18- to 29-year-olds claimed they had gone to services within the preceding week. The rate for those ages 65–74 was only 48%, and that for persons age 75 and older was 54%. Since no information was available on the health status of the older people, we might reasonably hypothesize that the lower numbers could reflect physical problems that confined these elderly in their homes or institutions. We obviously need to know more about relationships between age and religious practices.

Again, we should not overlook the fact that in their youth many of the elderly (particularly the oldest individuals) lived in an American culture in which religion was more prominent than it is today. Benson's (1988b) study of 5,000 Protestants supports this inference. When asked about the role of church and faith in their early life, those over 70 accorded them greater significance than younger adults did. The over-70 respondents also evidenced a higher level of congregational and denominational loyalty, which Benson termed "maturity of faith."

In another study, Koenig, Smiley, and Gonzales (1988) questioned four groups of geriatric patients and senior center participants, who illustrated both the relative strength of religion and the variability of research findings with different elderly samples. Possibly because of increasing infirmity, private religious activities such as prayer and reading religious material became of greater importance during old age than was true for those under 65. Again, clearly, we have to dig deeper into the meaning of religion for the elderly. Research Box 7.1 offers a good example of what may lie beneath the surface of religious expression for older people.

TABLE 7.2. Feelings of Closeness to God, and of Being Guided by God in Daily Activities, among Americans of Different Ages

Age group	% feeling very close to God	% feeling guided by God in daily activities
21–30	10.5	23.5
31–40	14.0	27.8
41–50	17.1	25.1
51–60	20.1	28.3
61–70	20.6	28.1
71–80	29.4	33.8
81–89	31.8	35.2

Note. Data for 1972–2014, from General Social Survey (2015).

RESEARCH BOX 7.1. Religious Involvement, Beliefs about God, and the Sense of Mattering among Older Adults (Schieman, Bierman, & Ellison, 2010)

Understanding the faith of any selected group of people without having available other groups for comparison opens the door to a continuing program of research—which, unhappily, is rarely pursued. Schieman and colleagues offered some well-thought-out possibilities that do not appear to have been followed up.

A sample of 1,167 whites and blacks 65 years and older were carefully selected, with subgroups balanced for gender, race, and locality where they were recruited. Respondents were administered questions defining their (1) sense of mattering to others, (2) frequency of attendance at defined religious activities, (3) prayer frequency, and (4) belief in divine control. In addition, indices for race, gender, education level, marital status, and religious group were provided.

A number of sophisticated analyses were performed, which indicated statistical significance for church attendance, prayer frequency, gender, education, race, sense of divine control, and sense of mattering. The authors stressed the meaning of connections between the last two variables. They made special note of what they felt to be a personal theology among African Americans, in which God is "active in all areas of life" (p. 530).

Even though much statistical significance was reported, its strength was often low, or at most middling. Still, this study demonstrates the complexity of religious beliefs and involvement among the elderly—matters that obviously merit considerable follow-up.

THE ROLES OF RELIGION IN LATE LIFE

Regardless of age, all of us want to feel secure and good about ourselves. These needs may be strongest among elderly individuals, for this is their time of greatest strain and probably of greatest social isolation. Physical and mental health problems are most likely to occur among the old, and these are frequently compounded by the loss of relationships as family members and friends die. Among aged persons, religion often counters these realities by helping them cope with life, offering meaning, and enhancing their sense of control and self-esteem.

Religion and Coping with Life

Recognizing church attendance as probably reflecting a connectedness to others, along with practical wisdom about life and the centrality and appreciation of the deity's roles ("awe of God"), Krause and Hayward (2015) focused on the coping feelings and responses of older whites and blacks. They hypothesized that religion, with an emphasis on God, is necessarily affiliated with claimed success in living. Support for their hypotheses was found, but correlational ties, though statistically significant, tended to be weak. Clearly sensitive to ethnic considerations, Krause and Bastida (2011) extended this research program to Mexican Americans. Other work of an overlapping nature emphasized prayer (Hayward & Krause, 2013). It should be noted that this research was part of a major effort by Krause and associates for over a decade to understand how the elderly integrate religion with their life circumstances. There is a breadth to their work from which the psychology of religion can learn much.

Despite a great deal of good thinking and the researchers' solid awareness of short-comings and difficulties, the statistically significant findings in favor of positive associations between religiosity/spirituality and coping were often weak, and alternative hypotheses such as social desirability responding need to be assessed. That this is an extremely complex realm goes without saying. Much more work is obviously needed to appreciate how religion and coping behavior are related. Pargament (1997) first opened this door to a large room, which to date is dimly lit. With regard to aging and faith, Krause and colleagues appear to be conducting much of the research needed to further our understanding of a complex realm.

Meaning and Religion

A noted psychologist of religion who was also theologically trained, Walter Houston Clark, stated clearly and simply that "religion more than any other human function satisfies the need for meaning in life" (1958, p. 419). Aldridge (2000) suggests that the search for meaning takes us to a different, probably higher level of understanding that calls upon an innate human capacity. He further claims that this is an essential aspect of spiritual development.

Recognizing the involved nature of the problem of meaning, Batson and his colleagues (Batson & Ventis, 1982; Batson, Schoenrade, & Ventis, 1993) emphasized how people approach their faith. They formulated the notion of a Quest orientation, in which cognition serves as a "way of being religious" that focuses on "complexity, doubt, and tentativeness" (Batson & Ventis, 1982, p. 149). In the course of developing this approach, Batson's group constructed a 12-item scale that assesses (1) "readiness to face existential questions without reducing their complexity," (2) "self-criticism and perception of religious doubt as positive," and (3) "openness to change" (Batson & Schoenrade, 1991b, p. 436). This is a rather sophisticated set of concepts for understanding and measuring faith.

Futterman, Dillon, Garand, and Haugh (1999) saw the potential of associating religion as Quest with elderly persons' search for meaning in their lives. This work is described in Research Box 7.2.

Krause (2003) examined the relationship between religious meaning and subjective well-being in a national sample of older persons. Participants had to be at least 66 years old; the average age was 74.4 years. There were 1,247 people in this sample, half of whom were white and half black. All were interviewed and given a brief survey to complete. Life satisfaction, self-esteem, and optimism were thus assessed. Religious meaning was defined as providing a direction and purpose in life—in other words, a reason for existence.

The results of this study indicated that older black persons attended church more often and more frequently engaged in private prayer than their white peers did. The former also manifested higher levels of religious meaning, self-esteem, and optimism. Religious meaning was found to be more pertinent than church attendance to life satisfaction. Self-esteem was correlated positively with religious meaning. An unexpected finding occurred with private prayer, which was associated with lower self-esteem and less optimism. This may have reflected a situation in which unhappiness over health or one's life situation elicited more praying in the hope that the wish for improvement might be granted. In sum, religious meaning was positively associated with life satisfaction, optimism, and self-esteem. It also played a greater role in the well-being of older black Americans than of elderly white Americans.

Krause (2004a) expanded this effort with additional attention to prayer expectancies in relation to race and esteem. This study is described in Research Box 7.3.

RESEARCH BOX 7.2. Religion as a Quest and the Search for Meaning in Later Life (Futterman, Dillon, Garand, & Haugh, 1999)

In this study, 342 elderly people with an average age of 72.3 years were administered Batson and colleagues' Quest Scale. Sixty-two percent of the sample were female, 48% were married, and 36% were widowed. Though 47% of the sample were Catholics, a broad range of Protestant denominations was represented. Two percent of the respondents were non-Christian. In addition to quantitative statistical analyses, qualitative information was gathered from interviews.

In contrast to the three scale dimensions defined by Batson and Schoenrade (1991), a factor analysis revealed primarily two factors. These stressed "questioning of religious meanings" and "religious doubt and willingness to change religious beliefs" (Futterman et al., 1999, p. 161). The interviews supported these themes. Questions were raised about Batson and Schoenrade's inference of the independence of Quest from the better-known Means (Extrinsic) and End (Intrinsic) forms of religiousness. These results indicate that religion among the elderly is too complex to be easily categorized.

There are two other lessons in this work, which must lead to additional research. First, we need to ask whether the difference between this study and those of Batson and colleagues is a function of the nature of the sample. The one used by Futterman et al. differs from the samples used by Batson's group. Second, it warns us to check on the measures we employ, no matter how popular they are or how often they have been used previously.

RESEARCH BOX 7.3. Assessing the Relationships among Prayer Expectancies, Race, and Self-Esteem in Late Life (Krause, 2004a)

In this study, Krause was not simply concerned with the act of praying, but with the expectancies it engenders. Such expectancies include beliefs about when and how prayers may be answered, as well as the nature of God's responses. Since the when, what, and how may not match what people have prayed for, they often express the view that they will trust in God to do what is best. These are termed "trust-based expectancies" (TBEs).

Approximately equal numbers of black and white participants were selected from a national sample for interviews, of which 1,500 were conducted. The mean age of the respondents was 74.3 years. In addition to demographic data, prayer TBEs, frequency of praying, and self-esteem were evaluated.

The elderly black participants were more likely than their white peers to rely on TBEs, and this tendency raised the self-esteem of the former more than the latter. It was further observed that self-evaluation was a function of the TBEs, not of the frequency of prayer.

This study demonstrates that research on prayer is probably insightful when other than simple frequency is considered. The complexity of prayer suggests that additional work in this area is merited.

Homan and Boyatzkis (2010) conducted a study with respondents 65+ years of age, which implied a connection among religiosity, meaning, and health behavior. Measures of the first and third elements were presented, but not a measure of meaning, which makes it difficult to see the link between religiosity and meaning.

The opposites of a meaningful faith are doubt, uncertainty, and confusion. These concerns have been addressed by Krause, Ingersoll-Dayton, Ellison, and Wulff (1999). Using a national sample of approximately 1,800 Presbyterians, Krause et al. found that the issue was much more complex than expected. The literature suggested that doubt could spur intrapersonal growth on the one hand, but might adversely affect well-being on the other. In this sample, religious doubt was associated with depression, and hence well-being suffered. Those over age 60 handled their religious questions better than younger individuals did. The wisdom of experience may have endowed these elderly persons with the knowledge and skills to cope more successfully with their faith.

Forgiveness

Forgiveness has only recently entered the psychology of religion as a research concern. Prior to the last 25 years, it rarely appeared as a topic for any psychological study. Johnson (1959) treated it in terms of theology, except for a brief mention of its psychotherapeutic potential. Pruyser (1968) peripherally wrapped it up in his psychoanalytic view of religion. Current approaches indicate that forgiveness is a surprisingly complex concept, and as such it has stimulated both research and clinical work.

In the main, most of this work has dealt with three forms of forgiveness "trait forgiveness," which is restricted to individuals; "state forgiveness," which is concerned with single offenses; and "self-forgiveness," which focuses on personal actions that are deemed undesirable (Davis, Worthington, Hook, & Hill, 2013). Generally, age is positively related to employing forgiveness. The elderly engage in it out of conviction that it is the necessary and appropriate thing to do (Girard & Mullet, 1997; McCullough, Bono, & Root, 2005).

Toussaint, Williams, Musick, and Everson (2001) compared three age groups (18–44, 45–64, 65+) on four forgiveness measures. These focused on self, others, and God, plus the feeling of being forgiven by God. Four measures of religiousness/spirituality dealt with church attendance, prayer, religiosity, and spirituality. Across the age groups, results were generally inconsistent and nonsignificant. On the average, there were more signs of greater religious commitment and activity with increased age, but again one cannot feel comfortable making inferences relative to age. The authors conclude that further study of age differences relative to forgiveness and health is merited.

Also emphasizing aging, Krause and Ellison (2003) examined the role of (1) forgiveness of others and (2) belief in forgiveness by God. Full forgiveness of others was more closely linked with psychological well-being than was forgiveness by God. Those who failed to extend unconditional forgiveness to others revealed more somatic symptoms of depression, plus signs of greater emotional depression, than their fully forgiving peers. These conditional forgivers expected transgressors to evidence contrition. Refusal or failure to forgive was also associated with more death anxiety than was true of forgivers. Such negative signs could be a function of feeling unforgiven by God. This study, along with the findings discussed in Chapter 3, reinforces both the spiritual and personal importance of forgiveness in the Western religious tradition.

Prayer and Aging

Well over a century ago, William James (1902/1985) stated that "Prayer is the very soul and essence of religion" (p. 464). Similar sentiments have been repeatedly offered (Krause, 2012), and Spilka and Ladd (2013) have attempted to review the massive amount of research that has been undertaken on this significant topic. In sum, there is probably no more personally significant religious or spiritual activity than prayer (Aldridge, 2000). Relative to the elderly, this is evidenced by the 1972–2014 GSS data (GSS, 2015). Those who claim they never pray are mostly found in the 21- to 30-year-old category while respondents who pray once a day or more are 71 or more years old. Again, these data provide evidence of the importance of faith to the oldest population segment.

If prayer is anything, it is an active coping strategy that is practiced by at least 90% of Americans (GSS, 2007). The GSS also showed that the percentage of those over age 65 who prayed ranged from 91 to 95%; 12% claimed that they pray several times a day. Resorting to prayer probably endows people with a heightened sense of control in problematic situations. Schulz and Heckhausen (1996) detail a lifespan theory of control that is pertinent to religion and aging. Another way of understanding what occurs to those who pray is offered by Krause (2004a), as described in Research Box 7.3. In sum, a number of studies show that the elderly pray more than their younger counterparts (Spilka & Ladd, 2013; Toussaint et al., 2001).

Krause (2011a) offers a descriptive analysis of "the prayer lives of older whites, older blacks, and older Mexican Americans" (p. 60). Explaining what is observed in research is often difficult, and Krause recognizes a number of problems with his. Researchers want to publish their findings and may not be willing to discuss possible measurement shortcomings. Krause does mention such difficulties: he uses rather large samples and finds statistically significant differences among his groups. Though noteworthy, these differences are numerically rather trivial.[2] Krause does his best to handle the problem of going from data to interpretation with a noteworthy issue of possible ethnic group variation among the elderly.

The complexity of religion–coping relationships in general (as discussed earlier), and prayer–coping links in particular, cannot be gainsaid. Research has consistently shown that religious coping mechanisms, especially prayer, are frequently employed by seniors dealing with health-related stress (Conway, 1985–1986; Manfredi & Pickett, 1987). In a national study, Gurin, Veroff, and Feld (1960) found that troubled older persons utilized prayer more than their younger counterparts did. Dunn and Horgas (2000) reported that 48 of their 50 respondents who were over 65 studied used prayer to cope with life's difficulties. Turning to the deity for support may appear to be the most effective strategy available to the elderly. This holds true for persons from different ethnic groups, of different socioeconomic status, and with varying levels of education (Koenig, George, & Siegler, 1988; Krause & Van Tranh, 1989). The data are clear: Religion in general and prayer in particular are powerful buffers against stress among the elderly. As Myers (1992) puts it, "the happiest of senior citizens are those who are actively religious" (p. 75).

---

[2]When the three groups in the Krause (2011a) study were compared on 12 items, 36 tests were conducted, which may be judged relative to the Bonferroni correction. In this instance, where statistical significance was reported at .001, the Bonferroni computation resulted in a level of .0014. Significance is borderline at this level. It should be noted that this correction tends to be conservative.

RELIGION AND HEALTH AMONG THE ELDERLY

Religion and Physical Health

Homan and Boyatzis (2010) state that "religious involvement is positively related to improved health and longevity" (p. 173). This positive relationship extends to cardiovascular conditions, hypertension, and even selected cancers; The immune system also benefits. At best, however, we are dealing with correlations, not specific and detailed cause-and-effect relationships between faith and physical health. In other words, we can easily understand the psychological benefits of having faith in old age, but a much more difficult issue comes to the fore when we study how physical health and religion are related for the elderly.

We have seen that faith can aid older persons who are under psychological stress, because it can remedy a lack of meaning, control, and social support. This is a realm that requires extra caution, and Harold Koenig (1997, 2000) has introduced such concerns into his writing and research. Recognizing the roles religion may play in mental and physical health, he appropriately adds that "these health effects do not depend on supernatural phenomena, but can be explained by behavioral, social, and psychological mechanisms acting through known physiological pathways" (Koenig, 2000, p. 90).

The mechanisms in question are broad in scope. Churches often actively sponsor a wide variety of healthful practices that are adopted by believers (King, 1990; Levin & Schiller, 1987; Sarafino, 1990). For example, the Mormons and Seventh-Day Adventists condemn the use of alcohol, smoking, and other self-destructive behaviors; in addition, they encourage constructive eating and health habits (Koenig, McCullough, & Larson, 2001). Moberg (2001) summarizes work showing that religious involvement relates negatively to hypertension, the occurrence of strokes, cancer pain, and the need for lengthy hospitalization. These findings may relate to religion's positive influence on attitudes, and in part to the effects of the health-promoting behaviors that churches and synagogues sponsor.

Congregations also often provide social connections and support for the elderly. Along with spiritual doctrines, these factors appear to counter depression and suicide, the rates of which are high among older persons (Plante & Sharma, 2001). Spousal loss and isolation, combined with illness and infirmity, are major factors in suicide in this group (Bock & Warren, 1972). Pastoral caregivers and counselors may help to alleviate these problems—which seem to be especially severe among widowers, who are often not skilled in caring for themselves (Aldridge, 2000; Kimble, 1995).

It is not really possible to distinguish between the effects of the health-promoting activities of churches and the influence that being religious per se has on people. Koenig (2000) has observed that religious patients with conditions that resist improvement adapt to their situations and resolve their depression faster than those low in religiosity. He reports similar findings in study after study. Asking why this occurs, he offers two possibilities: (1) The religious elderly have "a world-view in which suffering has meaning and purpose" (Koenig, 2000, p. 89), and (2) faith in God and the use of prayer heighten their sense of control through the idea that they may be able to influence the deity. Koenig further stresses the view that religion is a source of meaning; nothing is simply random, and hence coping is enhanced. The evidence of enhanced use of prayer in those over age 60 may also relate to increased health difficulties (Spilka & Ladd, 2013).

In general, faith is associated with lower reported rates of cardiovascular conditions, hypertension, stroke, and different forms of cancer, all of which are concentrated among the elderly (Colantonio, Kasl, & Ostfeld, 1992; Levin & Schiller, 1987). It is possible, however, that since religiosity correlates positively with optimism, life satisfaction, and purpose in life, more religious people could be less inclined to report symptoms of illness and therefore may downplay their possible significance (Kass, Friedman, Leserman, Zuttermeister, & Benson, 1991). Though this does not seem to be generally true, its potential should not be overlooked. Wotherspoon's (2000) research on a sample predominantly composed of people over age 80 indicated that both spiritual well-being and existential well-being were positively related to self-assessments of health.

Though researchers often make efforts here to distinguish among such concepts as prayer, coping, stress, and health among the elderly, it is obvious that they overlap. An appreciation of this reality is offered in the work of Ai and colleagues, an example of which is now offered in Research Box 7.4. Further work on the roles of prayer, spirituality, and religiosity in regard to physical health flourished as the 21st century opened (Spilka & Ladd, 2013).

Lastly, let us confront cancer—that terrible group of diagnoses so often found in old age. Though cancer occurs at all ages, the elderly constitute the majority of its victims. Recent work involving over 44,000 patients with cancer in relation to physical, mental, and social health tells us that those who were conceptually able to integrate their illness with their religious and spiritual stance were in relatively good physical health (Jim et al., 2015) In regard to patients' mental health, those who integrated the emotional aspects of faith and spirituality into their condition manifested less anxiety and depression (Sherman et al., 2015). Finally, people who were able to continue their "social health" (i.e., normal social activities and relationships) had more personally positive images of God plus a benevolent conception of their faith in general (Salsman et al., 2015). Work such as this demonstrates how complex the domains of both illness and religiosity/spirituality are.

RESEARCH BOX 7.4. The Role of Private Prayer in Psychological Recovery among Midlife and Aged Patients Following Cardiac Surgery
(Ai, Dunkle, Peterson, & Bolling, 1998)

This research paper was the first of several Ai and her coworkers offered in the area of religion—primarily prayer relative to coronary artery bypass graft (CABG) surgery. Without question, this procedure constitutes a major stressor and induces serious feelings of lack of control in patients undergoing it. The study concerned the use of prayer in postoperative recovery. The authors defined such prayer as a "tool of 'spiritual coping'" (p. 592).

The final sample consisted of 151 respondents, 74 under 65 years of age and 77 over 65. These patients completed two questionnaires—one given 6 months after the surgery, another 6 months later. Relative to coping, private prayer was the most common practice among a total of 21 assessed. Patient optimism both prior to and following CABG related favorably to prayer both pre- and postoperatively. Unexpected was the finding that the over-65 group engaged in significantly less prayer than their under-65 counterparts. Prayer was also employed most by those who were more depressed immediately after the CABG surgery. The authors suggested that prayer was largely used by these patients to suppress distress. It should not be surprising that the use of prayer was primarily a function of patients' level of personal religiosity. Research like this stimulated a variety of questions that these scholars followed up in other studies in the following decade.

Religion and Psychological Health: New Possibilities

A great deal of research has been undertaken on the psychological health of the elderly. A fair amount of this research has already been presented. Rather than draw more exhaustively on this literature, let us recognize a professional paper that, in our opinion, opens a door to some new possibility. Recognizing that different faiths may have different appeals to their troubled adherents and that different religious groups may vary in the meanings they bring to their religious and spiritual attachments, McGowan, Midlarsky, Morin, and Graber (2016) conducted a study in which they focused on Intrinsic religiosity in examining anxiety and depression among Christian and Jewish elderly individuals.

The participants in the study were "74 Christians (43 Catholics and 31 Protestants) and 69 Jews (predominantly Conservative and Reform Jews)" (pp. 4–5). Ages ranged from 65 to 94. A number of other controls and considerations were present. Similarities and differences were primarily observed relative to depression rather than anxiety, and the differences observed were not significant

Failure to find significant differences, for example, might mean that terms such as "religious coping" were not defined similarly by the two groups. Christians were said to stress personal "thoughts and intentions" (p. 12) in their coping, while Jews emphasized institutional involvement and practice. Other variations in the meanings of religious coping and engagement may have been present. Though such variations may be most apparent in denoting one as a Christian or a Jew, they may necessitate closer scrutiny when individuals from different denominations or from major and minor religious subgroups are studied. Given such possibilities, McGowan and his associates turn our attention to a number of different studies and publications that other scholars might overlook.

The Role of Stress

In order to understand the research on religion and both mental and physical health, we need to deal with the issue of stress. Old age is a particularly significant stressor for many people. Because youth, individuality, and progress are valued in Western society, those who have retired and/or developed the infirmities of old age usually find it difficult to avoid negative self-views and loneliness. Erik Erikson (1963), the first modern thinker to develop a lifespan developmental psychology, pictured the last years of life as a struggle between ego integrity and despair. The aging individual must confront a number of noteworthy changes and losses: Physical and often mental skills decline; personal significance through work is usually reduced after retirement; family members and friends die; and, finally, the knowledge that one's own life may shortly conclude is ever present.

Former capabilities are supplanted by weaknesses and the loss of muscle. Youthful beauty is replaced by wrinkles and white hair. Memories become tenuous. There is a growing susceptibility to illness, not the least of which is the heightened likelihood of cancer, heart disease, arthritis, and neurological disorders such as Alzheimer disease and other dementias. New aches and pains keep appearing as the years pass. These constitute additional sources of unavoidable stress.

With regard to stress and cancer, a study not immediately relevant to the present topic is nevertheless worth mentioning. McClintock (cited in Packard, 2007) noted that black women in Chicago who lived in poverty-stricken, high-crime neighborhoods moved frequently and tended to lose their social connections. A correlate of this isolating stress was "lethal breast cancer" (Packard, 2007, p. 42). Using an animal model (a strain of white rats prone to mammary tumors), McClintock created a combination of stress and isolation, and observed that rats subjected to these conditions developed more cancerous tumors faster than did control groups. Even though this work is distant from our immediate concern with aging and religion, it is suggestive.

RELIGION AND MORTALITY

Some impressive research has examined the relationship between mortality and religious involvement. Strawbridge, Cohen, Shema, and Kaplan (1997) collected data on more than 5,000 people over 28 years. The results showed that frequent church attenders lived longer than infrequent attenders. Apparently the former were more likely to cease smoking, engage in exercise, remain married, and maintain their social connections. In follow-up work involving over 2,600 people and covering the period from 1965 to 1994, Strawbridge, Shema, Cohen, and Kaplan (2001) confirmed their earlier findings. Those who attended religious services weekly in 1965 engaged in more positive health behaviors and manifested better mental health through 1994. Similar work from a different vantage point was undertaken by McCullough, Hoyt, Larson, Koenig, and Thoresen (2000): They conducted a meta-analysis of data from 42 studies (see below), and again observed a positive connection between religious involvement and living longer. Other work shows that church attendance, self-assessed religiosity, and the attitude that religion is a source of personal strength are all positively related to staying alive (Koenig, Smiley, & Gonzales, 1988).

Though all of these researchers are wary of explaining their findings as direct effects of faith, recent work suggests that loneliness—a common problem among older people—may adversely influence the body's immune system. In specific, being alone can turn over 200 genes on or off. Many of these genes control the function of white blood cells, possibly increasing the likelihood of infections and infirmity (Cole et al., 2007).

Many variables confound the religion–longevity relationship, and research findings have been neither clear nor consistent. For example, the tie between gender and faith shows that correlations between mortality and religion are stronger for women than for men (McCullough, 2001). We cannot take this finding at face value, because women tend to outlive men, so we must correct for gender. Moreover, indices of public religious organizational involvement such as church attendance (but not nonorganizational involvement) relate positively to the length of life, and women tend to be more religious than men. The probability is that among the elderly, many nonattenders have poorer health that prevents them from going to church. These are only two of many possible confounds; hence it is understandable why the more such variables are controlled for, the weaker the association between faith and a long life becomes (McCullough et al., 2000).

Recognizing the necessity for a meta-analysis of the data, McCullough et al. (2000) conducted such an analysis on studies that utilized almost 126,000 people. "Meta-analysis" is a methodological/statistical procedure in which researchers gather a great deal of what they hope are comparable data from different studies, and analyze these data in order to resolve discrepancies and conflicting findings. After considering some 15 possible confounding factors, these scholars found that religious involvement and longevity continued to be positively related. The association was, however, rather weak. For example, if we had two groups of 100 people each—one group being high in religiosity, the other less religious—in a later follow-up we could expect to find that 53 people in the less religious group had died, while only 47 in the more religious group had died. The positive association of longevity with church/synagogue attendance (but not with private devotions) held. Women also seemed to benefit more than men from attending services. Unfortunately, as indicated above, age, sickness, and disability go together, suggesting again that more and more older religious individuals may cease attending church because of home confinement. This group may show high mortality, leaving relatively healthy regular churchgoers who live longer. Still, for those at home, religious radio and television programs may serve as partial substitutes for church participation (Swatos, 1998; Wotherspoon, 2000).

Koenig et al. (1998) attempted to relate religion to survival among 1,010 hospitalized veterans between 1987 and 1989. Two-thirds of the sample died during this period. Despite an attempt to get information with sophisticated statistical techniques, the researchers acknowledged that mortality was largely a function of health indices rather than religious and social measures.

A more recent meta-analysis also deserves mention (Shor & Roelfs, 2013). Seventy-four publications reporting on more than 300,000 respondents were assessed on social participation and mortality. Prior analyses of 334 publications suggested that social participation was in essence the only variable distinguishing when mortality occurred: Those with low mortality tended to have higher rates of social participation. The authors discuss difficulties with making definitive inferences relative to religious participation because of a number of problems, such as private versus public participation possibilities.

Research on a sample of institutionalized chronically ill elderly persons claimed that those who died within a year were less religious (Reynolds & Nelson, 1981). This picture is muddied by the fact that these persons also had poorer prognoses and were more cognitively impaired. In a contradictory vein, Zuckerman, Kasl, and Ostfeld (1984) reported that religion was positively correlated with longevity, but only among elderly persons who were in poor health.

A. H. Richardson (1973) studied over 1,300 octogenarians and found religion to be unrelated to 1-year survival rates. Later work by Koenig (1995) confirmed this finding. Idler and Kasl (1992) also found that neither public or private religiousness predicted mortality; however, for both Christians and Jews, there were significantly fewer deaths in the 30 days prior to a major religious holiday than for the same period afterward.

Despite much work in these areas, the mechanisms through which faith may operate have yet to be identified. We also need studies that control for religious affiliation, cultural differences, and health-promoting/health-damaging behaviors (King, 1990; Levin & Schiller, 1987). In addition, issues of response biasing have yet to be addressed.

Finally, we see religion and spirituality in action in research on cardiac patients, often awaiting cardiac surgery (Ai, Dunkle, Peterson, & Bolling, 2000; Ai, Peterson, Bolling, & Koenig, 2002; Oxman, Freeman, & Manheimer, 1995). Though the age adjusted death rate for cardiovascular disease CVD) has remained the highest of all causes in the United States up to 2016, the rate of CVD increases with age in such a manner that by 65 years, it is the second leading cause of death in the United States; when Americans reach 75, it is the top killer (U.S. Bureau of the Census, 2007, Sydney et al., 2016). Ai et al. (2002) employed a sample ranging in age from 41 to 81 years old, with a mean age of 65. All participants were awaiting Coronary Artery Bypass Surgery (CABG) surgery (see Research Box 7.4). Private prayer was the most frequent supportive behavior practiced and was associated with a reduction in personal distress. Those engaged in spiritual coping also fared better 1 year following surgery than did their nonpracticing cohorts. The authors of this work suggest that prayer empowers those who pray. In other words, the patients enhanced their sense of control in this stressful situation. Another study of religion's positive effects on cardiac patients was conducted by Oxman et al. (1995).

Determined researchers attempt to counter criticism of their research on longevity and church attendance by doing two things: (1) controlling for possibly confounding variables, and (2) obtaining massive samples. We leave it to other researchers to attempt to top a Harvard professor of epidemiology, Tyler Vanderweele, who controlled over a dozen variables and collected a sample of 75,534 women (see Bakalar, 2016). We will say no more!

Though we have looked at the general tenor of theory and research on religion and mortality relative to aging, death per se has always been a central concern relative to faith on many levels, from the social-psychological to the theological. The latter approach must be left to the scholars of each faith; however, we must examine the former, as it has been a rich domain for creative research.

DEATH AND RELIGION: A COMPLEX RELATIONSHIP

We humans do not take kindly to death. Shakespeare (1604/1964, p. 81) called it "a fearful thing," and Matthew Arnold (1853/1897, p. 288) viewed death as "a hideous show." One may speak of "noble deaths," "death with dignity," "eternal paradise," "ultimate rewards," or may state that "nothing can happen more beautiful than death" (Whitman, 1855/1942, p. 18), but its immediate reality is terrifying to virtually all of us. We lament those who die, and dread the fact that we too, in time, will confront the end of our own existence. Many of us, however, refuse to come to terms with death. We repress, deny, shun, and withdraw where possible from reminders of death, and above all, we fight to delay death. If there is a basic purpose to medicine, it is to reduce mortality and increase longevity. And finally when we die, the customary North American way of death includes embalming, which Aries (1974) interprets as a "refusal to accept death" (p. 99). In other words, we wish to keep our bodies unchanged. Furthermore, our faiths inform us that we do not simply die; we move to another realm—heaven, hell, limbo, purgatory, or life with God. Finally, there is resurrection: We return to everlasting life. In sum, we never die; our destiny is immortality. Religion guarantees it.

Theologian Paul Tillich (1952) championed such an inference by claiming that "the anxiety of fate and death is the most basic, most universal, and inescapable" (p. 40). Reasoning further, the noted anthropologist Bronislaw Malinowski (1965) maintained that "Death, which of all human events is the most upsetting and disorganizing to man's calculations, is perhaps the main source of religious belief" (p. 71). In one study of clergy, only 2% felt that concern about death was not a factor in religious activity (Spilka, Spangler, Rea, & Nelson, 1981).

Even though Western religion assures us of our continuation, it often treats death as a correlate of evil. Scripture is replete with references to death as the appropriate punishment for sin. The Bible tells us that it all started with Adam and Eve, and has been our heritage ever since: "Wherefore, as by one man sin entered into the world, and death by sin; and so death passed upon all men, for that all have sinned" (Romans 5:12). Through death, therefore, religion engenders hope, guilt, and fear.

Religion has historically been our culture's dominant means of coping with the inevitability of our own demise. Religion makes death meaningful. Death is a mystery that we must unravel. It belies meaning and demands explanation. We have questions, and religion offers us the desired answers. Taken at face value, death implies a simple, final end to life. Understandably, we do not easily accept the prospect of ultimate extinction; it is not just that we want to live on indefinitely, but that we desire certainty that this will occur. Religion provides assurance that this will eventually take place. Unamuno (1921/1954) asserted that the theme of "immortality originates and preserves religions" (p. 41).

Institutionalized faith, as we have seen, plays many roles in life, but the issue of death lies at its core. Kearl (1989) got to the heart of the matter when he pointed out that "religion has historically monopolized death meaning systems and ritual," and helps "create and maintain death anxieties and transcendence hopes as mechanisms of social control" (p. 172). Social control easily translates into personal control, another major function of religion. Expectations of judgment in an afterlife can prompt socially conforming behavior and give people the feeling that they are in charge of their final destiny. Especially in individualistic, achievement-oriented American society, this means, as the historian Arnold Toynbee observed, that death is "un-American, an affront to every citizen's inalienable right to life, liberty, and the pursuit of happiness" (quoted in Woodward, 1970, p. 81). Religion, therefore, stands as the only major bulwark against the threat of death.

RELIGION, DEATH, AND IMMORTALITY

Belief in an Afterlife

Intellectually, we all know that everyone dies; emotionally, we are rarely inclined to accept that reality for ourselves. The result may be beliefs in an afterlife, heaven, and hell. These ideas have a strong grip on the minds of Americans. The GSS for the United States from 1972 to 2014 (GSS, 2015) indicates that 80.2% of the almost 16,000 respondents questioned believe in an afterlife. The specific percentages for the elderly are 78.7% for ages 81–89 and 80.2% for ages 71–80. International Social Survey Program data for 1998 reveal no European country with such a high proportion of its population holding these views (Greeley, 2002). And according to the National Opinion Research Center (NORC), between the 1970s and 1990s, belief in life after death increased in the United States from 19 to 56% among Jews and from 74 to 83% among Catholics (Morin, 2000).

Greeley and Hout (1999) present additional data suggesting that from 1900 to 1970, Catholic belief in an afterlife increased from 67 to 85%, and agreement by Jews went from 17 to 74% in the same period. Though a number of possibilities are offered in relation to Jews, these authors note that "the evidence of change is clear; an explanation of it is not" (p. 832). Actually, this statement holds true for all of these findings. Further understanding may come from an appreciation of the effects on individuals and groups of the rapid rate of technological development, national and international stresses, and a certain tenuousness to life (as shown by terrorist activities such as the attacks of September 11, 2001). Contexts also seem to be of considerable importance, as research suggests that persons who are socially and economically disadvantaged may believe more strongly in an afterlife than people who are in adequate cultural circumstances (Ellison & McFarland, 2013). We might hypothesize that for many people, the world has "gotten away from them." The search for immortality may be an attempt to regain the security that the "illusion of control" confers (Langer, 1983). Probably of considerable importance is the fact that one may intellectually conceive of an afterlife, but thinking about a time without consciousness is impossible.

Bering and Bjorkland (2004) undertook research on afterlife beliefs from childhood through adulthood, and though they speak of belief in an afterlife as a "developmental mechanism," implied in their work is the notion that it may be an evolutionary product. In other words, this is a phenomenon whose basic cognitive and neurobiological characteristics merit deeper examination.

For many if not most people, belief in an afterlife first brings to mind the ideas of heaven and hell—concepts that have been used in Western countries for centuries. Extremely widely accepted, they are found in popular songs and also well-known epithets (more for hell than, we believe, for heaven). Americans are less inclined to believe in hell than in heaven. Whereas 65.0% believe in the latter, only 53.2% accept the existence of the former (GSS, 2015). Given the religious criteria for being consigned to either realm, self-examination might prompt aversion on the part of most people to their potential for an afterlife in hell. A Harris Poll supports this hypothesis: 79% of this poll's respondents believed that they would go to heaven, and fewer than 2% felt that their final destination would be hell (Taylor, 1998).

A digression is in order. It is obvious that even though survey samples are large, there is often considerable variation in their findings. Hynson (1975) presents afterlife belief findings in consecutive years for Catholics of 75% and 48%, and for Protestants of 65% and 50%. Using Gallup Poll data, Hertel (1980) addresses some of these inconsistencies. Differences in questions and the selectivity of the samples studied may explain such discrepancies, but this information is rarely presented. Our suggestion is that readers keep open yet challenging minds when it comes to such reports.

The most current data on distribution of afterlife beliefs by faiths indicate more or less what we might expect. In the GSS (2015) percentages of such beliefs in the United States, Jews stand out as the only group scoring less than the 72.3% for Buddhists, the next closest group (see Table 7.3). Why? Conceptions of an afterlife are usually rather well developed and discussed in most major Western faiths. Though Judaism considers life after death a continuation of what existed before dying, there is surprisingly little theological speculation about the nature of an afterlife. In modern times, there is almost an element of denial: The one who dies is supposed to be buried within 24 hours of his or her demise. Maurice Lamm (1969) has written a clear exposition of Jewish death and mourning practices and the reasoning behind them.

An interesting earlier study of church members revealed that only 46% of Protestants and 71% of Catholics claimed that "what we do in this life will determine our fate in the hereafter" (Stark & Bainbridge, 1985, p. 53). In addition, there seems to be considerable

TABLE 7.3. Percentages of Major Religious Groups in America Believing in Life after Death

Religious group	%
Protestants	85.5
Catholics	79.8
Jews	44.3
Muslims	89.5
Buddhists	72.3
Hindus	84.3
Native Americans	78.3

Note. Data for 1972–2014, from General Social Survey (2015).

reluctance to change one's ways to avoid hell (Litke, 1983; Stark & Bainbridge, 1985). Since over half of the Protestants and almost a third of the Catholics surveyed by Stark and Bainbridge agreed that heaven and hell are our destiny for reasons other than the way we live, we might wonder whether we are seeing a return to Calvinistic predestination. Again, further investigation into afterlife beliefs is warranted.

These ideas tend to be vague, since personal continuation is usually viewed as applying to the spirit rather than the body. Still, for many believers, the afterlife is succeeded by resurrection of the body. Contemporary Christianity prefers to conceptualize this as a "spiritual" body rather than a physical one (Badham, 1976). Those desiring further details are often referred to faith and "trust in the Lord." Under such circumstances, this imagery becomes individualized. Nevertheless, the promise that one will not simply and totally cease to exist is present and widely believed.

Transcending Death

"Transcending death" means overcoming its existence as a simple and final termination of further life in any form. Afterlife beliefs interpret transcendence as a simple transition from predeath life to a postdeath form. Transcendence in a more general sense looks to a domain above that of humans—namely, the realm of a deity. Regarding transcendent goals, Emmons and Schnitker (2013) consider them to be idealistic and cite research indicating that they resolve uncertainty and aid individuals in working toward these goals. They thus support coping behavior. Piedmont and Wilkins (2013) claim that the issue is "how perceptions of the transcendent impact the texture, tenor, direction, and quality of people's inner lives" (p. 293). This is asking a lot of transcendent thinking, but Piedmont and Wilkins offer evidence in favor of it. These last references also tell us that transcendent notions may need clearer operational specification, as mental health issues plus possible religious confounds (e.g., church attendance) complicate the research

In a broader sense, Lifton (1973) speaks of a universal need to transcend death. Utilizing the rubric of "symbolic immortality," he suggests five ways of accomplishing such a goal. "Biological immortality" lets a person live on through offspring and descendants. This potential is further realized when the person continues through contributions to larger biosocial units, such as attachments to groups ranging from the family to the human species. "Theological immortality" or "religious immortality" stresses spiritual attachment, implying the triumph of spirit over bodily death. "Creative immortality" is attained through one's works and achievements—the lasting contributions one hopes to make to the future. "Nature immortality" deals with continuation as part of an undying, enduring, permanent nature. Lastly, there is a state of "experiential transcendence" or a mystical kind of immortality, "a state so intense that in it time and death disappear. . . . the restrictions of the senses—including the sense of mortality—no longer exist" (p. 7).

A few research efforts have related these modes of immortality to personal faith. Gochman and Fantasia (1979) found, as might be expected, that the religious form is strongest among devout persons, while the remaining types appear to be independent of religion. Religious immortality is also associated with short- and long-term life planning, implying a flexible time perspective—a tendency also noted in the positive relationship between time perspective and religion found by Hooper and Spilka (1970).

Utilizing a cognitive theoretical framework, Hood and Morris (1983) constructed a more rigorous quantitative assessment of Lifton's modes, relating these to forms of personal faith and death perspectives. This work is described in Research Box 7.5.

RESEARCH BOX 7.5. Toward a Theory of Death Transcendence
(Hood & Morris, 1983)

With sensitivity to the necessity of theoretically guided research, Ralph Hood and Ronald Morris denoted what they termed "transcendent" and "reflexive" facets of the self. The former is conceptually associated with immortality, in which the person "survives" this world. The reflexive self or selves, which exist in this world in a real sense, can also survive after bodily death. Cognitive issues come to the fore in thinking about transcendent–reflexive relations and the various forms of the latter. Robert Lifton's (1973) modes of biological, creative, and nature immortality/transcendence, described in the text, fall into the reflexive category.

Applying these ideas, Hood and Morris developed reliable measures of the Lifton modes from interviews with 39 persons averaging 65 years of age. Independent judges agreed 94% of the time on classifying the responses to the modes. In terms of the modes' presence or absence, 27 people were identified with nature transcendence, 30 with biological (now viewed as biosocial) transcendence, 31 with religious transcendence, and 33 with the creative mode. These people were then administered scales assessing death anxiety and death perspectives, as well as the Allport–Ross scales for Intrinsic and Extrinsic religious orientations. Patterns of meaningful relationships were obtained, suggesting the usefulness of both the Lifton modes and Hood and Morris's transcendent–reflexive distinction with elderly persons.

The religious mode was associated with perceptions of death as a test of courage, and belief in an afterlife of reward. It further countered not only fear of death, but perceptions of death as pain and loneliness, failure, the unknown, or a loss of experience and control—tendencies not found with the other modes. The experiential/mystical mode negated the idea of death as a natural end. The biological/biosocial mode shared the positive religious correlation with courage and an afterlife of reward, but added death as failure. The creative mode was tied to perceptions of death as pain and loneliness, the unknown, forsaking dependents, and failure, as well as to indifference toward death. These findings suggest that personal achievement is antithetic to ideas of death, which, of course, terminate individual accomplishment.

Searching for Evidence of Immortality

The idea of complete termination is terrifying to most people; hence the need to convince oneself that life never really ends is intensely pursued on all fronts from the humanistic to the scientific. When motivation is extremely high, we seek information to buttress our convictions, often making inferences that go beyond the pertinent data. This is probably nowhere more true than in the way we deal with death. An excellent illustration of this tendency may be seen in making a leap of faith from near-death experiences (NDEs) and possible contact with the dead to the existence of an afterlife. These phenomena imply that people do not simply cease to exist, but are transformed and have the potential of remaining connected to the living.

One or two distinctions need to be added. First, an NDE is not necessarily an out-of-body experience. A study of 2,060 cardiac arrest cases showed only a 9% overlap between these two types of experiences (Parnia & Fenwick, 2002). Moreover, 39% of those who survived cardiac arrests had a perception of events occurring that they witnessed but could not recall, and such incidents were often interpreted as occurring after death. Apparent consciousness occurred during a 3-minute period when there was no heartbeat. One proposed explanation suggests that this phenomenon results from oxygen deprivation to the brain.

Near-Death Experiences

Though the notion of the NDE has probably been around since humanity thought about predeath expressions, the concept was popularized during the 1970s. Rather easily, many people transformed the idea of "near death" to "after death." It was commonly believed that those undergoing NDEs had really died, entered an aspect of the afterlife, and then returned to tell what happened to them. The volume *Life after Life* by psychiatrist Raymond Moody (1976) supported such views, and Moody became quite popular. Criticality, logic, and alternative explanations were acceptable only in limited quarters.

Pollster George Gallup, Jr., and his associate William Proctor (1982) pointed out that NDEs (which they termed "verge-of-death experiences") have much in common with mystical and religious experiences, in that all may be triggered by threats to life. They even suggested seven different situations that can elicit these episodes. (Keep in mind, as discussed in Chapter 1, that at least a third of the U.S. population reports having had mystical experiences, and that among religious persons the percentage is far higher.) According to Gallup and Proctor, 15% of their respondents claimed to have had NDEs. The possible identification of religious encounters with NDEs suggests that those who report the former may be inclined to have the latter, and this appears to be true. Gallup and Proctor (1982) found that 23% of those claiming religious experiences also stated that they had had NDEs—a percentage 8 points above that for the general populace. Another variation on this theme found correlations between NDEs and belief in other extraordinary phenomena, such as unidentified flying objects (UFOs), reincarnation, and the likelihood that the living can contact the dead.

Turning to scientists (a group whose members are likely to question NDEs), Gallup and Proctor (1982) reported that 10% admitted personal involvement in an NDE. Though 32% believed in an afterlife, only 3% felt that they had actually had a supernatural encounter. The overall tendency of scientists was to separate NDEs from the idea of an afterlife, and many attempted theoretical explanations of these phenomena in terms of physiological changes related to brain chemistry and function under oxygen deprivation, anesthetics, or the operation of endorphins. It is also significant that many religionists are also reluctant to claim that NDEs represent proof of an afterlife.

Doubt is cast on the supernatural origins of NDEs by the fact that descriptions of these have changed over time, and are also affected by place (Osis & Haraldson, 1977; Zaleski, 1987). In addition to much individuality entering the picture, cultural influences are obviously present (Osis & Haraldson, 1977; Kastenbaum, 1981). To some religionists, the absence of religious content in most NDEs raises questions about their authenticity. Suggestions of increased social concern and compassion, less materialism, improved self-esteem, and greater internal control have been reported (Ring, 1984). These last possibilities are also correlates of religious experiences.

Concern with NDEs has resulted in the production of a *Journal of Near-Death Studies*. Authors of papers published in this journal have taken essentially every stance that can be conceived, from the paranormal and religious to the exclusively scientific. It goes without saying that proponents of each extreme fail to, or even vehemently refuse to, appreciate the position of those who differ. Gibbs (2005a) agrees with another thinker in this field, Michael Sabom, that "near-death experiences (NDEs) should not be used to promote religious agendas" (p. 105). Still, Gibbs (2005b) claims that NDEs promote spirituality relative to a form of Christianity. Research has found that NDEs do relate to an increase in religious importance and activity (McLaughlin & Malony, 1984). A variation on this theme interprets NDEs as mystical experiences. Pennachio (1986) explored this possibility, largely relying on a nine-aspect typology for mystical experience offered by Walter Pahnke (1969). Though Pennachio considered this framework "useful for understanding and interpreting the experience" (p. 71), he simply had to recognize that our knowledge is "limited" and "more research . . . is necessary" (p. 71).

The initial enthusiasm that greeted NDEs in the 1970s and 1980s has subsided. Interpretation of these experiences varies widely from their acceptance as "proof" of an afterlife, to the concept of NDEs as "spiritual experiences," to analyses in terms of consciousness and brain function. In this last category, we see research overlapping with that cited in Chapter 3. Britton and Bootzin's (2004) work on temporal lobe function parallels that of Persinger, Newberg, and d'Aquili, and Azari on religious experience, as described in Chapter 3. Britton and Bootzin suggest that NDEs involve altered function in the temporal lobe. In a controversial and complex area, this offers an objective research avenue that may provide additional insights into other psychological and phenomenological questions raised by NDEs.

In addition to nonreligious factors either causing or relating to NDEs, a fascinating situation arises when the result of a religious activity serves as the stimulus for an NDE. Hood and Williamson (2008b, pp. 170–184) undertook a highly creative research program on members of a serpent-handling sect who sustained bites from rattlesnakes and copperheads. (The prevalence of such bites may be low, but fatalities are common.) These researchers conducted in-depth interviews with 13 snake handlers who were bitten and were close to death before recovering. Religious attributions to God's will were employed by the victims to explain the experience of being bitten plus what followed, including final recovery.

An interesting large-scale cross-cultural study that bears on NDEs was conducted by Osis and Haraldson (1977). Research Box 7.6 shows the difficulties and hazards of conducting such research.

A very useful overview of thinking about NDEs ranging from the theological to the scientific has been offered by Gibbs (1988). As psychologists of religion, we look toward the critical scientific aspect of this troubled realm by also recommending that interested readers examine the strongly scientific work of Blackmore (1991).

Contact with the Dead

The idea of contact with the dead is very popular in Western society. In October 2015, one Internet browser, Google, listed 725,032,704 websites and contacts pertaining to this topic. This appeal to electronics may have originated in the 1920s, when Thomas Edison was reportedly working on a "spirit phone" with which to contact the dead. Though this story was widely believed, no evidence was ever found of plans or mock-ups for such a device. (Given *Edison's* reputation as an inventor, someone desirous of interacting with the deceased might have created this myth—or, as has been suggested, he himself may have proposed it as a joke (Zarrelli, 2016).

To be able to communicate with the deceased means that they are still somehow "alive," existing in a state that is "connected" to our life realm. Death thus suggests transformation, not termination. Krause (2011a) cites a number of studies claiming that anywhere from 36 to 63% of Americans believe in the likelihood of after-death communication.

RESEARCH BOX 7.6. At the Hour of Death (Osis & Haraldson, 1977)

These researchers conducted three major surveys: a pilot study, a U.S. survey, and a survey in India. The last two efforts constituted the final comparative study. The pilot work sampled 5,000 physicians and 5,000 nurses. We read that "640 medical observers returned their questionnaires. These reported a total of 35,540 observations" (p. 27). In other words, there was a 6.4% return rate, which was not further defined by the nature of the "medical observers." Still, an effort was made to imply validity with reference to the 35,000-plus pieces of data, but these too remain largely undefined. A respondent return rate as small as that obtained here casts considerable doubt on the generalizability of the information. Apparently 190 cases "of interest" were followed up with questionnaires and phone interviews, but again vagueness prevails. Given the use of questionnaires and the low return rate, one also wonders about the completeness of the returned forms. This is not discussed.

The real core of this work consisted of further studies in India and the United States. In the United States, mail questionnaires were sent to 2,500 physicians and 2,500 nurses. The return rate was 20%, or 1,004 responses. A more personal procedure was used in India: 704 medical professionals responded, which the authors indicate comprised almost all who were approached. Unhappily, again, an unscientific lack of precision is present in the descriptions of both the sampling and responses. Still, an attempt was made to provide data, some of which are interesting and possibly useful.

If we concentrate on the India–U.S. comparisons relative to religion, the categories employed often lack the desired exactitude. It makes good sense to see that only Indian respondents viewed the apparitional figures of Shiva, Rama, and Krishna, and a grouping of Mary, Kali, and Durga. If we interpret this latter grouping correctly, it mixes Christian and Hindu beings. The same is true of "saints and gurus" and of "demons and devils." Of special interest to us is the finding that of the 418 apparitional figures seen, only 140 were religious beings. Of the figures seen by the U.S. respondents, only 12% were religiously identified; the comparable proportion witnessed by the Indian sample was 37.5%.

This work is more useful for hypothesis construction and testing than it is for making reliable and valid inferences. Its subjectivity demands rigorous cross-checking. Considerable room is left for the expectations and values of researchers and interpreters of NDEs to introduce bias, while giving the impression that it is scientifically rigorous. A door has been opened to understanding a fascinating phenomenon. To date, however, there has been much more talk than solid research (Bailey & Yates, 1996).

GSS data from 1972 to 2006 suggest a tendency for more religious than nonreligious persons to claim contact with the dead (Spilka, 2007). Of those who feel that their faith is strong, 48% believe that they have experienced such contacts. Thirty-two percent who state that they are not at all religious feel similarly. Also supportive of this theme, 42% of persons who pray at least once daily report such contact; the percentage is 29% for those who pray less than once a week. With regard to religious groups, 38% of Protestants, 42% of Catholics, and 34% of Jews state that they have had contact with the dead. Utilizing other data, Kearl (1989) indicated that 66% and 68% of Catholics and Mormons, respectively, believe that "religious observances by the living" (p. 185) may benefit those who are deceased. Other Christian groups are considerably less likely to feel this way; nevertheless, such ideas keep alive the notion of a connection between the living and the dead.

Krause (2011a) focused on contact with the deceased relative to religious involvement and death anxiety. Using sophisticated statistical analyses, he found that religious activity and meaning seemed to be negligibly better related to each other than to contact with the dead. Relationships tended to be low, but were sometimes significant with the large samples used. Still, when we examine the intercorrelations among different kinds of contact, we see some impressive associations. For example, the belief that the deceased "look over" the living once in a while correlates .634 with the feeling that they are "in the same room." Having both seen and heard the deceased are even more strongly positively associated (.688). The profound significance of the dead to the living cannot be denied (N. Krause, personal communication, September 27, 2015). We agree with Krause that this is a fascinating topic to study and needs further work.

Recognizing that contact with the deceased has been identified by a number of different terms, McDonald (1992) adopted the esoteric label "idionecrophanies." He recognized that researchers often jump in with rather complex theories and variables, and create quite involved systems that require unusual explanations. Focusing on such basic variables as age, gender, race, and God image, McDonald found that all of these variables were significant predictors of reported contacts with the dead. Specifically, more females than males and more blacks than whites claimed to have more such contacts. The same was true of perceiving God as a "lover" as opposed to being a "judge." Again, we encounter mostly weak to middling coefficients with large samples, plus a lack of meaningful explanations for these observations.

Krause has pointed out the fascinating nature of work on contact with the deceased plus the need for a wide-ranging theoretical framework. Unfortunately, we are still awaiting the latter.

RELIGION AND FEAR/ANXIETY ABOUT DEATH

With the exception of some who may be mentally or physically deviant in some way, people prefer life over death. We all know that we will eventually die, though we probably unconsciously hope that we may be overlooked in the process. In fact, seriously thinking about death, particularly our own, makes us uncomfortable, fearful, and anxious. A great deal of research on these feelings has been conducted (Ellis & Wahab, 2013). Most, however, seems to have been undertaken on young people (largely college students). Since no one appears to escape death, culture and society have much to say about it, especially through religion.

Western civilization has a religious heritage that affirms ideas such as resurrection and life after death in the strongest terms. In one form or another, similar views exist worldwide. They offer much gratification, and they help to alleviate a basic source of fear and anxiety. This last concern has been central to those who study the association of religion and death.

Death continually surrounds us. The mass media reveal its presence in daily news accounts of accidents, crimes, natural disasters, and war; and more specifically in ever-present obituaries, death notices, and funeral announcements. Though death is usually distant from our everyday lives, we all personally encounter death—beginning in childhood with the loss of pets and the demise of elderly relatives. As already discussed, we seek explanations and solace in notions about the afterlife that family, friends, and religious authorities reinforce. The factor motivating such views has been variously termed "fear of death," "death anxiety," or "death concern," and it has been a fairly popular area for research.

Research Problems

Studies of relationships between religion and fear/anxiety about death have been confounded by measures from both areas containing similar items (e.g., belief in an afterlife). Second, various deficiencies have been identified, including poor experimental designs, weak measures, inadequate controls, inappropriate statistical analyses, and the use of questionable samples (Ellis & Wahab, 2013; Lester, 1967, 1972; Martin & Wrightsman, 1964). With respect to the last problem, most researchers have examined college students—a young population with limited experience of death. For most students, speaking of death, considering its likely temporal distance, is an unrealistic, intellectual exercise. Finally, we have described how measurement in the psychology of religion has gone from simple unidimensional scales to more refined multidimensional instruments. A parallel development has occurred in the assessment of death anxiety.

Despite these questions, it has been claimed that "one of the major functions of religious beliefs [is] to reduce a person's fear of death" (Groth-Marnat, 1992, p. 277). We may reasonably ask this question: Does faith lessen concern about death? Kalish (1981) simply affirms Feifel's (1959) view that "those individuals who are more afraid of dying are more likely to become religious" (Kalish, 1981, p. 115). Our own survey of this literature in the first edition of this book (Spilka, Hood, & Gorsuch, 1985) found that 24 of 36 studies evidenced negative relationships between fear on the one hand and faith and afterlife beliefs on the other. Another 7 studies suggested these domains were independent of each other while 3 showed an unexpected positive association. Two others demonstrated two of these results by assessing different levels of death fear such as conscious and unconscious expressions. Another examination of 16 studies indicated that 6 found a negative relationship, 3 a positive association, and 5 no connection between religion and death concern (Gartner, Larson, & Allen, 1991); there were also 2 studies with curvilinear patterns. The most recent work (Ellis & Wahab, 2013) surveyed 84 studies that yielded 108 results. Forty reported negative associations between "religiosity and fear of death" (p. 149). There were 9 curvilinear relationships, 27 positive correlations, and 32 nonsignificant ones.

Employing a sample of Israeli Jews, Lazar (2006) attempted to study death fear and religiosity when both domains were treated multidimensionally. Within and across these realms, intercorrelations above .50 and as high as .78 prevailed. This suggests to us that true multidimensionality is quite dubious in this research. One might, however, argue that the complexity of religious motivations and perceived personal meanings for death may be playing a role here, to the degree that these factors really constitute one overriding complex. In like manner, with understandable variations, death fears and religiosity have been studied among Christians in general and Buddhists (Wong, Fung, & Jiang, 2013). Similar work has been undertaken among members of the Presbyterian Church (U.S.A.) (Silton et al., 2011).

Research on different groups introduces a variety of new sociocultural variables into the mix. Unfortunately, it is too easy to leave these unaccounted for. Though it is relatively simple to denote sex and age, education is far more complex than simply how far one went in school. In a similar manner, socioeconomic status is commonly ignored. Still, the dominant inclination is to emphasize religious identification without paying too much attention to possible subgroups and differences among churches within a denomination, even though they may reflect (among other things) socioeconomic, ethnic, cultural, and regional factors (Pressman, Lyons, Larson, & Gartner, 1992). Despite a minority of discrepant findings, our overview of this literature suggests that the more exacting research argues for the reduction of death anxiety when religious commitment increases. Wink and Scott (2005) contend that differences in findings may be occurring because the relationship of death fear and religiousness is simply much more complex than usually thought (as we have just noted). They found a curvilinear relationship, replicated it, and finally felt that their findings "support the hypothesis that firmness and consistency of beliefs and practices rather than religiousness per se, buffers against death anxiety in old age" (p. 207).

The general label of "religiosity" may mask other factors that reduce death anxiety—for example, age. Long-lived elders are probably more appropriate to sample than only young people when the topic is death. Even though religion and afterlife beliefs correlate positively, especially among Christians, we need to consider the degree to which institutional faith in general includes belief in an afterlife. Thorson (1991) further points out that belief in an afterlife correlates more strongly in a negative direction with death anxiety than does religiousness. Others confirm the centrality of afterlife ideas in resisting death distress and related depression (Aday, 1984–1985; Alvarado, Templer, Bresler, & Thomas-Dobson, 1995). Confounding may well occur between religiosity and belief in an afterlife.

Rasmussen and Johnson (1994) bring another issue to the fore—namely, the question of spirituality versus religiosity. Their research showed no significant relationship between death anxiety and religiosity, but a noteworthy association with scores on a Spiritual Well-Being scale. Because of the often great overlap between spirituality and religiosity, this relationship needs to be explored further.

Breaking with the traditional sampling of American college students, Roshdieh, Templer, Cannon, and Canfield (1998–1999) were able to study death anxiety and death depression among almost 1,200 Iranian college students. The results were similar to what has been observed in the United States: Namely, religion countered both death depression and death anxiety. Again, the issue is age, and comparative research on these measures over different age groupings needs to be undertaken.

Though there is some disagreement among the rather large number of studies in this area, the dominant finding is that both religion and spirituality seem to oppose death anxiety and depression. Still, the referents of religion and spirituality may overlap considerably.

Experimenting with Death Fear

Despite the observations above, can we say that increasing concern with death may actually influence one's belief in an afterlife? In an ingenious experimental study, Osarchuk and Tatz (1973) found that inducing death fear could affect one's afterlife beliefs. This work is described in Research Box 7.7. When significant research findings such as those of Osarchuk and Tatz (1973) are obtained, their findings should be confirmed before congratulations are offered. Too often in psychology—or, for that matter, in all of the sciences—initial findings may be later contradicted. This is further suggested by a later study (Ochsmann, 1984). Differences in methods call for more research with new controls, in order to resolve the discrepancies between these studies.

The Influence of Circumstances: The Threat of AIDS as an Example

A particular type of life-threatening situation is still found among gay men and bisexuals. In this population in particular, the threat of AIDS is ever-present if one is sexually active. Research Box 7.8 details one significant study in this troubled area (Bivens, Neimeyer, Kirchberg, & Moore, 1994–1995).

RESEARCH BOX 7.7. Effect of Induced Fear of Death on Belief in an Afterlife
(Osarchuk & Tatz, 1973)

To test the hypothesis that making fear of death more salient would increase belief in an afterlife, these researchers constructed two equivalent and reliable 10-item scales of belief in an afterlife (Forms A and B). Two groups were created. Half of the people in each group received Form A initially; the other half received Form B first. From each group, 10 members were assigned to a death threat subgroup; 10 were assigned to a shock threat group; and 10 were designated as controls. Six subgroups were thus formed—three with high belief in an afterlife, and three with low belief. To the death threat subgroups, a taped communication was played giving an exaggerated estimate of the probability of an early death for individuals ages 18–22, due to accident or to disease caused by food contamination. The tape contained a background of dirge-like music. A series of 42 death-related slides was coordinated with the communication, including scenes of auto wrecks, realistically feigned murder and suicide victims, and corpses in a funeral home setting.

The members of the shock threat group were informed that they would receive a series of painful electric shocks (to which, of course, they never were subjected). The control groups engaged in ordinary play for the same amount of time that the other groups underwent the death or shock threats. All were then given the alternate form of the belief-in-afterlife scales that they had not taken earlier. The results were partially as predicted. Those with low belief in an afterlife, regardless of what group they were in, revealed no changes in their beliefs. In contrast, only those initially holding strong afterlife beliefs who were exposed to the death threat manifested a meaningful increase in these views. Apparently, heightening one's concern with death can influence belief in an afterlife. It would have been interesting to see whether other religious views (such as belief in God) were also similarly affected, but this was not examined here. The question is one of focus. As the 18th-century man of letters Samuel Johnson put it, "When a man knows he is to be hanged in a fortnight, it concentrates his mind wonderfully" (quoted in Boswell, 1791/n.d., p. 725).

This effort charts a path to even more complex and insightful work regarding how religion may be employed as a resource to reduce fear of death by individuals suffering from a life-threatening disease. Concurrently, religion may play a negative role. One can also read the punishment motif of orthodox Christianity in Bivens et al.'s findings. This last theme may also be seen in other work, which found that the more men with AIDS attended church, and the more similar this church was to the one in which they were reared, the more death anxiety they showed (Franks, Templer, Capelletty, & Kauffman, 1990–1991). In Franks et al.'s research, the greater death fear associated with religious activity in patients with AIDS does not necessarily point to the external stigmatizing role that religion may play. Churches are purveyors of community social values, and the prevailing levels of fear and rejection of AIDS and patients with AIDS are often internalized by these patients (Gilmore & Sommerville, 1994; Kegeles, Coates, Christopher, & Lazarus, 1989). The motivation to distance oneself from AIDS is illustrated by the Muslim denotation of AIDS as a Western disease that can be best avoided by complying with Islamic views and practices (Gilmore & Sommerville, 1994). Similar pronouncements by Christian ideologues are common.

RESEARCH BOX 7.8. Death Concern and Religious Beliefs among Gays
and Bisexuals of Variable Proximity to AIDS
(Bivens, Neimeyer, Kirchberg, & Moore, 1994–1995)

A sample of 167 gay or bisexual men was obtained; 24 were HIV-positive, and 19 had full-blown AIDS. These 43 were termed the "HIV+" group. The remaining men were HIV-negative ("HIV–"). Sixty-nine of the latter were defined as the "AIDS-involved" group, as they helped patients with AIDS in a variety of settings. The remaining participants were denoted "AIDS-uninvolved." All participants were administered a multidimensional scale that yielded eight measures of death fear/concern. An index of personally perceived threat from the potential of one's death was also used. Intrinsic and Extrinsic religious orientations were assessed by the Allport–Ross scales. Also included were a scale assessing Christian orthodoxy and a more general inventory of religious beliefs and practices.

The HIV+ group displayed greater fear than the other two groups with respect to the likelihood of a premature death. No difference on this measure was found between the AIDS-uninvolved and AIDS-involved groups. The AIDS-involved participants, however, (1) manifested less global threat and less threat regarding meaningfulness and survival concerns, and (2) were significantly more religious, than the AIDS-uninvolved participants. Intrinsic faith, belief in God, and church attendance were also associated with less global threat, threats to meaningfulness, survival concerns, and negative emotional appraisals. Literal Bible interpretations correlated positively with greater death fear, fear of personal destruction, and fear of consciousness in death.

The foregoing studies portray a negative role for religion in relation to AIDS, but there is research that indicates the opposite. Over the years, scientific progress has increasingly worked against the notion that AIDS is an automatic death sentence; newer treatments have provided hope. Moreover, the work of Hall (1994) with patients having end-stage HIV disease shows that a major source of hope is religion. Hope is generated through religious beliefs and faith-related rituals that reduce death anxiety and depression on the part of those facing AIDS, as well as friends and relatives of those who have died from AIDS (Jull-Johnson, 1995).

Virtually all of the research discussed above and much that follows stresses negative considerations relative to death. Most of what follows is in the same mode. An interesting variation that may aid the terminally ill handle their forthcoming demise has, however, been reported. Kerr and his coworkers (2014) daily interviewed 66 patients in their final weeks regarding their dreams and visions. These tended to be about deceased friends and relatives, and increased in frequency as patients approached death. They were said to be comforting, meaningful, and realistic, and hence largely positive to the dying patients.

RELIGION AND EUTHANASIA

"Euthanasia" is defined as "the act of killing a person painlessly for reasons of mercy" (Davis, 1976, p. 245). It is a troubled realm that is often simplified and euphemized by such terminology as "mercy killing," "physician-assisted suicide," "right to die," and "death with dignity." A distinction must, however, be made between "passive" and "active" euthanasia. The former usually implies the withholding of heroic measures to sustain life when death is imminent and the quality of life is very poor. In contrast, active euthanasia is the intentional termination of life under the same conditions, especially when great pain and suffering are present. This is probably practiced more often than we think when a patient makes an impassioned plea to die.

Getting information about attitudes toward euthanasia is surprisingly difficult. For example, among factors affecting information is the nature of the question asked. When physicians were asked about ending a terminally ill "patient's life by some painless means," 70% affirmed that it should be allowed. If, however, they were asked about "assist[ing] the patient to commit suicide," only 51% agreed (Saad, 2013). In a study where the respondents were Protestant and Catholic clergy and the issue was phrased as the "patient doesn't want to live any longer," passive euthanasia was acceptable to 34% of the former and 30% of the latter. For active euthanasia, approval dropped to 13% and 2%, respectively (Nagi, Pugh, & Lazarine, 1977–1978). Since these two studies were conducted 35 years apart, there is good reason to doubt their comparability. When the general public was asked about "physician-assisted suicide," 46% approved of it and 45% disapproved (Masci, 2013). We must remain aware of the fact that we frequently do not know the nature of the question asked, plus other factors such as respondents' gender and age, and a host of other considerations.

The Evaluation of Euthanasia: Political, Religious, and Medical

Euthanasia is illegal in most U.S. jurisdictions. It is currently (2016) approved in only five states: Oregon, Washington, Montana, Vermont, and California plus Washington, DC. Religious groups dominate the opposition, with the exception of the Unitarian Universalists and the United Church of Christ. The issue has generally been negated in the courts, with few exceptions, such as the approval in Montana (the decision in the other states was made by passing a state law).

Although we must keep in mind the questions and problems noted above, the overwhelming majority of medical professionals seem to favor passive euthanasia. Surveys reveal that from two-thirds to over 90% of health care practitioners approve passive approaches, whereas only 17% of physicians and 36% of nurses take positive views of active euthanasia (Carey & Posavec, 1978–1979; Hoggatt & Spilka, 1978; Lavery, Dickens, Boyle, & Singer, 1997; Rea, Greenspoon, & Spilka, 1975). The Gallup Poll organization (Gallup, 1992; *The Gallup Poll Monthly*, 1992) has taken a sophisticated view of the euthanasia issue, revealing how attitudes are dependent on a number of factors, such as severe pain, incurable disease, burden on the family, and the person's own judgment that life is meaningless. The Gallup figures also vary according to how euthanasia is defined (as "withholding of treatment," "doctor-assisted suicide," etc. A thoughtful and comprehensive current detailed definition has been offered by Moreland (2018).

Religious Perspectives on Euthanasia

Scripture and theology usually oppose euthanasia, but there is lay deviation from such a position. One study found that if euthanasia was approved by a physician, 61% of Protestants, 62% of Catholics, and 78% of Jews agreed with such a stance (Kearl, 1989). The strength of one's religious position affected these findings, as the comparable data for "strong" Protestants, Catholics, and Jews were 49%, 51%, and 67%, respectively (Kearl, 1989). Evidently euthanasia under certain circumstances is widely supported, regardless of religious affiliation. This support, however, decreases as religiosity increases. In addition, for over 50 years, approval of euthanasia has grown steadily among moderate and liberal religionists (Kearl, 2002). Such approval also accompanies belief in an afterlife (Klopfer & Price, 1979). In general, physicians and members of the public who are religious in general or Catholic in particular are less favorable to euthanasia (Emanuel, 2002); physician approval rates in Emanuel's study ranged from 33 to 66%.

Religion and Physician-Assisted Suicide

Opposition to physician-assisted suicide (hereafter abbreviated as PAS) has come more from formal religious organizations than from their individual members. Still, the more liberal Christian and Jewish groups are slowly increasing their support for PAS. The United Church of Christ already formally backs such action (Koenig, 1994a).

The increasingly favorable positions taken by clergy suggest that it is probably just a matter of time before more religious bodies justify euthanasia and PAS. In one investigation, Carey and Posavec (1978–1979) found that 96% of the clerics they sampled advocated passive euthanasia, and that 21% espoused its active form. Support for passive euthanasia varies with the reasons advanced for such action (Nagi et al., 1977–1978). Depending on the justification, Carey and Posavec (1978–1979) found that support ranged from 34 to 73% among Protestant clergy; the comparable percentages were 30 to 69% for Catholic priests. In regard to active euthanasia, the percentages were significantly lower: Only 13–25% of the Protestant clergy and 1–3% of Catholic priests countenanced such action. Even though Carey and Posavec's investigation did not designate the denominations sampled, approval of euthanasia grows with liberality of a cleric's theological position and group. Conservative clergy balance their opposition with strong beliefs in a rewarding afterlife (Spilka, Spangler, & Rea, 1981).

A word is in order regarding why there is religious opposition to euthanasia and PAS. In brief, a position derived from scripture simply avers that life and death are in "God's hands." That is, life can only be given and taken away by the deity. Other considerations are that the pain and suffering of the ill person is supposed to be experienced by that individual, and may benefit all concerned in the long run.

RELIGION AND SUICIDE

Institutionalized religion has uniformly treated suicide in negative terms. The Judeo-Christian tradition teaches that suicide is immoral and therefore sinful (Kastenbaum, 1981). Those who commit suicide may not be allowed burial with the faithful in religiously sponsored cemeteries, or are consigned to certain sections that signify condemnation and rejection. Because of the stigma that has traditionally been attached to suicide, medical, religious, and civil authorities are often reluctant to identify a death as a suicide. The more modern religious perspective is to consider these individuals as mentally disturbed—a diagnosis that removes the burden of sin and mitigates the opprobrium that surviving family members have often received from the religious community. The influence of religion on attitudes toward suicide has, however, lessened considerably in the contemporary world, especially in the United States over the last half century (Wasserman & Stack, 1993).

Religion and Suicide among the Elderly

In 2016, 44,965 people in the United States committed suicide. This was approximately 10,000 more than a decade earlier (American Foundation for Suicide Prevention, 2018). The highest suicide rate is found among white males 85 years old and older (Worthington, 2018). The National Institute of Mental Health tells us that approximately another half million people each year enter hospital emergency rooms as a result of attempting suicide (Brunner, 2003; Hoyert, Kochanek, & Murphy, 1999). Though women attempt suicide three times more often than men, the latter "are four times more likely to die than are females" (National Center for Injury Prevention and Control, 2015). Wu, Wang, and Jia (2015) did a meta-analysis of 9 studies and showed that religion exercised a protective effect against suicide in western cultures.

Kearl (1989) has suggested that "for some elderly individuals, suicide is preferable to loneliness, chronic illness, and dependency" (p. 145). This may be especially true for physically ill older men, the group with the highest suicide rate in the United States. Still, among elderly individuals, religion plays its traditional role in opposing self-destruction. Koenig (1994b) has suggested that faith suppresses suicidal thinking in this group. He found that 18% of his sample of physically ill older men experienced suicidal thoughts, and that these related to ineffective religious coping.

As already noted, elderly religious individuals were reared at a time when religion was a stronger cultural force than it is today. Because of this, they may identify with their faith's opposition to suicide, as well as with the promise of a happy afterlife. A related finding is that the recovery from bereavement of those who lose a loved one via suicide is enhanced by belief in an afterlife (Smith, Range, & Ulmer, 1991–1992).

We might argue that there are two dominant psychosocial approaches to understanding suicide, particularly among older individuals. The main, long-existing approach goes back to Durkheim (1915), who basically claimed that suicide relates to a failure to integrate into the local community and culture. This is basically a sociological approach. In contrast, Pargament (1997) emphasizes the inability of persons to cope with the immediate problems they confront. This looks to the psychology of the individual, and Pargament has developed three short scales to measure different forms of coping, which he terms "self-directing," "deferring," and "collaborative." Including the problems of the elderly, this work is detailed in Pargament's outstanding 1997 book, *The Psychology of Religion and Coping*. Without question, it should be in the library of every psychologist.

The idea (based on Durkheim's approach) that one form of protection against suicide could be social integration into a community, especially a religious community, has gained both support and contradiction (Stark, Doyle, & Rushing, 1983). Pargament's theory possesses solid psychological credentials, but should have direct research to back it up. For example, church attendance is negatively correlated with suicide rates (Martin, 1984). Investigators have observed that the highest suicide rates are among older, single, socially isolated men (Dublin, 1963; Stengel, 1964). Dealing with suicide ideology, Stack and Wasserman (1992) have noted three possibilities:

1. Religion fosters general social integration, which opposes suicide.
2. Specific religious views, such as belief in an afterlife, may contravene self-destructive impulses. (We add that it could support such tendencies.)
3. Religious organizations foster networking and social support, which should thwart suicidal inclinations.

Using sophisticated statistical techniques on national data, these researchers found evidence supporting all three views, especially for conservative religious bodies. Focusing on church attendance, Stack and Wasserman concluded that the social connections faith may create and strengthen could be the main elements hindering suicide. One can also make a case for both Durkheim's and Pargament's approaches from these observations.

Apocalyptic Suicide

Recent decades have witnessed a spate of mass suicides among members of religious cults. The cases of the Jonestown People's Temple, the Branch Davidians, and Heaven's Gate (among others) have shocked the world, and have left most of us without a satisfying explanation for these tragedies.

The rather bizarre forms religion has taken in several cults in which there were mass suicides have been analyzed by Dein and Littlewood (2000). Scholars have primarily examined these cults' leadership and group structure, searching for common personality factors or various forms of mental disorder. This approach has not been productive. The lack of hard data—specifically, too much clinical subjectivity and a dearth of confirmatory efforts—makes inferences in the realm of the individual rather tenuous. Vague allusions to paranoid traits, poor reality contact, or distressing early life conditions also do not appear useful. Previous work on mental disorders among cultists indicates that the rates of such problems are no higher in cults than in the population at large (Needleman & Baker, 1978; Richardson, 1980; Wright, 1987).

If generalizations can be offered, a number are in order. Cults are groups centered around charismatic leaders who want their members to be separate from society in general, from family members, and from anyone who might have divergent views. Absolute devotion to the leader's beliefs and teachings is reinforced in every manner possible. These doctrines may include notions that death is invariably a door to a future life; that the physical body is a hindrance; and that those who commit suicide never truly die, but continue on into a heavenly existence. These groups create the conditions that make suicide appear to be the only means of achieving ultimate happiness.

RELIGION, GRIEF, AND BEREAVEMENT

Living means that we will experience the deaths of loved ones, for there must always come that dreaded time when a beloved person "goeth to his long home, and the mourners go about the streets" (Ecclesiastes 12:5). When someone dies, the likelihood is high that family and friends will turn to religion for solace and understanding. Faith is often a basic part of the coping process, and death is frequently conceptualized in spiritual terms.

The process of grief and bereavement is surprisingly complex. The broadest perspective, that of culture, can influence the same religious framework, so that individual responses to death may be radically different (Loewenthal, 2013). "Grief" is an individual emotional process; "bereavement" is ambiguously defined as separate from grief, though it emphasizes the sense of loss that leads to grief. Another overlapping concept is "mourning," which refers to the combination of cognitive, emotional, and behavioral responses that one manifests in bereavement.

The literature offers discussions about stages of grief, models of grief, degrees of grief, ritual in grief, religion as a resource in bereavement, the grief of parents and grandparents for deceased children and grandchildren, the grief of spouses for deceased mates, and grief for other family members and loved ones. In all of these areas, the role of faith is significant. For example, Flatt (1987) suggests some 10 grief stages that range from "initial shock" to what he terms "growth." In most of these stages, God is given a role. It might be a questioning of how the deity could let someone die or how the divine actively brings about a death, or a place for "God's grace" in recovery from the depression resulting from grief. Another possibility is that recovery from grief may move the person toward new stages and tests, such that the deity is seen to care as the person is reintegrated into "God's world." This means that the bereaved gains new strength to realize "God's purpose" in his or her remaining life (Flatt, 1987). Here we observe how significant attributions to God may be when death is confronted. Some researchers claim that "the feeling of recovery following bereavement is enhanced by high belief in afterlife" (Smith et al., 1991–1992, p. 217). In other words, recovery may be promoted by the view that the deceased is only temporarily out of contact with the bereaved.

The central issue is "making sense" out of the loss, and religion is commonly the main source of meaning available to the survivors. Regardless of who dies, religious/spiritual commitments, doctrines, and ideas offer meanings that reduce symptoms of distress and engender hope (Dahl, 1999; Golsworthy & Coyle, 1999).

Though the majority of research on religion and bereavement points to the beneficial role of faith in such circumstances, it should be noted that not all work in this area supports such inferences (Sanders, 1979–1980). This is indeed an involved realm—one that requires more sensitivity to theory and the possibility of confounding factors.

Focusing on the elderly, Heyman and Gianturco (1973) studied the effects of loss of a spouse on a sample of individuals over 60 years old. Mean survivor age at the time of spouse death was 74.8 years. No change in religiosity or the overall level of activity was observed. Relationships with others and membership in clubs also showed little or no change. Women tended to be less happy and manifested mild depression. Only two males improved in mood, most likely because supportive actions and pressures before death reduced their distress. In sum, the overall feeling was that relatively little changed over the long run, and that religiosity had little to do with any changes.

Sanders (1979–1980) conducted an interesting study in which she compared grief reactions to the death of a spouse, a child, and a parent. Though the most intense responses occurred when a child died, church attendance was related positively to optimism, reduced anger, and a better appetite. When church attendance and family interaction were treated together, the findings even more graphically favored the religion–family combination. This may imply the significance of religion not only in terms of meaning, but in regard to a broader beneficial basis for social support from one's kin. Loveland (1968) supports the idea of a constructive role for religion in bereavement. Both subjectively and objectively, religious beliefs were felt by widows to place bereavement in a meaningful perspective that aided coping with the death of significant others. The first year of bereavement was a time for adjustment. In other research, whereas approximately 12% of bereaved widows had their faith in God shaken, the remainder maintained their religious commitment, and most saw it as offering them a constructive outlook (Glick, Weiss, & Parkes, 1974).

There is also evidence that bereavement varies as a function of the kind of death that occurred—in other words, whether it was natural, accidental, a result of violence, or a suicide

(Morin & Welsh, 1996; Sheskin & Wallace, 1980). Morin and Welsh (1996) interviewed urban and suburban adolescents. The urban adolescents were in a facility for adjudicated youths, and had experienced more violent deaths than the suburban groups had. Their views of death also involved violence and religion to a greater degree than those of the suburban teens. The latter emphasized the experience of suffering, while the urban juveniles were more concerned with the loss of loved ones. Both groups found that their grieving benefited from talking about their feelings and concerns.

Sheskin and Wallace (1980) studied widows, and observed that, regardless of the nature of their husbands' deaths, they usually needed to "unburden themselves" to good listeners. Theoretically, one might expect clergy to fulfill such a role, but this was not found. According to the studies reviewed by Sheskin and Wallace (1980), clergy were found to be particularly unhelpful by widows whose husbands committed suicide. The implication is that since organized religions oppose suicide, their representatives will have difficulty counseling the survivors of those who have committed suicide. Accordingly, the clergy, who should be understanding and sympathetic regarding death, may not be of much help in such cases. Clerics could respond like others who relate to the surviving family members of those dying by suicide. This group feels that they are less accepted by their communities than those whose relatives died accidental or natural deaths (Smith et al., 1991–1992).

Another consideration brings us back to the issue of meaning. Even though the meaning of death in the religious/spiritual sense is enhanced by devotion to one's faith, suicide poses additional explanatory problems. We may try to play word games and attribute the death to depression or some "psychotic break," but then we face the question of why this mental state was present. We struggle to make sense out of the tragedy, for our social order values individual worth and dignity, and taking one's own life often creates a deep and troubling dilemma.

Religious Schemas and Bereavement over Child Loss

A very significant concern for religion relative to death that usually does not involve the elderly concerns the death of children. When such occurs, it is likely to arouse a "sense of injustice"—it simply should not happen (Walsh, 2013). Among the religious, anger at the deity may occur, and pastoral therapy is a possible remedy.

One noteworthy theoretical treatment of bereavement has been advanced by Daniel McIntosh and his colleagues (McIntosh, Silver, & Wortman, 1993). McIntosh (1995) has extended this approach to religion in general and its role in life. Noting that "a schema is a cognitive mental structure or representation containing organized prior knowledge about a particular domain, including a specification of the relations among its attributes" (1995, p. 2), McIntosh observes that "people have different schemas for many domains." Schemas influence what is perceived, speed up cognitive processing of information, and offer meaning in difficult situations by filling in the gaps in our knowledge. In sum, they orient us to the world and the problems with which we must cope. They can help us adapt to problematic circumstances. With respect to death and bereavement, one salient aspect of a religious schema might be belief in an afterlife. Apparently such belief is "associated with greater recovery from bereavement regardless of the cause of death" (Smith et al., 1991–1992, p. 222). In contrast, bereaved persons with little belief in an afterlife evidence less well-being in general, and poorer recovery from the bereavement in particular. Such people also make greater efforts to avoid thinking about the death in question.

For many reasons, primarily culturally based, most people possess religious schemas that may be called upon when ambiguity and threat become troublesome. In their significant work on how parents cope with the death of an infant from sudden infant death syndrome (SIDS), McIntosh et al. (1993) demonstrated how parents' faith, through the use of religious schemas, indirectly facilitated their adjustment. The schemas both made the death meaningful and supported efforts to come to terms with the loss. Religious participation and social support promoted the acquisition of helpful religious explanations. Cognitively, religious importance contributed to constructive mental processing and helped reduce distress.

The work of McIntosh et al. (1993) explains similar findings in other studies that have dealt with parental and grandparental bereavement (Bohannon, 1991; De Frain, Jakub, & Mendoza, 1991–1992). Studying the influence of church attendance, Bohannon (1991) showed that it was inversely related to anger, guilt, helplessness, obsessive thoughts about a child's death, somatic complaints, and death anxiety on the part of grieving mothers. Similar effects were found for paternal anger, guilt, and death anxiety. De Frain et al. (1991–1992) found that religious beliefs were strengthened for 46% of the grandparents of children who died of SIDS, and 90% felt that their faith aided them in coping with the SIDS death.

Further work by Gilbert (1992) stressed the perceived role of God in this situation. When religion was a resource, bereaved parents felt that (1) God did not do bad things; (2) God was in control and could be relied on to make the wisest decision; (3) God had good reasons for the child's death; (4) God inflicted this tragedy upon the parents because they had the strength to deal with it; (5) God wanted them to appreciate life more; and (6) God desired that they change their lives for the better. Interestingly, those who claimed that religion was not initially helpful acquired a more positive outlook over time. Lastly, those who claimed that religion was irrelevant tended to be extrinsically oriented. The implication is that for faith to be significant in this kind of tragedy, it must have an intrinsic, not superficial or utilitarian, quality.

An excellent example of theoretically guided and methodologically sophisticated work in this area is presented in Research Box 7.9.

Conjugal Bereavement

The demise of a spouse is extremely distressing to the widow or widower. No one has yet assessed all of the factors that may affect the surviving mate. For an older couple, separation after a half-century or more of living together may be extremely wrenching and painful. Often we read that the passing of an elderly husband or wife is shortly followed by the death of the other spouse, as if their link in life must continue indefinitely. The issue of an expected death versus an unexpected one must also be considered. If a wife's death is not anticipated, the level of somatic symptoms and depression is greater in the husband than if the death has been expected for some time (Winokuer, 2000). In the latter instance, anticipatory grieving may take place and reduce the overall amount of physiological disruption that occurs.

The classic research of Glick et al. (1974) stressed the benign effects of faith on bereavement when a spouse dies (see also Parkes, 1972). In this research, to the extent that widows were devout, they were described as turning "to the formal doctrine of their religions for explanation" (Glick et al., 1974, p. 133). Again we see the significance of spiritual meaning and understanding in alleviating depression and the sense of loss. In other work, social and religious support appeared to operate independently, both working to counter depression

RESEARCH BOX 7.9. The Stress-Buffering Role of Spiritual Support: Cross-Sectional and Prospective Investigations (Maton, 1989)

Maton theorized that religion may mitigate the effects of stress through the use of cognitive and emotional pathways. Specifically, he defined these as "cognitive mediation" and "emotional support." The former implies a positive reframing of negative life events, while the latter comprises perceptions of God as valuing and caring for the distressed individual. Treating these as independent, Maton assessed the contributions of each with two samples: (1) bereaved parents who had lost a child, and (2) college students. In the first sample, 33 parents who had been bereaved within the preceding 2 years constituted a high-stress group, and 48 whose child had died more than 2 years previously made up a low-stress group. Measures of spiritual, social, and friendship support plus depression were completed by the respondents.

Spiritual support countered depression and aided self-esteem for the high-stress group, but not for the low-stress sample. A similar pattern was noted for support provided to the former group, but not to the latter. A prospective study with college students ruled out the likelihood that spiritual help followed rather than contributed to well-being. Maton concluded that "spiritual support may influence well-being through directly enhancing self-esteem and reducing negative affect ('emotional support' pathway) or through enhancing positive and adaptive appraisals of the meaning of a traumatic event ('cognitive mediation' pathway)" (p. 320). He went on to theorize various forms of spiritual support, suggesting research possibilities for exploring this domain further.

and subjective stress (Levy, Martinkowski, & Derby, 1994). Research in the United Kingdom further demonstrates that coping with conjugal bereavement by the elderly is especially difficult when there has been loss of faith (Coleman, 2001). Study after study confirms these findings: Personal adjustment and religious commitment and activity go together. As might be expected, religious involvement is likely to increase following the death of a spouse (Bahr & Harvey, 1980; Haun, 1977; Loveland, 1968).

An interesting study of older widows and widowers brought to the fore the question of religion and adjustment to past and recent death of a spouse (Meusner, Davies, & Marwit, 1994–1995). Unhappily, the fact that the total sample consisted of only 51 respondents means that the study must be considered as really preliminary and necessitating further work. The mean age for the 34 widows was 63.5 and for the 17 widowers was 67. Though the passage of time did not fully resolve grief symptoms, it was implied that a kind of possibly protective repression defensiveness might be present to a greater degree among those who lost spouses in the past as opposed to the recent present. One might argue that religion aids in this form of adjustment. It certainly offers those in grief potentially soothing explanations.

The Significance of Ritual

As described in Chapter 3, ritual has roots deep within our human and animal past. It performs many functions, not the least of which is to establish and maintain control over our personal world and ourselves, especially when we feel pressured. Rites and ceremonies are integral to religion; they bring us psychologically closer to others and to our common cultural heritage. Ritual is a core feature of faith that plays a constructive role in grief. Variously said to create a sense of safety and impart new constructive meanings, it may also distance a person from disturbing emotions. Reeves and Boersma (1989–1990) thus maintain that "rituals can provide a sense of positive personal power for an individual who is feeling out of control and clarify and provide meaning to an issue so that it is easier to work on" (p. 289). In sum, rituals, according to Pargament (1997), are an essential group of coping behaviors. He notes further that religious rituals mark major life transitions (p. 187). Catton (1966) cited the noted sociologist Robert K. Merton as pointing out that rituals perform latent group functions: They reinforce "group identity by bring the scattered members of the group together periodically to participate in collective activity" (Catton, 1966, p. 78).

Rituals thus serve many purposes; they are important to people and are often rigorously observed. Pruyser (1968) states that "it is possible to do these things without conceptual grasp of the grounds or reasons for doing them, and without explicit justification . . . and the doings often become ritualistic, self-perpetuating, a doing for doing's sake" (p. 90). Brown (1991) adopts the phrase "innate urge" (p. 69) in his volume *Human Universals.* Tying rituals to beliefs, Pargament (1997) states that "they add gravity and deeper meaning to [an] event" (p. 174). The probability is rather high that the tendency toward ritual has an evolutionary biological basis, although we have yet to learn its foundation. Here is a feature of the psychology of religion with roots throughout the social and probably biological sciences. In the present context, we must think about the role of rituals as funerary and allied practices relative to death and dying.

On another level, rituals introduce structure, elicit social support, and may serve as a distraction from grief itself. Formal ceremonies allow bereaved individuals to work through the pain of loss. Death is a disruption in the survivors' lives, and religious ideology and ritual may help restore stability to those who are bereaved (Honigmann, 1959).

Illustrative of this principle is the Jewish practice of *shiva,* a 7-day, repetitive set of mourning rites that evokes community support in the form of a group whose members often bring food to the griever's home and participate in a well-established set of ceremonies. It has been compared to group therapy (Kidorf, 1966). Gerson (1977) describes in depth the formalized mourning process in Judaism, and notes how it is designed to thwart the development of pathological grief by specifying degrees of return to normal social interaction. Even though the Jewish *shiva* remains the accepted practice, some Jews feel that a new ritual for the terminally ill should also be created (Millenson, 2015). Given the therapeutic role of ritual, the possibility seems ever present to argue that there is always room for another beneficial ceremony.

For these reasons, the symbolic power of religious rituals has become part of the psychotherapeutic armamentarium of pastoral counselors. The San Francisco gay community, for instance, has created a set of rituals to commemorate those who have died of AIDS (Richards, Wrubel, & Folkman, 1999–2000). Though many of these ceremonies are privately designed, the majority (69%) contain formal or informal religious content. Multiple rituals may be carried out over a number of months, and possibly years.

All known societies have their death rituals. Whatever biopsychological resonances these represent, their significance is buried in cultural practice. Rituals do, however, reflect much elemental psychology—communication, emotional control, and the fostering of group cohesion (Lorenz, 1966; Wulff, 1997).

DEATH AND THE CLERGY

Even though we now emphasize the traditional clerical roles when death enters the picture, let us first recognize that clergy confront the same human issues as everyone else. Facing a fate largely dominated by unknowns, people usually call upon beliefs that deny the possibility of absolute terminality. History and culture readily provide ideas and images that have been with humans for untold millennia, and that we all learn from early childhood. These are continually reinforced by parents, relatives, friends, and social institutions. Unlike the rest of us, however, the clergy are trained in pastoral skills to deal with terminally ill patients and their families, naturally in terms of the faiths with which they are affiliated. Furthermore, once death has occurred, they conduct the approved final rituals that consign the souls of those who have died to their ultimate divine destiny. Here a significant distinction occurs between hospital chaplains and home pastors (i.e., people's regular clerics making home visits): The latter particularly turn their attention to grieving family members and friends, attempting to bring solace to them. This may include such practices as praying with bereaved individuals, reading scripture with them, interpreting theology, discussing spiritual and practical matters, conducting home visits, and whatever else may help to alleviate the pain of loss. The pastoral goals are to engender hope in the face of death, and to assist bereaved persons through the process of recovery. Given these responsibilities, it is understandable why White (1991) perceives clerics as "primary caregivers" (p. 4). Leane and Shute (1998) define all aiding clergy as "gatekeepers," a first line of help to those who grieve.

As noted above, pastoral training and personal experience do not free clerics from anxiety and concern when they are involved with death. One study of 273 pastors revealed that "the death and dying situation is troubling to most pastors" (Spilka, Spangler, Rea, & Nelson, 1981, p. 303). This was especially evident among the younger and least experienced clerics.

The relatively recent development of modern hospice programs and facilities has greatly extended the role of clergy in the period before death. In the hospice context, a cleric provides friendship, and becomes a good listener to the patient and to visiting family members and friends (Dubose, 2000). The need for psychological understanding and clinical skills is overwhelmingly evident in these situations.

Three aims may be posited in work with dying persons and their survivors: (1) to make the death meaningful through a religious or spiritual system; (2) to transform the distress of the death and dying process into a vista of personal strength, self-identity, and a natural closing to an existence in which one has contributed to a better future; and (3) to attempt to convince all that death is not an end, but a new beginning—a doorway to immortality, a personal permanence, a new kind of life (Cook & Oltjenbruns, 1989). We have already shown how clergy may do these things by strengthening spirituality, offering hope, and enhancing the sense of death as meaningful beyond the immediate situation. Research Box 7.10 anchors some of these considerations with actual findings from a study of home pastors and hospital chaplains.

Training the Clergy to Deal with Death

Even though clergy overwhelmingly feel that they have a responsibility to deal with those who are dying (91%) and bereaved (89%), they find performing these duties difficult and anxiety-producing (White, 1991). However, an increased emphasis on death education for prospective clergy has sometimes imparted a heightened sense of competence in dealing with terminality. In one study, 64% felt moderately to well educated in this area (Spilka, Spangler, & Rea, 1981). In contrast, older clergy had to learn about death and dying through direct experience in the pastorate. Today these important skills can be acquired both in seminaries and through internships prior to ordination. Opportunities are currently provided for neophyte clerics to model themselves after mentors who have been engaged with dying people and their families for long periods of time.

With relatively little variation, those to whom the clergy provide their services are pleased with the pastoral efforts of hospital chaplains and home pastors (Brabant, Forsyth, &

RESEARCH BOX 7.10. Spiritual Support in Life-Threatening Illness
(Spilka, Spangler, & Nelson, 1983)

In the last analysis, the effectiveness of clerics must be determined by those who receive their ministrations. This was assessed in a study of 101 patients with cancer and 45 parents of children with cancer. All were questioned about their interactions with home pastors and hospital chaplains. The participants were generally quite religious. All respondents were administered a 55-item questionnaire, in which 6 items were open-ended, permitting a free response.

Twenty-nine percent of the patients were visited at home by their pastors, and 66% received hospital visits. With regard to the families of the children with cancer, 42% had home visits and 56% hospital visits. About 56% of both the patients and parents saw hospital chaplains. From 78 to 87% of the patients and parents were satisfied with the home and hospital visits. Most satisfaction was expressed in cases where the home clergy actually prayed with the patients and the family. Engaging in religious reading was also positively regarded. In the hospital, the families approved discussions of the future by the chaplain. Finally, the willingness of a cleric simply to be present and to devote time to this troubling situation was considered most desirable.

The respondents were often clearer about the undesirable characteristic of clerics than those they found positive. Most that was displeasing was attributed to poor communication and lack of understanding by a pastor. Specifically, conveying the impression of visiting out of a sense of duty alone, or failing to appreciate or be sensitive to the pain of the circumstances, was upsetting to these people. Extremely distressing were efforts (fortunately rare) to obtain "deathbed conversions." For example, one cleric harangued a patient to "change his pagan ways." Much more common were indications of the pastors' own discomfort—looking at their watches, acting "nervous," verbalizing clichés, standing at a distance from patients, being painfully silent and unresponsive, and finally being in a rush to leave.

Pastoral identity was also a problem. A fair number of patients and parents (14% and 12%, respectively) reported difficulty discovering who was and was not a chaplain. This resulted from the wearing of informal sports clothes, the absence of a badge that defined one as a chaplain (or the use of a badge too small to read at any distance), and/or a person's failing to state that he or she was a chaplain.

The many things pastors do can bring comfort and solace to those greatly in need of such aid. In most instances, this is what takes place. Still, clergy sometimes convey a lack of feeling and compassion without intending to do so. There is clearly a need for "on-the-job" training in these critical situations.

McFarlain, 1995; Johnson & Spilka, 1991; Spilka, Spangler, & Nelson, 1983). An interesting exception occurred in one study of patients with breast cancer: Both male and female clerics usually avoided discussing some of these women's central concerns about their identity as females and the surgical mutilation of their bodies (Johnson & Spilka, 1991). Obviously, there is still a need for pastoral training to deal with such sensitive personal issues.

Another approach revolves around the concept of a "good death." Utilizing focus groups of clergy and congregants, Braun and Zir (2001) found agreement on a number of criteria that pastoral education might emphasize for a terminally ill patient to have a "good death." The implication is that clerics should (1) be involved in pain management; (2) see that the dying process is not inappropriately prolonged; (3) work to encourage a supportive family atmosphere at the bedside; (4) try to resolve conflicts and introduce the potential of forgiveness, when desirable; (5) aid not only the terminally ill patient, but grieving family members; and (6) where proper, bring in theology and rituals to lighten the burden of mourning and bereavement.

Other troubling areas for which clergy feel unprepared are infant deaths and youth suicides (Strength, 1999; Thearle, Vance, Najman, Embelton, & Foster, 1995; Leane & Shute, 1998). With regard to adolescent suicide, an Australian study revealed low levels of knowledge about risk signs for such an eventuality. This is believed to handicap clerical efforts to counteract such suicidal inclinations (Leane & Shute, 1998).

Pastoral education might also look more closely at the problems children have when loved ones die. Inaccurate, distorted, and troubling magical fantasies need to be confronted in order to resolve a child's grief (Fogarty, 2000).

Theology, Personal Faith, and Clergy Effectiveness

Spilka, Spangler, Rea, and Nelson (1981) found that among clergy dealing with death and dying, two-thirds claimed that the theology of their church was "very helpful," while only 2–3% felt that it was of little or no use. Surprisingly, these numbers held whether the clerics were affiliated with a conservative or a liberal religious body. An interesting variation on this theme suggests that clerics' own personal faith is of greater importance than their church's theology as 83% regarded the former as providing them with the most support in their death work (Spilka, Spangler, & Rea, 1981).

There is little doubt that working with terminality is a very trying experience for clerics. Almost 70% of those surveyed were less than "very satisfied" with their efforts, and 11–14% were quite unhappy with themselves. Some 43% of these pastors described themselves with qualifying adjectives such as "frustrated," "inadequate," "apprehensive," and the like (Spilka, Spangler, & Rea, 1981).

That bereaved people consider the clergy helpful at this troubled time is abundantly evident. Carey (1979–1980) compared the satisfaction of widows and widowers with physicians, nurses, chaplains, social workers, and family members. Although family members were viewed as most helpful, hospital chaplains came in a close second.

Like virtually everyone who confronts death, clergy probably never become immune to the feelings that death and dying engender. They have entered a profession in which they must continually confront these hard realities. Undoubtedly, pastoral effectiveness is a function of experiences that force clerics to face their own mortality while expressing the empathy and humanity these situations call for. Fortunately, most clergy acquire the skills, compassion, and understanding to handle these trials.

OVERVIEW

Much of this book is about you, the reader. In particular, this chapter touches upon elements of your future. When we are busy with our current lives, we rarely contemplate our *probable* future of job, family, old age, retirement, and of course death. In these pages, we have tried to show you some of these complexities.

Until fairly recently, psychology paid little attention to older individuals. The fact that people are living longer and that the elderly population is growing at an extremely rapid rate has awakened the social-scientific community to the necessity of understanding this population. Similarly, religious institutions have found that the average age of congregation members has increased. As churchgoers grow older, new psychological and faith needs arise. The significance of religion in these circumstances cannot be ignored or minimized. Growing isolation, mental and physical infirmities, and the loss of friends and family create new functions for church and faith.

Overall, we have seen a major development in research in this area—namely, from the use of unitary notions of aging and death to multidimensional conceptualizations in both domains. Even though more sophisticated instrumentation is now available, too much work still relies on simplistic measures of death fear/anxiety. Part of this may be due to the fact that researchers are much more knowledgeable in the coping realm than they are about advances in the psychology of religion. Convenience samples in which testing must be kept to a minimum may also be impeding the use of more sophisticated measurement of religious perspectives; however, we now see multiform trends in work on religiosity relative to coping with AIDS, bereavement, euthanasia, and such phenomena as NDEs and contact with the dead.

Our position is that the deaths of others and the prospect of one's own death raise for each individual two very basic coping issues we have often referred to in this volume: the issues of meaning and control. Both aging and death arouse these concerns in their most intimate and ultimate forms. It is here that faith probably makes its greatest adaptive contributions.

CHAPTER 8

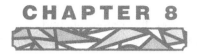

Conversion, Spiritual Transformation, and Deconversion

Riding home with a friend that evening in the back seat of a car, I listened incredulously as my companions spoke glowingly about the message that they had just received. In fact, they were so moved by the guru's words that they made tentative plans to return the next day to pay homage to him by kissing his feet. I was flabbergasted, stunned. How could anybody have thought this guy was a spiritual master?

There are two lives, the natural and the spiritual, and we must lose the one before we can participate in the other.

He was down and out, the Catholics took him in and before he knew it, he had faith. So it was gratitude that decided the issue most likely.

But the Muslim believes that the propositional tenets of his faith are self-evident if they are properly presented and understood, and the focus of his proselytization is the proclamation of these tenets rather than the experiences of human beings.

All conversions (even Saul's on the road to Damascus) are mediated through people, institutions, communities, and groups.

And Priests in black gowns were walking their rounds, And binding with briars my joys & desires.[1]

In the early months of 1881, G. Stanley Hall delivered a series of public lectures at Harvard University. His topic was religious conversion, and much of the material he covered was later incorporated into his classic two-volume study of adolescence (Hall, 1904). Advocates for the young science of psychology were courageous enough to tackle some of the most profound and meaningful religious phenomena of the times. Because the emerging psychology was linked in the popular mind with religious and parapsychological phenomena (Coon, 1992), some of the first North American psychologists divided along lines claiming to debunk or support such phenomena (Hood, 1994). Hall eventually went on to write a two-volume treatise with the title *Jesus, the Christ, in the Light of Psychology* (1917). The title reveals the Christian bias of the emerging science of psychology: When they said "religion," most psychologists meant Christianity. Furthermore, when they said "Christianity," most

---

[1]These quotations come, respectively, from the following sources: Kent (2001, p. xvi); James (1902/1985, p. 139); Kundera (1983, p. 308); Poston (1992, p. 158); Rambo (1993, p. 1); and Blake (1789/1967, Plate 44).

psychologists meant Protestantism. Thus, not surprisingly, the North American psychology of religion emerged as a psychology of North American Protestant Christianity (Gorsuch, 1988). However, today studies of conversion are placed within a global context, and they focus upon in-depth appreciation of diverse traditions. An inclusive handbook of religious conversion (Rambo & Farhadian, 2014b) includes specific chapters devoted to not only the Abrahamic faiths (Christianity, Islam, and Judaism), but others, such as Buddhism, Confucianism, Daoism (Taoism), Hinduism, Jainism, and Sikhism. However, as we shall see below, how one studies conversion is a major factor in determining what kinds of conclusions can be drawn about conversion. As Paloutzian (2014) has emphasized, there is more than just a linguistic difference between conversion and transformation.

At the turn of the 20th century, religious revivals were common in North America, especially in evangelical Protestantism (Gaustad, 1966; Taves, 1999). Evangelicals focused upon the "born-again" experience. In his Gifford Lectures, James distinguished between those "once-born," who are cultivated within their faith and gradually socialized to accept it unproblematically, and those "twice-born," with more melancholy temperaments, who are literally compelled through crises to accept or realize their faith within an instant (James, 1902/1985, Lectures VI through VIII). Not surprisingly, North American psychologists were fascinated by this predominantly Protestant phenomenon, and conversion became the earliest major focus of the psychology of religion.

Sociologists were also concerned with conversion. Jackson (1908) chose conversion as his topic when he gave the Cole Lectures at Vanderbilt University. James (1902/1985) devoted two of his Gifford Lectures in Edinburgh to the specific topic of conversion (Lectures IX and X). James's lectures relied heavily upon the research of his contemporaries, especially Edwin Starbuck and James H. Leuba. Both had been students of Hall's at Clark University. Leuba (1896) published the first psychological journal article on conversion; this was rapidly followed by Starbuck's (1897) article on conversion and by his first book-length treatment of the topic (Starbuck, 1899). Not surprisingly, Leuba's and Starbuck's research methods paralleled Hall's, including the use of questionnaires and personal documents. Despite James's aversion to questionnaire studies, he utilized material supplied by Starbuck from his questionnaire studies of religious converts. Another early investigator, Coe (1916), added quasi-experimental techniques to the investigation of religious converts.

Whereas these early investigators tended to focus upon dramatic cases of sudden conversion, others argued against the selection of such extreme cases as the basis for developing a general model of conversion. For instance, Pratt (1920), a student of James's at Harvard, focused upon gradual converts, whose experiences were less dramatic, required intellectual seeking, and were hypothesized to be more genuinely characteristic of conversion within both Christianity and other religious traditions. As we shall soon see, from the beginning of the study of conversion, fundamental issues were identified and debated that continue to characterize the contemporary study of the subject. Yet as the psychology of religion waned in North America, conversion was ignored by psychologists. By the late 1950s, W. H. Clark bemoaned the fact that psychology had all but abandoned the study of conversion:

> For students of religion and religious psychology there is no subject that has held more fascination than the phenomenon called conversion. Yet of recent years a kind of shame-facedness becomes apparent among those scholars who mention it. . . . among the more conventional psychologists of the present day, who infrequently concern themselves with the study of religion and practically never with the subject of conversion. It is quite obvious

that the latter is regarded as a kind of psychological slum to be avoided by any respectable scholar. (Clark, 1958, p. 188)

Even now, critical reviews of the literature on conversion reveal that there are no systematic programs of methodologically sophisticated research on conversion. The necessary longitudinal studies are nearly nonexistent. As Paloutzian, Richardson, and Rambo (1999, p. 1048) note, "most of the research is retrospective and cross-sectional, and no systematic program of research has ever been sustained." Paloutzian (2005) has proposed placing the study of conversion within an analysis of meaning systems, which could produce programmatic research. Likewise, Streib and his colleagues have recommended using mixed methods (qualitative and quantitative) to study deconversion systematically within a narrative framework linked to biographical analyses (Streib, 2008; Streib, Hood, Keller, Csöff, & Silver, 2009; Streib & Hood, 2016). Thus the future promises more systematic programs of empirical research on conversion, spiritual transformation, and deconversion, consistent with the call for a new paradigm that is multilevel and interdisciplinary (Hefner & Koss-Chioino, 2006; Gooren, 2007; Paloutzian, 2005; Streib et al., 2009; Streib & Hood, 2016).

CONVERSION AND SPIRITUAL TRANSFORMATION: DEFINITIONS AND APPROACHES

A distinction can be made between "spiritual transformation" and "conversion," given the distinction between "spirituality" and "religion" that now dominates much of the scientific study of religion. As we discuss in Chapter 9, most persons in the contemporary United States identify themselves as both spiritual and religious. However, a stable minority identify themselves as either *more* spiritual than religious (Zinnbauer, Pargament, & Scott, 1999) or spiritual but *not* religious (Marler & Hadaway, 2002). Several investigators have noted that this latter group asserts an independence from, and often even hostility to, religious institutions (Hood, 2003, 2005b; Streib, 2008; Streib & Hood, 2016). However, insofar as individuals alter their spirituality, they may do it either in association with religious institutions or in opposition to them. Consistent with Paloutzian (2005, pp. 333–334), we refer to the former alteration as "conversion" and the latter as "spiritual transformation." Thus spiritual transformation expressed in conventional religious language and associated with religious institutions is conversion in the classic sense. Spiritual transformation is expressed in nonconventional religious language and often in opposition to religious institutions from which the individual has deconverted (Streib et al., 2009; Streib & Hood, 2016). Although there may be overlap between religion and spiritual self-identification, Schlenhofer, Omotto, and Adelman (2008) noted in an in-depth qualitative study of older adults that spirituality is a more abstract concept than religion and includes nontheistic notions of a higher power. Religion, on the other hand, is more closely associated with community participation, specific beliefs, and organized practices.

Social psychologists have produced the majority of the empirical measurement-based research to date in the psychology of religion. Social psychology can be divided into sociological social psychology and psychological social psychology (Stephan & Stephan, 1985). Although contemporary research on conversion is rapidly increasing in volume, the clear tendency has been for sociological social psychology to dominate the field. Much of this can be attributed to the sociological interest in new religious movements, discussed in Chapter 9.

For instance, a major bibliography on new religious movements by Beckford and Richardson (1983) contained at least 145 references pertinent to conversion, only 5% of which appeared prior to 1973. An earlier bibliography specifically on conversion literature prepared by Rambo (1982) listed 252 references, only 38% of which were published prior to 1973. Despite the claim of Beit-Hallahmi and Argyle (1997, p. 115; emphasis in original) that conversion has been "*the* classical topic in the psychology of religion," we see a reemergence of studies of conversion as a major focus for the contemporary social psychology of religion, but with a distinctive sociological rather than psychological emphasis reflecting what Gooren (2007, p. 347) has aptly identified as "disciplinary biases." Furthermore, as Rambo and Farhadian (2014a) note, conversion, whether religious or spiritual, is embedded in a global context. While within specific cultures the focus is more upon spiritual transformation than upon religious conversion, this is not the case in a global context, where conversion to religious groups that endorse terrorist tactics has become of immense concern. (For an extended discussion of such groups, see Chapter 9.)

Quite naturally, then, we can focus upon three major approaches to conversion and transformation—roughly identified with what we term the "classic" (psychological) focus, the "social-scientific" (sociological) focus, and the "global" (interdisciplinary) focus. The classic approach, influenced primarily by psychological social psychology, has been dominated (as noted above) by a concern with North American Protestantism. Many different techniques and methods characterize this research, but the focus is primarily upon intraindividual processes in conversion. The social-scientific approach is influenced primarily by sociological social-psychological studies of conversion and transformation. This research is focused upon new religious movements, or varieties of communal Christian groups; it is less likely to be strongly measurement-based, and the focus is upon interpsychological processes. The global approach is multidisciplinary and embeds the study of conversion within a historical perspective that includes not only individual conversion but mass conversion, in which entire cultures are converted. To some extent, both the social-scientific and global paradigms suggest that exclusive reliance upon quantitative measures is too limiting to capture the complexity of conversion and the nuances of individual converts' narratives of transformation. However, just as there is no singular definition of religion, neither is there of science (Ryle, 1954). Conversion studies, like many contemporary studies in the psychology of religion in general, are no less scientific if they lack a firm quantitative basis. The global paradigm promises to transform the study of conversion by focusing upon mixed research methods, balancing quantitative studies with qualitative research. A review of leading publications in psychology of religion and spirituality over a 25-year period (1978–2003) revealed that only 22 out of the 2,726 articles described qualitative or mixed-methods research (Aten & Hernandez, 2005). Likewise, Leach and Soto's (2013) analysis of the first 4 years of the *Psychology of Religion and Spirituality* (2008–2012), the official journal for the American Psychological Association's Division 36, indicated that only 8 of the 77 published studies were qualitative research. This situation, though, is likely to change in the near future.

It is also likely that a shift to a global paradigm will force psychologists to recognize that there are psychologies that are functionally incommensurate in epistemology, methods, and practices (Pickren, 2009, p. 88). The exclusive focus upon the classic psychological paradigm is recognized from both the social-scientific and global perspectives as an American anomaly. Pickren prophetically warns that not only with respect to conversion, but with respect to the exclusive reliance on quantitative methods, "the 21st century is unlikely to be another American century in psychology" (2009, p. 87).

These three major paradigms are not exclusive and overlap in significant ways, but as we shall see, they provide differing (and to some extent even contradictory) views of conversion and spiritual transformation. The extent to which the differences among the three approaches are confounded by claims about the nature of conversion and transformation processes is an open question.

THE CLASSIC RESEARCH PARADIGM: PSYCHOLOGICAL DOMINANCE

What we have chosen to call the classic research approach to conversion is not merely of historical interest. The early psychologists utilized a variety of methods to study conversion. They also accepted as raw data for analysis various types of material; these included personal documents such as private letters and confessions, as well as autobiographical and biographical materials. Questionnaires, interviews, and public confessions were employed as well. Although contemporary psychology tends to minimize the use of many of these sources, especially personal documents, their value can be immense (Capps, 1994; Capps & Dittes, 1990). They cannot be used to identify the causal processes in conversion, but they are essential and valid as rich descriptions of the process of conversion as a human experience. They also provide a richness of detail that moves beyond single-cause explanations of what are clearly complex processes of social and personal change (Kwilecki, 1999; Streib et al., 2009).

Classic Conceptualizations of Conversion

Snow and Machalek (1984) have appropriately noted that any effort to understand the causes of conversion presupposes the ability to identify converts. However, they have also noted that few investigators have bothered to give clear conceptualizations of conversion. Most psychologists define "conversion" as a radical transformation of self; these definitions emphasize intrapersonal processes. Furthermore, early psychologists such as Cutten (1908) and Pratt (1920) emphasized that such definitions rely heavily upon a Protestant understanding of Saul's (Paul's) conversion on the road to Damascus as typical of all conversion (Richardson, 1985b).

The use of Paul's conversion as prototypical so dominates the classic paradigm of conversion research that Richardson (1985b) refers to the "Pauline experience" as the exemplar for conversion research in an article contrasting the classic paradigm with an emerging contemporary paradigm. Ironically, contemporary views echo Pratt, who argued that the fascination of psychologists with Paul's conversion as a model for all crisis-precipitated sudden conversion accounted for its overrepresentation in textbooks on psychology of religion. In Pratt's own words, "I venture to estimate that at least nine out of every ten 'conversion cases' reported in recent questionnaires would have no violent or depressing experience to report had not the individual in question been brought up in a church or community which taught them to look for it if not to cultivate it" (1920, p. 153).

As was the case with psychology at the beginning of the 20th century, much of the contemporary psychology of religion is really a study of Christianity, particularly Protestantism (Gorsuch, 1988; Taves, 1999). Gorsuch (1988, p. 202) has appropriately cautioned against extending the psychology of Christianity to other religions. However, social psychologists have not been appropriately cautious in this respect: They have generalized from Paul's conversion not only to all conversion within Christianity, but even to conversion experiences in other religions as well.

Defining conversion as a radical alteration in the self is probably itself heavily influenced by the conversion of Paul. Even sociologically oriented investigators tend to define conversion in terms that imply radical change in the self, even if these terms are deemphasized or if conversion is empirically assessed by other indicators as well. For instance, in an often-cited definition, Travisano (1970, p. 594) refers to conversion as "a radical reorganization of identity, meaning, life." Heirich (1977, p. 674) refers to conversion as the process of changing one's sense of "root reality," or of one's sense of "ultimate grounding." After critical analysis of definitions of conversion as radical personal change, Snow and Machalek (1984) define conversion in terms of a shift in the universe of discourse, which carries with it a corresponding shift in consciousness. However, as Coe (1916, p. 54) long ago noted, if self-reorganization is used to define conversion, "Conversion is by no means co-extensive with religion." Indeed, most psychologists are likely to focus upon changing the self outside religious contexts (Brinthaupt & Lipka, 1994). What then makes conversion, contextualized as a radical self-change, distinctively religious?

It does little good to define conversion in distinctively religious terms, by imputing causal power to a deity to distinguish religious from nonreligious conversions. For instance, Rambo (1993, p. xiii) admits his own predilection to define as genuine only conversions as alteration of the person by the power of God, though he recognizes that this is not a useful definition for empirical psychology. However, it is clear from Rambo and Farhadian's (2014b) recent handbook that especially in more radical conversions, facilitated by Internet sources, sudden conversions perceived by the converts to be due to God or Allah are increasingly common and problematic within a global perspective that must balance absolutist claims against religious tolerance.

Furthermore, whether or not one makes attributions to the self-altering power of God is problematic. But with appropriate methods, this can be empirically investigated (Moghaddam, 2006). The use of religious attributions or a religious universe of discourse is what makes conversion *religious* conversion (Snow & Machalek, 1984). It is also what makes conversion to extreme groups such as cults, and groups that advocate terrorist tactics, legitimate targets for psychological analysis within a global perspective (see Chapter 9). After conversion, religious attributions defining and identifying the new self become "master attributions," replacing secular attributions or religious attributions that were peripheral prior to conversion (Snow & Machalek, 1984). In this sense, early clarifications of conversion mesh nicely with contemporary considerations. Coe (1916, p. 152) spoke of "self realization within a social medium" as defining conversion. James (1902/1985, p. 162) noted that "To say a man is 'converted' means . . . that religious ideas, peripheral in his consciousness, now take a central place, and that religious aims form the habitual center of his energy." Paloutzian (2005) explores the shifts in meaning systems following conversion, especially meaning expressed in classical religious language.

Most empirical studies of conversion implicitly, if not explicitly, utilize criteria that correspond to Coe's analysis of conversion. First, conversion is a profound change in self. Second, the change is not simply a matter of maturation, but is typically identified with a process (sudden or gradual) by which the altered self is achieved. Third, this change in the self is radical in its consequences—indicated by such things as a new centering of concern, interest, and action. Fourth, this new sense of self is perceived as "higher" or as an emancipation from a previous dilemma or predicament. Thus conversion is self-realization or self-reorganization, in that one adopts or finds a new self. The process also occurs within a social medium or context. Specifically, in religious conversion this entails a religious framework within which the altered self is described, acts, and is recognized by others. The fact that conversion may result in new habitual modes of action links any purely *intrapsychological* processes of conversion to the *interpsychological* processes that maintain them. Long ago, Strickland (1924) argued against James's distinction between once-born and twice-born believers, on the grounds that anyone who consciously adopts a religious view (whether gradually or suddenly), is twice-born: "And if action from new ideals and changed habits of life do *not* follow, there has been no conversion" (p. 123; emphasis in original).

Although admittedly some change must occur in conversion, the nature of that change must be carefully delineated. Psychologists frequently focus upon personality change. Paloutzian et al. (1999) argue that the two distinct literatures on conversion and personality change ought to be related. Adopting contemporary views of personality that recognize levels or domains to personality (Emmons, 1995) suggests that one can organize the empirical literature on conversion by the extent to which it produces changes in particular domains or levels of personality. For instance, research at the basic personality level, using such indicators as a measure based on the five-factor model of personality (McCrae, 1992), has produced little if any evidence that conversion changes basic personality. However, at other levels of personality functioning, changes resulting from conversion can clearly be identified. Research Box 8.1 summarizes the conversion literature with respect to the changes conversion produces in various levels of personality functioning.

RESEARCH BOX 8.1. What about the Personality Changes in Conversion?
(Paloutzian, Richardson, & Rambo, 1999)

The empirical study of conversion interfaces two bodies of literature in psychology: the literature on conversion, a perennial topic in the psychology of religion, and that on personality change, a topic of renewed interest in personality theory. Paloutzian, Richardson, and Rambo have reviewed and organized these two literatures according to levels of personality. Identifying three levels or domains of personality and the accompanying empirical literature of the effects of conversion reveals a fairly consistent picture. The magnitude of the effects of conversion across these three levels or domains of personality is consistent, whether conversion is sudden or gradual, or whether it is active or passive. They also appear to hold regardless of whether conversion is to a Western or Eastern faith tradition. We can summarize these findings as follows:

Personality level or domain	Effects of conversion
Level I: Basic functioning	No or minimal change
Level II: Midlevel functions (attitudes, feelings, behavior)	Significant change[a]
Level III: Self-defining personality functions (purpose in life, meaning, identity)	Profound change[a]

[a]Change may not be permanent if continual conversions occur (this is common among active seekers).

Efforts to Explain Conversion and Spiritual Transformation

Perhaps the two most empirically studied correlates of conversion (and, more recently, of spiritual transformation) are linked to temporal issues. One is the age at which conversion or spiritual transformation is most likely. (In Chapter 5, we review the typical finding that religious conversion is most common in adolescence. However, as we note in a later section, spiritual transformation is likely to occur and continue after adolescence.) The second temporal issue related to conversion and spiritual transformation is the rate of change: Is it sudden or gradual?

Sudden Conversion

Early investigators did not fail to classify conversion types into simple dichotomies. The most obvious was derived from a continuum of duration. Some persons convert quickly, appearing suddenly to adopt a faith perspective previously unknown (conversion) or to make a faith that was previously of peripheral concern suddenly central (intensification). Other people seem to mature and blossom gradually within a faith perspective that in some sense has always been theirs. We have already noted the dispute surrounding James's once-born and twice-born types. James (1902/1985) acknowledged the possibility of gradual conversion, but he focused upon sudden conversion, probably precipitated by crises. Many of James's examples of crisis-precipitated conversion are what Rambo (1993) identifies as intensification experiences.

In his fascination with sudden conversion, James was not alone. Starbuck (1899) focused upon "conversions of self-surrender" and "voluntary conversions." The former were thought to be elicited by a sense of sin, suddenly overcome; the latter by a gradual pursuit of a religious ideal. Ames (1910) favored restricting the term "conversion" to sudden instances of religious change associated with intense emotionality. Coe (1916) noted at least six senses of conversion, but likewise favored limiting the term to intense, sudden religious change. Johnson (1959, p. 117) later echoed these views succinctly when he stated, "A genuine religious conversion is the outcome of a crisis." Sudden conversion facilitated by the Internet and social media is a recent phenomenon and seems characteristic of conversion to extreme groups within a global perspective (Rambo & Farhadian, 2014a), suggesting that contemporary researchers ought not to ignore the considerable research on sudden conversion that has dominated much of the early psychology of religion.

So influential were the early psychologists in focusing conversion upon sudden, intense experiences of religious self-reorganization that Richardson (1985b, p. 164) summarizes their implicit conceptualization as the "old conversion paradigm." The prototype is the conversion of Paul in the Christian tradition. It suggests what Miller and C'deBaca (1994) refer to as "quantum change."

Richardson emphasizes that what we have called the classic model implies a passive subject transformed by forces that may be differentially identified. However, whether these forces are identified as "God" or "the unconscious" makes little difference. The convert is not seen as an active agent; instead, emotion dominates the irrational alteration of self that suddenly changes belief, and subsequent behavior change follows.

Richardson's model has similarities to Strickland's (1924) summary of the success of sudden conversions common among evangelical and fundamentalist Protestant groups in North America, including those that occurred during revivalist meetings. Strickland also emphasized the institutionalization of Paul's conversion as the valued form of entering the

Christian faith, with the emphasis upon sin and guilt as eliciting conditions joyously relieved in the emotionality of a sudden conversion. Strickland's perspective thus adds a more dynamic understanding to Richardson's assertion that the classic conversion paradigm is facilitated by emotional factors that are likely to erupt suddenly in late adolescence.

Not surprisingly, several empirical studies have related emotional states to sudden conversions. For instance, in a classic study by E. T. Clark (1929), 2,174 cases of adolescent conversions were classified as either sudden or gradual. Approximately one-third were sudden and were precipitated by either emotion or crisis; they also tended to be linked with a stern theology. Starbuck (1899) studied adolescent conversions and found that two-thirds were at least partially triggered by a deep sense of sin or guilt. However, he found that in later adolescence, conversion was likely to be more gradual. Pratt (1920) went so far as to identify the view that prior to their conversions, twice-born individuals wallow in extreme feelings of unworthiness, self-doubt, and depreciation that are released or overcome via conversion, as in the James–Starbuck thesis. The James–Starbuck thesis recognizes conversion as a functional solution to the burdens of guilt and sin, which are found to be unbearable prior to conversion. Research Box 8.2 presents a more detailed analysis of Clark's (1929) classic study of conversion, which supports the James–Starbuck thesis.

In light of the James–Starbuck thesis, we must be cautious not to interpret negative emotions such as guilt, sin, and shame as necessarily psychologically unhealthy. Watson and his colleagues have provided a series of studies relevant to this thesis (Watson, 1993; Watson, Morris, & Hood, 1993). Watson argues that negative emotions such as shame and guilt can function positively when interpreted within an "ideological surround" that provides a context for both their meaningfulness and their resolution. Clearly, one individual's personal

---

RESEARCH BOX 8.2. The Psychology of Religious Awakening (Clark, 1929)

In this classic study, E. T. Clark classified 2,174 conversions as to whether they were sudden or gradual. Sudden conversions (32.9%) were subdivided into two types: (1) "definite crisis awakening," in which a personal crisis was suddenly followed by a religious transformation (6.7%, majority males); and (2) "emotional stimulus awakening," in which gradual religious growth was interrupted by an emotional event that was suddenly followed by religious transformation (27.2%, equal proportions of males and females). Gradual conversions were described as "gradual awakening," a steady, progressive, slow growth resulting in gradual religious transformation (66.1%, slightly more females). A stern theology was associated with sudden conversions, equally distributed between crises and emotional awakenings. This was as would have been predicted from the James–Starbuck thesis. Almost all gradual conversions were associated with compassionate theologies that emphasized love and forgiveness.

Clark suggested that sudden conversions were associated with fear and anxiety. In addition, 41% of these conversions occurred during revivals, which were likely to be highly emotional settings. The dominant emotional states reported were joyful reactions, assumed by Clark to result from the alleviation of negative feelings that occurred prior to conversion, which were elicited by stern theologies emphasizing sin and guilt. This study suggests that negative emotional states can precipitate experiences within a religious setting, and that conversion then provides positive relief of these negative feelings.

religious reactions may be another's madness. Just as many people refuse to experience the necessity of salvation from sin insisted upon by some fundamentalist groups, so may others perceive fundamentalists to be encased in a rigid, outmoded religious framework. Nevertheless, the functionality of sin, shame, and guilt within fundamentalism is hard to dispute (Gordon, 1984; Hood, 1992b). As Hood and his colleagues have noted (Hood, 1983; Hood, Hill, & Williamson, 2005), the empirical issues involved in studying fundamentalist religious groups are clouded by differences (often value-based) between investigators and those who are investigated.

That sudden conversion is often correlated with emotionality seems well established. However, such correlations do little to provide meaningful causal claims, such as that emotional feelings trigger conversions or that guilt and sin are resolved by such conversions. Nevertheless, essentially correlational studies can be suggestive. A classic study by Coe (1916) compared 17 persons who anticipated striking conversions that actually occurred with 12 persons anticipating striking conversions that did not occur. Emotional factors were dominant in the group for which striking conversions occurred; cognitive factors were dominant in the group for whom striking conversions did not occur. In addition, the actual converts were more suggestible than the other group. Although Coe's research suggests that emotional factors may be causally involved in sudden conversions, no true experimental studies or longitudinal studies documenting this claim exist. However, more recent research in cognitive psychology suggests a reason to link emotionality and sudden dramatic conversions. McCallister (1995) has noted that emotional situations such as dramatic conversions may restrict the encoding of knowledge about experience, leading dramatic converts to utilize narrative formats to reconstruct their experience.

Still, in many studies it may be that emotionality and sudden conversions are merely correlated phenomena. For instance, Spellman, Baskett, and Byrne (1971) divided persons in a small Protestant town into sudden or gradual converts and compared them to nonconverts. They found that sudden converts scored higher on an objective measure of anxiety than gradual converts or nonconverts did. Yet this difference found was *after* conversion; there was no evidence that greater emotionality differentiated the groups prior to their conversion, as postulated by the James–Starbuck thesis. Furthermore, as Poston (1992) has noted, emotional and crisis-triggered conversions are uncommon in many non-Christian religions; they do not, for instance, characterize conversion to Islam. Woodberry (1992) notes that traditional Islamic thought does not even have a term for "conversion." Finally, the specific case of sudden conversion associated with claims to mind control and "brainwashing" is discussed in Chapter 9.

There is considerable research relating attachment theory to religious conversion. Attachment theory has been discussed more fully in Chapters 3 and 4. Here we simply note that insofar as sudden religious conversion is concerned, a meta-analysis based on almost 1,500 participants strongly supports an association with early parental insensitivity, consistent with the theory that God serves as a compensatory attachment figure (Granqvist & Kirkpatrick, 2004). Likewise, even dramatic increases in religious commitment have been shown to be precipitated by emotional turmoil among individuals whose parents were judged to be insensitive, again supporting the compensatory hypothesis (Granqvist, Ivarsson, Broberg, & Hageskull, 2007). In light of the new paradigm proposed for the psychology of religion, the relationship between the compensatory hypothesis and conversion is strengthened by the fact that it has been demonstrated in research using a variety of methods and measures of attachment (Granqvist & Kirkpatrick, 2004).

Gradual Conversion

Like sudden religious conversions, gradual conversions result in a major change of self within a religious context. Yet gradual conversions occur almost imperceptibly; they are usually distinguished empirically by not being identified with a single event. Some investigators have argued that gradual conversions need not result in radical shifts in personality, self, or even religious beliefs. These researchers have essentially redefined conversion or have accepted as empirical criteria such things as merely joining a new religious group. Scobie (1973, 1975) even argues for "unconscious conversion," referring to persons who cannot recall *not* having been religious. Clearly, characteristics associated with joining a new religious group need not precisely parallel those defining conversion in the classic sense. Neither do continual faith commitments without an intensification experience. We must note in each case the empirical criteria used to assess conversion, and must keep these in mind when comparing individual empirical studies.

Strickland (1924) contrasted gradual and sudden conversions. In gradual conversions, the emphasis is upon conscious striving toward a goal. This is consistent with Paloutzian's (2005) emphasis on meaning, and with the summary of Paloutzian et al. (1999) in Research Box 8.1 that changes in personality occur with respects to attitudes and behaviors (Level II) and in terms of purpose in life and meaning (Level III). The convert is not likely to experience a single decisive point at which conversion is either initiated or completed. There is an absence of emotional crises and of feelings of guilt and sin. The process is cognitive rather than emotional, and if it occurs in opposition to religion, it is best viewed as a spiritual transformation.

THE SOCIAL-SCIENTIFIC RESEARCH PARADIGM: SOCIOLOGICAL DOMINANCE

Strickland's distinction between gradual and sudden conversion laid the foundation for the emergence of what we term the social-scientific paradigm of conversion and spiritual transformation. The focus upon an active agent, seeking self-transformation, has become the target of extensive research among more sociologically oriented investigators. No single theory dominates this research literature, but most theories share enough common assumptions to contrast them with the classic psychological paradigm.

Five characteristics of the social-scientific paradigm are notable. First, the research is done primarily by sociologists and anthropologists or sociologically oriented social psychologists, rather than by psychologists or psychologically oriented social psychologists. Second, the research focuses upon new religious and spiritual movements, many of non-Western origin or influence (or, if Christian, often fundamentalist groups of a sectarian nature). Third, the research is often participatory in nature, with single groups studied over a period of time. Investigators are less likely to take a single set of measurements on a group, as is typical of classic research by psychologists on conversion. Both structured and unstructured interviews with research participants are common. Fourth, almost by definition, the research focuses upon gradual rather than sudden conversion or transformation. Finally, the process of deconversion is investigated, in which individuals who have converted and then left new religious movements are studied. (We cover deconversion in greater detail later in this chapter.)

THE GLOBAL RESEARCH PARADIGM: INTERDISCIPLINARY DOMINANCE

Perhaps no topic best responds to the call for a new multilevel interdisciplinary paradigm in the psychology of religion (Emmons & Paluutzian, 2003) than contemporary studies of conversion within a global perspective. The key resource here is the handbook by Rambo and Farhadian (2014b), and the implicit paradigm we have derived from their text suggests major changes in the breadth and scope of research on not only religious but spiritual conversion. However, a cautionary note here is that for some, this exemplar of the new paradigm remains problematic from what one reviewer has called a "*prototypical* 'social scientific'" perspective (Acevedo, 2014, p. 854; emphasis in original). The options for a psychology of religion raised by us in Chapter 1 are relevant here precisely with respect to how far psychology can address conversion from a truly multilevel and interdisciplinary perspective and still be "scientific."

We cannot address this issue more fully here; we only note that the global paradigm is truly interdisciplinary, and as such can be contrasted with both the classic psychological and social-scientific paradigms.

MAJOR DIFFERENCES AMONG THE THREE PARADIGMS

Richardson (1985b) has been the most articulate theorist arguing that the classic paradigm, based upon the "Pauline experience," has been abandoned in favor of a social-scientific paradigm. Some have debated the claim that there are contrasting paradigms; they argue instead that perhaps the nature of conversion itself has changed over time (Lofland & Skonovd, 1981). It is difficult to compare paradigms empirically, given differences in research methods and the nature of religious groups studied. This is especially true with the global paradigm, which places conversion within a worldwide historical perspective and pays careful attention to how converts narrate their own transformations, whether these are defined as religious or spiritual.

What undoubtedly differentiates the social-scientific and global interdisciplinary paradigms is the use of typologies, often based upon assumed contrasts widely acknowledged in the classic paradigm. In the classic paradigm, sudden change was contrasted with gradual change, and associated with this distinction were other contrasts (such as passive vs. active and emotional vs. intellectual). The three paradigms are contrasted in Table 8.1. It is noteworthy that all these contrasts were noted by early investigators (Starbuck, 1899), as well as emphasized by later investigators (Richardson, 1985b; Granqvist, 1998; Gooren, 2007).

The classic paradigm acknowledged a series of contrasts between sudden and gradual conversion, although empirical research was focused upon the more dramatic case of sudden religious conversion. Perhaps it was this narrowed focus in the empirical literature that allowed the social-scientific paradigm to emerge. In addition, the emergence of new religious movements and their obvious appeal to converts altered that typical pattern of research, almost by definition. Thus intensification experiences within traditions that focused upon intrapsychological processes (studied by psychologists) gave way to conversion to new religious movements focused upon interpersonal processes (studied by sociologists and social psychologists). This in turn has given way to placing conversion within a broad historical perspective, in which a focus is upon the way in which complex motivations are expressed in narratives that are both embodied and diverse (Rambo & Fahadian, 2014a). Thus, as several

TABLE 8.1. Conversion: The Classic, Social-Scientific, and Interdisciplinary Global Paradigms Compared

Classic paradigm	Social-scientific paradigm	Interdisciplinary global paradigm
Sudden change	Gradual change	Continual change
Middle to late adolescence	Late adolescence to early adulthood	Placed in historical context
Emotional, suggestive motivations	Intellectual, rational motivations	Complex motivations
Stern theology	Compassionate theology	Emphasis on embodiment
Passive process	Active process	Active process
Release from sin and guilt	Search for meaning and purpose	Diverse conversion careers
Emphasis on intraindividual psychological processes	Emphasis on interpersonal psychological processes	Emphasis on narrative analyses

investigators have noted, the distinction between sudden and gradual religious conversion is partly due to the fact that temporality is confounded with two different definitions of "conversion"—one that we define as "religious conversion" (or simply "conversion"), and the other that we define as "spiritual transformation" (Granqvist, 1998, 2003; Paloutzian, 2005; Zinnbauer & Pargament, 1998). The focus on sudden religious conversion has reemerged within the global perspective in contemporary studies of converts to groups that endorse terrorist tactics, and of converts whose conversion is facilitated by the Internet and social media (there is considerable overlap between these types of converts; see Chapter 9).

Spiritual transformation is different from intensification experiences within a religious tradition that typify the psychological conversion paradigm. Spiritual transformation is associated with many of the new religious movements, as well as with deconversion from mainstream religious traditions (Hood, 2003; Streib et al., 2009; Streib & Hood, 2016), and is freed from the classic Protestant conversion model that dominated the early study of religious conversion as described above.

It is readily apparent, however, that Richardson's claim to primacy for the social-scientific paradigm ironically meshes quite closely with earlier psychological research on spiritual transformation. Perhaps appropriate is the fact that the Lofland and Stark (1965) model, seen by Richardson (1985b) as transitional between the classic and social-scientific paradigms, is still useful insofar as it permits identification of both predisposing psychological factors (typically studied in religious conversion) and situational and contextual factors (typically studied in spiritual transformation). This model is based upon Lofland's (1977) provocative research in what was then only a minor new religion. He was one of the earliest investigators to study the Unification Church (popularly known as the "Moonies"), at a time when it was a minor cult and had not yet gained prominence on the world scene. As discussed in Chapter 9, research on the Unification Church, like research on many religious cults, is often dichotomized into psychological and sociological studies. In the former, sudden conversion is associated with denigrating popular metaphors, such as "brainwashing" and "mind control." Yet more sociologically oriented studies of the gradual and voluntary process of conversion to the Unification Church are consistent with empirical findings concerning a variety of new religious movements, and are not compatible with denigrating models of conversion or transformation as pathological (Barker, 1984). Long and Hadden (1983) have argued for a "dual-reality" approach, in which conversion may involve either sudden, emotional processes (associated with intrapsychological processes, which can be denigrated in terms of a "brainwashing" metaphor) or more gradual processes (associated with interpsychological processes). However, we need not assume conversion/transformation to be an either–or process, based upon dichotomies such as sudden–gradual or passive–active.

Conversion (and Transformation) Motifs

Among those studying conversion to new religious movements or spiritual transformation, the emphasis upon gradual processes has suggested a variety of empirical phenomena operating over time. Several investigators have attempted more diversified classifications of conversion types, identifying various possible "conversion careers" (Richardson, 1978b). It is undoubtedly true that personal accounts of conversions often reflect biases elicited by investigators who rely upon interviews and observation after the fact to assess which factors are operating, as Beckford (1978) has noted. Classifications of conversion that rely upon psychological dispositions and intrapsychological processes ought not to be simply opposed to those that rely upon social contexts and interpsychological processes. The union of both is needed.

One classification system admirably linking the classic and social-scientific models, the psychological and the sociological, is that of Lofland and Skonovd (1981). These scholars coined the concept "conversion motif" to take account of the "phenomenological validity" of "holistic subjective conversion experience" (p. 374). They have postulated six conversion motifs, and five major dimensions that apply to each motif. These are presented in Table 8.2.

The Lofland and Skonovd typology allows for variations in conversion without forcing arbitrary dichotomies. It permits a distinction among basic objective phenomena, identified along the five dimensions; it also respects the subjective account of conversion by the

TABLE 8.2. The Lofland and Skonovd Conversion Motifs

	Intellectual	Mystical	Experimental	Affectional	Revivalist	Coercive
Degree of social pressure	None or low	None or low	Low	Medium	High	High
Temporal duration	Medium	Short	Long	Long	Short	Short
Level of affective arousal	Medium	High	Low	Medium	High	Low
Affective content	Insight	Awe or love	Curiosity	Affection	Love and fear	Fear and love
Belief–behavior sequence of change	Belief first	Belief first	Behavior first	Behavior first	Behavior first	Behavior first

Note. Adapted from Lofland and Skonovd (1981). Conversion motifs. *Journal of Scientific Study of Religion, 20,* 373–385. Copyright © 1981 the Society for the Scientific Study of Religion. Adapted by permission.

convert. Thus their six conversion motifs provide "phenomenological validity" to the objective factors (dimensions) postulated to be operative in conversion (Lofland & Skonovd, 1981, p. 379). Their motifs are capable of operationalization and empirical study. They also cut across the psychological and sociological concerns that mediate between the classic and social-scientific paradigms of conversion discussed above. For instance, their mystical motif fits the classical Pauline prototype of conversion, emphasizing intrapsychic factors; by contrast, the experimental motif focuses upon the processes by which "seekers" creatively transform themselves, often by interacting with others who model proper converted behavior, as in the social-scientific paradigm (Straus, 1976).

Embedded in the conversion motif typology is the assumption that there are three levels of reality to consider. The first is what Lofland and Skonovd (1981, p. 379) call "raw reality," or the actual truth of conversion, which is only imperfectly available to the social scientist. The second level is the convert's experience and interpretation. The third is the analytic interpretation provided by the social scientist. The change in conversion motifs over time may reflect a change in any one or all of these levels of reality. Obvious examples are the clearly historical contingency of coercive motifs (discussed in detail in Chapter 9) and the revivalist motif (now less common among nonevangelical forms of Protestantism).

The processes of conversion within each motif need to be empirically researched. Once again, psychological and sociological social psychologists actually parallel one another in their analyses. For instance, whereas sociological social psychologists tend to focus on accounts (Beckford, 1978; Snow & Machalek, 1983), a parallel literature exists among psychological social psychologists in terms of attributions (Spilka & McIntosh, 1995; Spilka, Shaver, & Kirkpatrick, 1985). To a large extent, various conversion motifs exist because of the linguistic frameworks within which conversion is understood. These include biographical reconstructions, the adaptation of master attribution schemes, and various rhetorical indications that one has indeed been converted. Mafra (2000) has even argued that conversion can be treated as a narrative genre in its own right.

Much of the sociological literature on the process of conversion emphasizes how people behave in such a way that they essentially "convert themselves." Whereas classic conversion research focused upon what happens to passive converts, the contemporary research focuses upon what converts actively do to produce their conversions. For instance, Balch (1980) has emphasized how individuals must learn to act like converts by performing particular role-prescribed behaviors expected of people who have been converted. Thus behavior change occurs before an individual internalizes beliefs and perceptions characteristic of a convert. Perhaps actual perceptual changes require a reconditioning of habitual patterns of perception, aptly captured by Deikman's (1966) notion of "deautomatization." However, it is only after participating in activities associated with new religious groups that such alterations in perceptions can occur. Thus behavior change precedes belief change. Several investigators have documented this via participation research with new religious groups. For instance, Wilson (1982) has demonstrated such a process with converts to a yoga ashram, and Preston (1981, 1982) has demonstrated this same tendency among converts becoming Zen practitioners.

In terms of empirical assessment, it is important to note that the use of either behavior change or belief change as an indicator of conversion will determine at what point conversion occurs (if at all). The two types of change need not occur at the same time. In addition, the temporal duration of conversion may be different for belief change and behavior change, even within a single conversion process. An individual may gradually be socialized into a new religious group and at some point suddenly experience a deautomatization, resulting in new perceptions congruent with the group's world view. This is apparently particularly true of some Eastern traditions that emphasize practice over belief, such as Zen and yoga (Preston, 1981, 1982; Wilson, 1982; Volinn, 1985). In this sense, a person may not be able to actively pursue deautomatization as a goal; it is a product of successful socialization into religious groups, and becomes possible once proper techniques and practices are mastered (Balch, 1980; Deikman, 1966). Much of the research literature has reintroduced classic cognitive dissonance theory (Festinger, 1957; see below) to provide theoretical justification for a sequence of behavior change → belief change. The focus has been upon maintenance of conversion within groups when prophecy appears to fail.

Finally, the distinction we have made between conversion and spiritual transformation is associated with distinctions firmly rooted in mainstream social science. To cite but one example, Granqvist (2003) has noted that conversion is likely to be associated with previously insecure attachment in those for whom conversion is a compensation and effective means of controlling distress, and is likely to occur suddenly. On the other hand, spiritual transformation is associated with those with continual secure attachment and is more involved with socialization processes and the quest for meaning.

Support for both conversion and spiritual transformation is provided by the National Spirituality Transformation Study (NSTS; Smith, 2006). With funding from Metanexus and support from the University of Pennsylvania, three items were added to a random half of the 2004 General Social Survey (GSS). The NSTS used a full-probability sample of 1,328 adults living in American households. The personal interviews conducted with these adults included qualitative explorations of the triggers and consequences of experiences of spiritual transformation. The percentages of reported experiences agreed well with similar reports of mystical experiences (discussed in Chapter 11). However, with respect to conversion and spiritual transformation, several points can be emphasized. First, of three questions asked, two focused upon conversion. One focused upon "born-again" experiences common to Protestant fundamentalists and evangelicals, and its constant response rate mirrored the percentage of persons identifying themselves as evangelicals in America. Question 1 referred to an intensification experience, and focused upon renewed commitment to one's religion. Only Question 2 referred to change that could pertain to spiritual transformation, but unfortunately the wording of the question confounded spirituality with religion. This, we suspect, may have been responsible for the decline in positive responses to this question over the years: There was a 10-point decline from 1991 to 2004, which we suspect could be accounted for by persons who were now likely to be identifying themselves as more spiritual than religious.

The interview data focused upon triggers of the experiences as well as their consequences. Here, consistent with the data on mysticism discussed in Chapter 11, the widest possible nature and types of triggers were cited. However, relative to the issue of distress, approximately half who indicated that they had had a religious or spiritual experience that changed their lives indicated that a personal crisis had triggered it, while the remaining half indicated that the experience was a result of gradual and routine religious practices. Thus the NSTS data support the distinction between conversion (or intensification) as likely to be sudden and stress-induced, and spiritual transformation as likely to be more gradual and unassociated with distress. This latter point is supported by the fact that experiences perceived to have changed respondents' lives were moderately related to switching religions, even for those interviewees who did not indicate that they changed their religion because of their experience (Smith, 2006, p. 287).

As further support for spiritual transformation being less related to institutional religious involvement than conversion, we can note data from the 1988 GSS as summarized by Streib and his colleagues. Streib et al. (2009, p. 32) note that 64% of the respondents answered "no" to the question "Have you ever had another religious preference?" However, of the 36% who answered "yes," the vast majority had had only one (24%). Fewer than 1% had had four or more previous preferences. Thus conversion and intensification experiences are associated with limited religious exploration.

Streib et al. (2009, p. 36) also provide data from the 2006 GSS results asking persons whether they were "more religious than spiritual," "equally both," "more spiritual than religious," or "neither." Here we simply note that among persons with no religious affiliation, the majority (49%) indicated that they were "more spiritual than religious." Within religious groups, the percentages of believers responding that they were more spiritual than religious were equal for the Protestants and Catholics (both 22%) and higher for Jews (30%). Yet we suggest that these data overall are most consistent with the move from conversion and intensification experiences to spiritual transformation that largely is focused outside institutional religion. This is also consistent with our discussion of the emergence of mystics outside the church (see Chapter 11).

Maintenance of Conversion When Prophecy Appears to Fail

One theory that has had considerable influence in the study of conversion is the theory of cognitive dissonance, first proposed by Festinger (1957). Basic to his theory is the notion that cognitions more or less map reality. Hence there is pressure for individual beliefs to be congruent with reality—whether physical, psychological, or sociological (Festinger, 1957, pp. 10–11). This has led some researchers to puzzle over how individuals can maintain membership in religious groups when prophecy fails. Indeed, the classic study by Festinger and his colleagues was titled *When Prophecy Fails* (Festinger, Riecken, & Schachter, 1956). This participant observation study of a group that believed in flying saucers and predicted the end of the world began a series of participant observation studies of religious groups whose success in maintaining converts is paradoxically linked to failed prophecies. Part of the appeal of Festinger's theory is undoubtedly due to its counterintuitive claim—that prophecies proven to be incorrect result both in maintenance of conversion and in efforts to convert others. How is this possible?

Central to Festinger's theory is that cognitions can be dissonant. Dissonance exists if the obverse of one belief follows from the other. When this is the case, the believer is motivated to reduce this dissonance. However, since the dissonance of two cognitions is defined by psychological as well as logical means, Festinger's theory has undergone a series of modifications as investigators have continued to study religious groups and what perhaps are only apparent prophetic failures. As in much of the literature on conversion, the more psychologically oriented and the more sociologically oriented social-psychological studies yield different results.

Psychologically Oriented Social-Psychological Studies of Failed Prophecy

Festinger et al. (1956) infiltrated a religious group in which a housewife began experiencing automatic writing that revealed to her the coming end of the world. Included in this prophetic claim was that superior beings would come in flying saucers and save those who, like this housewife, believed in them. Festinger and his colleagues infiltrated this group and, as participant observers, sought to test their own prophecy—namely, that when this group's prophecy of the world's destruction failed, the group would both continue in its beliefs and attempt even greater proselytization. Simply put, in Festinger's theory of cognitive dissonance, proselytization increases when prophecy fails. Why?

Festinger's theory requires five basic conditions: First, the belief must be sincere and held with one's "whole heart"; second, and closely related, the person must be committed to this belief; third, he or she must actually take "irrevocable action" based upon it; fourth, the individual must be presented with "unequivocal and undeniable" evidence that the belief is wrong; and, finally, there must be social support subsequent to disconfirmation (Festinger et al., 1956).

Festinger's theory seems straightforward enough and is uniquely relevant to religious groups for two basic reasons. First, religious groups do seem to make predictions and assert beliefs that from other perspectives seem disconfirmed. This is especially the case when clear prophecies are made that do not come true. Second, Festinger sidetracked the issue of pathology by noting that the beliefs are shared among individuals: There is social support. In Festinger et al.'s (1956) classic study, the predicted date came and passed, apparently falsifying the prophecy. Nevertheless, Festinger and colleagues claimed that the group did not disband because of the failed prophecy, but continued—renewed in its faith commitment, and passionate in its efforts to convince others of the truth of its beliefs. Although this has been widely reported by psychologists as a positive test of Festinger's theory, we shall shortly note that more sociologically oriented social psychologists have criticized this claim.

Festinger's claim to have identified the consequences of failed prophecy has been applied to many historical examples of failed prophecy, such as the Montanists, the Millerites, and even Christianity itself. For instance, it is claimed that the 2nd-century failure of Montanus to predict the return of Jesus led to renewed commitment and the success of the Montanists (Hughes, 1954). Similarly, William Miller's mid-19th-century prediction of the end of the world never materialized, and yet the Millerites prospered as a consequence (so we are led to believe) of their failed prophecy (Sears, 1924). Perhaps most dramatic is the interpretation that Christianity itself succeeded largely because of the failed prediction of Christ's second coming (Wernik, 1975). Although Festinger and his colleagues were careful only to suggest that historical examples of failed prophecy can be explained by cognitive dissonance, specific historical studies of the prophetic traditions of the Bible have considerably modified their claims—particularly their claim to have objectively identified actual failed prophecies (Carroll, 1979). However, psychologically oriented social psychologists continue to interpret dissonant beliefs objectively, offering even quasi-experimental support for Festinger's basic theory (see, e.g., Batson, Schoenrade, & Ventis, 1993, pp. 210–216). Thus psychologically oriented social psychologists have tended to see in Festinger's theory a classic model of theory construction that has allowed specific empirical tests, which are viewed as largely supportive of the theory. However, sociologically oriented social psychologists have argued quite the opposite.

Sociologically Oriented Social-Psychological Studies of Failed Prophecy

Sociologically oriented social psychologists have found major flaws in cognitive-dissonance-based interpretations of failed prophecy. First, Festinger et al.'s (1956) classic study has been faulted on methodological grounds. Bainbridge (1997) has noted that often almost one-third of the members were participant observers, and that the group members were continually badgered by the press to account for their commitment. Thus the increased proselytizing and affirmations of faith may have been influenced by media pressure. Others have noted that Festinger's interpretation of historical cases in the light of dissonance theory is flawed. For instance, Melton (1985) has argued that the Millerites were not simply focused upon prophecy and did not disband in the manner Festinger claimed in order to provide support for his theory. Melton (1985, p. 20) further notes that "within religious groups prophecy seldom fails." Likewsie, Van Fossen (1988) has noted that the continual citation of Festinger et al.'s (1956) classic study provides a deficient guide to the study of prophetic groups. Bader (1999, p. 120), after critically reviewing his own and Festinger et al.'s study, concludes: "Nevertheless[,] no study of a failed prophecy, the current research included, has provided support for the cognitive dissonance hypothesis."

How can psychologically and sociologically oriented social psychologists have such different evaluations of dissonance theory? The answer is largely methodological. Psychologically oriented social psychologists tend to take an outsider's perspective—as if they could identify dissonant beliefs by more objective criteria, or could identify "unequivocal and undeniable disconfirmation of a prophecy" (Festinger et al., 1956, p. 3). Yet as Coyle (2001, p. 150) notes, the term "religious gap" has become common with reference to the difference between mental health professionals and the general population in regard to religious beliefs. Table 8.3 shows the nature of this gap.

The religious gap hypothesis is relevant when it is recognized that researchers tend to describe for themselves when beliefs are dissonant or when prophecy has failed. This is crucial, since Festinger's theory requires that beliefs must be *proven* false—in his group's own words, that the disconfirmation must be "unequivocal and undeniable." However, as Carroll (1979) noted when applying cognitive dissonance theory to Biblical prophecy, there are no simple objective criteria by which one can identify failed prophecy. What outsiders (especially researchers!) see as failed prophecy is seldom seen that way by insiders. Tumminia (1998, p. 165) notes that "what appears to be seemingly irrefutable evidence of irreconcilable contradictions to outsiders, like Festinger, can instead be evidence of the truth of prophecy to insiders." Carroll (1979) observes that among the faithful, there is a transcendental dimension to prophecy, securing it from failure. Sociologically oriented social psychologists have noted

TABLE 8.3. Religious Gap between Mental Health Professionals and the General Population

Group	Religious	Nonreligious
General population	72%	19%
Family therapists	62%	15%
Social workers	46%	19%
Psychiatrists	39%	24%
Psychologists	33%	31%

Note. Religious respondents endorsed the statement "My whole approach to life is based upon my religion." Nonreligious respondents identified themselves as atheist, agnostic, humanistic, or otherwise nonreligious. Data from Coyle (2001, p. 150).

this as well, recognizing that failed prophecy entails hermeneutical considerations that make claims to "unequivocal and undeniable" falsification problematic.

Sociologically oriented social psychologists have tended to take an insider's perspective and to focus upon interpersonal processes that maintain a socially constructed reality incapable of any simply falsification. "Failed prophecy" is thus a negotiated term and depends upon negotiated claims to reality (Berger & Luckmann, 1967; Carroll, 1979; Pollner, 1987). Furthermore, among prophetic groups, prophecy is less central than outsiders assume. The exclusive focus upon prophecy leads outsiders to assume that the major concern of the group is prophecy; it ignores the complex cosmology that serves to integrate the group (Melton, 1985). Participant observation studies of prophetic groups have begun to show how rare increased proselytization is as a reaction to what is only apparently failed prophecy (Stone, 2000). Zygmunt (1972, p. 245) defines "prophecy" as a prediction that a "drastic transformation of the existing social order will occur in the proximate future through the intervention of some supernatural agency." The recognition of the transformation is socially constructed, and hence it cannot be unequivocally or undeniably disconfirmed. Thus, from the insider's perspective, prophecy cannot fail.

The denial of failure of prophecy is the most common response from within prophetic groups, as members struggle to stay within the group and to seek a proper interpretation of what must be only an apparent failure (Carroll, 1979; Dein, 1997, 2001; Melton, 1985; Tumminia, 1998). Again, increased proselytization is actually an uncommon response to failed prophecy (Stone, 2000). As Dein (2001) notes, dissonance theory is utilized too often to persuade others that those who stay within prophetic groups are irrational and driven by forces they do not understand. Such claims are possible only when researchers assume an objectivist stance and can claim that in fact prophecy has failed. However, researchers who adopt the perspective of the insider avoid committing what James (1890/1950) identified as the "psychological fallacy"—assuming that others must experience the world as psychologists do. The task is to understand how believers confront a more spiritual understanding of prophecy, rather than a simple literal understanding of its "failure" (Carroll, 1979; Dein, 2001). For instance, Dawson (1999) notes that increased proselytization is only one way to decrease dissonance, and that it is not at all a common way in the face of failed prophecy. More common than increased proselytization is the denial of failed prophecy (Zygmunt, 1972). This can take the form of "spiritualization"—a reinterpretation of the prophecy so that it has been fulfilled. For example, Bainbridge (1997) notes that when Charles Taze Russell of the Jehovah's Witnesses apparently failed to predict Christ's return in 1874, he argued that Christ had indeed returned invisibly. Likewise, Tumminia (1998) studied the Unarius Academy of Science in El Cajon, California, over a period of 5 years (1988–1993). Failed prophecies were reinterpreted in terms of past lives and reincarnation, thus allowing denial of the failure of prophecy in terms of experiencing its fulfillment in a more spiritual sense. Both historical and more recent participant observation studies of diverse prophetic groups—such as the Baha'i sect (Balch, Farnsworth, & Wilkins, 1983), a Mormon sect called the Morrisites (Halford, Anderson, & Clark, 1981), and the contemporary Lubavitcher Hasidic movement (Dein, 2001)—reveal that members continue to struggle with their beliefs and membership within groups, sometimes become disillusioned, and occasionally leave groups. However, they always rationally struggle with the meaning of prophecies that become not simply false, but problematic.

One common interpretation is that failed prophecies are tests of faith (Hardyck & Braden, 1962; Tumminia, 1998). Again, however, the struggle is always rational and meaningful from an insider's perspective. As Dein (2001, p. 399) notes, individuals within a prophetic religious group "are not a group of fanatics who follow doctrine without question. They are sane people trying to reason their way through facts and doctrine in the pursuit of understanding." Finally, as Bader (1999) has noted, the theoretical task is to propose testable hypotheses that not only clarify under what conditions failed prophecy will have specific effects, but also specify which members will leave a group if they perceive prophecy to have failed. Research Box 8.3 presents the results of a contemporary study of a religious group, Lubavitcher Hasidism, in which the complexities of apparently failed prophecy are explored in the tradition of Festinger's classic study.

RESEARCH BOX 8.3. What Really Happens When Prophecy Fails? (Dein, 2001)

Simon Dein, a nonreligious Jew, lived in the Stamford Hill Lubavitcher Hasidic community in England over a 3-year period (1992–1995). While working part-time as a physician, he studied the ways in which Lubavitchers dealt with illness. Beginning in 1993, intense messianic fervor emerged in the community. Dein interviewed 30 Lubavitchers (24 were males, and the majority of these were rabbis).

The Lubavitcher movement is a worldwide movement of Hasidic Jews who emphasize feelings over intellect and emphasize that one's thoughts should be continually upon God. They believe that their spiritual leader (*zaddik* or *rebbe*) is a perfectly righteous man. In accordance with traditional Jewish teachings, Lubavitchers believe that in each generation there is a potential messiah (*moshiach*). However, although each *zaddik* is a potential messiah, the *zaddik* himself may not realize this potential because the generation is unworthy of him.

Rebbe Menachem Mendel Schneerson became the leader of Lubavitcher Hasidism in 1951. He has been described by Lubavitchers as the "most phenomenal Jewish personality of our time" (quoted in Dein, 2001, p. 390). He became an intense focus of the Lubavitchers, many of whom suggested that he was the messiah. Rebbe Schneerson (or simply "the Rebbe," as he was called) did little to diminish this expectation. For instance, in April 1991 he stated, "Moshiach's coming is no longer a dream of a distant future, but an imminent reality which will very shortly become manifest" (quoted in Dein, 2001, p. 391).

The Rebbe's statements had profound effects on the Stamford Hill Lubavitchers. A "Moshiach Awareness" caravan that toured Britain was held; public discussions were held on messianic issues; and, while never publicly identifying the Rebbe as the messiah, many Lubavitchers privately acknowledged that he was. Others expressed doubt. As one Lubavitcher told Dein, "The Rebbe may be Moshiach, but I am unsure. I hope he is" (p. 393). The Rebbe died on June 12, 1994, having been comatose after a stroke and on a respirator since March 1994. His death was widely reported in the news media. After his death, several themes arose among the Lubavitchers. Many believed that he would be resurrected. Others emphasized his continual spiritual presence in the world. All continued to hope and pray for the messianic arrival. Lubavitchers began to visit the Rebbe's tomb, and miracle stories continue about people who have visited his grave. Some Lubavitchers noted that although the Rebbe was a potential messiah, the generation did not possess enough merit to warrant his coming. Others simply admitted that they had been wrong— that only God knows when the messiah will come. Dein notes that the Lubavitchers have adapted an apparently failed prophecy in complex ways that have not only preserved, but enhanced, their commitment to messianic prophecy.

PROCESSES INVOLVED IN CONVERSION AND SPIRITUAL TRANSFORMATION

Social-scientific research has been guided by a focus upon gradual conversion to new religious movements and to spiritual transformation outside of religious institutions. In addition to typologies, numerous investigators have presented models of the process of conversion or transformation. Some are formal in scope and propositional in nature (Gartrell & Shannon, 1985). The majority are qualitative models that have been inductively arrived at and used to organize the empirical literature (Kwilecki, 1999; Lofland & Stark, 1965; Rambo, 1993); it is not clear that such models can be easily submitted to empirical tests capable of falsifying them (Kilbourne & Richardson, 1989; Kuhn, 1962; Masterman, 1970; Richardson, 1985b). Most models share a recognition that conversion and spiritual transformation involve complex processes in which a variety of factors must be considered. In general terms, we can identify these factors under four headings: context; precipitating events; supporting activities; and finally participation/commitment. This is obviously an area in which the social-scientific paradigm needs to be embraced, especially in terms of interdisciplinary cooperation utilizing longitudinal methods.

Context

Conversion and spiritual transformation always take place within a context. The term "context" is broad and vague enough to incorporate historical, social, cultural, and interpersonal situations that make conversion or transformation possible. For instance, Wallace (1956) noted that historical figures such as Jesus, Muhammad, and Buddha have become foci of revitalization movements. Within varieties of North American Protestantism, we have already seen how Paul's conversion has served as a prototype for a model of transformation that permits the expected "born-again" experience associated with conversion or intensification experiences. Yet the cautionary note that this is only one model of conversion/transformation is now well substantiated by empirical research. Research Box 8.4 presents a study of

---

RESEARCH BOX 8.4. An Empirical Study of Conversion to Islam (Poston, 1992)

Poston attempted to obtain questionnaire responses from 20 Muslim organizations. Only 8 of these 20 responded at all, and from these 8, only 12 completed questionnaires were obtained. Poston notes that this is typical of Muslims (at least in North America), who are suspicious of research into their beliefs and practices. By contrast, Christians and members of many new religious movements in North America readily cooperate in completing questionnaires on reports of their conversion experiences.

Reverting to reports of conversion experience in Islamic publications, Poston was able to obtain 72 testimonies of conversion, 69% of which were from males. Classifying these testimonies, Poston found that most converts (57%) had been raised as Christians. Only 3 of the 72 converts reported an emotional, Pauline-type conversion in which supernatural factors were perceived to account for the conversion. All but one of the converts were seekers who sought out a variety of religious options before becoming converted to Islam, with 21% stating the reasonableness of the faith as the motive for conversion, and 19% giving the universal brotherhood of all as the reason.

conversion within Islam, in which emotional, Pauline-type experiences are neither modeled by the religion nor typically reported by converts. Clearly, the context of Islamic culture does not facilitate such experience.

Included among the contextual factors facilitating religious conversion are purely social and cultural phenomena that alter the probability of conversion. For instance, Bulliet (1979) has argued from a historical perspective that conversion to new religions follows the typical S-curve established to characterize diffusion of innovation in cultures. Psychologists will readily recognize the S-curve as a summated normal "bell curve." What is important for studies of conversion is Bulliet's classification of those who converted at various points in history along the curve. Using the history of Islam as his example, he described the first 16% who converted as the "innovators" (2.5%) and "early adopters" (13.5%). Then came the 34% constituting the "early majority," followed by the next 34%, the "late majority." Finally, the remaining 16% who converted were described as the "laggards" (Bulliet, 1979, pp. 31–32). Figure 8.1 illustrates Bulliet's classification curve.

Bulliet's theory has been operationalized and tested for the historical dominance of Islam in various cultures, but this model could be empirically tested within other historical contexts as well. What is important is the fact that the social-psychological processes of conversion may vary, depending upon the historical moment at which one converts to a religion and its dominance at that time in the culture. The kinds of persons and the processes by which they convert to new religious movements may vary as such movements gain ascendancy within the culture. Bulliet's historical perspective can be linked to other models of conversion, particularly those sensitive to the varieties of conversion motifs. Research Box 8.5 presents a study of British converts to Islam, interpreted in terms of the conversion motifs of Lofland and Skonovd (1981).

Precipitating Events

The effort to dichotomize theories of conversion/transformation often focuses upon whether or not precipitating events can be identified, and if so, within what time frame they operate. We have seen how proponents of sudden conversions often cite crises or emotional events as

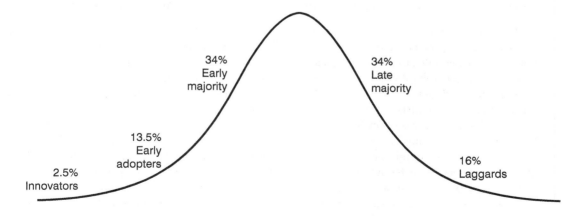

FIGURE 8.1. A bell curve model of conversion types based upon time of conversion relative to percentage of population converted. Data from Bulliet (1979, pp. 31–33).

RESEARCH BOX 8.5. Conversion Motifs among British Converts to Islam
(Köse & Loewenthal, 2000)

Köse and Loewenthal studied 70 contemporary British converts to Islam. Köse, a male Muslim, interviewed each convert; both he and a female psychologist then independently rated the interviews in terms of the six conversion motifs of Lofland and Skonovd (1981). Their results are summarized in the following table.

Motif[a]	Males	Females	Factors significantly associated with conversion motif
Intellectual	38	12	Cognitive concerns before conversion
Mystical	9	1	Sufism; new religious movements
Experimental	28	14	None
Affectional	28	18	Sufism; marriage; being female
Revivalist	0	0	(Not applicable)
Coercive	3	0	None

[a]Motifs are not mutually exclusive; actual numbers, not percentages, are reported in this table. These investigators note that the conversion motifs of Lofland and Skonovd (1981) allow for a shorthand representation of complex religious autobiographies that permits them to be linked to normative features of conversion. They also note that the antecedents of conversion vary with conversion motifs. It is also noteworthy that revivalist conversion, which is associated with the classical paradigm largely derived from Christianity, does not apply at all to converts to Islam.

the turning point. Yet as Rambo (1993) has noted, crises can vary in length, scope, and duration. Proponents of gradual conversion/transformation emphasize interpersonal processes and the active seeking of meaning and purpose over a longer time interval as key factors (Gerlach & Hine, 1970).

The use of the conversion/transformation motifs discussed earlier allows for many variations, compatible with the existing empirical literature. There are many pathways to conversion and transformation, varying in length, scope, and nature (Heirich, 1977). For instance, crisis-precipitated conversions, including the affective and coercive motifs, vary widely among themselves in terms of duration, intensity, and scope (Straus, 1979). Furthermore, a crisis may be intrapsychic or interpsychic; the former often refers to some variety of personal stress, the latter to some variety of social strain (Seggar & Kunz, 1972). Likewise, actively seeking meaning and purpose (as in the experimental and intellectual motifs) varies in the range and nature of meaning sought, as well as in the motivation for seeking such meanings (Rambo, 1993). It may be, as Gerlach and Hine (1970) have shown, that some individuals gradually employ new systems of rhetoric that allow them to see themselves and the world transformed. Similarly, in a study that employed a comparison group to look at differences among Catholic Pentecostals, Heirich (1977) found that converts were most likely to be persons introduced to the group by friends or spiritual advisors who facilitated the gradual use of new religious attributions in the process of conversion. Nonconverts were not introduced to the group by friends or spiritual advisors and failed to acquire the appropriate language (attributions or rhetoric) of conversion. Thus mundane and even chance factors can precipitate conversion (Gooren, 2007, p. 351). Straus (1979) has documented how several converts to Scientology managed to seek and find beliefs, and to enter groups that allowed them to convert themselves by "creative bumbling."

Thus no one process of conversion applies to all conversion motifs. Generalizations concerning the conversion process are highly suspect if proffered as other than hypotheses for empirical investigation. Furthermore, it is not clear how the nature of the religious group to which a person has converted interacts with whatever general conversion processes have been empirically proposed. For instance, Seggar and Kunz (1972) found that one widely cited process model of religious conversion accounted for only 1 of the 77 cases of conversion to Mormonism in their study. Likewise, compensatory models of religious conversion must be tempered by the empirical assessment of the consequences of conversion, which are typically positive (Richardson, 1995). This is the case even when the conversion is to religious groups that remain marginal to the larger culture. Research Box 8.6 reports a study evaluating the legitimacy of conversion based upon the factors that precipitated conversion.

Ullman (1982) made empirical comparisons of conversion processes across different religious groups. Emotional factors, rather than cognitive factors, differentiated converts to all four religious groups from nonconverts. This was not a direct test of the relative contribution of cognitive and emotional factors in conversion, given that all converts were selected according to criteria that included actual changes in religious identity but excluded such changes when they were made for interpersonal reasons, such as marrying a spouse in the new faith. We have already noted the role of interpersonal factors in some conversion motifs, especially

---

RESEARCH BOX 8.6. Evaluating the Legitimacy of Conversion Based upon the Five Signs in Mark 16:17–18 (Hood, Williamson, & Morris, 1999)

Judgments regarding the legitimacy of conversion experiences can be expected to be based either upon prejudice or upon reasoned, rational rejection of certain practices. The serpent-handling sects of Appalachia practice all five signs specified in Mark 16:17–18— casting out demons, laying hands upon the sick, speaking in tongues, handing serpents, and drinking poison. A sample of 453 undergraduate psychology students was asked to evaluate the legitimacy of individuals' hypothetical conversion experiences, in terms of each of the five signs. As anticipated, results indicated that both prejudiced and rational rejection of conversion was associated with the two most extreme signs—serpent handling and drinking poison. Prejudiced rejection included stereotyping, negative affect, and specific behavioral intentions to avoid associating with converts.

However, when the effects of rational rejection were controlled for, there remained a strong relationship between prejudice and the evaluation of the legitimacy of conversion, including stereotyping. Conversion based upon serpent handling and drinking poison was still less accepted than conversion based upon casting out of demons, speaking in tongues or the laying of hands upon the sick. The relevance of separating prejudice from rational rejection is important, given the legal repercussions for serpent-handling sects in many states. It may be the case that even reasoned disagreement with serpent-handling sects masks an underlying prejudice, especially since knowledge of this tradition is largely available only from stereotyped presentations of these sects in the mass media.

RESEARCH BOX 8.7. Emotional versus Cognitive Factors
in Precipitating Conversion (Ullman, 1982)

Ullman studied 40 white, middle-class individuals raised as Jews and Christians, who had converted from 1 to 10 months previous to the study. Half the converts were male and half female. They were compared on the basis of both objective measures and in-depth interviews to each other and to 30 controls (nonconverted subjects). All converts actually changed religious denomination. The four converted groups consisted of 10 subjects each, who were now Orthodox Jews, Roman Catholics, Hare Krishnas, and Baha'i adherents. The major differences between converted and nonconverted groups were on emotional, not cognitive, indices. Among the major significant differences between all converts and the control group were a greater frequency of both childhood and adolescent stress, as well as a greater frequency of prior drug use and psychiatric problems, among the converted subjects. Converts recalled childhoods that were less happy and filled with more anguish than those of nonconverts. The emotions recalled for adolescence followed the childhood patterns, with the addition of significant anger and fear in adolescence for the converts but not the nonconverts. Converts also differed from nonconverts in having less love and admiration for their fathers, and more indifference and anger toward them. Differences among the converted groups were less relevant than the consistency across all converted groups, suggesting that similar processes operated regardless of the faith to which a subject converted.

---

those unlikely to be precipitated by crises or emotional factors. In addition, all four of Ullman's groups cultivated intense emotional experiences, perhaps biasing the sample toward an affective conversion motif. Still, Ullman's study is one of the few empirical studies that have used appropriate measurement procedures to compare converts to a variety of religious groups with matched controls. Some highlights of this research are presented in Research Box 8.7.

Supporting Activities

The classification of conversion motifs is helpful in directing research into factors in the conversion process that have long been ignored. Among these are interpersonal relationships between a potential convert and what Rambo (1993) refers to as the "advocate." The advocate is often a friend who initiates and sustains the potential convert in the group. Sometimes simple factors (such as marriage) convert one partner. Much of the literature has documented the importance of social networks in facilitating conversion, especially among noncommunal religions. For instance, Snow and Machalek (1984, p. 182) found that the vast majority (59–82%) of Pentecostals, evangelicals, and Nichiren Shoshu Buddhists that they studied were recruited through social networks.

Much of the research has focused upon how social networks may facilitate gradual emotional conversions by the mere fact that intensive interaction among group members increases the likelihood of affective bonding among the members (Galanter, 1980; Snow, Zurcher, & Ekland-Olson, 1980, 1983; Stark & Bainbridge, 1980a; Straus, 1979). Jacobs (1987, 1989) has reintroduced the analogy of conversion and falling in love into the contemporary literature on conversion to groups with charismatic leaders. William James (1902/1985) used the same analogy, as did Pratt (1920), who went so far as to state that "In many cases getting converted means falling in love with Jesus" (p. 160). Cartwright and Kent (1992) have noted that new religious movements provide alternative pathways to intimacy and love within a familial perspective.

More psychologically oriented social psychologists have also focused on affective bonding, operationalized more rigorously in terms of attachment theory (discussed in Chapters 3 and 4). Individuals with the less secure types of attachment may exhibit higher rates of sudden conversions in adolescence or adulthood, regardless of the religiosity of their parents (Kirkpatrick, 1992, 1995; Kirkpatrick & Shaver, 1990). Kirkpatrick (1997) has provided one of the few longitudinal studies of this issue, in which he demonstrated that women readers of a Midwest newspaper surveyed approximately 4 years apart were more likely to report a changed relationship to God at the second assessment if they had insecure rather than secure attachment styles. Women with insecure-anxious attachments were most likely to report a conversion experience within this 4-year period. Granqvist (2002a) has suggested that the attachment literature can clarify some of the relationships between gradual conversion (or the social-scientific paradigm) and sudden conversion (or the classic paradigm). Secure attachment leads to the gradual acceptance of the religiosity or nonreligiosity of parents. When there are religious changes, they are likely to be gradual and associated with loving and intimate God images. However, among persons with the insecure attachment types, the influence of parental religiosity is minimal. Religious changes are likely to be sudden and associated with a distant and unloving image of God. In these types, the image of God serves as a compensatory attachment figure. Thus much of the attachment literature parallels the sociological literature of relationships. Once again, the literatures of sociological and psychological social psychology have focused upon similar concerns, although unfortunately these are not often cross-referenced. In addition, Beit-Hallahmi and Argyle (1997, p. 120) have noted how the attachment literature "seems to lend clear support to the psychodynamic view of religious conversion."

Thus various theories converge to suggest that religious conversion can be compensatory for psychological deficiencies linked to childhood experiences. For instance, Oksanen's (1994) meta-analysis of 25 studies sampling a total of over 4,500 converts found considerable support for the view that, however interpreted, conversion can be seen as serving a compensatory function for difficulties in interpersonal relationships with significant others (in either adulthood or childhood). However, as the data reviewed earlier suggest, by no means are all conversion experiences compensatory. Furthermore, qualitative studies often suggest correctives to exclusively quantitative research. For instance, Streib (2001b) has used qualitative/biographical research to study both converts and deconverts to new fundamentalist religious movements. He has found "no typical sect biography and no typical set of motivational factors" (p. 235). Furthermore, although childhood trauma and anxiety were identified in fundamentalist biographies, they were found in nonfundamentalist biographies as well (Streib, 2001b). Likewise, Zinnbauer and Pargament (1998) found that persons reporting spiritual conversions were similar to nonconverts who had become more religious. The only difference between the two groups were that spiritual converts reported more postconversion life transformation. Thus psychologists ought to be sensitive to the extent to which qualitative studies may add depth and clarification to purely measurement-based approaches (Streib, 2001a; Zinnbauer & Pargament, 1998). What is clear is that various theoretical and methodological orientations are beginning to converge and to clarify how individual differences in interpersonal styles (whether attachment-based, psychodynamically based, or sociologically based) may affect the conditions under which conversion may be sudden or gradual, and compensatory or not.

Social networks may also function to facilitate more cognitively motivated conversions, by providing interpersonal support for world views associated with what amount to cognitive reformulations of converts' sense of themselves and others. Religious converts not only use more religious attributions, but use those associated with their new group. For instance, Beckford (1978) has demonstrated the process by which Jehovah's Witnesses converts gradually come to cognitively assess the world in light of a master attribution scheme consistent with Jehovah's Witnesses' theology. One rhetorical indicator that conversion is occurring is the utilization of such a master attribution scheme, which both defines and produces conversion. Interacting within a given social network supports the scheme and serves to differentiate the newly emerging convert. It is the new religious attribution scheme that permits a biographical reconstruction of the transformed self. Often such reconstructions are solidified by participation in appropriate rituals confirming one's conversion (Boyer, 1994; Morinis, 1985).

The more sociologically oriented research on rhetorical indicators of conversion meshes nicely with psychologically oriented measurement-based research on cognitive change among converts. For instance, Paloutzian and colleagues have demonstrated an increase in scores on a measure of purpose in life for converts, as compared to nonconverted controls or controls who were unsure they were converted (Paloutzian, 1981; Paloutzian, Jackson, & Crandell, 1978).

Participation/Commitment

It is not likely that conversion as a process can be identified in temporal terms as having been completed once and for all. After conversion, commitment and participation can be expected to vary. It is not uncommon for converts to new religious movements to follow "conversion careers," joining and leaving a variety of religious groups over time (Richardson, 1978b). Bird and Remier (1982) note that only a small percentage of converts to new religious movements remain members of one movement. Furthermore, participation in religious groups is not necessarily higher among converted individuals than among those born and socialized into the groups (Barker & Currie, 1985).

DECONVERSION AND RELATED PHENOMENA

The concept of "conversion careers" makes it clear that for some converts, a variety of conversion experiences can be expected. This especially characterizes converts to new religious movements, the majority of whom can be expected to leave within a few years. "Deconversion" is the term most typically used to identify this process, although Gooren (2010) prefers "disaffiliation." However, empirical investigators believe that whatever term is used, disaffiliation or deconversion entails permanent abandonment of a religious group through processes that constitute more or less a mirror image of conversion (Gooren, 2010; Streib et al., 2009; Streib & Hood, 2016). Given the complexity of conversion as described above, deconversion is no less complex.

Compared to the massive research literature on conversion, few studies of deconversion exist, and the few existing studies are of fairly recent origin. For instance, Wright (1987) could document only three studies of deconversion published prior to 1980. Furthermore, a criticism of deconversion studies is that to a large extent, the deconverts who are empirically studied are like the researchers who study them (Gooren, 2011). This bias must be acknowledged, and caution must be exercised in extrapolating what is known about deconverts from studies conducted in largely Western cultures and heavily biased toward samples of university students to other cultures and samples. As Shweder et al. (2006) remind us, "The Western institution of the university carries with it many features of an elite cosmopolitan culture wherever it has diffused around the world" (p. 722), and hence university students and those researching them are more like one another than like their respective societies.

Not surprisingly, the literature on deconversion parallels that for conversion and spiritual transformation. With the exception of the special case of "brainwashing" discussed in Chapter 9, most studies of deconversion have been conducted by sociologists using participant observation or descriptive research strategies. Assessment is often carried out via interviews, either structured or open-ended, with former members. Most studies of deconversion have focused upon defectors from new religious movements, paralleling the tremendous literature on new religious movements and conversion discussed above. Unlike the literature on apostasy, the deconversion literature focuses upon the processes involved in leaving religious groups, not simply correlates and predictors of leaving. Heinz Streib and his colleagues have begun the cross-cultural study of deconversion in a series of ongoing studies at the University of Bielefeld, Germany (Streib et al., 2009, pp. 43–48). Before we present this group's work, however, we need to explore its roots in the study of new religious movements, largely in the American context.

Deconversion within New Religious Movements

Skonovd (1983) studied former members of fundamentalist Christian groups, as well as of Scientology, the Unification Church, the People's Temple, and various Eastern groups. He identified a process of deconversion consisting of a precipitating crisis, followed by review and reflection, disaffection, withdrawal, and a transition to cognitive reorganization. His model, however, does not distinguish between voluntary and involuntary leaving—an issue of concern, given the debate on deprogramming discussed in Chapter 9.

Wright (1986) studied matched samples of those remaining in and those voluntarily defecting from the Unification Church, Hare Krishna, and a fundamentalist Christian group. He focused upon precipitating factors that initiated the process of deconversion. Among those identified were breakdown of insulation from the outside world, development of unregulated interpersonal relationships, perceived lack of success in achieving social change, and disillusionment. Wright's research parallels conversion research, in that both emotional and cognitive factors can trigger the process of deconversion, and the process itself can be sudden or gradual. Furthermore, he identified different modes of departure, based upon the length of time people had been committed to a group. Most of those who had been members for 1 year or less (92%) left by quiet, covert means. Those who had been members for more than a year left by either overt means or direct confrontations, often emotional and dramatic in nature ("declarative" means).

Downton (1980) has documented the gradual process of deconversion from the Divine Light Mission (the sect associated with Guru Maharaj Ji). Intellectual and social disillusionment predominated. The breaking of bonds within the group occurred only as new bonds were established outside the group. Galanter, Rabkin, Rabkin, and Deutsch (1979) found that converts to the Unification Church who had not completely severed nonsanctioned emotional attachments within the group were likely to deconvert even when they believed in the doctrine of the group.

Jacobs (1989) studied 40 religious devotees, most of whom were involved in either charismatic Christian, Hindu-based, or Buddhist groups. All groups had charismatic leaders, were patriarchal in orientation, and had structured hierarchies with rigid disciplines of behavior and devotion. The 21 male and 19 female participants were predominantly middle-class, white, and well educated. Among the 40 deconverters, both social disillusionment and disillusionment with the charismatic leader were major reasons cited for discontent leading to deconversion, as noted in Table 8.4. Jacobs (1989) notes that the total process of deconversion for these individuals required severing ties both with the group and with the charismatic leader. The total process of deconversion included a period of initial separation, often accompanied by an experience of isolation and loneliness; this was followed by a period of emotional strain and readjustment, culminating in the reestablishment of identity outside the group.

Descriptive studies of deconversion, like those of conversion, run the risk of confounding the natural history of groups with causal processes assumed to operate in them (Snow & Machalek, 1984). Furthermore, investigators tend to avoid measurement in favor of utilizing subjective accounts of deconversion, placed within descriptive systems proposed by the investigators as explanatory. Few tests of these models have been undertaken. Longitudinal research is virtually absent. Finally, no studies have compared individuals who have deconverted from several religious groups to see whether the same process of deconversion occurs each time.

As described briefly in Chapter 5, Altemeyer and Hunsberger (1997) studied 24 "amazing apostates" and "amazing believers." They referred to them as "amazing" because they were selected from extremes in a sample of over 4,000 college students. The amazing

TABLE 8.4. Sources of Disillusionment among 40 Deconverters

Source	%
Disillusionment with a charismatic leader and his actions	
Physical abuse	31
Psychological abuse	60
Emotional rejection	45
Spiritual betrayal	33
Social disillusionment	
Social life	75
Spiritual life	50
Status/position	35
Prescribed sex roles	45

Note. Based on Jacobs (1989, pp. 43, 92).

believers came from nonreligious or religious backgrounds; the amazing apostates came from religious backgrounds and turned to agnosticism or atheism. The apostates had deconverted gradually and, unlike the believers, felt no need to proselytize about their newfound unbelief (Altemeyer & Hunsberger, 1997, p. 232). Hunsberger (2000) characterized the apostates as having succeeded in a hard-won fight for autonomy and personal identity—a finding with remarkable parallels in a study by Davidson and Griel (2007, p. 213) on the exit narratives of ultra-Orthodox Jews who took pride in their courage to leave a tradition into which they had been born. Unlike conversion to fundamentalist groups, deconversion offers no "scripts" that those who deconvert can follow as they struggle to transform themselves outside of clear religious norms. They are part of what Heelas, Woodhead, Steel, Szerszynski, and Trusting (2005) identify as a spiritual revolution where religion is yielding to spirituality.

Streib and Colleagues' Bielefeld Deconversion Project

Heinz Streib and his colleagues have taken the lead at the University of Bielefeld, Germany, in making deconversion a recognized area of research in the social-scientific study of religion. In two complementary studies conducted over a 4-year period with research teams in two countries, Streib and his colleagues used mixed methods to compare deconverts from new religious movements with those who stayed within religious traditions in North America and Germany (Streib et al., 2009). Among the objective measures used were an instrument based on the famous five-factor model of personality (McCrae, 1992), and the Well-Being and Growth Scale developed by Ryff and Singer (1996). Also administered to all participants were independently derived measures of fundamentalism. Qualitative measures included open-ended interviews with in-tradition members, and faith development interviews with all deconverts and a matched sample of in-tradition members from the same group.

The use of mixed methods allowed comparison quantitative and qualitative data to complement one another in illuminating the complex dynamics of deconverting from relatively new (in German culture) religious groups. From the qualitative data, Streib and his colleagues identified four major types of deconversion narratives: (1) "the pursuit of autonomy," primarily motivated by seeking independence, personal freedom, and growth; (2) "debarred from paradise," primarily characterized by an original crisis-precipitated conversion now followed by disillusionment and abandonment; (3) "heroes, survivors, and victims," primarily characterized by a crisis and associated with increased self-reflection; and (4) "finding a new frame of reference," similar to intensification experiences in conversion. Like spiritual transformation, then, deconversion appears to be a process that occurs gradually over time. Deconverts in both Germany and America were characterized by low authoritarianism and an openness to experience that led them to identify themselves as more spiritual than religious.

A provocative summary of the quantitative data reveals cultural differences suggesting that deconversion is a growth-oriented process for Americans, who in this research sought autonomy and personal growth (as indicated by higher subscale scores on the Ryff–Singer measure) in a more open religious "marketplace." However, for Germans, deconversion was associated with lower scores on the Ryff–Singer subscales measuring environmental mastery, personal relations with others, purpose in life, and self-acceptance. The combined results suggest that for Germans, given Germany's more limited religious "marketplace," deconversion may be associated with a more problematic status—indicative, perhaps, of personal crises associated with deconversion. In the United States, given the different religious culture, deconversion may be (as shown in other studies cited above) associated with positively evaluated aspects of personal growth and freedom of religious choice, including identification as spiritual but not religious. These data are consistent with research indicating that authoritarianism is associated with religion but not with spirituality (Wink, Dillon, & Prettyman, 2007). Perhaps if spirituality is linked to openness (Saucier & Skrzypińska, 2006), religion may be linked to both conscientiousness and agreeableness in the five-factor model, as well as a need for closure (Saroglou, 2002a). Furthermore, it is not the case that individual spirituality is narcissistic, insofar as those who identify themselves as more religious than spiritual are also socially compassionate (Wink, Dillon, & Fay, 2005). Table 8.5 summarizes six types of deconversion and five reasons most commonly noted for deconversion, based upon the research of Streib and his colleagues.

The Streib-headed Bielefeld deconversion project best parallels Rambo's (1993) model of conversion and spiritual transformation discussed above. Both Streib and Rambo accept the complexity of the processes involved in conversion, spiritual transformation, and deconversion, and refuse to proclaim a single overarching narrative or causal mechanism. This is in the best spirit of the call for a new paradigm, of which mixed methods are one essential component. Both Germans and American deconverts scored low on measures of religious fundamentalism and high on openness to experience in the five-factor model. On the other hand, one must not underestimate the psychological value of remaining within a faith tradition. For instance, in Germany, in-tradition members most clearly showed high scores on the Ryff–Singer subscales measuring purpose in life, positive relations with others, and environmental mastery, while their higher scores on all aspects of the five-factor model except

TABLE 8.5. Six Types of Deconversion Trajectories and Five Reasons for Deconversion

Deconversion to other religious groups

- *Religious switching:* Migrating to a religious organization with a similar system of beliefs, rituals, and practices
- *Oppositional exit:* Affiliating with a higher-tension, more oppositional religious organization, such as conversion to a fundamentalist group
- *Integrating exit:* Adopting a different system of beliefs and engaging in different ritualistic practices, while affiliating with an integrated or more accommodating religious organization

Deconversion from religion

- *Privatizing exit:* Disaffiliating from and terminating membership in organized religion, but continuing private religious belief and private religious praxis
- *Heretical exit:* Disaffiliating from a religious organization and terminating membership, but with individual heretical appropriation of new belief system(s); or engaging in different religious praxis but without new organizational affiliation
- *Secularizing exit:* Disaffiliating from organized religion altogether

Five reasons for deconversion

1. Loss of specific religious experiences
2. Intellectual doubt, denial, or disagreement with specific beliefs
3. Moral criticism
4. Emotional suffering
5. Disaffiliation from the community

Note. Based on Streib (2014, pp. 272–273); Streib, Hood, and Keller (2016, p. 21).

openness suggested a stability and meaning provided by those who remain committed to a faith tradition, even one that is authoritarian in nature.

The balance between tradition and transformation is an integral part of any religious dynamic (Peterson, 1999), and the two-factor solution of the five-factor model measure has direct relevance to the current debate between religion and spirituality (Streib, 2008). For instance, generally values relate to religion more powerfully than personality factors do (Saroglou, Delpierre, & Dernelle, 2004; Saroglou & Muñoz-García, 2008; Schwartz, 1992). Personality as measured by the five-factor model does show a fairly consistent pattern across many studies (Saroglou, 2002b). Openness is most consistently unrelated or negatively related to religion, while agreeableness and conscientiousness are positively related to religion. Also, religious fundamentalism tends to be negatively correlated with openness (Saroglou, 2002a). The possibility of a higher-order two-factor solution to the five-factor model measure suggest why this pattern exists. Agreeableness, conscientiousness, and emotional stability (neuroticism reverse-scored) form one factor associated with stability, and openness and extroversion form another factor associated with plasticity (DeYoung, 2006; DeYoung, Peterson, & Higgins, 2002). Streib et al. (2009) identify the factors as "traditionalism" and "transformation." They postulate that religion is more associated with traditionalism, while spirituality is more associated with transformation. Further empirical support for this distinction can be gleaned from comparing deconverts from a specific tradition with members who stay within that tradition. In the Bielefeld cross-cultural study of deconverted individuals in the United States and Germany, individual identification on the spiritual–religious binary classification revealed interesting patterns, which are identified in Table 8.6.

The tension between maintaining tradition and encouraging transformation is likely to be part of the personality substrate that may provide the motivational basis for conversion and spiritual transformation. For instance, Streib et al. (2009) suggest that persons high in openness in more restricted religious traditions explore the limits of the tradition and then are motivated to begin a (probably gradual) process of deconversion associated with slightly elevated faith development scores. On the other hand, those lower in openness find satisfactory meaning and purpose in life within a tradition. This interpretation is not inconsistent with numerous studies relating the five-factor model to religion, but provides a dynamic model for the tension between tradition and transformation that has been masterfully explored by Peterson (1999) as the personality basis for what he terms the "architecture of belief."

TABLE 8.6. In-Tradition and Deconverted Respondents' Religious and Spiritual Self-Identification

Sample	n	R > S	S > R	R = S	Neither
United States					
Deconverted	66	6.1	63.6	13.6	16.7
In-tradition	356	43.3	18.3	32.6	5.9
Germany					
Deconverted	52	19.2	36.5	23.1	16.7
In-tradition	649	10.2	37.0	46.8	6.0

Note. R > S, more religious than spiritual; S > R, more spiritual than religious; R = S, equally religious and spiritual; Neither, neither religious nor spiritual. Data from Streib, Hood, and Keller (2016, p. 22).

Finally, the measure of the five-factor model employed in this research is a complex instrument that, in addition to the commonly employed five domains or factors, allows the identification of six facets to each domain; in turn, each facet is related to eight basic behavioral, affective, and cognitive tendencies. This results in 240 items, which can yield a more nuanced understanding of personality correlates of religiosity, as Aguilar-Vafaie and Moghanloo (2008) have demonstrated with a sample of Shiite Muslims. None of the studies of conversion, deconversion, or spiritual transformation that have employed this instrument have yet focused upon the more subtle and nuanced use of the measure when facets and the full conceptual basis of the five-factor model are utilized. Streib et al.'s finding that deconverts had slightly elevated faith development scores is also consistent with Jindra's (2008) finding, using Oser's stages of development of religious judgment (discussed in Chapter 4), that conversion and deconversion narratives follow trajectories of religious judgment closely.

Disengagement within Mainstream Religious Groups

Although most of the research on deconversion has focused upon new religious movements that are sectarian or cult-like in nature, most religious participation in North America is within denominational religious groups. The Streib et al. (2009) study described above is the most ambitious study to date of deconversion from what, in the United States at least, are largely mainstream religious groups. However, these groups have long been noted to have transitional memberships. As a general pattern, participation in religious groups waxes and wanes. Probably 80% of denominational members withdraw at some point in their lives, only to return at some later point (Roozen, 1980). Thus only a minority of persons socialized into religious groups in North America ever truly reject religious identity or participation. As we have noted, the percentage of apostates in the United States has remained fairly constant at about 7%. This means that well over 90% of the U.S. population belonging to a religious group engages in some form of religious participation, whether this takes place at a church, mosque, or synagogue.

However, the frequency of this participation fluctuates. For instance, Albrecht, Cornwall, and Cunningham (1988) mailed questionnaires to a stratified random sample of 32 active and 45 inactive families in each of 27 different Mormon wards (similar to congregations). Seventy-four percent of the active families and 44% of the inactive families responded. Phone follow-ups to the inactive families raised their participation rate to 64%. Two measures of disengagement were used: (1) behavior (a period of 1 month or more of no church attendance), and (2) belief (a period of at least 1 year when the Church of Jesus Christ of Latter-Day Saints was not an important part of a family's life). Summarizing the results for every 100 families revealed that 74 became disengaged in terms of either behavior (55) or belief (19). Only 4 families remained engaged nonbelievers; only 22 remained engaged believers. Of the 55 families that were disengaged nonbelievers, 31 returned to church participation (Albrecht et al., 1988; see also Albrecht & Cornwall, 1989). These data are consistent with studies of disengagement and reengagement among Catholics (Hoge with McGuire & Stratman, 1981). They are also consistent with the studies of denominational switching and the cycling of religious participation discussed in Chapter 9. However, in light of the historical context within which new religious movements have emerged, it appears that many disengaged from mainstream religion have explored new religious movements as one form of reengagement.

Baby Boomers and Disengagement/Reengagement

As noted in earlier chapters, several investigators have been concerned with what has been called the "baby boomer" generation. Although not precisely defined, this generation includes those raised in the 1960s in North America during a period of intense social upheaval (Roszak, 1968). Associated with this upheaval was the emergence of new religious movements, competing with and often congruent with a variety of countercultural movements (Tipton, 1982). Participants in these countercultural movements were largely youths reared in mainstream religious traditions. For instance, Roof (1993) found that two-thirds of all baby boomers reared in mainstream religious traditions dropped out or disengaged from mainstream religious participation in their late adolescence or early youth.

Roof used a commercial firm to conduct focused group interviews with individuals from randomly digit-dialed samples. Households in four states (California, Massachusetts, North Carolina, and Ohio) were sampled. A 60% participation rate was obtained from an initial sample of 2,620 households. Baby boomers were defined as those born between 1946 and 1962 ($n = 1,599$; 61% of sample). The sample was further divided into older boomers (1946–1954; $n = 802$) and younger boomers (1955–1962; $n = 797$). Follow-up interviews were conducted with older boomers, and eventually 64 in-depth, face-to-face interviews and 14 group dialogues were conducted with these participants (Roof, 1993).

As discussed in Chapter 5, religious disengagement tends to follow a pattern that includes religious socialization and participation, followed by youthful rebellion and departure, and subsequently by return. Thus high rates of disengagement among boomers would not be surprising; nor would a return of most of these to mainstream religious participation. Indeed, Roof found that a return to mainstream religion occurred as expected for many of those who were disengaged. Furthermore, categorizing participants by the extent to which they were part of the mainstream culture (in terms of having settled into a community, married, and had children) indicated that the more normalized a participant's current lifestyle was in terms of the dominant culture, the more likely the person was to have returned to religious involvement.

The fact that those who disengaged from religion tended to return as they participated more fully in the dominant culture is readily understandable in terms of life cycle theories of socialization. As noted in earlier chapters, youth is a time for exploration and rebellion—or, in more psychological terms, a time in which one searches for identity (Erikson, 1968). However, it is also the case that theories of social change suggest the relevance of youthful participation in radical social movements aimed at altering society (Keniston, 1968, 1971; Roszak, 1968). Kent (2001) has marshaled considerable empirical evidence to support the thesis that youthful political protest is often followed by attraction to mystical religions.[2] Whereas religious denominations tend to be at ease with the dominant culture, religious sects and cults are at tension with at least some aspects of this culture, as discussed in Chapter 9. New religious movements are likely to appeal to individuals not committed to the dominant culture, and thus may recruit members whose initial protest was expressed in political terms (Kent, 2001). Montgomery (1991) has argued that the spread of new religions is facilitated when the new religions either constitute a threat to society or come from a source other

---

[2] However, the conversion to religious frames may have been only temporary for many boomers who were protesters. For instance, Whalen and Flacks (1989) studied 17 political activists convicted for a Bank of America bombing in 1970. The majority did turn temporarily to countercultural religions, but eventually resumed political activities, although in a less extreme form.

than the society; they provide sources of identity and resistance for those alienated from the dominant culture. Although Montgomery's theory applies to the emergence of new religions within a historical context and focuses upon macrosocial relations, it also applies to the emergence of new religions within a culture where a dominant culture opposes a subculture—a phenomenon characteristic of the 1960s in North America (Tipton, 1982). The subculture is likely to accept new religious movements that promulgate behaviors and beliefs at odds with the dominant culture, as sects and cults do.

One empirical prediction congruent with these macrosocial assumptions is that exposure to countercultural values should make a person more susceptible to new religious movements and/or to disengagement from mainstream religion. Roof's research provides data relevant to this claim. Using an index of exposure to the 1960s counterculture, Roof found that the preference for sticking to mainstream cultural expressions of faith varied as a function of such exposure, as did willingness to explore other teachings and religions.

The high rate of former drug use among members converted to new religious movements is well documented. In some new religious movements, the rate of former drug use has been reported to be almost 100%. For instance, Volinn (1985) used in-depth interviews and extensive participatory observation to study 52 members of an ashram in New England. Forty-seven of these admitted to smoking marijuana, and 46 had used it 50 times or more. Likewise, all but 8 admitted to using LSD, but only 6 had used this more than 50 times, and 14 had used it only "once or twice" (Volinn, 1985, p. 152). Other investigators have documented former drug use among converts to new religious movements. Among new religious movements, Judah (1974) has documented abandonment of drug use among converts to Hare Krishna; Galanter and Buckley (1978) have obtained similar results for converts to the Divine Light Mission; Anthony and Robbins (1974) have documented abandonment of drug use among converts to Meher Baba; and Nordquist (1978) also found such outcomes for converts to Ananda, a "New Age" community in Sweden.

The low rates of illicit drug use among members of mainstream religions have long been established (Gorsuch, 1976), and both mainstream religions and new religious movements discourage the use of illicit drugs. However, it appears that prior drug experience varies according to whether one is a member of a mainstream denomination or a new religious movement, whether sect or cult. In denominational religion, norms and beliefs serve to decrease the probability of illicit drug use among participants. However, among those who use illicit drugs, spiritual seeking can result in conversion to new religious movements that then discourage illicit drug use. Several investigators have described new religious movements as providing an alternative to drug experiences. Some argue that conversion can even be a new form of addiction (Simmonds, 1977a); new religious converts may simply substitute one addiction for another. Others, such as Volinn (1985), have focused upon the spiritual experiences of converts to new religious movements as meaningful alternatives to illicit drug "highs."

It would appear that with few exceptions, institutional forms of religion—whether denominations, sects, or cults—tend to discourage drug use. An interesting exception is the Native American use of peyote (LaBarre, 1969). Yet many who utilize drugs outside of religion define themselves as spiritual seekers. Roof (1993) noted that among his baby boomers, those most exposed to the counterculture of the 1960s were least likely to be conventionally religious, but most likely to define themselves as spiritual. Eighty-one percent of those scoring highest on his index of exposure to the 1960s defined themselves as spiritual, whereas 92% of those who scored zero on his index defined themselves as religious. Not surprisingly, 84% of those scoring highest on the exposure-to-the-1960s index were religious dropouts (Roof, 1993).

THE COMPLEXITY OF CONVERSION, SPIRITUAL TRANSFORMATION, AND DECONVERSION

It has been almost 70 years since Allport (1950, p. 37) claimed that "no subject within the psychology of religion has been more extensively studied than conversion." However, despite the massive empirical literature—first from psychologically oriented and more recently from sociologically oriented social psychologists—no simple conclusion can be reached that has any degree of empirical validity. Clearly, conversion, spiritual transformation, and deconversion all can entail significant changes in persons, even if changes in basic personality functions are unlikely. The questions of precisely how and why these changes occur demand systematic programs of research (Paloutzian et al., 1999, p. 1048). Such programs are unlikely to be useful if they are not guided by theories or models as complex as the empirical realities they hope to illuminate. In this sense, the call for a new paradigm in the psychology of religion (noted throughout this text) is once again to be emphasized.

With this complexity in mind, Rambo (1993) has proposed the integrative model most consistent with the call for the new paradigm. His model utilizes insights from anthropologists (Berkhofer, 1963), missiologists (Tippett, 1977), and sociologists (Lofland & Stark, 1965). It is not simply developmental, although it does propose stages or sequences that can serve as a heuristic model. Unlike those of many purely psychological approaches, the stages or

TABLE 8.7. An Integrative Model for Conversion/Transformation

Stages or facets of the process	Factors that must be assessed in this stage
Stage 1: Context	Factors that facilitate or hinder conversion/transformation. These include cultural, historical, personal, sociological, and theological factors.
Stage 2: Crisis	May be personal, social, or both.
Stage 3: Quest	Intentional activity on part of individual.
Stage 4: Encounter	Recognition of alternative spiritual or religious option. May be facilitated by individual ("advocate") or institution (missionary activity).
Stage 5: Interaction	Extended engagement at many levels with new religious/spiritual option.
Stage 6: Commitment	Identification with new spiritual or religious reality.
Stage 7: Consequences	Conversion/transformation as a result of new commitment, including beliefs, behaviors, and identity.

Note. See Rambo (1993) and Paloutzian, Richardson, and Rambo (1999).

sequences are neither unidirectional nor invariant. The stages are interrelated in complex dialectical ways that allow them to be interactive, so that not only can early stages influence later stages, but these in turn can influence earlier ones (Paloutzian et al., 1999). Finally, we have added spiritual transformation to Rambo's single use of conversion, as it is implicit in his model. The model is summarized in Table 8.7.

OVERVIEW

Conversion has occupied the interest of social scientists since the beginning of the 20th century. The early research was dominated by psychologists, who focused upon adolescence and sudden emotional conversions. The classic paradigm for conversion was fashioned after Paul's experience. Gradual conversions were recognized to occur and were linked to an active search for meaning and purpose, but were seldom studied except to be contrasted with sudden conversions.

In the early 1960s, sociologically oriented social psychologists began to study conversion and spiritual transformation as a phenomena linked to new religious and spiritual movements. They have focused upon gradual conversion/transformation, postulating models of the conversion/transformation process most typically derived from participant observation or interview studies.

The emergence of a global perspective can be dated from 2000 and was heavily influenced by the destruction of the World Trade Center towers in New York on September 11, 2001. Concern shifted to a focus on major faith traditions and how they interact with the politics of nations. Immigration on a global scale has led to studies of how individuals merge their faith commitments with the political realities when faced with relocation. How the faith traditions of individuals and cultures interact in the face of global migrations will continue to be a focus of conversion research in the future.

Studies employing cognitive dissonance theory have shifted the focus from researchers' and outsiders' claims about failed prophecy to insiders' perspectives on how such prophecy becomes interpreted in ways to maintain group commitment and cohesion. Studies are beginning to look at the conditions under which different individuals may leave prophetic groups to which they have converted.

Deconversion is emerging as a phenomenon closely linked to conversion. In the United States, relatively few individuals remain apostates without any institutional religious involvement; most who leave return to religion at some point in the life cycle. This typically occurs when they are married, have children, and settle in an established community. However, spiritual seekers may remain outside religion altogether and identify themselves as either "more spiritual than religious" or "spiritual but not religious." Deconversion from a new religious movement is likely to be a gradual process of disillusionment, both with the religious group and with its leader, but can occur suddenly as well. The extent to which deconversion is a mirror image of conversion, spiritual transformation, or both remains to be explored.

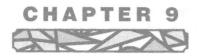

CHAPTER 9

Relationships between Individuals and Religious Groups

Religious revelation aims to liberate the world from the night in which it appears to be immersed; it would appear that one now welcomes, however, the inverse revelation.

Between you and God there stands the church.

Amish values, Amish limits, and the Amish definition of success cannot be grafted onto American culture. It would be pointless to imitate their use of bonnets, buggies, and kerosene lamps. The value of the Amish lies, rather, in making clear limits of some kind and in their insistence in defining for themselves the limits within which they will live.

Muslim traditionalists are not fantasizing when they identify divorce, abortion, more open sexual experimentation, sexually transmitted diseases, and women's demands for equality in the workplace and in decision-making as threats to traditional values.

When a society would turn its eyes away from the deepest questions of responsibility, brainwashing becomes an explanation that avoids the responsibility of looking inward.[1]

The process of becoming religious continues to intrigue social scientists and to foster both theoretical and empirical debate. The simple fact that persons are not born religious means that they must become religious if they are to be religious. The process of becoming religious entails numerous possibilities. Persons may be born into a family with a particular faith commitment and may simply be socialized to adopt that faith as their own. These individuals are those whom William James (1902/1985) dubbed the "once-born," as discussed in Chapter 8. On the other hand, persons may be born into one faith tradition and later change to another. Those born outside any faith tradition may later choose to commit to one. Those previously committed may fall away. Persons may have a series of different faith commitments throughout their lives. Some may simply engage in an interminable quest, in which spiritual issues absorb their interest but never find a resolution. And some may reject or abandon religion altogether. Much of this flux is the subject matter of religious conversion; converts are James's (1902/1985) "twice-born."

---

[1]These quotations come, respectively, from the following sources: Vergote (1997, p. 240); statement attributed to the bishop presiding at the trial of Joan of Arc, quoted in Stobart (1971, p. 157); Olshan (1994, p. 239); Awn (1994, p. 76); and Scheflin and Opton (1978, p. 50).

Yet this individual religious change does not take place in a vacuum. The maintenance of faith, as well as conversion, is not an individual affair. Those with faith tend to seek companions in a social context within which their faith may be both shared and practiced. In this flux of individual religious change also lie the rise and fall of churches and the growth and decline of denominations. In addition, the emergence of novel religious forms from within established groups creates sects, and from without creates cults. James (1902/1985) typifies the psychologist's propensity to emphasize religious experience in individual terms, as we have discussed in Chapter 8. The renowned philosopher Whitehead (1926) even went so far as to define religion in terms of what individuals do with their solitude. There is a rich conceptual literature linking spirituality and solitude (Koch, 1994; Storr, 1988). Yet it remains true that religion has an inherently social dimension, and as Taylor (2002) has argued, James must be revisited in terms of the social and political context of the variety of religions that exist today. As Streib, Hood, and Keller (2016) have demonstrated, religion is a dynamic process and both conversion and deconversion take place within a religious field.

THE CLASSIFICATION OF RELIGIOUS ORGANIZATIONS

Although it may be true that psychologists are particularly prone to define religious commitments in terms of individuals, it remains abundantly clear that these are shared and under varying degrees of organizational control. Whitehead's (1926) focus on the great solitary images of religious imagination—Muhammad brooding in the desert, Buddha resting under the Bodhi tree, and Christ crying out from the cross—is balanced by the fact that such solitary religious figures maintain their importance within great traditions maintained by generations of the faithful, organized into "churches" or "denominations" and "sects." Furthermore, novel forms of religious commitment centered upon newly identified charismatic figures are likely themselves quickly to take an organizational form, however unstructured, if they are to survive. These are the religious "cults."

Closely linked to cults is a relatively new phenomenon: the emergence of groups that advocate terrorism as a tactic (GATTs). Such groups most often utilize terror as a means for political ends (Pape, 2005). However, GATTs become genuine religious groups when they utilize terror for sacred ends that outsiders may see as only political, but that the group itself perceives as religious (Jones, 2008, p. 27). GATTs seldom if ever identify terrorism as an end, but only as a means to an end (Pape, 2005). Hence GATTs are identified by the tactics they use, often in opposition to nations who have access to superior force. Thus, like Jones (2008, p. 27), we find "terrorist" an inappropriate term to define a group—insofar as there are no terrorist groups, but only GATTs. Whether a group is religious or not depends upon whether or not the group advocates terrorism as a means to achieve sacred ends. No major faith tradition can alone be identified as a "terrorist group."

Therefore, to be either traditionally or innovatively religious is to be related in some fashion to a religious group. The solitary religious figure is a myth reconstructed and abstracted from the organizational forms that both define this figure and give him or her meaning. The classification of these religious forms has been of much interest to the more sociologically oriented psychologists of religion. Of the various classification schemes proposed, the most influential has been "church–sect theory."

CHURCH–SECT THEORY

Church–sect theory was never intended as a theory of origins, and hence it is a bit surprising that it has so dominated the empirical literature on both established and new religious movements. Furthermore, as Dittes (1971b) has noted, the careers of Troeltsch's church–sect theory and of Allport's theory and measures of Intrinsic versus Extrinsic religion (discussed in Chapter 2) have numerous parallels. Recently, Streib and Hood (2016, p. xi) have noted parallels to the religious–spiritual binary (discussed in Chapter 10). All three theories have dominated their conceptual and empirical literatures, and all have numerous critics. Dittes (1971b) said of the initial Troeltsch and Allport parallels that they have "some considerable promise of surviving their obituaries" (p. 382). This statement remains true today and applies to the religious–spiritual binary as well.

A common criticism shared by these three theories is the confounding of evaluation with description. This often entails implicit claims to "good" and "bad" forms of religion (Troeltsch, 1931), of religious motivation (Kirkpatrick & Hood, 1990), or of being more religious than spiritual (Streib & Hood, 2016). As we note later in this chapter, religious cults initially shared the burden of various pejorative connotations that for many have now shifted to GATTs (Galanter, 2013). They are typically perceived as "bad" religions. As psychologists, we must explore the empirical reasons for such connotations, and (as difficult as it may be) must understand that the members of such groups can be sincerely motivated, act rationally, and are seldom pathological (Galanter, 2013; Horgan, 1999; Moghaddam, 2006). Thus descriptions such as "suicide bomber" and "martyr" are not the same, and empirical studies that cannot distinguish between the two do little to help us understand GATTs in terms of the dynamics of the now-globalized religious field (Streib & Hood, 2016).

Understanding more extreme forms of religion requires an empirical grounding in the relationship between forms of religious organizations and their dominant or host cultures. In this section, we draw upon the roots of church–sect theory and attempt to show how these have influenced the sociologically oriented social-psychological literature. Only a few would argue against the importance of church–sect theory (Robertson, 1975; Snook, 1974). We hope that our discussion of this theory's roots in the work of Troeltsch will demonstrate both its relevance and its usefulness in organizing contemporary empirical studies on the social psychology of religious organizations, whether these are considered religions, sects, cults, or GATTs (Hood, 2003; Streib, 2008; Streib & Hood, 2016).

Origins of Church–Sect Theory

The main source of church–sect theory in modern social psychology has been H. Richard Niebuhr's (1929) work on the social sources of denominationalism. Denominations are what many persons think of as "churches"—groups commonly accepted as legitimate religious organizations within their host cultures. Most people identify themselves by reporting their denominational membership (if they are Christians) when asked for their religious identification. Thus, as Wimberley and Christenson (1981) have noted, individual religious identity is largely synonymous with group religious membership.

Niebuhr's work is a modification and popularization of church, sect, and mysticism—three types of religious organizations articulated in Troeltsch's (1931) classic work *The Social Teachings of the Christian Churches*. Niebuhr's popularization significantly altered Troeltsch's conceptualizations. As discussed in Chapter 11, Niebuhr ignored Troeltsch's three-part typology (church–sect–mysticism) in favor of a two-part typology (church–sect). Furthermore, Niebuhr added a dynamic tendency to the theory: He suggested that persons who are dissatisfied with the commonness and permissiveness of churches as they successfully appeal to the masses seek more demanding criteria for membership. This exclusiveness creates a sectarian movement and implicitly implies a more positive evaluation, due to more rigorous criteria for membership than those for membership in churches (denominations). Although Niebuhr thought that sects are unable to gain control from elites within churches— and hence that the direction of change is from church to sect, but not from sect to church— others argued against this. Johnson (1963, p. 543) argued that a shift from sect to church is theoretically "conceivable." Eister (1973) argued more forcefully for what he referred to as the "paradox of religious organizations": Dynamic processes produce sects from churches, but sects then tend to become like the churches they once criticized. However, in more extreme groups such as cults and GATTs, there may be a pattern to membership that is irreversible, such as when GATT members commit acts of martyrdom that outsiders are unlikely to see as other than acts of senseless violence or suicide (Hall, 1989; Moghaddam, Warren, & Love, 2013; Zaehner, 1974).

For our purposes, it is important to emphasize that the Troeltsch theory includes a crucial defining criterion that differentiates churches (denominations) from sects: Churches are inclusive, while sects are exclusive. By focusing upon the single criterion of degree of exclusiveness, church–sect theory can contribute to organizing the empirical literature in value-neutral terms. The criterion of exclusiveness is easily operationalized, and it permits us as social scientists to sidestep issues of evaluating "good" and "bad" religion.

The Empirical Tradition Influenced by Church–Sect Theory

Not surprisingly, contemporary social scientists have divided into two camps regarding church–sect theory. One camp continues the classical tradition of modifying church– sect theory and of debating its validity and value, mainly at the conceptual level (Eister, 1973; Johnson, 1963, 1971; Wilson, 1970). Most of the resulting classification systems are qualitatively derived, relying upon appeals to face validity. Few in this camp seek empirical verification of predictive consequences for their typologies. In the rare instances when these classifications have been empirically assessed, they have been found to be less than adequate. As Welch (1977, p. 127) has noted, "Few existing set classification schemes—both unidimensional and multidimensional varieties—are able to offer true discriminatory power when put to the empirical test."

Members of the other camp have opted for more precise operationalization of their typologies, often employing quantitative procedures to construct their typologies (Eister, 1973; Finke & Stark, 2001; Johnson, 1963, 1971; Stark & Bainbridge, 1987; Wilson, 1970), and seeking systematic testing of hypotheses derived from these classifications. One of the most systematic efforts has been made by Stark (1985), whose model has moved the debate beyond mere conceptual criticisms to the testing of empirical hypotheses based upon operational measures.

Stark owes much to a now-classic paper by Johnson (1963), who first operationalized the essential difference between church and sect that he felt Troeltsch set forth with varying degrees of explicitness. Churches are inclusive (e.g., accepting infant baptism) and are widely accommodating to their host cultures, seldom being at significant odds with their major values. On the other hand, sects are exclusive (e.g., often demanding adult baptism) and seek a religious purity that often puts them at odds with their culture. The universalizing tendency of the church type accommodates to the host culture, accepting many persons who meet only minimal criteria for membership. The perfectionist tendency of the sect type sets rigorous criteria for membership; as such, it is less accommodating to the host culture as it limits membership. Johnson (1963) operationalized these tendencies as follows: "*A church is a religious group that accepts the social environment in which it exists. A sect is a religious group that rejects the social environment in which it exists*" (p. 542; emphasis in original). Johnson further restricted church and sect to religious groups, stopping by definitional fiat the efforts to extend church–sect typologies to other groups (such as political ones) that some theorists have found useful (Robertson, 1975). In a similar vein, some theorists have argued that extreme religious groups, especially those that either direct others to kill or endorse acts of terrorism, ought not to be included in the psychology of *religion*. For instance, both Hoffman (2006) and Pape (2005) define terrorism in essentially in political terms. However, as noted above, when GATTs seek to sacred goals, terrorism has religious significance as a means to achieve or defend perceived threats from outside—including, as we discuss below, threats from nation-states that often themselves can be classified as GATTs.

Stark and Bainbridge (1979, 1985, 1987) have refined Johnson's definition by further operationalizing acceptance and rejection according to degree of difference, antagonism, and separation between a religious group and its host culture. In our view, the most fruitful operational indicator is the degree of difference, indicated by beliefs and behavioral norms, between sects and the dominant host culture. Moghaddam et al. (2013) have used the "staircase" metaphor to argue that in extreme groups, a final, irreversible act can be martyrdom or suicide. This suicide may be a group act of withdrawal from this world, as in the case of Jonestown (Hall, 1989), or may be directed to elicit terror and mass death in the service of sacred goals perceived as meaningful within the groups that endorse them, as with the Manson cult (Buglios & Gentry, 1974). Furthermore, as the long history of Milgram's obedience experiments and the debates surrounding various replications of these reminds us, the violence is typically used in response to an order from a leader who does not him- or herself commit any direct act of violence (Hood, 1987). Salient differences are likely to lead to mutual rejection, but whether or not they do is an independent empirical question. Furthermore, antagonism is largely a corollary of different beliefs and behavioral norms. Difference itself can be operationally equated with subcultural deviance when the beliefs produce tension between religious groups and their host culture. Low-tension beliefs are congruent with being part of mainstream culture and are characteristic of denominations (churches). Streib, Hood, Keller, Csöff, and Silver (2009) have classified religious groups as "oppositional," "integrative," or "accommodating," depending on the extent to which they accept dominant/host culture norms.

Given this operationalization of church and sect along a continuum of tension, embedded within a more general theory of religion, numerous novel hypotheses have been generated and empirically tested (Stark & Bainbridge, 1980b). Perhaps the most hotly disputed among these is the concept of a general religious economy, in which religious views must compete in an open market. As such, extreme sects become more successful (gain members) by reducing their tension with the host culture. Over time, sects tend to shed their other-worldly and perfectionist tendencies as they accommodate to the culture. They may, but are unlikely to, remain isolated instances of subcultural deviance. Thus, in the Stark and Bainbridge theory, churches reemerge from sects as essentially secularized religious groups—insofar as secularization is recognized to be a process of accommodation to the dominant host culture. In other words, they become acceptable forms of denominational religious expression.

Finke and Stark (2001) have refined this theory to argue that under conditions of free competition, religious organizations can gain membership by moving to increase or decrease tension with their host culture. Their argument rests on the assumption that participation in religious organizations approximates a bell-shaped curve. Degree of tension, defined as the degree of distinctiveness, separation from, and antagonism with the host culture, ranges from very low ("ultraliberal") to very high ("ultrastrict"). Organizations at the extremes can only grow by moving toward the center; thus increasing tension facilitates growth at the more liberal end, whereas decreasing tension facilitates growth at the more sectarian end. Figure 9.1 presents the bell curve model of Finke and Stark.

As Finke and Stark (2001, p. 176) note, "To the extent [that] people seek religion . . . the demand is highest for religions that offer close relations with the supernatural and distinctive demands for membership, without isolating individuals from the culture around them." Thus, in North America, most religious people are members of congregations that fall somewhere between the extremes of the ultrastrict religious sects and the ultraliberal New Age and Unitarian–Universalist groups (Finke & Stark, 2001). Denominations predominate in the middle of the curve. However, this does not mean that only a "middle-of-the-road" religion can be successful. For instance, Williamson and Hood (2004) have documented that as the mainstream Church of God grew into denominational status, it abandoned its endorsement of serpent handling. However, the groups in Appalachia that refused to abandon the practice survived as "renegade" Churches of God. A similar process occurred with fundamentalist Mormon groups that refused to abandon the practice of polygamy, as did the mainstream Church of Jesus Christ of Latter-Day Saints (Quinn, 1993).

Another novel hypothesis derived from Stark and Bainbridge's general model of religion is that in similar religious markets, novel forms of religion can be expected to thrive. As we shall soon see, if cults are defined as novel religious organizations, cults can be expected to thrive precisely where churches or denominations are weak. This follows from the hypothesis that churches have already accommodated to the mainstream culture and that sects are unlikely to maintain for long a novel stance vis-à-vis the larger host culture, to which they also must accommodate to be successful. The hypothesis that weak church environments lead to increased probabilities of cult formation has yet to be fully empirically substantiated, but it remains as viable a hypothesis as it is controversial (Bibby & Weaver, 1985; Bruce,

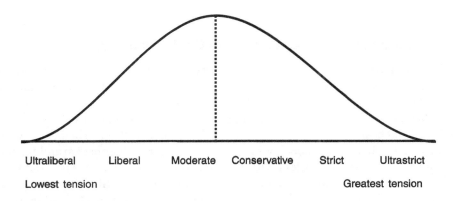

FIGURE 9.1. Hypothetical bell curve distribution of religious organizations. Data from Finke and Stark (2001, p. 177).

1999; Wallis, 1986). Similar reasoning applies to more extreme religious groups that endorse terrorism. For instance, Pape (2005) argues that the choice of martyrdom for some GATTs is a rational strategy for groups that perceive their countries or territories as occupied by foreign forces whose own cultural commitment is to a religion other than that of the lands they occupy. Likewise, efforts to define terrorism as violence directed toward the innocent or noncombatants fails to consider GATTs that deny these distinctions and settle for simply "us" versus "them" (Jones, 2008; Moghaddam et al., 2013).

Exclusivity both defines and characterizes sects as they emerge from churches. Yet they tend toward universality as they survive. Furthermore, religious subcultures, if sufficiently at odds with their host cultures and not in a process of accommodating to them, are likely to be targets of legal retaliation and control—something that has characterized the history of sects in the Western world (Johnson, 1963). It has also become a major issue with respect to the contemporary analysis of cults, as we shall shortly note. Likewise, for GATTs, universalization on a global scale is an often-stated sacred goal legitimating terrorism in the face of superior nation-states with powerful militaries (Jones, 2008; Moghaddam et al., 2013). For now, it is sufficient to note that religious organizations are continually in dynamic processes of change, with individuals joining and leaving religious groups partly on the basis of their appeal to either sectarian (high-tension) or denominational (low-tension) characteristics.

With church–sect theory, the useful empirical indicator is not simply a religious group's accommodation to or rejection of the host culture, but how the host culture in turn reacts to the religious group. What empirically distinguishes churches and sects is the degree to which their host cultures seek to control and minimize the influence of particular religious groups. In many Western cultures, especially North America, the generally favorable attitude toward "religion" suggests that both churches and sects are likely to do fairly well. Churches, or what we might call mainline denominations, are likely to fare better than sects, but both accommodate enough to their host cultures to be acceptable in varying degrees. As Redekop (1974) has emphasized, the useful empirical task is to identify the specific aspects of tension with the host culture that create problems of retaliation. The bell curve model illustrated in Figure 9.1 places tension along a single dimension, but tension with the host culture is clearly a multidimensional construct. We first focus upon this issue in terms of denominational and sectarian forms of religion. In a later section, we explore it in terms of cults—the area where it has generated the majority of empirical research in the face of popular controversies.

Operational Indices on the Church–Sect Continuum

Johnson's operationalization of church–sect theory in terms of degree of tension with the host culture permits Troeltsch's typology to be placed upon a continuum. Religions enforcing norms that are sharply distinct from the more generally accepted norms of the host culture are relatively sectarian; those permitting members to participate freely in all aspects of secular life of the host culture are more church-like (Johnson, 1963). They occupy the large middle range of the bell curve model of Finke and Stark (2001). Bainbridge and Stark (1980b) have provided survey data consistent with Johnson's operationalization. Their data are taken from a sample of church members in four counties of northern California; our focus is upon responses from 2,326 members of different Protestant denominations. Denominations "intuitively" identified as sects included the Church of God, the Church of Christ, the Church of the Nazarene, Assemblies of God, and Seventh-Day Adventists (Bainbridge & Stark, 1980b,

TABLE 9.1. Comparison of Mainstream Protestant Denominations and Five Protestant Sects on Selected Behaviors and Beliefs

	Percentage of respondents endorsing behavior/belief					
	Mainstream Protestant (n = 1,032)	Church of Christ (n = 37)	Church of God (n = 44)	Church of the Nazarene (n = 75)	Assemblies of God (n = 44)	Seventh-Day Adventist (n = 35)
Behaviors						
Disapprove of gambling	62	100	89	92	98	97
Favor censorship	31	57	57	73	82	66
Disapprove of dancing	1	95	77	96	91	100
Beliefs						
Reject Darwin	11	78	57	80	91	94
Believe Devil exists	14	87	73	91	96	97
Believe Jesus will return	22	78	73	93	100	100

Note. Percentages must be cautiously interpreted, given the variation in sample sizes. Based on Bainbridge and Stark (1980b).

p. 107).[2] Mainstream Protestant denominations were classified into those more compatible (low-tension) and those less compatible (high-tension) with their host culture. Our focus is only upon low-tension denominations contrasted with high-tension sectarian groups. We have selected from the survey data certain behaviors permitted by most of secular society but differentially forbidden by religious groups. It ought to be the case that the more sectarian groups should more frequently forbid behaviors permitted by the host culture than more church-like religious groups (denominations) should do. Table 9.1 compares results from the low-tension mainstream Protestant denominations (grouped together) and the five Protestant sects on differences in some common cultural behaviors and beliefs.

The fact that more sectarian groups hold beliefs at odds with the dominant culture simply indicates one dimension of tension. To oppose dancing or drinking within the host culture, where they are approved and considered normal, separates sect members by belief and behavior from certain cultural activities. Likewise, to oppose such beliefs as the theory of evolution puts sect members at odds with normative educational forces in the culture. Even the support of more literal religious beliefs, such as the reality of the Devil or Christ's return, may put sect members at odds with other, more culturally congruent religions. In the comparisons in Table 9.1, the differences among the sectarian groups are never as large as those between all sectarian groups and mainstream Protestants. This supports the contention that sects are at odds with the dominant culture and with denominations within that culture.

Additional evidence for the usefulness of operationalizing sectarian religions by belief tension with their host culture can be gleaned from Poloma's (1991) interesting study of Christian Scientists. Here a single axis of tension, appropriate medical care, is of overriding importance. It is clearly the case that medical perspectives on physical illness dominate

---

[2]Certain groups (Gospel Lighthouse, Foursquare Gospel Church) classified as sects had too few respondents to be included in the statistical tables. We focus upon mainstream denominations only, contrasted with sects for which the sample size is sufficient. For additional details on the sample, the research instrument, and groups we have excluded, see Glock and Stark (1966, pp. 86–122).

modern cultures; most persons seek medical treatment for illness. However, many persons use religious techniques such as prayer to facilitate healing. Several investigators have emphasized that spiritual healing is not as marginal in modern society as one might expect from the official dominance of medical perspectives. For instance, Johnson, Williams, and Bromley (1986) found that 14% of their sample of 586 adults claimed to have experienced a healing of a "serious disease or physical condition" as a result of prayer. Likewise, Poloma and Pendleton (1991) found that 72% of randomly chosen respondents from a Midwestern U.S. population believed that persons sometimes receive physical healing as a result of prayer. Nearly one-third of these (32%) claimed a personal experience of healing, and a third of this subsample (34%) claimed that the healing was of a life-threatening accident or medical problem. It is clear that spiritual healing is a widely diffused belief and practice through a broad range of the general population (Poloma, 1991; Johnson et al., 1986).

Although Poloma (1991, p. 337) is correct in her general assessment that religious healing is widely practiced, it is important to note that prayer as an adjunct to orthodox medical treatment is not a significant source of tension with the dominant culture. For instance, Trier and Shupe (1991, p. 355) have shown that among participants randomly selected from telephone numbers in the Great Lakes area, prayer was commonly used as an adjunct to traditional, mainstream medical care. They found no evidence that prayer was used in lieu of traditional medical treatments. Furthermore, frequency of prayer was correlated positively with consulting a physician. Prayer is most frequently used in conjunction with and not in opposition to orthodox medical treatment (Gottschalk, 1973). As such, prayer for recovery is hardly sectarian in nature.

However, the use of prayer as an adjunct to medical treatment is a far cry from the articulation of a religious ideology that argues against both the concept of disease and the relevance of medical treatment to a cure. Christian Science is one religion that argues for healing in opposition to, not in conjunction with, orthodox medical treatment (Gottschalk, 1973). This is clearly a belief at odds with the dominant host culture, and even with mainstream Christian interpretations of spiritual healing by faith or miraculous intervention (Peel, 1987). Thus the sectarian nature of Christian Science can best be revealed when comparisons are made between the beliefs of Christian Scientists and mainstream Protestant Christians who claim to have experienced a spiritual healing.

In a follow-up study of the 1985 Akron Area Survey, Poloma and Pendleton (1991) contacted 97 of 179 potential participants who had agreed to be interviewed for another study. These were those who reported having "experienced a healing of an illness or disease as a result of prayer" (Poloma, 1991, p. 339). They were interviewed this time on the topic of spiritual healing. The vast majority of participants were "born-again" Christians (82%) and identified themselves as charismatic, Pentecostal, or both (86%). Two were Christian Scientists, who were later used to obtain an additional sample of 42 members of the Church of Christ, Scientist (Christian Science). Comparisons between the 95 mainstream Protestants and the 44 Christian Scientists on beliefs regarding spiritual healing revealed expected differences, as noted in Table 9.2.

It should be stated that these differences in beliefs in spiritual healing between Christian religious groups were found despite similarities in beliefs on other religious matters. For instance, the majority of both Christian Scientists and mainline Christians in Poloma's (1991) sample agreed that Jesus healed in order to show compassion and divinity, as well as to gain followers and to glorify God. Furthermore, in terms of actual reported medical practices, the majority of both mainline Christians and Christian Scientists practiced their beliefs—the

TABLE 9.2. Differences between Mainline Christians and Christian Scientists in Beliefs about Spiritual Healing

Belief	Percentage of respondents endorsing belief	
	Mainline Christians (*n* = 44)	Christian Scientists (*n* = 95)
God always heals if faith enough	57	85
God withholds healing for spiritual good	72	10
Healing operates with fixed laws	69	95
God punishes evil with illness	24	0
God usually heals through doctors	73	12
God usually does not use divine healing	47	3

Note. All differences were significant at $p < .01$. Based on Poloma (1991).

former seeking and utilizing orthodox medical care, the latter much less likely to do so. Some comparisons are reported in Table 9.3.

As can be seen from Table 9.3, neither Christian Scientists nor mainstream Christians acted perfectly in conformity with their stated beliefs: 10% of Christian Scientists reported visiting a doctor within the last year, while an almost equal percentage of mainline Christians failed to visit one. Still, the Christian Scientists' rejection of orthodox medicine was related to very high rates of nonparticipation in its practices. Clearly, rejecting orthodox medicine is a point of tension that separates Christian Scientists from other Christians and from the mainstream culture as well.

ORGANIZATIONAL DYNAMICS

The operationalization of tension with the host culture along a single continuum is useful, but it also can be misleading. Cultures are not homogeneous entities; they are not defined by a single set of norms. Cultures are heterogeneous, with conflicting and often incompatible

TABLE 9.3. Differences between Mainline Christians and Christian Scientists in Reasons for Seeking Medical Care and Medical Visits

	Percentage of respondents endorsing belief	
	Mainstream Christians (*n* = 95)	Christian Scientists (*n* = 44)
Likely would seek help for:		
Relief of headache	100	0
Flu-like symptom	5	6
Severe chest pain	76	10
Severe injury	76	5
Visited doctor within last year	88	10

Note. All differences were significant at $p < .01$. Based on Poloma (1991).

norms existing simultaneously. In a word, cultures are pluralist. Some social scientists refer to this as "postmodernism" (Rosenau, 1992). Although little consensus exists on the meaning of this term, the fact that no single perspective dominates postmodern cultures suggests that tension with a culture must be defined in terms of opposition arising in significant power groups within the culture, which have vested interests in the support of particular norms. Deviation from norms whose enforcement is of little concern is less crucial than norm deviation that arouses reactions from those with significant power within the host culture. More sectarian groups arouse reaction from the powerful, not simply because they harbor different beliefs, but because they harbor different beliefs on a continuum considered salient or important to the powerful within the culture (Becker, 1963).

To take an obvious example, Christian Science, in opposing modern medical science, raises concern among the powerful in a culture dominated by belief in modern medicine. Numerous instances arise when parents from belief traditions such as Christian Science or the Jehovah's Witnesses, which oppose some or all of orthodox medicine, have children in need of medical care. Here, the confrontation between orthodoxy in medicine and the opposition to these powerfully sanctioned norms within sectarian traditions illustrates a significant tension. Outside of particularly specified religious alternatives, it is simply "common sense" that one treats disease by orthodox medical procedures. Yet common sense is but the culturally shared knowledge of reality defined within a tradition (Berger & Luckmann, 1967). The criteria for assessing claims to truth are often incommensurate between traditions. The very specifications of the criteria of judgment are themselves contextually bound. Thus the claim that medical treatment is "obviously" necessary for diseases does not simply affirm one reality, but rejects others, such as those articulated within Christian Science. The question of how to treat these issues empirically without imposition of value claims has long plagued the social sciences.

Before we address one possible resolution to this problem, we simply emphasize that the existence of differences between reality claims in which groups within the culture have dominant interests is not simply a source of identity, but one of conflict as well. To identify oneself as a Christian Scientist is both to belong to a group at odds with orthodox medicine and also to be at odds with the educational elite of the culture, who support and defend the perspective of orthodox medicine. It is almost axiomatic in the social sciences that strong identification of members with divergent groups increases prejudice, as measured by the social distance groups attempt to maintain from one another (Beit-Hallahmi, 1989; Tajfel & Turner, 1986).

Defining Sects versus Denominations in Terms of Change

All groups are in a continual process of change—denominations no less than sects. Cultures are in a continual process of change as well. However, the issue is whether changes within religious groups are in a direction compatible with those in the dominant culture (denominations) or not (sects). In most cases, the issue of congruence is a function of the meanings involved. We can identify this dynamic tension as a ratio between "restorative" and "transformative" efforts to maintain a tradition or shared system of meaning. Meanings are seldom if ever merely personal or idiosyncratic; they are almost always shared by some group, and at odds with those differentially shared by other groups (Berger & Luckmann, 1967). Religions groups undergoing either restorative or transformative changes become sectarian if the dominant culture's commitments remain fairly constant or shift in a direction opposite to the religious group's concerns, respectively.

Both restorative and transformative tendencies exist in all organizations. Within religious organizations, the crucial social dimension is whether the norms that are maintained by either of these processes are sufficiently congruent with the norms that are strongly supported by the host culture. If they are congruent, the religious group has a church (denominational) form, which assures that its members are nonproblematic to the host culture. If they are not congruent, the group has a sectarian or cult-like nature, which assures that its members are problematic to the host culture. Buxant and Saroglou (2008, p. 39) refer to such groups as "contested religious movements." Of course, the issue is complicated by the fact that cultures are changing along with and in opposition to religious groups. Yet it is always the position of religious groups' norms relative to cultural norms on issues of great salience that is the key to defining sects and denominations, and that probably conforms to the bell curve model presented in Figure 9.1.

The Position of Sects within the Host Culture

Sects persist—but, as Bainbridge and Stark (1980b) have noted, an ongoing, functioning group that is problematic to the host culture is a deviant subculture by definition. Thus sects are best viewed as tolerable forms of religious deviance, created when religious groups differ significantly from their host culture on salient values. Sects are problematic to the dominant host culture's interests, but are of the acceptable forms of religious identity characterized by the tolerance for diversity that is common in postmodern cultures (Rosenau, 1992).

Occasionally, sectarian practices become targets of legal sanction; however, within a culture that cherishes religious freedom, efforts to constrain sectarian religious practices are likely to meet with serious obstacles. This is particularly likely to be the case where religious freedom is a strong cultural tradition and where religion is a valuable label. As Richardson (1985a) has noted, being identified as a religion in the United States has numerous benefits, not the least of which is protection from government regulations that would prohibit otherwise problematic behaviors. Benefits include tax exemptions, as well as exemptions from civil rights legislation and many laws that govern business. For instance, religions can refuse to ordain women even in the United States, where women have achieved additional legal protection from discrimination based upon gender. No Catholic woman can bring a lawsuit on discrimination because she is refused the right to be a priest; nor can a fundamentalist woman appeal on legal grounds the refusal of ordination by her church. Yet religions risk losing their religious identification if they deviate too far from cultural norms for what constitutes a "religion." As Greil and Robbins (1994) have noted, the law does not concern itself with claims to religious heresy, at least in the United States; this indicates that within broad limits, religious norms, even those at odds with the dominant culture, are to be protected. However, being protected by the law does not mean that tension with the host culture is minimized. In the United States, the legal acceptance of religious diversity knows few limits. Sectarian groups are allowed to exist and even to flourish as pockets of subcultural religious deviance, characteristic of the religious pluralism and dynamism of postmodern culture. Among the more curious of sectarian religious practices is the handling of serpents among the Holiness sects of Appalachia, as noted in earlier chapters of this book and described in more detail in Research Box 9.1.

When tensions are extreme and reactions to religious subcultures become more intense, tolerance for diversity is likely to find its limit. In India, fundamentalist Hindus, who continue the practice of *sati* despite its illegality, support a restorative sectarian movement unlikely to find sympathy from either men or women influenced by modernity. Yet the practice of *sati*

RESEARCH BOX 9.1. Serpent-Handling Sects
(Hood, 1998; Hood & Williamson, 2008b)

Early in the 20th century in the rural South, George Hensley (and probably others independently) picked up a serpent in reaction to Mark 16:17–18: "And these signs shall follow them that believe; In my name shall they cast out devils; they shall speak with new tongues; They shall take up serpents; and if they drink any deadly thing, it shall not hurt them; they shall lay hands on the sick, and they shall recover." Hensley is widely credited with initiating the practice of serpent handling, unique as a form of religion in the United States. For a while the practice was normative in the Church of God, where Hensley was licensed. Later rejected as a practice by the Church of God, it became normative for Holiness sects in Appalachia. Often identified as "sign-following" sects and long predicted to disappear, these sects continue to outlive their obituaries. Preachers, with their serpent boxes ever present, handle deadly snakes—either when faith alone dictates it or, for some, when they feel they have a special experience of being "anointed." Associated with serpent handling but less common is the drinking of poison, often strychnine or lye. Ninety deaths have been documented from serpent bites (Hood & Williamson, 2008b, pp. 239–244). Henley himself was a victim, dying of a snake bite in 1955. Serpent bites are common, and among serpent-handling sects, opinions differ on whether one ought to seek medical aid if bitten. Although many Protestant sects practice some of the signs specified in Mark 16:17–18, only the Holiness sects of Appalachia follow all five signs. For instance, many Pentecostal groups speak in tongues (glossalalia) but reject serpent handling. The tension that serpent handling presents to a modern culture is obvious. Legal sanctions have been directed against the practice in some states, such as Tennessee. In other states, such as West Virginia, the practice carries no sanction. (For a listing of laws against serpent-handling sects, see Burton, 1993.) To the outsider, this obedience to the literal Biblical imperative is the major defining characteristic of these sects.

---

is rooted in the belief that the untimely death of a husband is due to the failure of his wife to protect him, and hence she must sacrifice herself on his funeral pyre. Cases of the reemergence of *sati* and its defense by Hindu fundamentalists have generated much social-scientific commentary and analysis (Hawley, 1994a, 1994b). Here the tension with most cultural views is extreme, despite the long tradition of *sati* as a minority movement within Hinduism. Legal repercussions in the interest of the dominant culture suggest a retaliation and an appeal to a higher standard unlikely to be heard within the "ideological surround" of *sati* and its defenders. (We discuss the "ideological surround" model more fully in Chapter 12.)

CULTS

If tension with the host culture on salient values best empirically defines a church–sect continuum, what about cults? The term "cult" has such a pejorative quality, especially in the popular media, that some investigators who have profitably utilized the concept in the past have begun calling for the elimination of the term "cult" altogether (Richardson, 1993). In one sense, it has become the sociological equivalent of psychopathology in the popular mind. Even the sociological literature on cults tends toward the dramatic and extreme, despite wide variations in the nature of cult beliefs and practices (Eister, 1973). Empirical studies of attitudes toward cults indicate that the majority of respondents have heard of Jonestown and Charlie Manson—names linked to the term "cult" in the popular media (Pfeifer, 1992, p. 538). It is as if all sects and cults were identified with the Hindu ritual of *sati*, or as if the sensationalized press descriptions of those who advocate Islamic *jihad* as mere "terrorists" were to be taken at face value. Yet death and violence are no more essential to cults than to other social groups.

Comparing Cults and Sects

Despite the fact that the cult type was never part of the theoretical development of church–sect theory, it is probably most useful to compare cults and sects. As Stark and Bainbridge (1979, p. 125) have argued, sects tend to rise from within existing religious groups and to move toward a new religious form. Schisms create sects by what we have termed either restorative or transformative movements. Hence sects are inherently religious protest movements. On the other hand, cults lack prior ties with religious bodies and tend to emerge afresh, often under the direction of a single charismatic leader. Cults are novel forms of religion, which, not surprisingly, are likely to emerge in tension both with established religious groups (such as churches and sects) and with the host culture. As such, we can expect that sects and cults share a rejection of their host culture or at least some aspects of their host culture, and are likely to be rejected by their host culture in turn.

As with sects, there are belief differences between cults and their host culture. There are also likely to be close patterns of interaction among cult members, as well as retaliatory actions on the part of the host culture toward them—all of which create an even more clearly defined religiously deviant subculture for cults than for sects. This occurs not only because cults are novel and hence lack previous religious legitimation, but also because their leader is likely to be a solitary, powerful, charismatic figure. Indeed, many characterize cults as lacking a formal organizational structure and as largely controlled in an authoritative manner by their leaders (Ellwood, 1986; Wallis, 1974). Cults are often defined and identified by the names of their leaders, at least in the popular media. Hence we have the "Charlie Manson cult," the "Jim Jones cult," and the "Moonies" (after the Reverend Sun Myung Moon). As Barnes and Becker (1938, p. 22) have noted about charismatic figures in general, "Charismatic domination is established through the extraordinary qualities (real or supposed) of the leader. . . . Law is not the source of authority; on the contrary, he [or she] proclaims new laws on the basis of revelation, oracular utterance, and inspiration."

Given the charismatic nature of cult leadership combined with the fact that cults (like sects) are in opposition to salient cultural values, there is often some confusion as to whether or not cults are truly "religions." The distinction between religious and secular groups has become blurred in the modern world. As Greil and Rudy (1990) have noted, many organizations are best conceived as parareligious or quasi-religious because they have mixed characteristics, some of which are sacred and some of which are secular. This applies, for example, to Alcoholics Anonymous, astrology, and many healing movements (Greil & Robbins, 1994; McGuire, 1992). In congruence with postmodern analyses, we should note that "religion" can be conceived as a category of discourse, negotiated by groups that would either desire to obtain or wish to refute the label. Although there are often benefits to the label (as noted above), there can be liabilities as well. For instance, Transcendental Meditation (TM) was successfully excluded from schools in the United States on the basis of a claim Maharishi

Mahesh Yogi denied—namely, that TM was a religion (Greil & Robbins, 1994). Hence efforts to include TM as a secular activity in schools were rejected, based upon a court ruling that such practices were in fact religious in nature. Thus the category of religion must be negotiated between groups and a culture; some groups desire the label, but others do not want it (Greil, 1993).

However, as novel forms of religious identity, cults are likely to be severely challenged by mainstream culture. Pfeifer (1992) found that the vast majority of college students in his sample (82%) described "an average cult member" only in negative terms; not a single student used positive terms. He also randomly divided his participants into three equal groups and had them respond to one of three vignettes describing three groups. None of these three groups were identified as cults, but each was selected based upon popular notions of alleged authoritarian structures and near-total environmental control of members, who are kept isolated from the wider society. The vignettes were identical except for the groups specified—either "Marines," "Moonies," or "priests." The vignette described a typical recruit, "Bill," at the relevant group facility (with only the identification of the persons surrounding him changed across the three vignettes) as follows:

> While at the facility, Bill is not allowed very much contact with his friends or family and he notices he is seldom left alone. He also notices that he never seems to be able to talk to the other four people who signed up for the program and that he is continually surrounded by (Moonies, Marines, priests) who make him feel guilty if he questions any of their actions and beliefs. (Pfeiffer, 1992, p. 535)

Among several assessments in this study, participants were asked to select the term that best described the process Bill had undergone in order to reach the facility from among these terms: "initiation," "conversion," "brainwashing," "basic training," "resocialization," or "religious education." The most common term used to describe the process by which Bill was surrounded by Moonies was "brainwashing" (22 of 31, or 71%), whereas this term was used much less frequently to describe joining the Marines (15 of 34, or 44%) or the priesthood (10 of 34, or 29%). Still, as we shall see later in this chapter, "brainwashing" as a term to describe conversion—especially conversion to unpopular groups—has become a major issue, dividing even professional psychologists. Likewise, when participants were asked to characterize cults on the basis of the degree to which they foster "psychological growth," "community programs," "child abuse," or "brainwashing," Pfeifer (1992) found that negative descriptive terms ("child abuse" and "brainwashing") were seen to characterize cults, whereas neither positive term was seen as characteristic of cults.

In addition, the participants rated Bill on various indices on a bipolar scale. Bill was generally perceived as less happy and responsible if he joined the Moonies, as well as likely to have been coerced into joining them and to be powerless to leave. Overall, he was also perceived to have been treated unfairly by the Moonies.

Pfeifer's study paints a negative picture of the perception of both cults and cult members that is supported by previous research. Zimbardo and Hartley (1985, p. 114) found that the most typical descriptions of cults obtained from students using a semantic differential scale tended to be those with strongly negative connotations, such as "not worthwhile" (64%) and "crazy" (60%). Consistent with the need for cults, as novel forms of religious organization, to negotiate for the validity of their label as "religious," more than one-fifth of these subjects identified cults as "nonreligious."

In a more recent study, Olson (2006) utilized data from the Nebraska Annual Social Indicators Survey, a telephone survey of 2,426 adults conducted from December 2003 to May 2004. He asked the respondents, "Would you be comfortable if your neighbor joined a cult, a new religious movement, or a new Christian church?" The results for the 44% who responded revealed that these Midwestern Americans held negative views of cults and positive views of a new *Christian* church, with their views of new religious movements in between. Olson also found that the Nebraskans who responded to the interview felt that the government should have the right to regulate cults (56% "very" or "somewhat" agreed), but felt much less strongly about this for new Christian churches (13% "very" or "somewhat" agreed). Again, their views on regulation of new religious movements were in between (26% "very" or "somewhat" agreed). Olson's findings are consistent with those of Pfeifer (1992), who argues that people hold schemas that stereotype cults and cult members. However, this does not mean that such schemas cannot be changed, as noted in Research Box 9.2 (dealing with schemas of serpent handlers).

The problem of novel groups' negotiating to be labeled as "religious" is accentuated when these groups combine charismatic leadership with authoritarian structures that tend toward withdrawal from the dominant culture. For instance, Galanter (1989a) emphasizes the strong influence on behavior by norms supported by the attribution of divine powers to a cult leader. Richardson (1978a) emphasizes the oppositional nature of cults, which is exacerbated

---

RESEARCH BOX 9.2. Changing Views toward Serpent-Handling Sects
(Hood, Williamson, & Morris, 2000)

It is well documented that serpent handlers have been stereotyped in the popular media, which provide the basis of most persons' "knowledge" about this tradition (Brickhead, 1997). In a quasi-experimental study, college students were presented with contemporary tapes of serpent-handling services—one in which serpent handling was both demonstrated and defended, and a comparison tape in which services were shown but handling was neither defended nor demonstrated. Participants were assessed before and after viewing the tapes on a measure of prejudice that included stereotyping, negative affect, and behavioral intentions. It also included three items to assess whether respondents thought the practice of serpent handling to be "unfortunate," whether they believed that those who practice serpent handling are sincere, and whether respondents supported laws restricting the practice. Results indicated that prior to viewing the tapes, all participants held generally prejudiced attitudes toward serpent handling, thought the practice to be unfortunate, thought the handlers insincere, and favored laws against handling serpents in church. Analysis showed that viewing a videotape of serpent handling and hearing the practice explained and defended influenced attitudes. All participants in this study continued believing the practice unfortunate and holding negative affect about it, as well as not wanting to be with handlers, regardless of which tape they viewed. However, only those who actually witnessed handling and its defense decreased their stereotyping and changed their views; they now expressed beliefs that serpent handlers are sincere and that they ought to be allowed to practice their faith without legal constraint. Thus factual presentation of information regarding religious groups can reduce stereotyping and change attitudes toward them.

by the fact that they often derive their inspiration and ideology from outside the predominant religious and secular culture. Wallis (1974) has emphasized that cults need not always take their ideology from outside the dominant culture. Yet, as novel religious forms, cults clearly have an ideology at least distinct from the dominant culture. As Ellwood (1986) emphasizes, cults present a distinct alternative to dominant patterns in society, and the tension this creates is exacerbated when they are also led by charismatic persons who demand high degrees of commitment. Swatos (1981) emphasizes that the cult leader may be an imaginary figure, not a real one. Yet to focus religious novelty on a single figure, cultivating fierce commitment from members willing to withdraw from significant aspects of both religious and secular culture, is likely to create a powerful deviant subculture that must fight to be recognized as legitimately "religious." There is considerable evidence that in western Europe, without the long tradition of separation of church and state that characterizes the United States, cults and new religions must struggle even harder to be recognized as legitimate religious groups (Richardson & Introvigne, 2001). For instance, in historically Roman Catholic Belgium, even Protestant groups are "contested religious movements" (Buxant & Saroglou, 2008, p. 268).

Thus models of sects as deviant religious subcultures may actually apply more forcefully to cults than to sects. As innovative deviant subcultures, cults stand in opposition to both the host culture and sects. Both sects and cults share the fact of tension with the dominant host culture, but cults more frequently emphasize separatist tendencies from a novel base and hence are more likely to attract intense cultural rejection in turn. As we have seen, sects tend to emerge out of religious organizations. They are likely to find some support for their aims, whether restorative or transformative, from others within the dominant culture. By contrast, cults arise as original movements within the culture and are likely to solicit opposition both from established religions and from the secular host culture.

In a postmodern culture, the acceptance of pluralism creates some added degree of tolerance—a milieu somewhat favorable to both sects and cults (Kilbourne & Richardson, 1984; Rosenau, 1992). However, tolerance has its limits. This is especially the case in light of two factors. First, as Stark (1985) has emphasized, cults tend to appeal for recruits to members of weakened churches or to unchurched individuals. Thus, in terms of the religious marketplace, denominations are either losing members to cults or failing to attract as members those individuals from the secular culture who join cults. Second, the oppositional nature of cults is directed not only against the churches' claims to appropriate accommodation to the world, but against the sects' claims to renewed efforts to maintain an exclusive religious purity. Not surprisingly, these rejections of both churches and sects as well as secular culture foster retaliation in turn. Cults are unlikely to have an easy birth or a long life. As we shall see, retaliatory efforts have created recent "anti-cult" movements, both in the United States (Shupe & Bromley, 1985; Shupe, Bromley, & Oliver, 1984) and in Europe (Richardson & Introvigne, 2001; Robbins, 2001). Much of this movement has been aided and abetted by psychologists and psychiatrists who support the claims that cults utilize "brainwashing" to convert members against their will. We confront both of these issues, after we first give some consideration to the axis along which tension is likely to occur.

Bainbridge and Stark (1980a) have properly noted that the nature of a cult's dominant activity is likely to define its source of tension with the dominant culture. For instance, "client cults" provide personal growth and treatments for their members. Hence they are likely to be opposed by established groups that claim to provide the only legitimate avenue for these services. To give an analogy, Bergin (1980) has noted that psychiatrists and psychologists provide competing services long claimed to be the proper domain of the clergy, including the claim to be authoritative moral agents. Similarly, both London (1964) and Gross (1978) note that in secularized societies, mental health personnel often take the role previously reserved for religious healers. Likewise, Frank (1974) and Ellenberger (1970) have provided authoritative historical analyses of numerous similarities between religious and psychological systems of healing. Illich (1976) has documented the expropriation of health by orthodox medicine. Thus competition between client cults providing unorthodox treatments is likely to create significant tension with powerfully established medical and mental health groups, both of which are heavily sanctioned by the dominant culture.

Further exacerbation is readily understandable in light of the research of Kilbourne and Richardson (1984), indicating that both established therapies and new religious movements attract persons seeking to change identities and to find new meanings in life. However, cults seek to produce more radical change than orthodox therapies, adding to tension (Kilbourne & Richardson, 1984; Schur, 1976). In terms of an ideological surround, the very success of cults is likely to be seen as pathological by representatives of orthodox therapies. To cite but two extreme cases, who would argue for the validity of mass suicide indelibly associated with Jonestown, or the violent murders associated with the Charlie Manson "family"? Yet even in these cases, serious scholars have raised significant questions beyond the stereotype of madness and cults presented in the media. For instance, Zaehner (1974) has argued that Manson's crimes were not merely expressions of psychopathology, but had religious significance as well: "Charlie Manson was sane: he had been *there*, where there is neither good nor evil, and he had read and reread the Book of Revelation. These two facts explain his crime" (p. 18). Likewise, Hall (1989) notes that Jim Jones, who led the mass suicide in Jonestown, cannot simply be understood in psychopathological terms:

> Ironically, Jones has become far more important for the society at large as a symbolic personification of evil than he has in any way to those who share some of the concerns that animated his movement. It is the opponents of Jim Jones who infused him with a charisma powerful enough to make him play the mythic role of scapegoat that cleanses the world of sin, even if they failed to acknowledge that the sin-offering of Jonestown had wider sources than the evil in Jones. (p. 311)

Thus we cannot ignore the religious relevance of even the most extreme of cult leaders. Feuerstein (1992) documents the relevance of madness as a category of the holy, especially for cult leaders. It is important to remember that religious extremism is also a normative part of religious history. We must be cautious not to identify all religion with cultural accommodations and compatibilities. Studies of contemporary militant movements worldwide under the broad umbrella of "fundamentalism" have shown that under appropriate conditions, militant action by religious groups is normative and cannot be attributed to the psychopathology of either leaders or followers (Marty & Appleby, 1994).

Using client cults as an example of an axis of tension identifies conflict between cults and orthodox healers that is not likely to engage massive cultural concern, except in isolated and highly publicized cases. However, an area of tension that cuts across diverse cultural groups and is perpetually a matter of intense concern is sexuality. A cult's violation of sexual norms is likely to elicit retaliatory responses from the dominant culture. We focus upon the social control of sexuality, since claims to legitimate forms of sexual expression have varied and continue to vary immensely, both within and between cultures. Yet few people have no opinion about what is appropriate.

Cults and Sexuality

Relating the control of sexuality to varieties of group formation and cohesion has a long history and firm theoretical grounding. Much of the social psychology of classical Freudian theory identifies group formation as being rooted in the control of sexuality and dyadic intimacy. As an inevitable dimension of tension with society, any form of sexuality can become problematic. The social and cultural history of sexuality is largely a religious history (Parrinder, 1980; Steinberg, 1983; Tennant, 1903/1968). Gardella (1985) has shown how Christianity, especially in North America, promoted a view of sexuality that required it to be both innocent and ecstatic. In English-speaking North America, the celibacy of Catholic priests and nuns has been challenged as abnormal, as was that of the early Shaker communities in the United States (Foster, 1984). The polygamy of early Mormons was violently criticized by a monogamous culture that was also equally opposed to what was perceived as the sexual permissiveness of the early Oneida community, which fostered free sexuality between its members (Foster, 1984).

Although monogamy has been challenged by many religious groups, retaliation is often swift, especially toward groups that put their alternative sexual beliefs into actual practice. Lewis (1989) recounts many instances of carefully constructed cultural atrocity tales directed at Catholics and Mormons, who were accused of using many different techniques of mind control to force persons to be either celibate (in the case of Catholics) or polygamous (in the case of Mormons). As we shall see, these historical instances applied to what are now mainstream religions have numerous parallels in contemporary retaliation toward cults. Lewis's discussion of atrocity tales directed at Catholics and Mormons is described in greater detail in Research Box 9.3.

Even mainstream religions have accommodated themselves to the acceptance of divorce and hence to a form of serial monogamy, seen by some as a form of polygamy. As Freud (1930/1961a, p. 61) noted, there is an antithesis between sexuality and civilization, given that "sexual love is a relationship between two people, in which a third can only be superfluous or disturbing, whereas civilization is founded on relation[ships] between large groups of persons."

Not surprisingly, theorists influenced by Freud have argued for the crucial importance of sexuality in all forms of group formation, not simply religious ones (Badcock, 1980; Marcuse, 1955). Thus we should not be surprised that religious cults are likely to arouse cultural wrath if they modify established norms of sexuality. Likewise, insofar as conversion to a mainstream religious commitment is one of the best predictors of delayed loss of virginity (as noted in Chapter 12), modification of sexual norms within cults is likely to incur retaliation from mainstream churches heavily involved in the sexual socialization of adolescents. For example, the Unification Church has been accused by Horowitz (1983a, p. 181) of being a collectivist organization, and chided in particular for supporting arranged marriages in which persons were married who were "in some cases unfamiliar with each other up to minutes prior to the ceremony." Yet there is firm theological justification for such marriages within the Unification Church (Barker, 1984). Moreover, Lewis (1989) has shown that dyadic intimacy is a factor in cult defection, insofar as among spouses joining cults, the best predictor is that if one partner leaves the cult the other will also leave. Not surprisingly, then, the Unification Church attempts to exert control over dyadic matching in terms of the larger group's interests, as do other religious groups such as the Hare Krishna (Judah, 1974). However, in a culture in which both free choice and romanticism are presumed to direct dyadic selection,

---

RESEARCH BOX 9.3. Catholic and Mormon Atrocity Tales
(Lewis, 1989; see also Gardella, 1985)

The most popular book written in the United States before *Uncle Tom's Cabin* was a pseudoautobiography by one "Marie Monk" titled *Awful Disclosures of the Hotel Dieu Nunnery of Montreal.* With more than a quarter of a million copies sold between 1836 and the Civil War, the book told of licentious sex between priests and nuns; it also told of babies born to nuns and quickly baptized after birth, and bodily dissolved in lye. Despite being thoroughly discredited, this fraudulent text was part of an anti-Catholic genre fueled by exaggerated tales of genuine ex-nuns and of fallen priests that continues today. For instance, tales of priests forcing ladies to confess sexual sins in order to seduce them were common in English-speaking North America before and during the 19th century. *The Priest, the Woman, and the Confessional,* an 1880 book by C. P. T. Chiniquy, is an example of this genre.

If "unnatural" celibacy fueled atrocity tales against nuns and priests, "unnatural" polygamy fueled atrocity tales against Mormons. Paralleling Marie Monk's book was another fabricated story by Marie Ward entitled *Female Life among the Mormons.* Assuming that no conscientious females would accept polygamy, the text accused Mormon males of using hypnotic techniques to force females to accept a presumably unnatural wedded life. Like ex-nuns, ex-Mormon women told elaborately embellished stories accentuating the misery of women under Mormonism. These helped to enrage the larger culture to action against Mormons, ranging from vigilante justice to government action directed against Mormon leaders and practices.

The insistence by a culture that only wedded monogamy is sanctioned by God provides a context within which advocates of other religious sexual practices, whether celibacy or polygamy, must fight to gain legitimacy for these practices.

---

such novel controls on sexual expression are likely to be serious sources of tension (Gardella, 1985). Similar tensions have emerged in studies of celibacy within the Catholic Church. Sipe (1990, p. 293), based upon a limited study of priests who failed to maintain their vows of celibacy, rashly concluded that the Catholic Church supports an archaic anthropological model inappropriate in light of modern understandings of human sexuality. (See Chapter 12 for a discussion of clergy sexual abuse and scandals within the Catholic Church.)

When sexuality is controlled in a manner permitting multiple partners (often several partners are sexually active with a cult leader), the challenge to sexual and religious cultural norms is even more obvious. Wangerin (1993) has documented how "flirty fishing," or the use of sexual favors to gain adherents, created significant tension for the otherwise fundamentalist Children of God/Family of Love. Further confounding their otherwise fundamentalist beliefs is the confusion they have created within fundamentalist circles by supporting masturbation and a generally masculine point of view regarding sexuality (Wangerin, 1993). Chancellor (2000) has written an oral history of this movement, based upon interviews with over 700 members; he has documented the tempering of their sexual views as they continue into subsequent generations. Jacobs (1984, 1987) has documented the fact that some male cults foster romantic idealization of the cult leader by female followers. This leads to what some perceive as sexual abuse and exploitation for those who fail to carry through their attachment to the cult leader. Then, much as in a more normative love relationship, the socioemotional bonds with both the group and the leader must be broken for defection from the cult to occur (as we will see in Chapter 12). With a charismatic male leader and a female follower, the process is accentuated, but similar processes operate in male followers as well.

THE ANTI-CULT MOVEMENT

In a partly tongue-in-cheek paper (a rarity in scientific journals), Kilbourne and Richardson (1986) described a new mental illness, "cultphobia." Although perhaps not to be taken seriously as a claim to defining a pathology, their effort was directed at "putting the shoe on the other foot" (Kilbourne & Richardson, 1986, p. 259). Richardson, a prominent sociologist and a lawyer involved in the study of new religious movements, has been a leader in arguing for researchers to abandon the term "cult" altogether, opposing his own earlier view in support of the concept (Richardson, 1978a, 1979, 1993). More recently, Woody (2009) has argued against the use of the term "cult" in the teaching of the psychology of religion and spirituality. Likewise, there is a huge contemporary debate on how to identify GATTs and whether or not some should be identified as explicitly linked to a particular faith tradition (Byman, 2015). Much of Byman's concern centers upon the well-documented fact that attitudes toward new religious movements are heavily influenced by the mass media, whose presentation of cults has been largely sensationalistic and heavily slanted in a negative direction (van Driel & Richardson, 1988). Few if any distinctions are made among cults. For instance, Patrick and Dulack (1977, p. 11), activists in the anti-cult movement, have stated: "You name 'em. Hare Krishna, the Divine Light Mission, Guru Maharaj Ji, Brother Julius, Love Israel, The Children of God. Not a brown penny's worth of difference between any one of 'em."

The Empirical Study of Resistance to Cults

Empirically, the identification of resistance from groups within the culture is worthy of study. Thus we consider the pejorative connotation cults have acquired within the mass media an important empirical issue—one that is integral to the operationalization of cults as novel forms of subcultural religious deviance. The refusal to differentiate among cults is also worthy of empirical study. As Zimbardo and Hartley (1985) have noted, similar negative views of cults are held by adolescents, regardless of whether or not they have ever had any contact with recruiters for various cults. Yet, as Wallis (1976) has rightly noted, not all authoritative groups are the same. For instance, Scientology has authoritarian features, but most members hold full-time jobs and limit their involvement in terms compatible with their occupation and domestic responsibilities.

The empirical study of hostility toward cults is only one aspect of general tolerance for deviance, which is often examined in political science studies of civil liberties (McClosky & Brill, 1983; Stouffer, 1955; Wilcox et al., 1992). Perhaps the most consistent finding is that education and tolerance are positively correlated. Although numerous challenges and modifications of this finding have been made in specific cases, it remains as a "most durable generalization" (Sullivan, Pierson, & Marcus, 1982, p. 29).

The study of tolerance for new religious movements is almost by definition the study of tolerance for cults. Despite a relatively small literature, empirical studies are congruent with the research on support for civil liberties (Bromley & Breschel, 1992; Robbins, 2001). Within a democratic culture, retaliation against new religious movements can be expressed by attitudes in favor of legal restrictions on cults (Delgado, 1982; Galanter, 1989b; Lifton, 1985; Stander, 1987). Several studies have used this operational indicator in either general or specific cases. For instance, Richardson and van Driel (1984, p. 413) found substantial agreement with the statement that "Legislation should be passed to control the spread of new religions or cults" in a telephone survey of 400 randomly selected voters in Nevada. However, they also noted that some respondents were confused by the phrasing of the question, wanting to control cults but not new religions (Richardson & van Driel, 1984, p. 417). This confusion is consistent with the problem already discussed of negotiating a religious identity for a novel group. Cults are often refused such a label, as many do not perceive them as legitimate religions (Greil, 1993). Thus, while there is generally strong support for the right of freedom of worship for all religions, the support is strongest among educated elites rather than the mass public; it is also tempered when the religions are seen to be too extreme, including cults, which may not be perceived as religious at all (McClosky & Brill, 1983).

When questions are more specific, the attitudes toward legal restrictions on cults are more illustrative. For instance, Bromley and Breschel (1992) utilized four specific issues to assess favorable attitudes toward cult legislation: a ban on cult recruitment of teenagers; the necessity for Federal Bureau of Investigation (FBI) surveillance of cults; the desirability of restricting solicitation by Hare Krishnas at airports; and the question of preventing the Reverend Moon from publishing a newspaper. Overall, they found that a majority of the mass public (66%), but a minority (25%) of the elites, approved of most items. Furthermore, the more religiously involved respondents were more likely to support legislation to control cults. This is consistent with the tension that cults as novel religious forms are likely to have with both secular and sacred groups within mainstream culture. In addition, it is often claimed that claims of "brainwashing" and sexual abuse (especially of children) are often used without empirical documentation, in efforts to discredit cults (Richardson, 1999).

O'Donnell (1993) utilized a similar measure to assess attitudes toward restrictions on new religions. He added an item indicating opposition to Satan worship. Opposition to Satan worship is an important indicator of media influence on cult perception, since empirical research has failed to establish either that there is a large Satanic movement in North America or that Satan worship has any significant following or influence among adolescents (Richardson, Best, & Bromley, 1991; Swatos, 1992). O'Donnell's sample included a mass survey of 1,708 persons and an additional sample of 863 elites, selected from business, government, education, media, and religious leaders. O'Donnell used the five items as a single scale. The responses for the various groups indicated that the academics within the elites had the greatest tolerance, but that among the mass group, education was the best predictor of tolerance. Thus, within the study of new religious movements, tolerance has been found to follow the similar pattern of the "most durable generalization" noted for civil liberties in general.

Still, we must confront a curious phenomenon proposed by some members of intellectual elites—one that medicalizes religious deviance and also suggests a basis for discounting much of the tolerance expressed by both elites and the educated masses toward religious cults. That phenomenon is coercive persuasion, or, in the inadequate vernacular of the popular media, "brainwashing." Here there has clearly been a clear advancement based upon empirical research, which, in Goldman's (2006) opinion, has reached at least "widespread agreement" (p. 89) if not unanimity.

The Question of Cults and Coercive Persuasion

The Medicalization of Deviant Religious Groups

The tendency for educated persons to be tolerant of new religious movements is confounded by controversies surrounding cults and the "medicalization of deviance." Although varying in precise meaning, this term generally refers to efforts to explain commitment to deviant groups in terms of dysfunctional or pathological processes (Conrad & Schnelder, 1980; Kittrie, 1971; Szasz, 1970, 1983, 1984). Thus individuals are assumed to be unable to commit themselves freely to a new religious group. Conversion to cult beliefs and adherence to cult norms are interpreted as symptoms of illness or pathology. Not surprisingly, much of the support for this position comes from clinical psychologists and psychiatrists. For instance, in a series of papers, Clark and his colleagues (Clark, 1978, 1979; Clark, Langone, Schacter, & Daly, 1981) have claimed to clinically identify powerful mental coercion used by cults to create pathological commitments in converts. Likewise, Shapiro (1977) has claimed to have clinically identified a syndrome of "destructive cultism," which includes such phenomena as loss of identity, behavioral changes, estrangement from one's family, and mental control by the cult leader. Finally, Singer and her colleagues (Singer, 1978a, 1978b; Singer & West, 1980; Singer & Ofshe, 1990) have gained a considerable reputation for the clinical treatment of former cult members, whom they have described as "psychiatric casualties."

In opposition to clinical claims are the claims of most empirical researchers, who have found no evidence that cults use unique methods or techniques in order to alter normal psychological processes. Some have seen the empirical response to exaggerated clinical claims as itself overstated. As a result of all this, much of the study of new religious movements has become highly politicized. The process has forced serious debate and disclaimers among investigators as to hidden motives involved in the study of new religious movements (Barker, 1983; Friedrichs, 1973; Horowitz, 1983a, 1983b; Robbins, 1983). This has led to concerns regarding the academic integrity of research on new religious movements in general (Wilson, 1983), as well as challenges to the integrity of researchers personally committed to controversial religions such as Wicca, often simply identified as "witchcraft" (Scarboro, Campbell, & Stave, 1994). In an article title, Segal (1985) has asked this serious question: "Have the Social Sciences Been Converted?" Others have noted that contemporary perspectives in the philosophy of science make distinctions between religious and scientific methods of knowing less distinct, blurring the boundaries of what many have tried to separate (Jones, 1994; Miles, 2007). The debate is most heated when claims to have identified a process of coercive persuasion unique to cults are linked to the popular but scientifically unwarranted concept of "brainwashing," which is perhaps the one term that contributes most to the misunderstanding of cults (Zablocki & Robbins, 2001).

A History of the Concept of Brainwashing

The term "brainwashing" has entered the popular language as a summary term for some loosely defined techniques of coercive persuasion that presumably can make persons adopt beliefs and conform to behaviors they would normally reject. Anthony and Robbins (1994) note that the term was first popularized by Hunter, a U.S. journalist who worked for the Central Intelligence Agency (CIA). This journalist claimed to have identified powerful techniques of thought reform utilized by the Chinese Communists, for which he coined the word "brainwashing" (Hunter,

1951). Research agencies of several governments—including the Nazi SS and Gestapo; the U.S. Office of Strategic Services, forerunner of the CIA; and investigators in Stalinist Russia and Communist China—had been involved in research programs to find effective procedures to obtain information from interrogation of prisoners of war, and to find ways to alter the beliefs of individuals so they would be cooperative with captor governments.

Despite widely exaggerated popular press accounts of the effects of brainwashing techniques, it was quickly recognized that no government had discovered any such techniques that were truly effective. Most efforts to alter beliefs utilized varieties of deception, often combined with the administration of drugs, or with techniques of coercion and force. Although compliance was easily produced by these crude techniques, true belief change was virtually nonexistent. "Compliance" simply means that persons conformed to demands to avoid pain and suffering within a totally controlled environment; however, their true beliefs did not change. Evidence for this was that behavioral compliance disappeared upon release from the environment. Of approximately 7,000 Korean prisoners of war subjected to harsh treatment techniques by the Chinese Communists, 30% died. Of the remainder, only 21 refused repatriation after secession of hostilities, and of these 21, 10 later changed their minds. Hence only 11 cases of over 4,500 survivors actually adopted Chinese Communist beliefs and refused ultimate repatriation (Anthony & Robbins, 1994). Not surprisingly, researchers given access to CIA material concerning all claims to brainwashing noted that no effective techniques existed, and that compliance produced by physical coercion, isolation, propaganda, peer pressure, and intense torture—in a context of total control combined with uncertainty about the future—involved no unknown social-psychological principles (Hinkle & Wolff, 1956). Indeed, the desired effects of mind change measured at repatriation indicated the complete failure of the presumed brainwashing. Thus responsible reviews of the facts indicate that no evidence exists for a technique using advanced psychological knowledge to alter a person's thoughts against his or her will.

Another phrase closely associated with brainwashing is "thought reform," a more adequate description of the Chinese Communists' intent. The term is closely linked to the research of Lifton (1961), a psychiatrist who studied Korean prisoners of war. Both thought reform and brainwashing are linked to what Schein, Schneier, and Barker (1971) have called "coercive persuasion." Although a scientifically inadequate popular literature extols the unlimited power of coercive techniques, the responsible scientific literature is consistent in agreeing (1) that such techniques can produce only limited attitude change, and (2) that such change is highly unstable when controls on the immediate environment are lifted.

Two major varieties of coercive persuasion have been utilized in recent history, the Chinese and the European. Although the two forms overlap, as Somit (1968) has noted, their differences are evident in the extreme forms of expression. European-oriented techniques primarily emphasize obtaining confessions of guilt from presumably innocent persons, typically singly and in isolation. Chinese-oriented techniques focus upon efforts to change a person's total ideological orientation, typically in group situations where many are solicited as volunteers. The Chinese-oriented techniques have much in common with "totalism." Totalism seeks ultimate control of the individual through actual or threatened physical techniques of coercion and torture (see Arendt, 1979; Friedrich & Brzezinski, 1956). It is most often associated with totalitarian states. Totalism assumes the freedom of individuals to resist, and it does not postulate a unique technique or method that can make anyone (regardless of predisposing factors or strength of will) change ideological orientation. As such, it is what

Anthony and Robbins (1994) refer to as a "soft determinism," quite compatible with theories of modern social science. Cults, like many other groups (both religious and secular), seek to attract persons with identifiable predispositions that can be manipulated in such a manner as to persuade the persons to become converts. Of course, such conversions remain intentional actions. They are not the process of some "hard determinant" such as brainwashing that abolishes the capacity to choose (Robbins, 2001). Although American social scientists have thoroughly discredited the concept of "brainwashing," it continues to be utilized as a legitimate concept in some western European countries to control contested religions (Richardson & Introvigne, 2001). This is particularly the case when religion is defined narrowly, so that new religious movements can be denied the label "religion" (Soper, 2001).

The popularization of a brainwashing model is compatible with neither the European nor the Chinese model of coercive persuasion, each developed independently. Although brainwashing is a thoroughly discredited concept, the broad basis of processes involved in coercive persuasion can be readily identified. They are empirically established and have removed the claim of "brainwashing" from contemporary concern with cults (Goldman, 2006, p. 90). Furthermore, the techniques of coercive persuasion that occur in some religious groups characterize any high-commitment group, whether religious or not.

Processes of Coercive Persuasion

Since techniques of coercive persuasion have developed from pragmatic sociopolitical concerns, they have not often been linked to broader theoretical views. Overstated efforts to link a particular technique to a theory, such as Sargent's (1957) appeal to Pavlovian theory, are neither adequate to the totality of coercive persuasion nor supported by sufficient empirical evidence to be generally acceptable. Our summary of the components involved in coercive persuasion focuses only upon what is shared across several responsible efforts to reconstruct, from historical and personal accounts, the processes involved in this kind of influence (Anthony & Robbins, 1994; Bromley & Richardson, 1983; Lifton, 1961; Robbins & Anthony, 1980; Somit, 1968).

1. *Total control and isolation.* Persons are isolated (individually or in small groups), under the absolute control of authorities.
2. *Physical debilitation and exhaustion.* Persons are physically exhausted and debilitated. Causes can include constant interrogation and/or continual prodding from peers, as well as sleep and food deprivation. In extreme cases, physical torture and starvation may be used.
3. *Confusion and uncertainty.* Personal belief systems and entire ideological orientations are challenged. Persons' uncertainty about their own fate is linked to uncertainty concerning their beliefs and values.
4. *Guilt and humiliation.* A sense of guilt and personal humiliation is induced by a variety of techniques. All are directed at making a potential convert feel unworthy if he or she persists in maintaining present commitments.
5. *Release and resolution.* An absolute framework provides only a single "out." Suicide is prohibited unless it is a collective action of the group. Only by compliance or full conversion can individuals gain release from the isolation, pain, guilt, and confusion induced in them by their persuaders.

It is readily apparent that coercive techniques of persuasion are seldom of an all-or-none nature. It is best to talk about degrees of coercive persuasion, ranging from the extremes of the techniques applied to prisoners of war, to the middle-range examples of draftees into the military, and then to the minimal extremes (say, a religious summer camp to which parents may send a reluctant child). Although the degree of compliance is rather straightforwardly linked to degree of control, actual conversion or internalization of beliefs is less clearly empirically understood. What is certain is that conversion is much rarer than compliance under any system of coercive persuasion. However, as Somit (1968) has noted, compliance achieved by extreme coercive persuasion has its own limits:

> To be successful it demands a uniquely structured and controlled environmental setting and an inordinate investment in time and manpower. Despite the cost entailed, its effectiveness is limited to individual subjects or, even under the optimum conditions, to a small group of persons. (p. 142)

Coercive Persuasion/"Brainwashing" and Cults: A Contemporary Appeal to a Discredited Process

It is readily apparent that popular interest in new religious movements and cults cannot be explained by such pseudoscientific concepts as brainwashing. Nor has the term been thoroughly discredited in the contexts within which it was first applied, since no powerful psychological technique to mandate beliefs or behaviors exists. Techniques of coercive persuasion are readily identifiable and work by methods well established in the social sciences. Yet these techniques are variously associated with a variety of groups and in no sense differentially or uniquely characterize cults.

For some, the popularity of new religious movements to which close friends or relatives convert is troublesome. Yet serious issues of value and lifestyle differences are sidestepped by essentially rhetorical schemes directed at delegitimizing cults. The Unification Church has been a particular target of such schemes (Robbins, 1977). For others, new religious movements can be discredited if an explanation for conversion can be offered that denies it was voluntary. Pseudoscientific terms such as "snapping" (Conway & Siegelman, 1978) and "mentacide" (Shapiro, 1977, p. 80) have been coined. Not only do such terms lack real scientific credibility; claims to a "cult syndrome" have never been substantiated, even in terms of the data provided by the most passionate champions of the claim. For instance, despite the popular appeal of one text—*Snapping: America's Epidemic of Sudden Personality Change* (Conway & Siegelman, 1978), which claims to document a "cult withdrawal syndrome"—few of the claims have withstood scientific scrutiny (Kilbourne, 1983; Kirkpatrick, 1988; Lewis & Bromley, 1987). Yet such claims are widely reported in the popular media, paralleling for new religious movements what historically occurred in terms of political ideologies (Verdier, 1977). This medicalization of the process of conversion is only part of the larger issue of the medicalization of deviance, which Robbins and Anthony (1979) have termed the "medicalization of religion." In a word, however thoroughly discredited the concept of brainwashing may be, the acceptance of brainwashing is the major way in which those who oppose conversion to cults have attempted to circumvent what would otherwise be rights of choice protected by the First Amendment to the U.S. Constitution (Anthony & Robbins, 1992).

This contemporary appeal to a discredited process follows the similar fallacious reasoning used previously to discredit political views. Applied to cults, as novel (and hence, to some, threatening) religious views, brainwashing or "snapping" implies that a person's ability to withstand such practices is severely limited. Comments offered to support a person's conversion to cult beliefs and practices are used as criteria for mental aberration, rather than as evidence of a successful search for an alternative religious view by a competent individual. When doctrines are viewed as symptoms of pathology, the process by which the individual was coerced to adopt such views is the target of concern, not the content of the beliefs or the religiously informed lifestyle the beliefs support. The right to choose even unpopular alternatives is denied to converts if the rhetorical strategies of those who would pathologize the process are successful (Robbins & Anthony, 1979).

Ironically, a largely self-fulfilling prophecy of what the rhetoricians of brainwashing fear most is realized in the anti-cult movement, portions of which support "deprogramming." Deprogrammers utilize many of the techniques of coercive persuasion to undo the presumed effects of brainwashing. The fact that cults appeal disproportionately to the young, and to others who are often in opposition to mainstream culture, fuels the anti-cult movement (Barker, 1986). Almost by definition, youths who join cults are abandoning the faiths of their parents (whether these are secular or religious). As discussed in Chapter 5, interpersonal factors are an important factor in religious conversion among youths. Not surprisingly, then, parent–youth conflict is both a motivating factor for conversion to cults and often a consequence of such conversion (Pilarzyk, 1978).

Parent–youth conflict plays a major role in deprogramming controversies, in which often parents must be granted legal rights to remove their children forcefully from cult groups. These legal issues are complex in their own right, and are confounded by the courts' need to evaluate scientific claims that are hotly disputed among those who defend or oppose cults as expert witnesses (Beckford, 1979; Delgado, 1977; Lemoult, 1978; Robbins, 1985; Zablocki & Robbins, 2001). Paradoxically, this has led to several studies of the process of deprogramming, as there are no identifiable studies on the processes of "brainwashing" presumably utilized by some of the more controversial cults (Kim, 1979). Although some have tried to sensationalize deprogramming as a new rite of exorcism (Shupe, Spielman, & Stigall, 1977) and to depict anti-cultists as themselves pathological (Kilbourne & Richardson, 1986), such rhetoric among researchers is best taken as empirical evidence for the necessity of paying serious attention to issues of the ideological surround, which inevitably inform social-scientific research. The actual empirical techniques of deprogrammers are no less mysterious than are coercive persuasive techniques. The ability of deprogrammers to isolate their subjects, with extensive control over their environment, permits them to utilize established procedures to reconvert cult members. Kim (1979) has summarized this process as involving three steps: (1) motivating the persons to "unfreeze" their commitment to the cult; (2) providing information that requires the reevaluation of cult beliefs in light of the beliefs to which the persons are to be "reconverted"; and (3) obtaining a "refreezing" of the supported perspective to which the persons are now recommitted.

Cults' Actual Ability to Retain and Recruit Members

Ironically, despite controversies surrounding cult practices, the majority of cult members are not likely to stay converted. As we have noted in Chapter 8, most converts to new religious groups are "seekers" who explore a variety of beliefs and lifestyles, many associated with the new religious movements. Most cults, by their very nature, can be expected to appeal permanently only to a minority of followers. The inability of any group in a pluralist society to maintain complete social isolation, totally regulate its members' lifestyles, channel dyadic intimacy, and articulate and defend one authoritative ideology (to cite but a few examples) assures that cults will have high rates of turnover (Wright, 1987). Furthermore, most voluntary defectors from cults feel neither angry nor duped over the experience. Most feel wiser for the experience, even though they were unwilling to stay cult members.

Not only do cults have significant voluntary turnover of members; their ability to recruit members through coercive techniques is severely limited, especially in a society where civil liberties are protected. For instance, in Galanter's (1989a) study of Unification Church induction workshops, those who agreed to attend were followed in terms of the success of eight of these workshops to persuade attendees actually to join. Of 104 participants in the workshops, 71 dropped out within 2 days; another 29 dropped out between 2 and 9 days; and an additional 17 dropped out after 9 days. Only 9 workshop participants actually stayed over 21 days to join the Unification Church. Thus Galanter (1989a) found that even among persons self-selected to be receptive to recruitment workshops where mild degrees of coercive persuasion were used, the vast majority failed to join. Barker (1984) replicated Galanter's findings with a sample of over 1,000 workshop participants in London 1 year later. She noted that after 2 years, far fewer than 1% of workshop participants were associated with the Unification Church, despite the fact that workshop participants were likely to be favorably predisposed to the Unification Church and presumably were the targets of powerful coercive techniques (Johnson, 1979). Contrary to media claims, the failure to successfully recruit large numbers of persons who voluntarily stay with deviant religious groups is typical of all cult recruitment and retention efforts.

Part of the consensus of research on contested religious groups is that most persons who are recruited by such groups never actually join, and that the majority of those who do leave within a year (Goldman, 2006). Thus Goldman (2006, pp. 91–92) recommends that social scientists reclaim "cult" as a legitimate term and educate the public about the factual characteristics of such contested religious groups. Likewise, Stark (1996) has emphasized that insofar as cults are cohesive spiritual groups that demand personal sacrifice and are in high tension with their host cultures, it is easy to dismiss them by claiming they have powers over members that in fact they do not possess. Voluntary submission to high-commitment groups that utilize coercive techniques has long characterized religious groups. Sorokin (1954/2002, pp. 309–355) has described how these techniques were effectively utilized in medieval monastic communities. Poloma and Hood (2008), in a 4-year study of a contemporary cult group in Atlanta, Georgia, demonstrated the failure of the cult to produce changes in homeless persons (except for limited behavioral compliance when the homeless individuals were voluntarily confined in order to receive shelter and food).

Cults: Discussion and Summary

The research on cult recruitment suggests that the controversy surrounding new religious movements is not simply an issue of the processes employed to attract and convert members. It is more likely one of the significant tensions that mainstream religious and secular groups have with novel religions, which solicit and legitimate diverse interpretations and modes of confrontation with sacred and symbolic realities. Hence, even in the most extreme cases, we must be careful not to naively utilize and uncritically accept delegitimizing modes of explanation for perspectives different from our own (Barker, 1984). The tendency to explain away beliefs and practices distant from our own through labels for the processes presumed to be operating, which need not take the content of beliefs into account, is a pervasive tendency in the social sciences.

Yet, as Kroll-Smith (1980) has shown, even the most private experiences of members of deviant religious groups are influenced by normal social-psychological processes. Several studies show that conversion to new religious groups helps individuals adapt to social and cultural change, of which these groups by definition are a part (Lebra, 1970; Turner, 1979; Weigert, D'Antonio, & Rubel, 1971). Even converts to deviant religious groups are often socialized by the process of conversion to accept other mainstream cultural values (Johnson, 1961). In addition, deviant religious groups socialize people into subcultures within which otherwise maladaptive behaviors are functional (Lewellen, 1979). Also, we cannot underestimate the power of such variant religious bodies to reconceptualize commonly accepted social realities, so that they both justify participation in, and legitimate the continuance of, what to mainstream culture are at best puzzling but acceptable instances of subcultural deviance (Festinger, Riecken, & Schachter, 1956; Weiser, 1974). This is particularly true of many of the practices of cult leaders, whose behaviors to an outsider appear to be no more than trickery, chicanery, or pathology (Feuerstein, 1992).

The failure of cults to be differentially associated with pathology must be emphasized. It has not yet been confirmed empirically that cults either attract or produce pathology when pathology is judged independently of the cults' own behavioral norms. For instance, Galanter (1983, 1989a) notes that deviant sects actually avoid recruiting persons who show obvious pathological characteristics. Likewise, Ungerleider and Welish (1979) have documented the absence of obvious pathology in former and current members of a variety of cults. Finally, Taslimi, Hood, and Watson (1991) failed to substantiate previous claims to pathology in a follow-up study of former members of a fundamentalist Jesus commune, Shiloh. Furthermore, the earlier claims about the presumably maladaptive characteristics of these members while in the Jesus commune failed to account appropriately for the fact that objective indices of maladaptive behavior must be judged within the particular context; behaviors that were otherwise less functional outside the commune may have been adaptive for members inside the commune (Richardson, Stewart, & Simmonds, 1979; Simmonds, 1977b). In fact, Robbins and Anthony (1982) have critically reviewed the relevant empirical literature and concluded that members of deviant religious groups are socially integrated on many criteria:

1. Likely termination of illicit drug use.
2. Renewed vocational motivation.
3. Mitigation of neurotic distress.
4. Suicide prevention.
5. Decrease in anomie/moral confusion.
6. Increase in social compassion/responsibility.
7. Decrease in psychosomatic symptoms.
8. Improved self-actualization.
9. Clarified sense of identity.
10. Generally positive problem-solving assistance.

Finally, it must be emphasized that judgments of the relative value of identities and lifestyles are inevitably beyond the ability of social sciences to resolve factually. Efforts to set criteria for authentic spiritual choices must be individually and collectively made, but their existential base is never simply resolved by factual descriptions or explanations of the processes by which such choices are made. Although research clearly demonstrates that identities linked to divergent social groups increase the prejudice of such groups toward one another, the ability of groups to identify superordinate goals (which can only be achieved by the cooperation of all groups) reduces conflict and prejudice (Sherif, 1953). Thus the seeking of superordinate goals that transcend religious groupings and require the collective effort of all to achieve is a worthwhile project, however ambitious it may be, if prejudices and conflicts among religious groups are to be reduced (Anthony, Ecker, & Wilbur, 1987).

GROUPS THAT ADVOCATE TERRORIST TACTICS

Much of the concern with cults has shifted in the last few years to a concern with terrorist groups. Much of what is known about joining and resisting cults applies to GATTs. However, as Jones (2008, p. 8) has argued, terrorism is best conceived as a tactic and not as a defining characteristic of a group. Terrorism as a tactic links GATTs to the Allport tradition, in that terror as a means (extrinsic motivation) may be used for intrinsic ends, and thus GATTs become religious cults. The disjunction between means and ends characterizes not only terrorism, but the response to terrorism as well (Hood, 2011). Thus the effort to restrict terrorism to purely political groups (Pape, 2005) or to only political aims and motives (Hoffman, 2006) is too limiting. Terrorism as a technique can be and is used to achieve sacred ends, and, again, this links GATTs to established research on cults (Hall, 1989; Moghaddam et al., 2013). Galanter (2013) identifies GATTs as cults; he sees them as a subset of charismatic groups that are characterized by a shared belief system, a high level of social cohesiveness, and strict behavioral norms centered upon a perceived charismatic leadership (which may be perceived to be divine). Thus more and more GATTs are now classified as religious, as the leaders and aims of these groups are embedded in a search to defend or implement sacred goals.

As Moghaddam et al. (2013, p. 632) have noted, the U.S. State Department's list of foreign terrorist organizations now describes only about 40% of these groups as being *non*religious organizations. However, it is often hard to separate political from religious ends, especially in traditions and groups that view their cultures as driven by and committed to religious values. The distinction between terrorism as an end and terror as a means in the service of achieving religious ends should also caution us against identifying terrorism with any particular religious tradition. For instance, efforts to identify Islam with terrorism are simply erroneous. To speak about "Islamic terrorism" is to imply that Islam as a faith tradition is more prone to violence than other faith traditions are. However, terrorism and violence have been associated with many religious traditions, as documented by the six-volume series known as *The Fundamentalism Project*, beginning with *Fundamentalism Observed* (Marty & Appleby, 1994) and ending with *Strong Religion* (Almond, Appleby, & Sivan, 2002). Even identifying fundamentalism with militancy conceptually forestalls asking the appropriate empirical question as to the conditions under which various fundamentalist religious groups are willing to use violence as a means to achieve their religious ends (Hood, Hill, & Williamson, 2005, pp. 2–3). As we shall shortly note, the use of violence as an end rarely characterizes any religious group. Likewise, nonviolence rarely characterizes any religious group as well, and rarely any nation-state (Hood, 2011). Thus we speak of religious groups that endorse terrorism and or violence as a means, and not of "terrorist religious groups," much less of any specific faith tradition as inherently "terrorist."

As noted above in regard to cults, most members of extreme religious groups are neither pathological nor committed to violence as an end. Hoffman (2006) has stated that violence or the threat of violence is a necessary defining condition for GATTs—but its aim, as Pape (2005) has noted, is a specific strategy that in terms of our discussion become not simply a set of secular acts, but acts of martyrdom. Members of GATTs are notoriously hard to study. Groebel (1989, p. 25) has observed that such "groups are rarely open to direct observation and do not usually volunteer for scientific interviews." However, Moghaddam (2006) has broken through this barrier and has presented an illuminating portrait of members of GATTs. His portrait is congruent with most research, in that it depicts members of GATTs as nonpathological (Horgan, 1999; Pape, 2005; Jones, 2008; Moghaddam et al., 2013). Within GATTs, terrorism is often viewed as necessitated by resistance to what is perceived as an occupying army from a foreign nation, especially when that nation is committed to a religion not indigenous to the country or region occupied. Under such circumstances, even suicide bombings are seen as rational acts of martyrdom (Pape, 2005).

The Staircase Model

Moghaddam (2005) has initially developed a "stairway" model used not as a conceptual model to be empirically tested, but rather as a helpful metaphor. It suggests a gradual process whereby, in a similar fashion of coercive persuasion models associated with cults, individuals can reach a final "stair" where they comply with the demands of martyrdom in terms of the internalized goals of the group. His model has a "foundational" ground floor occupied by most individuals, where the focus is on perceived fairness and justice. The quotation marks around "foundational" are used in Moghaddam's initial presentation of his model (2005, p. 162). However, in a presentation of his model in a handbook chapter, the emphasis in the description of those on the ground floor is upon fundamentalists, who are seen as particularly likely to be threatened by existing conditions (Moghaddam et al., 2013, p. 638). Likewise, the discussion in the handbook chapter focuses upon Muslims, whereas in the initial article the staircase model is kept general, although there is reference to anti-Americanism in the Middle East and North Africa (Moghaddam, 2005, p. 164). While the staircase model can be applied in reference to specific faith traditions, the linkage of Muslims, fundamentalism, and violence must be carefully circumscribed. The initial presentation of the model as a more general model of coercive processes may be the more appropriate, lest the impression be given that somehow a particular faith tradition is more prone than others to use terrorism as a means, when this is decidedly not the case. Our own summary of Moghaddam's general staircase model is presented in Figure 9.2 and can be compared to Moghaddam et al.'s (2013, p. 638, Figure 32.1) more specific rendering of the model.

Stair 5: Sidestepping of inhibition to allow terrorist acts

Stair 4: Categorical thinking and perceived legitimacy of group

Stair 3: Moral engagement

Stair 2: Displacement of aggression

Stair 1: Perceived options to fight unfair treatment

Ground Floor: Psychological interpretation of material conditions

FIGURE 9.2. Heuristic model of the "staircase to terrorism." Based on Moghaddam (2005, pp. 162–168) and Moghaddam, Warren, and Love (2013, p. 638).

Examining Religious Traditions of Violence and Nonviolence in Context

Even if we explore Muslim groups that use violence as a means, we must be sensitive to the fact that Islam has a long tradition of *jihad*, or holy war (Ruthven, 1984). Furthermore, few religious groups renounce all violence as a means; even states with religious diversity reserve the right to utilize violence in defense of the state. It is a mistake to think that Islam is inherently a violent religion, and it would be inappropriate to fail to understand the conditions under which believers might feel justified in acting violently against those whom their tradition feels must be opposed. For instance, it is often claimed that violence in the expression of one's faith (as in Islamic fundamentalist protest movements that utilize force) is necessarily fanatical and fueled by only negative characteristics, such as paranoia and authoritarianism (Dekmejian, 1985). However, empirical studies of actual violent protesters who are still alive and imprisoned fail to support such claims. For example, a well-known study by Saad Eddin Ibrahim (1980, 1982) focused upon participants imprisoned for Islamic militancy. Ibrahim (1980, p. 427) defined Islamic militancy as "actual violent group behavior committed collectively against the state or other actors in the name of Islam." Members of two militant Islamic groups in Egypt (the Islamic Liberation Organization and Repentance of the Holy Flight) who had actually been imprisoned for Islamic militancy failed to confirm stereotypes related to any supposed personality characteristics of religious fanaticism. The prisoners were predominantly students or recent university graduates in the sciences and medicine, with median ages in the mid-20s, and clearly had achieved greater educational success than their parents. They were motivated by Islamic ideals and felt justified in the use of force to obtain these ideals.

Similar justifications were claimed by Malcolm X in his quest for social justice as framed within the Black Muslim religion. Research Box 9.4 presents a study comparing attitudes toward Malcolm X and Martin Luther King, Jr. among lower-socioeconomic-status black and white males.

Hoffman (1995, p. 225) has presented a summary of Muslim fundamentalists' psychosocial profiles and concluded that the resurgence of Islamic fundamentalism often leads to the discounting of its more violent sects as "crazy," even though such claims lack empirical grounding. It is unlikely that the willingness to use force to achieve one's aims is likely to be other than a source of tension with the host culture or the global community at large. However, such aims and their forceful means can have meaningful religious justifications and make sense to some. Within the notion of an ideological surround (again, see Chapter 12 for a fuller discussion of this concept), every action motivated by faith must be understood from the perspective of the actors involved, and not by some standard outside their perspective. Moghaddam et al. (2013) have provided a useful exposition of the beliefs and motivations of members of GATTs, supporting the consensus of most researchers that psychopathology plays a minimal role (if any) in contributing to our understanding of these members. Clearly, one major source of tension is the claim of GATTs to a legitimate use of violence to achieve their aims, even when this is framed within a religious perspective (Jones, 2008; Kressel, 2007; Moghaddam, 2006).

However, we should also note that few faith traditions unequivocally endorse the use of nonviolence (such as that of Martin Luther King, Jr.) as the only means to achieve or defend sacred goals—even though, as Miles (2004) has argued, it may be that nonviolence is an evolutionary preadaptation. The pivotal issue is that evolutionary preadaptive traits developed in one context may prove to be adaptive in unanticipated future environments. While we are not exclusively committed to an evolutionary model, it is useful, in that it highlights

RESEARCH BOX 9.4. Malcolm X and Martin Luther King, Jr. as Cultural Icons
(Hood, Morris, Hickman, & Watson, 1995)

Malcolm X and Martin Luther King, Jr. (hereafter referred to as "Malcolm" and "Martin") both framed their protests against perceived injustice in religious terms. A major difference in the means they advocated to achieve their visions was in the justification of violence. Malcolm, taking the Black Muslim view, refused to reject violence as a means; Martin, taking the Christian view, did reject it. Hood and his colleagues reasoned that the acceptance of Martin and Malcolm would differ among culturally alienated lower-socioeconomic-status black and white males.

Using a semantic differential scale to measure both evaluative assessments (i.e., approval) and potentiality assessments (i.e., estimates of power) of Malcolm and Martin, they found that black and white males did differ as predicted. The following table presents the most relevant summary of these results.

	Evaluating rating		Potentiality rating	
	Martin	Malcolm	Martin	Malcolm
Black males				
Mean	36.19	44.66	33.02	46.17
SD	9.95	6.96	9.35	5.79
White males				
Mean	32.13	24.87	30.49	47.28
SD	9.81	7.76	8.06	5.26

Analyses of these data indicated that black males evaluated Martin more highly, and Malcolm much more highly, than did white males. On potentiality, both black and white males thought Malcolm much stronger than Martin. The investigators suggested that these data are consistent with the grudging preference of Martin over Malcolm among whites, precisely because Martin's rejection of violence made him less of a threat than Malcolm's willingness to use violence if necessary. Thus the justification of violence as a means is a clear source of tension for cults within their host cultures.

that nonviolence may be a necessary adaptation for humankind's survival. If nonviolence is seen as preadaptive, we can seek exemplars in modern history in such figures as Mahatma Gandhi and Dr. King. Both actively opposed evil, and each demanded the use of nonviolence, refusing to make a distinction between the means used to eradicate evil and evil itself. Perhaps this was most evident in Gandhi's commitment to *satyagraha*—a concept with no easy English equivalent, but one perhaps best summarized as "the force of nonviolence." Hence *satyagraha* is far from passive, seeking to eradicate evil by means that themselves are not tainted with evil (Bondurant, 1965). Perhaps in Western Christianity the Quakers have most forcefully expressed this view. It is well over 300 years since the Quakers declared to King Charles II of England, "We utterly deny all outward wars and strife, and fighting with outward weapons, for any end, or under any pretense whatever; this is our testimony to the whole world" (quoted in Olson & Christiansen, 1966, p. 141). Still, this total commitment to nonviolence remains the exception rather than the rule.

Thus, few groups, religious or not, categorically reject the use of violence—and while terrorism is seldom an end in and of itself for any group, its use as a means is perceived as necessary in some contexts. Indeed, some groups even applaud suicide as martyrdom. As Galanter (2013, p. 731) notes, "Even if a terrorist attack is the goal, this act can be justified as serving the needs of the group, needs that take primacy over the individual's basic desire for a longer life." It may be that GATTs are more productively contrasted with those few groups that deny the use of violence as a means under all conditions than with other groups in general. In the face of ultimate perceived threats, incongruent means and ends seem to characterize most groups, religious or otherwise (Hood, 2013). In another line of research, studies are beginning to explore the effect of terrorism on believers within countries in which GATTs operate in the name of those countries' own faith traditions (Khan, Watson, & Chen, 2016).

GATTS: Discussion and Summary

We have deliberately interwoven our discussion of more extreme religious groups such as cults and GATTs with general processes well documented in the psychology of religion. We do so in order to suggest that what is already known about social-psychological processes in religious participation is likely to be the best starting point for extrapolating studies from within cultures to a more global dimension. Differences will probably emerge, but only if they are examined in the light of established processes that have already been well documented empirically, If there is a generalization that most clearly emerges, it is in the dynamics of the embrace of "more spiritual than religious" identifications among those for whom religious beliefs are more fluid and negotiable, as opposed to those for whom religious beliefs are foundational and seen as absolute and non-negotiable—even to the extent that terrorism emerges as a significant force on a global scale.

SOCIAL-PSYCHOLOGICAL PROCESSES IN RELIGIOUS PARTICIPATION

Are Religion and Mainline Religious Groups Doomed to Extinction?

It has been 50 years since two of the major researchers in the sociology of religion raised the issue of whether or not North America was entering a post-Christian era (Stark & Glock, 1968). A major factor in their questioning was survey research documenting a decline in what many perceived as core Christian beliefs—most centrally, the belief in the divinity of Christ. Stark and Glock (1968) provided a pessimistic prediction for mainline Christian denominations:

> As matters now stand we can see little long-term future for the church as we know it. A remnant church can be expected to last for a long time if only to provide the psychic comforts which are currently dispensed by orthodoxy. However, eventually substitutes for even this function are likely to emerge leaving churches of the present with no effective rationale for existing. (p. 210)

In a similar vein, the renowned anthropologist Wallace (1966) argued that all supernatural beliefs are doomed to extinction, presumably along with the churches that rely upon such beliefs for the effectiveness of their rituals.

However, associated with predictions of the eventual extinction of churches and supernatural beliefs are two assumptions that can be seriously questioned. One is that religious beliefs and church attendance are heavily correlated, and hence that changes in the one can be used to infer changes in the other. It is assumed that people who change religious beliefs are likely to lower their rate of church attendance, or that persons who lower their rate of church attendance have probably changed beliefs. Yet belief and attendance are far from perfectly correlated, and one can be a very poor predictor of the other (Demerath, 1965). Second, the evidence (largely derived from Gallup Poll data) suggesting declines in church attendance is confounded by variations within denominational groups. For instance, Greeley (1972) documented an increase in church attendance among Catholics, associated with a decrease in commitment to orthodox Catholic beliefs. There is no paradox in these findings when we realize that persons attend churches for a variety of reasons, many of which are only marginally related to belief issues. Furthermore, we have noted earlier that as denominational attendance falters, sectarian and cult commitments are likely to increase, so that overall levels of religious group participation may remain strong. Yet before we accept evidence for the decline in mainstream denominations, it behooves us to consider denominations that are similar to the sects and cults in terms of ideological and behavioral strictness, even though their norms are less in tension with the dominant culture than are the more extreme norms of either sects or cults.

The Kelley Thesis and Iannaccone's Modification of It: Strictness Contingencies

While many social scientists were predicting doom for traditional Christian denominations, one investigator burst onto the scene with a book that stimulated much controversy and continues to generate empirical research. Kelley (1972) argued that overall decline in church attendance, especially among North American Protestants, masked two contradictory trends: The more liberal and ecumenical denominations were declining in membership, while the more conservative and fundamentalist denominations were increasing in membership. Ironically, then, the more a religious group was accommodating itself to mainstream culture, the less effectively it was maintaining its membership.

Strict groups are likely to be sectarian in nature, demanding a purity that the more lenient denominations relax as they universalize and welcome a diverse membership, which itself is accommodating to the pluralism of mainstream modern or postmodern culture. Like sects, both cults and groups that endorse terrorism demand seriousness and strictness that are inappropriate to broader universalizing tendencies. Hence Kelley's thesis is compatible with our earlier discussion of sects as acceptable forms of subcultural deviance, and of cults and GATTs as more problematic forms of religious deviance that elicit cultural retaliation. Kelley's thesis is strongly stated. Though it needs conceptual refinement, it does have the merit of identifying the postulated determinants of church growth in terms capable of empirical investigation (Bouma, 1979; Perry & Hoge, 1981). However, this thesis is far from a general covering law (Tamney, 2002).

Still other investigators have focused upon a modification of Kelley's thesis. Unlike Kelley, Iannaccone (1994) focused upon organizational strength rather than simply growth. He also operationalized strictness in terms of the costs of organizational membership, and avoided a potential tautology by using as indicators of "cost" only activities defined as being outside normal church activities. Furthermore, Iannaccone (1996) persuasively described the methodological limitations of testing the Kelley thesis across denominations, arguing instead that a fair test of the thesis requires comparing strictness within groups of the same denomination. Olson and Perl (2001) found support for Iannaccone's modification of the Kelley thesis across five different denominations. Although strictness did not systematically correlate with measures of religious commitment within denominations, it did across denominations.

Although empirical investigation is continuing, Kelley's thesis and especially Iannaccone's modification of the theory (in terms of both its conceptualization and the most appropriate statistical procedures to test the theory) suggest that strictness does indeed lead to greater religious commitment, if not simply church growth. However, growth and strictness are not unrelated. Research Box 9.5 indicates that in the Amish tradition, growth and strictness are dynamically interrelated, insofar as strictness may aid in retaining children within the tradition and hence may contribute to church growth (Kraybill, 1994). Hood and Williamson (2008b) have documented the same for the serpent-handling sects of Appalachia.

RESEARCH BOX 9.5. Four Amish Traditions (Kraybill, 1994)

The Amish are not simply a homogeneous group, and their tension with modern culture varies among the different Amish affiliations. Ninety percent of all Amish belong to one of four affiliations. Three of these emerged from the original Old Order Amish, founded in 1809. Kraybill identifies the first of these newer affiliations, the Swartzentrubers, as "legendary for their stubborn traditionalism" (1994, p. 55). For instance, indoor bathrooms are still strictly forbidden in this order of the Amish, founded in 1913. A dispute over the shunning of Andy Weaver for affiliating with a Mennonite group led to a second new Amish affiliation in 1952. In 1968, a third new affiliation emerged, whose members were more accommodating to modern culture. In Kraybill's terms, these New Order Amish developed "a more rational and individualist understanding of Christian faith" (1994, p. 57). Where reliable data are available, they support the fact that the stricter the Amish affiliation, the greater the ability to retain children, as noted in the following table.

	Swartzentruber	Andy Weaver	Original Old Order	New Order
Degree of traditionalism	Extreme	High	Moderate	Low
Estimated no. in affiliation	2,500	2,750	14,400	2,750
Average no. of children	*a*	5.9	5.1	4.9
Percentage of children affiliated with Amish	90	95	86	57
Percentage of families retaining all their children	*b*	95	88	72

Note. Data from Kraybill (1994, pp. 57, 73).
*a*Not reported, but estimated to be generally larger than in the other three affiliations.
*b*Not reported, but estimated to be 90–95% by local informants.

ATHEISTS, AGNOSTICS, AND SECULARISTS

It would be a mistake to think that individuals who, to use Wuthnow's (1998) terms, either "dwell" within religious groups or become spiritual "seekers" exhaust the possible dynamics of the relationships between individuals and religious groups. Fuller (2001) reminds us that there have always been people whom he identifies in modern terms as "neither religious nor spiritual." Fuller estimates their total in the contemporary United States to be about 15%. These persons include atheists, agnostics, and secularists. In many European countries, their numbers are larger than in the United States; psychologists should thus be cautioned against a too-easy reductionism of religious experiences to built-in biological tendencies (Chapter 3) or to natural tendencies selected by evolution (Chapter 8).

Streib and his colleagues have taken the lead in identifying variations in nonbelief as a dynamic process associated with changes in the religious field (Streib, 2008; Streib & Klein, 2013; Streib & Hood, 2016). Rather than focusing upon substantive definitions of atheism, agnosticism, and apostasy, these investigators contend that "Each concept is dynamic and includes experiential, moral, ritual, and participatory dimensions" (Streib & Klein, 2013, p. 714). One simple descriptive fact emerging from this research is that persons raised in homes where religion is absent tend to remain unaffiliated with religion when they mature (Streib, 2007).

However, the fact that persons are unaffiliated with any religion does not necessarily mean that they are not spiritual seekers. Those identified as "spiritual but not religious" have always played a role in American culture. Fuller (2001) refers to them as the "unchurched" and estimates their present proportion of the U.S. population at about 21%. He also notes that the recent "discovery" of these groups by social scientists fails to take into account that they have always been integral to U.S. religious history. By contrast, genuine atheists, agnostics, and secularists are rare in America but fairly common in many western European countries (Streib & Klein, 2013; Streib & Hood, 2016).

In their ongoing study of the dynamics involved in the spiritual landscapes of Germany and the United States, Streib et al. (2009) noted that among deconverts (defined as those who had left a religious tradition), 172 out of 1,113 in the United States identified themselves as being "spiritual rather than religious" (15.5%), while 171 of 773 in Germany so identified (22%). However, this does not mean that those who self-identify as "more spiritual than religious" are atheists or nonbelievers. Even when they deliberately sampled those identifying themselves as "neither religious nor spiritual," Streib and Hood (2016) found that 107 of 1,110 Americans (9.65%) also identified as atheists or nonbelievers, but that 65 of 1,110 (5.8%) explicitly did not identify themselves as such. The corresponding figures for their German sample were 94 of 763 (12.2%) identifying as atheists or nonbelievers, and 77 of 763 (10%) explicitly not identifying themselves as such. Thus it is crucial, to focus upon the dynamic nature of atheism, agnosticism, and apostasy. Moreover, efforts to illuminate changes in the dynamics of the religious field are limited if only cross-sectional data are interpreted; longitudinal data are sorely needed.

Keysar and Kosmin (2007, p. 18) noted that from 1999 to 2001, the number of Americans reporting no religious identification doubled. They reported statistics from the 2001 American Religious Identification Survey (ARIS), a nationally representative telephone survey of over 50,000 Americans, described in Chapter 6. The ARIS data revealed that 14% of these Americans claimed "none" when asked for their religious identification, and that only 1% of those rejecting religion gave a positive secular alternative such as "humanist." In addition to this 14%, 5% of the respondents refused to answer the question about religious identification, summing to 19%. Of this 19%, 5% either agreed or strongly agreed that God does not exist (Keysar & Kosmin, 2007, p. 19). However, persons who self-identified as atheists accounted for only 1%, suggesting that persons who do not believe that God exists nevertheless do not necessarily identify themselves as atheists. For some, it is not necessary to reject a belief in God; they are simply socialized not to believe.

Pasquale (2007) studied persons in the U.S. Northwest who were unchurched but defined themselves in a variety of ways. Table 9.4 provides the descriptors with which Pasquale's respondents chose to identify themselves. It also indicates for each group the extent to which they rated themselves as "spiritual" and "religious" on a 9-point scale. Inspection of Table 9.4 reveals that, first, regardless of self-identification, all groups rated themselves as more spiritual than religious; however, all groups were low on both ratings. Second, Pasquale (2007, p. 53) notes that members of these groups used the term "spirituality" in a nontranscendent sense. This is important, as we can identify two dimensions of spirituality. One affirms what we might call "vertical transcendence," while the other affirms "horizontal transcendence." For instance, persons who reject God may nevertheless be involved in ecological movements, indicating an interconnectedness that is purely horizontal or immanent. Whereas Kalton (2000) has focused upon "green spirituality" as a form of purely horizontal transcendence, S. M. Taylor (2007) has demonstrated in her study of Catholic nuns involved in the environmental movement that there can be a simultaneous affirmation of both vertical and horizontal transcendence.

In a survey conducted between August 2007 and January 2008 in India, 1,100 persons (predominantly male) who held doctorates from 130 universities and research institutes were studied by Keysar and Kosmin (2008). As would be expected in Indian culture, the majority (66%) were Hindu. Only 10% described themselves as atheist, agnostic, or secular (Keysar & Kosmin, 2008, p. 268). Despite this, only 26% agreed with the statement "I know God exists and I have no doubts about it." When asked, "To what extent do you think of yourself

TABLE 9.4. Self-Rated "Spirituality" and "Religiosity" among Variously Identified Unchurched Persons

Descriptors respondents applied to themselves	Mean self-description as "spiritual" (0 = not at all; 8 = very much)	Mean self-description as "religious" (0 = not at all; 8 = very much)
Naturalistic (*n* = 38)	2.46	0.84
Agnostic (*n* = 33)	2.09	1.0v3
Scientific (*n* = 58)	2.05	0.95
Humanist(ic) (*n* = 89)	2.03	0.97
Secular(ist) (*n* = 56)	1.97	0.89
Atheist(ic) (*n* = 58)	1.60	0.81
Anti-religious (*n* = 27)	1.56	0.78
Skeptical (*n* = 44)	1.43	0.86

Note. Adapted from Pasquale (2007, p. 53). Copyright © 2007 the Institute for the Study of Secularism in Society and Culture. Adapted by permission.

TABLE 9.5. Responses to the Question "What Does 'Spiritual' Mean?" by Predominantly Male Hindus Holding Doctorates

Response	%
Commitment to higher human ideals, such as peace, harmony, or well-being	34%
A higher level of human consciousness or awareness	31%
Sensitivity to a force that connects all (living) things	16%
Contact with forces or entities that exist beyond nature	10%
A purely emotional or psychological sense of connection with others and/or nature	9%

Note. N = 1,100. Adapted from Keysar and Kosmin (2008, p. 14). Copyright © 2008 the Institute for the Study of Secularism in Society and Culture. Adapted by permission.

as spiritual?", only 11% responded "not at all," while 57% rated themselves as 5 or above on a 7-point scale. However, when the respondents were asked what "spiritual" meant, there were wide variations, indicating both vertical and horizontal transcendence. Table 9.5 presents the categories into which responses were coded.

Thus, in cultures as diverse as the United States and India, there is evidence that identification as "spiritual rather than religious" is on the rise and that, as Charles Taylor (2007) has recently argued, we are in a secular age. Secularism characterizes much of western Europe, but is an emerging force in the United States as well (Houtman & Aupers, 2007; Keysar & Kosmin, 2007). Although to be secular is not necessarily to be an atheist, "atheist," "agnostic," and "secular" are all ways in which individuals identify themselves as neither religious nor spiritual in a vertically transcendent sense. As Keysar (2007) has cautioned, social scientists must be careful not to lump all who identify themselves as "unchurched" or religious "nones" into one homogeneous group. In a secular age, they are all worthy of study in their own right.

A FOCUS ON ATHEISM

According to Bullivant (2013), atheism is best identified as "an absence of belief in the existence of God or gods" (p. 12). However, as Martin (2007) notes, there are as many varieties of atheism as there are of theisms being rejected. Furthermore, complexity is added when the degree of certainty of belief denial is considered: "Positive" atheists are more certain of their denial, while "negative" atheists are less certain and shade into forms of agnosticism (Streib & Klein, 2013; Streib & Hood, 2016).

The psychological study of those who never develop a belief in God, or who come to reject a belief in God, is just beginning (Bullivant & Ruse, 2013). Despite the fact that estimates of the number of atheists worldwide vary significantly, figures of over half a billion are generally considered conservative (Zuckerman, 2007). Gervais (2013b, p. 386) argues that atheists are certainly the fourth largest "religious" group after Christians, Muslims, and Hindus. However, it is not obvious that atheism should be classified as an expression of religion—especially given the variety of atheisms discussed below, all of which are worthy of study in their own right (Bullivant & Ruse, 2013). As we note below, while some atheists can be defined by the theisms they reject, not all can. Likewise, the claim that some atheists must have a God representation (Rizzuto, 1979, p. 42) must be tempered by cultural considerations. As Farias (2013, p. 46) has cautioned, scientific studies of atheism in the United States are heavily influenced by America's religious culture, in which atheists are an "exotic group."

Lepp (1963, p. 11) reminds us that atheists tend to be absolute in their lack of belief, rejecting not just God, but all gods, spirits, or higher beings. For instance, in their study of adult atheists in the San Francisco Bay Area, Hunsberger and Altemeyer (2006, p. 35) asked the participants whether or not they believed in seven classic attributes of divine beings. The 253 respondents responded "no" to 1,758 of 1,771 possibilities (7 × 253)! Hunsberger and Altemeyer were also surprised that, like fundamentalists, atheists could be ethnocentric and dogmatic (depending on the measures used). However, the novel dogmatism measure of Hunsberger and Altemeyer (2006, p. 136) was rejected by some atheists who had a chance to comment on the study, and the results for ethnocentrism probably reflect no more than individuals' general tendency to favor people who believe as they do. One distinction that separated these atheists from a comparative sample of Manitoba fundamentalists was their lack of a need to proselytize. Obviously, Christian fundamentalists have a textual mandate to spread the Gospels (Hood et al., 2005), so this difference is to be expected. However, one must be careful not to conclude that atheists are necessarily different from believers on all spiritual matters. For instance, in their study of over 16,000 youths between 13 and 15 years of age in England and Wales, Kay and Francis (1999) noted that while only 4% of the atheists believed agreed with the statement "I believe that Jesus really rose from the dead," as compared to 67% of the theists (p. 15), nearly identical percentages (30% and 31%, respectively) agreed with the statement "I believe it is possible to contact spirits of the dead" (p. 16).

Varieties or Types of Atheism

Given the dynamic nature of the religious field, it is not surprising that efforts are underway to produce a more complex typology of the varieties of atheism. Silver, Coleman, Hood, and Holcombe (2014) have proposed six types of atheism, based upon in-depth qualitative interviews with nonbelievers in the United States. A sample consisting of 59 nonbelievers (37 males, 22 females) was selected from all regions of the United States, and this sample not restricted to nonbelievers who identified with organizations advocating forms of nonbelief (only 17 admitted to membership in such groups). Based upon extensive interviews (at least 1 hour long), and using a modified version of Fowler's Faith Development Interview (see Chapter 4 for discussion), Silver and colleagues constructed a typology of atheism. This was then used in an online survey as part of a quantitative exploration of psychological correlates of the typology (Silver et al., 2014, pp. 996–1000). The typology is presented in Table 9.6.

If we assume that at least in the United States, most types of nonbelievers have deconverted from a faith tradition (see Chapter 8), some important findings are worth noting here. First, it is likely that some reasons for deconversion can be associated with emotional distress and may involve struggles with God (Exline & Rose, 2013; Exline, 2013), whereas others may be simple consequences of rational doubt (Caldwell-Harris, Wilson, LoTempio, & Beit-Hallahmi, 2011). Indeed, the focus on varieties of atheism suggests that, as with theism, reasons for belief or unbelief vary. For instance, Silver et al. (2014) found that only their anti-theist group differed significantly from their intellectual atheist/agnostic group on a multi-dimensional measure of anger, suggesting that anti-theists are as dogmatic as some religious

TABLE 9.6. Six Types of Nonbelief in an American Sample

Identification of type	Dynamic characteristics
Intellectual atheistic/agnostic (38%)	
Intellectual denial of or debate over existence of God or gods. Debate is philosophical and/or scientific.	Enjoyment of intellectual arguments. May join discussion groups with other intellectuals.
Activist atheistic/agnostic (23%)	
Motivated by belief in secular rather than religious values. May be spiritual (horizontal rather than vertical transcendence).	Likely to get involved with specific groups to advance their perceptions of social justice (e.g., gay or environmental issues).
Seeker–agnostic (8%)	
Uncertain of any claims to ultimacy. Doubtful of any person or group claiming to possess certain knowledge. Focus upon the journey, not the destination.	Privatized doubt; likely to be uninvolved in either social action or formal believing groups.
Anti-theist (15%)	
Seeking to end religion, which is viewed as either immature thought or simply scientifically falsifiable. Often affectively driven.	Actively seeking out religious people to disabuse them of their beliefs and all forms of religious instruction.
Non-theist (4%)	
Simply not thinking about or endorsing any religious beliefs.	Seeking to associate with like-minded persons for whom religion or belief in God is not an issue.
Ritual atheist/agnostic (13%)	
Rejecting belief in God, but continuing to participate in religious rituals. Participation may be ethnically or culturally based.	Continued religious participation for extrinsic personal and/or social reasons. May selectively hide atheism.

Note. Sample characteristics: $N = 1,153$; 50% female, 49% male, 1% other; mean age = 36.14 years ($SD = 12.94$). Percentages are rounded and are descriptive only of this sample. Based on Silver et al. (2014, pp. 993–996).

fundamentalists are authoritarian. Other patterns of difference among atheistic types on a variety of measures suggest that not all theistic types can be lumped together under any single explanation (see Silver et al., 2014, p. 999). This is consistent with evidence suggesting that atheism can be treated partly as an individual-difference variable, often associated with openness (Caldwell-Harris et al., 2011; Saucier & Skrzypińska, 2006).

Atheism and the Cognitive Science of Religion

As discussed in Chapter 4, the cognitive science of religion (CSR) is heavily influencing the contemporary psychology of religion. If we can identify a single basic assumption of CSR, it is that religious ideas are natural by-products of ordinary, universal human cognitive processes. In addition, many CSR studies use other than Western samples, and thus expand the psychology of religion beyond its usual North American/European base.

At first, it may seem counterintuitive to examine atheism (the absence of belief in a God or gods) from a CSR perspective, and much of this research is still in its infancy (Coleman, Hood, & Shook, 2015). Still, there are strong arguments for this approach. In many countries, the vast majority of atheists are deconverts (Fazzino, 2014; Streib & Klein, 2013), meaning that they have left and now stand in various forms of opposition to their former faiths (Streib et al., 2009). There are also "hidden" atheists who are active in churches (Dennett & LaScola, 2010) and in synagogues (Shrell-Fox, 2015). Secular and atheistic individuals can even be found in predominantly Muslim countries such as Turkey (Sevinc, Hood, & Coleman, 2017). Atheists and the nonreligious constitute some of the fastest-growing "religious" demographics (Twenge, Exline, Grubbs, Sastry, & Campbell, 2015) and are projected to maintain this growth (Stinespring & Cragun, 2015). Therefore, taking a CSR approach to atheism appears not only justifiable but potentially illuminating.

Despite the fact that the population of atheists is growing steadily, perceptions of atheists are negative and often juxtaposed with the religions they have abandoned. Thus one might reasonably expect tension between believers and atheists, and prejudice from faith groups toward atheists and nonbelievers in general has been well documented (Cragun, Kosmin, Keysar, Hammer, & Nielsen, 2012; Edgell, Gerteis, & Hartmann, 2006; Mann, 2015). Despite the findings that atheists lead lives as normal and moral as those of members of any other religious group (Coleman & Arrowood, 2015; Zuckerman, 2014), much research suggests that discrimination against atheists is primarily based upon a perceived lack of "moral trust" (Gervais, 2013a), and that even exposing individuals to information suggesting that the human moral sense is innate does not reduce this view (Mudd, Naijle, Ng, & Gervais, 2015). A particularly interesting area of this research involves the atheists identified by Silver et al. (2014) as "anti-theists," or by more popular media in the Western world as the "new atheists" (Zenk, 2013).

The Anti-Theist Movement

The anti-theists have much in common with the anti-cult movement discussed above. However, they differ in that they are not simply opposed to particular forms of religion, but stand in opposition to all religion. Another similarity to the anti-cult movement is that the anti-theist or new atheist movement is associated with charismatic individuals who have popularized their opposition to religion. Often referred to as the "Unholy Trinity" (Zenk, 2013, p. 234), they include Daniel Dennett, a cognitive scientist, author of *Breaking the Spell* (2006); Sam Harris, a neuroscientist, author of *The End of Faith* (2004); and Richard Dawkins, a philosopher, author of *The God Delusion* (2006). Perhaps an exception is the late Christopher Hitchens, another philosopher, author of *God Is Not Great* (2007), who spoke positively of Buddhism; however, when Hitchens is added to the others, they are often referred to in a term borrowed from the Book of Revelation (Revelation 6:1–17) as the "four horsemen" (Zenk, 2013). The religious metaphors are appropriate, as these individuals have argued that while religion is natural and science is not, it is the very naturalness of religion that must be overcome by a scientific and naturalistic critique. Furthermore, their claims often are phrased as if they supported metaphysical claims, such as the scientific overcoming of natural tendencies to produce the "ontological commitments to non-existent agencies and powers" that religion demands (Bulbulia, 2005, p. 91). Overcoming the naturalness of such delusions is a task that Dawkins (2006) refers to as the "brights campaign" (p. 280).

Atheism, Education, Intelligence, Gender, and Science

The unnaturalness of science versus the naturalness of religion is a mainstay of many CSR claims, as we have noted in Chapter 4. However, among the anti-theists, opposing this naturalness is itself a passion (Zenk, 2013). The overall claim they make is that those more committed to science in opposition to religion are of higher intelligence (Zukerman, Silberman, & Hall, 2013), have more education (Streib & Klein, 2013, pp. 719–721), and are male (Beit-Hallahmi, 2015, pp. 89–108). However, these claims must all be viewed with caution. Although the most widely cited meta-analysis of religion and intelligence revealed a negative correlation between religious *belief* and intelligence of –.24, the relationship was weaker for religious *behavior*. In addition, one cannot assume that those scoring lower on measures of religion are necessarily atheists (Farias, 2013, p. 48). Also, as with relationships between atheism and health/well-being, curvilinear relationships between atheism and intelligence or education are likely (Streib & Klein, 2013, pp. 721–723). Still further complicating the picture is that even linear relationships established in studies in one culture may be curvilinear in another. For instance, Farias (2013, p. 469) has noted that the often-cited positive correlation between atheism and education was based almost exclusively upon studies done in the United States. However, when these studies were replicated in the United Kingdom, the relation was curvilinear. Finally, the consistent finding that males are more likely to be atheists and females religious is deserving of a bit more elaboration.

When pushed, those committed to the naturalness of religion (again, see the discussion of CSR in Chapter 4) argue that failure to believe can be viewed almost as a disability. Barrett (2012, p. 203) has suggested precisely this: "Not believing in any sort of gods may prove to be a trait that is analogous to not being able to walk." It is precisely such claims that the anti-theists want to discount. Rather than a disability, they see not believing as an insight, and argue for an overcoming of all religion rooted in the belief of God or gods; they view the defense of one religion over another as illusory, since in fact religious difference and religion itself are simply illusions (Bulbulia, 2005, p. 92). One of the most important theoretical assumptions within the CSR literature is that variations in mentalizing abilities can explain diminished or absent God beliefs (i.e., can explain atheism). In short, it has been suggested that atheists may not believe in God because they are "socially disabled" (Barrett, 2012, p. 85) or "mind-blind" (Norenzayan, Gervais, & Trzesniewski, 2012).

However, there is little consensus in the massive literature on CSR that allows us to rise above what also characterizes the literature on cults: Each side seems to find a way to marshal evidence and provide studies to support its own hypotheses. On one side are religion and intuition; on the other, analytic thinking and science. At best, it seems that for American psychologists at least, science appears less natural than religion (Barrett, 2010), but the evidence is far from conclusive. As Jong (2014) has observed in his critical review of a text claiming to criticize CSR and its application to atheism, there is little consensus on methods or measures, and if there is any consensus at all, it is only that religion is a socially constructed topic for academic study. Part of the difficulty is conceptual. As both Ruse (2013) and Watts (2014) have noted, most CSR adherents are methodological naturalists, and hence are rooted in the long tradition of the methodological exclusion of the transcendent (noted in Chapter 1). However, methodological naturalism need not entail metaphysical naturalism (Ruse, 2013), although it limits the range of possible explanations. Likewise, one ought not to confuse science with scientism and the necessary exclusion of the transcendent as a metaphysical dogma (Haught, 2005; Hood, 2013). Watts (2014) notes that those who do not exclude the transcendent can provide alternative explanations for the explanation of agreed-upon empirical facts.

At the present stage of our knowledge, it appears that religion and science serve similar functions for many people—an idea coming to be known as the "replacement hypothesis" (Farias, 2013, pp. 471–474). An example of a study testing this idea is presented in Research Box 9.6. Given this hypothesis, combined with the evidence that rational acceptance of equally valid beliefs (and evidence?) for the existence or nonexistence of God (Tobias, 2015) is likely to be determined by prior implicit beliefs, the debate over the relative merits of science and religion remains open. While most types of atheists are open to dialogue with religion when not indifferent to it, it is worth noting that among the six types of atheists identified by Silver et al. (2014, p. 998), only anti-theists differed from all other atheists by scoring higher on a widely used measure of closed-mindedness.

RESEARCH BOX 9.6. The Compensation Hypothesis:
Can Belief in Science Serve the Same Function as Belief in Religion?
(Farias, 2013; Farias, Newheiser, Kahane, & de Toledo, 2013).

The compensation hypothesis is a simple assertion that the belief in either science or religion can serve the same psychological function. The focus is upon *belief*, in which science and religion are seen as mutually exclusive, and thus a person believes in either one or the other. In a field study, 100 rowers (46 women, 54 men; mean age = 23 years, SD = 4.18; ages ranging from 16 to 43) of amateur international standing were compared in two conditions. In one condition, assumed to be high-stress, 52 rowers were tested just prior to competing in a regatta; in the other condition, assumed to be low-stress, 48 rowers were tested at a training session. In both conditions, rowers indicated stress (from 1 = "none at all" to 7 = "very much"); rated how religious they were on a similar scale; and rated their belief in science on a specially constructed 10-item, single-factor scale. Results were as follows:

	High-stress (regatta) (n = 52)		Low-stress (training) (n = 48)	
	Mean	SD	Mean	SD
Reported stress	4.04	1.36	3.02	1.76
Belief in science	4.03	0.87	3.54	0.86

As predicted, there was a significant difference between the regatta condition and the training on reported stress, t (98) = 3.26, p = .002, d = 0.65, and on belief in science, t (98) = 2.82, p = .006, d = 0.57. The entire sample was low in religiosity (M = 1.86, SD = 1.69), with no difference between groups. However, as anticipated, religiosity was negatively correlated with belief in science, r (98) = −.29, p = .004.

One interpretation of these data is that for less religious individuals, belief in science rather than religion provides compensation under high-stress conditions.

Scientists, Religion, and Atheism

In a classic study clearly related to the contemporary research just described, Leuba (1916, 1934) presented data indicating that successful biological and physical scientists (the latter included physicists and mathematicians) tended toward atheism. Using data randomly selected from *American Men of Science*, Leuba demonstrated that scientists had high rates of disbelief in God and immortality. Furthermore, such disbelief was higher among the more eminent or "greater" scientists. Many years later, Larson and Witham (1998) replicated Leuba's study, using a sample of eminent scientists as operationalized by membership in the prestigious U.S. National Academy of Sciences. Leuba's data and Larson and Witham's replication are presented in Table 9.7.

What is most striking about the data in Table 9.7 is that disbelief in a personal God continued to rise among eminent scientists. Most of the 1998 respondents clearly rejected belief in a personal God. If we define this as atheism, then eminent American scientists are outliers with respect to the American public. In a nationwide survey conducted from May 8 to August 13, 2007, by the Pew Research Center's Forum on Religion and Public Life (Pew Research Center, 2008) among a representative sample of more than 35,000 adults in the United States, 98% of Protestants and 97% of Catholics affirmed belief in God. Although for most Protestants and Catholics this belief was in a personal God, for a significant minority the belief was in an impersonal force, not a personal God (19% of the Protestants, 29% of the Catholics). Contrary to Beit-Hallahmi's (2007) equation of Jewish self-identification with atheism, the Pew Research Center's (2008) survey indicated that 83% of Jews believed in God, but that at least 50% saw God as an impersonal force; the latter figure was similar to that for Hindus.

However, the results of the Leuba (1916, 1934) and Larson and Witham (1998) surveys are difficult to interpret without further information, especially qualitative data. First, it would be interesting to look at the eminent scientists who did believe in a personal God and compare them to those who did not. Although these data suggest mean trends, they mask and

TABLE 9.7. Comparison Data for Eminent Scientists: Leuba Data (1916, 1934) and Larson and Witham Replication (1998)

Belief	1914	1933	1998
Belief in personal God			
Personal belief	28%	15%	7%
Personal disbelief	53%	68%	72%
Agnosticism	21%	17%	21%
Belief in immortality			
Personal belief	35%	18%	8%
Personal disbelief	25%	53%	77%
Agnosticism	44%	29%	23%

Note. Percentages are rounded to nearest whole number and thus need not total 100%. Adapted from Larson and Witham (1998, p. 313). Copyright © 1998 the Nature Publishing Group. Adapted by permission from Macmillan Publishers Ltd: Nature, Larson and Witham (1998). The sums in excess of 100% are possible because doubt and personal disbelief are not treated as mutually exclusive.

ought not to be confused with longitudinal data, including data on eminent scientists who maintain their faith. Second, the rejection of a personal God does not necessarily entail a rejection of an impersonal force that many identify with the term "God." Although the implication is that education, especially scientific education, may negate belief in God, the issue is too complex to resolve simply with survey data. Third, asking scientists about belief in a personal God may be a psychologically loaded question. As one participant in the Hunsberger and Altemeyer (2006, p. 136) study commented, the denial of a belief in God may be no more than disillusionment with a naively theistically conceived God. We need to understand more fully exactly which definition of "God" these scientists were rejecting.

From 2005 thorugh 2007, the Religion Among Academic Scientists (RAAS) survey explored religious beliefs among scientists at 21 elite universities—includng Harvard, Stanford, Princeton, Yale, and Duke, as well as some top-ranked public universities (Ecklund & Park, 2009, p. 292). The sample included scholars both from the social sciences (sociology, economics, political science, psychology) and from the natural sciences (biology, chemistry, physics). The RAAS survey obtained a respectable 75% response rate from the 2,198 scientists who were originally approached ($n = 1,646$). Using data from 2005, Ecklund and Park compared social scientists ($n = 761$) to natural scientists ($n = 761$) and found that the conflict between religion and science was not as sharp as might have been expected. While more elite scientists in both groups did not believe, and while those who were religious were more likely to be liberal or spiritual in their beliefs, the majority (63%) did not see an "irreconcilable conflict between religious knowledge and scientific knowledge" (Ecklund & Park, 2009, p. 291). Results relative to belief in God are presented in Table 9.8.

These data suggest the complexity of any simple statement of the relationship between religion and science, and even more with respoect to elite scientists who either remain or become religious.

The Negative Case against Atheism

It is not surprising that challenges to the faithful in terms of claims that they exhibit psychological deficiencies have been met by not only contemporary cognitive scientists, but by psychologists whose work predated CSR. Lepp (1963) made a case for the multidimensional

TABLE 9.8. Belief in God among Social and Natural Scientists at Elite American Universities

	Social scientists ($n = 761$)	Natural scientists ($n = 627$)
Do not believe in God	31%	37%
Believe in a higher power, but it is not God	7%	9%
Believe in God	26%	21%
Some doubt	16%	13%
No doubt	10%	8%

Note. Data from Ecklund and Park (2009, p. 285). Percentages do not add up to 100%, as some options have been omitted.

nature of atheism we have noted above. To cite but two of his examples, atheism can be the result of principled reason (such as in Marxism) or the result of a neurotic denial of God. Hunsberger and Altemeyer (2006, p. 53) noted that 76% of their San Francisco Bay Area atheists once believed in God. However, many simply came to see such beliefs as false, as documented in the same authors' study of "amazing apostates" (Altemeyer & Hunsberger, 1997). Thus, as with conversion and spiritual transformation, we can postulate at least two ways to reject belief in a personal God. One is a neurotic denial of God, linked to the same type of attachment issues that characterize conversion. Such denials are likely to be stress-related and sudden, paralleling religious conversion (Buxant & Saroglou, 2008). Koster (1989) made the case for a neurotic denial of God in his psychohistorical study of four great atheists (Charles Darwin, Aldous Huxley, Friedrich Nietzsche, and Sigmund Freud). In each case, he found a consistent pattern of a weak, submissive son, unsure of his goals and desires. The victimized son attempted to flee from his unhappy family situation and, in so doing, shook off apathy and confusion. In maturity, he saw himself becoming like his father and thus turned to self-hatred and self-destruction. All this was seen as dynamically involved in the denial of the father.

Although Koster's thesis was speculative, it has been supported by clinical studies of neurotic atheism's being associated with defective fathering (Vitz, 2000). Vitz applies the theory of absent or defective fathering to numerous historical exemplars of atheism. Thus, just as insecure attachment histories may characterize belief in God (Buxant & Saroglou, 2008), they may also play a role in disbelief in God. Novotni and Petersen (2001, p. 171) suggest a dynamic model in which an option in the recognition of difficult situations is to blame God, then to recognize that one must not blame God; this is followed by repression and emotional distancing, resulting in the denial of God. Such models are empirically testable and suggest a form of "emotional atheism" (Novotni & Petersen, 2001, p. 38). Exline and her colleagues (Exline & Martin, 2005; Exline & Rose, 2005) have taken the lead in the empirical study of anger toward God and of spiritual struggles that can lead to atheism or at least to doubts about God's existence. Their research in many ways is an empirical complement to the psychoanalytic work of Vergote (1997, pp. 207–278) on varieties of belief and unbelief associated with the Christian notion of God.

Comparative studies of the psychological processes involved in belief and denial of God are appropriate and seem to remind social scientists of the dangers of the genetic fallacy: Psychological factors involved in the acceptance or rejection of belief in God are incapable of answering the ontological question of God's existence. However, a criticism of most current theories of neurotic atheism is that they focus upon males and their fathers, with little theoretical speculation concerning females. In addition, the theories are more advanced than the empirical data that might support them.

Moreover, as with deconversion, denial of belief in a personal God may be a function of principled reason that simply finds no need for a personal God. Atheism is positively associated with education and tolerance, and need not imply a neurotic denial of God (Beit-Hallahmi, 2007; Caldwell-Harris et al., 2011). Rejection of a personal God can thus be a gradual process of education or of socialization within a culture in which secularism is dominant, such as parts of western Europe. Thus, as with conversion, deconversion need not at all involve a personal crisis resulting from a neurotic rejection of God (Hunsberger & Altemeyer, 2006; Streib et al., 2009). Atheism as a result either of primary socialization or of secondary socialization (i.e., a previous belief in God is rejected) can involve a gradual spiritual transformation without vertical transcendence (Comte-Sponville, 2007; Elkins, 2001).

For many, "science" stands as an alternative to "religion." Current debates often associated with "cultural wars" pit metaphysical options against one another. We have warned our readers in Chapter 2 against reducing belief (or disbelief) in God to simply psychological processes. It is likely that the same processes that operate in belief operate in disbelief. Furthermore, it is obvious that culture cannot be ignored. It is a simple fact that cultures that minimize belief in God socialize individuals to seek meaning in other ways, some of which are clearly purely secular (C. Taylor, 2007). If many people are both spiritual and religious, and others are spiritual but not religious, it is likely that more research will have to focus upon the emerging group that is neither religious nor spiritual in any vertical transcendent sense (Kosmin & Keysar, 2007). These are the atheists, agnostics, and secularists. However, of interest are what have become outliers among eminent men and women of science—those who maintain their religious faith. Only at the cost of falsifying data can these scientists be excluded from analysis.

OVERVIEW

The contemporary debate over forms of religious expression is as old as religion itself. The long tradition of church–sect theory suggests that religious organizations are in a constant process of change—some adapting to cultural changes, and others trying to resist change. The temptation to postulate unique psychological processes involved in religions distant from one's own is unlikely to be fruitful. Individuals committed to cult and sect forms of religion struggle no less for significance and meaning in their lives than do those committed to more mainstream forms of religious faith. This, combined with the discussion in Chapter 10 on the emergence of forms of spirituality in opposition to religion, suggests that the empirical study of the dynamics within and between religious groups has a certain future.

The claim that unique psychological processes must be involved in the maintenance of religious groups in tension with their culture is as conceptually unenlightened as it is empirically ungrounded. Polemical terms such as "brainwashing" are clearly less than useful. If we maintain the concept of "cult," it is because accurate descriptions of phenomena are crucial in science, and perhaps even more so in the social-scientific study of less popular forms of religion. We ought not to abandon terms whose usefulness is only threatened by popular ignorance. The fact that, in the end, evaluations must be made is all the more reason to make them only with descriptions of religious groups that are fair and accurate.

The extension of research on cults to GATTs must be cautious, but has clearly established empirical parallels that must be acknowledged. How psychology will change in the face of globalization is uncertain. However, as noted in Chapter 8, Pickren (2009, p. 87) warns that "the 21st century is unlikely to be another American century in psychology." This is not to dismiss the methods and procedures currently in use, but only to suggest that in a global environment other approaches must emerge. As we focus upon religion in a more global perspective, we are reminded that much of the psychology of religion has been focused upon and studied by WEIRD people—the acronym for "Western, educated, industrialized, rich, and democratic" societies (Henrich, Heine, & Norenzayan, 2010). When American psychologists confront more extreme religious groups, especially GATTs, the limitations of the WEIRD perspective have clouded their ability to understand such groups, but a clearer understanding is sorely needed. Even the American Psychological Association (APA) itself has recently been chided for its clandestine support for of the Bush administration's use of torture and similar tactics in the wake of 9/11. What is widely referred to as the "Hoffman report" (Hoffman et al., 2015) forced resignations at the APA, as well as a clear affirmation of an ethics rule that forbids American psychologists to play any role in what are perceived by some to be terrorist tactics.

Finally, psychologists of religion can no longer ignore the rising numbers of persons who are neither religious nor spiritual. Although self-identified atheists remain rare in the United States, they are more frequent among eminent scientists and in western European cultures that are already strongly secularized. The psychological processes involved in the rejection of God are likely to mirror those involved in the acceptance of God; however, the ontological question of God's existence cannot be answered by those whose task is purely psychological.

CHAPTER 10

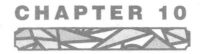

Religious and Spiritual Experience

If any one individual ever personified what is means to be "spiritual but not religious," it was William James.

The very beginning, the intrinsic core, the essence, the universal nucleus of every known high religion . . . has been the private, lonely, personal illumination, revelation, or ecstasy of some acutely sensitive prophet or seer.

Belief, ritual, and spiritual experience: these are the cornerstone of religion, and the greatest of them is the last.

Therefore, let's consider the proposal that when our volunteers journeyed to the further bonds of DMT's [N,N-dimethyltryptamine's] reach, when they felt as if they were *somewhere else,* they were indeed perceiving different levels of reality. The alternative levels are as real as this one. It's just that we cannot perceive them most of the time.

I'd see serpent handling, and . . . I thought, "Oh, Lord, I'd like to feel that. I'd like to feel what they're feeling."

If humans were no longer taught any religions, they would, I think, spontaneously create new ones from the content of ecstatic experiences, combined with bits and pieces transmitted by language and folklore.[1]

WHAT MAKES AN EXPERIENCE RELIGIOUS OR SPIRITUAL?

The study of religious experience can be perplexing, partly because so much time and effort can be wasted on defining precisely what is meant by "experience." Gadamer (1986, p. 310) argues that the concept of experience is "one of the most obscure we have." At a common-sense level, we are aware that experience is something other than mere action or behavior. Yet it would be odd indeed to think of experience without any action involved—for even to do nothing is to do something. Similarly, experience is not simply thought or belief, even though we are often thinking when we have an experience. Finally, many people try to equate experience with emotions or feelings. Yet feelings and emotions are only part of what we sometimes mean by experience; they cannot be equated with the experience. We refer in this chapter to "experience" as a total way of reacting or being that cannot be reduced to its parts, even if such parts could be identified.

---

[1]These quotations come, respectively, from the following sources: Fuller (2001, p. 130); Maslow (1964, p. 19); Lewis (1971, p. 11); Strassman (2001, p. 315; emphasis in original); Rachelle ("Shell") Martinez Brown, quoted in Brown and McDonald (2000, p. 73); and Goodman (1988, p. 171).

For instance, Taves (2009) calls for a reconsideration of religious experience from a "building-block" approach, which essentially places such experience within a social-constructionist perspective. An example is the debate within Pentecostalism as to whether or not Mark 16:17–18 is to be followed in its plain meaning when it says, "They shall take up serpents." Most Pentecostals reject the handling of serpents; some doubt the legitimacy of the longer endings of the Gospel of Mark; others argue that the passage in question refers to Paul's accidental bite from a serpent, not to an imperative to handle serpents deliberately (Hood & Williamson, 2014). Thus whether or not handling a serpent is a religious experience depends on many contextual factors, so that what is deemed religious by some is seen as fanaticism or foolishness by others.

One of the most ambitious empirical projects employing a building-block approach to religion and spirituality has yet to be adequately acknowledged by mainstream psychologists of religion. Based upon decades of empirical research with over 7,000 participants, Reiss and Havercamp (2005) created a scientifically derived list of 16 basic human desires or strivings constituting the Reiss Motivation Profile (RMP), which includes neither religion nor spirituality as a basic human motivation (see also Reiss, 2013; Reiss, 2015, pp. 34–35). Consistent with Taves's approach, but empirically derived, the model proposed by Reiss and his colleagues uses these 16 universal motives (which Reiss also calls "strivings") as the basic building blocks from which experiences can be deemed religious and/or spiritual (Reiss, 2004). Reiss's 16 motives or strivings range from the desire for acceptance and honor to the desire for power and vengeance (for a complete list, see Reiss, 2015, pp. 17–18). In one study (Reiss, 2000), it was found that very religious Christians had a particular set of composite scores on the RMP, with the strongest desires being those for eating, family, honor, idealism, and order, and the weakest desires being those for independence, romance, and vengeance. Other desires were intermediate. According to Reiss (2004, 2013, 2015), the entire range of things deemed religious can be catalogued according to various combinations of the 16 basic strivings.

However, we must caution our readers that while a building-block approach seems simple, it is really not. In the example cited above for the composite strivings of very strong Christians, there are 4,368 possible combinations for 5 of the 16 strivings. This is the number of ways one could combine any possible 4 by selecting from 16 strivings. There are 560 possible combinations possible for the weakest 3 of the 16 strivings. It is not clear whether the precise strivings empirically determined would consistently be replicated in these precise combinations, such that any particular set of building blocks would result in a religious experience. To give another example, if one wanted to see which of 7 strivings could best be combined to deem something religiously or spiritually significant, there are 11,440 combinations possible. After the fact, any combination can be seen as forming a meaningful pattern, even if the 16 strivings are empirically substantiated as fundamental blocks from which to create religious and or spiritual experiences. The empirical issues are, first, whether or not such blocks exist (and, if so, what their precise number is); and second whether or not things deemed religious actually emerge out of such fundamental blocks (Coleman & Hood, 2015).

An alternative to a building-block approach is that to have any experience is to identify some totalizing aspect that is directly recognized—an event or episode that is "experienced" in response to a sense of ultimacy and transcendence (Streib & Hood, 2016). This experience is often contrasted with being dogmatic, in the negative sense of the mere insistence on particular beliefs, and it is likely to be identified as being "spiritual but not religious" (Streib & Hood, 2016). Gadamer (1986) argues:

> The experienced person proves to be . . . someone who is radically undogmatic; who, because of the many experiences he [or she] has had and the knowledge he [or she] has drawn from them is particularly well equipped to have new experiences and to learn from them. The dialectic of experience has its own fulfillment not in definitive knowledge but in the openness to experience that is encouraged by experience itself. (p. 319)

Gadamer more than anticipated the distinction between religion and spirituality that characterizes much of the contemporary psychology of religion, as we have noted throughout this book. Religion provides meaning and closure for many persons (Saroglou, 2002a). Thus the range of specifically religious experiences is more restricted than the diversity that characterizes spiritual experiences (Streib, 2007). For most of this chapter, when we speak of religious experience, the context will make it clear whether the experience has a specifically religious framing (and hence is a *religious* experience) or is not specifically religiously framed (and hence is a *spiritual* experience). This parallels the distinction between religious conversion and spiritual transformation discussed in Chapter 8, and anticipates the distinction between religious and spiritual mysticism discussed in Chapter 11.

Although Gadamer speaks of experience in general, it would appear that religious experience identifies something particular. Religious experience distinctively separates, from the vast domain of experience, that which is perceived to be *religious*; spiritual experience separates that which is perceived to be *spiritual*. Both of these refer to ultimacy that is revealed in experience and to which individuals can respond. Once the whole is comprehended, we can focus upon its parts; but without the prior comprehension of the whole, the parts do not exist (Polanyi, 1958, p. 29). In this view, in other words, the building blocks are recognized only after the whole is experienced to be what it is. Thus psychologists are free to identify religious experience as experience that is acknowledged within a faith tradition as religious. Religious traditions define the distinctively religious for the faithful. What is religious within one tradition may not be so within another. With the possible exception of mystical experience (discussed in Chapter 11), it is probably not fruitful to define religious or spiritual experiences by their inherent characteristics. The issue of a distinctive religious or spiritual experience—one that is religious or spiritual in and of itself—is only partly an empirical issue (Jones, 2016). Streib and Hood (2016) have argued that spirituality as an "emic" term (i.e., one defined from within a social group) shows great individual variation, but as an "etic" term (i.e., one defined from an outsider's perspective) it functions as an implicit religion. Thus whether an experience is religious or spiritual depends partly on the context and the interpretation of the experience. It is in this sense that even if what is experienced is both immediately present and unquestionable to the experiencing individual, the epistemological value of the experience is dependent upon discursive meanings that entail public interpretations (Sharf, 2000; Taylor, 2002). Interpretations provide meanings not inherently obvious to those outside the tradition that provides the context for meaningfully identifying any particular episode as religious.

As psychologists, we often study retrospective accounts of experience that are linguistically framed as religious. Almost any experience humans can have can be interpreted as an experience of God (Leech, 1985). As Yamane (2000) notes, narration is dependent upon a loose relationship between experience and its linguistic representation, so that an experience not initially described as religious may be so described on subsequent reflection. However, it is within a linguistic community that claims to religious experiencing are ultimately judged (Williams & Faulconer, 1994). The ultimate judgment is linked to that which is not simply deemed religious, but is an object of ultimate concern (Neville, 2001; Streib & Hood, 2016). Spiritual experiences are less dogmatically framed and open to a wide variety of subjective interpretations; however, insofar as they reference ultimacy and transcendence, they can be considered at least implicitly religious (Streib & Hood, 2011, 2016) In this sense, both religious and spiritual experiences are not simply constructions of things that can be deemed religious, but also responses to ultimate realities (Neville, 2001; Wildman, 2011). It is part of the task at the intersection between psychology and related disciplines, such as philosophy and theology, to determine the ontological and even metaphysical claims regarding responses to and constructions of experiences of ultimate reality (Hood, 2012b; Jones, 2016; Wildman, 2011). Robinson (2002) reminds us that psychologists are less than honest when they simply declare certain metaphysical options absolutely binding, such as naturalism, which some of the historically most influential psychologists (e.g., William James) adopted as only provisional assumptions (Hood, 2012b).

The subjective nature of spiritual experience has led some to argue that the quest for spiritual experiences outside of religious traditions is motivated only by narcissism. The highly popular *Habits of the Heart* (Bellah, Marsden, Sullivan, Swidler, & Tipton, 1996) became the second-best-selling sociological work in history (Yamane, 2007). In it, the pseudonymous Sheila Larson gave rise to the term "Sheilaism," used by Larson to describe her own faith. Yamane (2007) has noted that if she had today's language available to her during the interview, she "surely would have offered up the contemporary mantra, 'I'm spiritual, not religious'" (p. 183). However, Wink and his colleagues have shown that spiritual but not religious persons have a healthy narcissism that includes an acceptance of others (Dillon & Wink, 2007; Wink, Dillon, & Fay, 2005; Wink, Dillon, & Prettyman, 2007). Likewise, in-depth phenomenological studies of "New Age" believers revealed that one of the consequences of their spiritual seeking was the realization of a greater capacity of love (Bloch, 1988; Norlander, GÅrd, Lindholm, & Archer, 2003). Greenwald and Harder (2003) found that self-effacing altruism and a loving connection to others were two of four factors that emerged from ratings of 122 adjectives to describe spirituality. Thus, it appears from research using a variety of methods that the individuality associated with spirituality is not a selfish narcissism focused upon the self, but rather a quest for self-realization that includes acceptance and concern for others, without a need to impose a single consistent set of beliefs to frame one's spirituality. The individuality associated with spirituality is one that fosters acceptance of self and others.

CONCEPTUAL CONSIDERATIONS IN DEFINING RELIGIOUS AND SPIRITUAL EXPERIENCE

As we have noted in Chapter 2, James's (1902/1985) classic work *The Varieties of Religious Experience* has continued to influence psychologists since it was initially delivered as the Gifford Lectures at the beginning of the 20th century. Although we can speculate about the varying reasons why this book has remained in print since its first publication, the simple fact remains that James set the tone for contemporary empirical work in the psychology of religious *experience* that is nonreductive (Hood, 2000a). More than one psychologist has noted that if James were writing today, his lectures would undoubtedly have been titled *The Varieties of Spiritual Experience* (Gorsuch & Miller, 1999). Likewise, as noted at the start of this chapter, Fuller (2001, p. 130) holds William James to be the exemplar of what it means to be "spiritual but not religious."

James's Formula for Religious and Spiritual Experience

James's definition of religious experience for the purposes of the Gifford Lectures clearly revealed his sympathy for the extreme forms of religious experience. James defined "religion" as "*the feelings, acts, and experiences of individual men, in their solitude, so far as they apprehend themselves to stand in relation to whatever they may consider the divine*" (James, 1902/1985, p. 34; emphasis in original). The presence of something divine within all religious traditions can be debated. Buddhism is often cited as an example of a faith tradition without a god (Hong, 1995). However, one need not equate something divine with belief in God or in supernatural beings. James's clarification of what he meant by "divine" makes the case for the near-universal application of this concept. As he saw it, the divine is "such a primal reality as the individual feels compelled to respond to solemnly and gravely, and neither by a curse nor a jest" (James, 1902/1985, p. 39). Thus, influenced by James's notion of divinity, religious experience—ultimately, the experience of the solitary individual—is placed at the forefront of the psychology of religion. James's Gifford Lectures minimized both belief and behavior. Yet in these justly famous lectures, James was parsimonious in his conclusion regarding the value of religious and spiritual experiences in general. As he perceived it, the infinite variety of religious and spiritual experiences can be subsumed under a simple formula: discontent and its resolution. Placed in the context of individual lives, responses to the divine are resolutions.

Taylor (2002) argues that James's Protestant biases minimized the social aspects of religion inherent in Catholicism, but that James's intent was to open metaphysical options. Wildman (2011) has emphasized that both supernaturalism as a belief in disembodied intentionality and supernaturalism as a belief in the ultimate reality of a god as a personal being are viable metaphysical options to naturalism. James's effort in *The Varieties* was to deny that psychologists must adopt Flournoy's (1903) methodological exclusion of the transcendent as the only option for the psychology of religion, as we have discussed in Chapter 1. To dogmatically adopt this principle is, in the words of Wildman (who is committed to naturalism), to be forced to reduce religious experience to "improperly anthropomorphic projections of human experience onto a universe that is not scaled to human interests and concerns" (2011, p. 23). Studies derived from documents similar to those solicited and used by James focus upon experiences that elicit ontological wonder and cannot be easily dismissed. They suggest, as we shall see, that the realities engaged in by those who have religious or spiritual experiences cannot be easily dismissed by the naturalistic assumptions of many who seek knowledge about experiences that they have no personal acquaintance with (Hood, 2012b). However, as we shall see, the issue may be confounded by the methodology of focusing upon personal declarations of religious and spiritual experience. As noted in Chapter 1, the resolution of discontent is an appealing formula that can mask the often complex relationships between religion and coping, as well as religion and mental health.

Varieties of Spiritual Experience: Research from the Hardy Centre

Perhaps most congruent with the Jamesian tradition of the use of personal documents to understand religious experience has been the work associated with what was originally known as the Religious Experience Research Unit of Manchester College, Oxford University. Alister Hardy achieved scientific accolades as a renowned zoologist. Yet his lifelong interest in religious experience led him upon retirement from his career in zoology to form a research unit in 1969 devoted to the collection and classification of religious experiences. For this work, he was awarded the Templeton Prize for research in religion. Hardy's basic procedure, stemming from his zoological training, was to solicit voluntary reports of religious experiences and to attempt to classify them into their natural types. Typically, these reports were solicited via requests in newspapers, as well as newsletters distributed to various groups, mostly in the United Kingdom. Requests were not simply for the more extreme and intense types of experiences favored by James, but for more temperate religious experiences as well. Often individuals simply submitted experiences unsolicited. In *The Spiritual Nature of Man,* Hardy (1979) published an extensive classification of the major defining characteristics of these experiences from an initial pool of 3,000 experiences. Thus we have significant data on the range of experiences individuals respond to as religious, spiritual, or both.

At present, much of the demand is not for more data, but for a meaningful way to frame the data we already have. For instance, Taylor (2002) notes that both Hardy and James reached similar conclusions from the study of personal documents, and both accepted the claim that there is something "more" than what can be captured by reductive naturalism. Likewise, James's own insistence on intuition as a valid form of knowing has been supported by Wiebe (2015), who has used data collected by the Hardy Centre to support the claim that religious and spiritual experiences are valid forms of intuitive knowing. Research in the Hardy tradition continues at the Centre's current home at the University of Wales, Trinity Saint David (see *www.uwtsd.ac.uk/library/alister-hardy-religious-experience-research-centre*). The important issue here is that many of the basic data relevant to producing a theory of religious and spiritual experience are available.

For instance, many of the "blocks" for research taking a building-block approach are readily available. Hardy's own major classifications included sensory or quasi-sensory experiences associated with vision, hearing, and touch; less frequent, but still fairly common, were reports of paranormal experiences. Most common were cognitive and affective episodes, such as a sense of presence or feelings of peace (Hardy, 1979, pp. 25–29). It seems that there is little agreement about exactly what might constitute the common characteristics of religious and spiritual experience if one works from the building-block perspective. There may be no common elements that all religious or spiritual experiences share unless they are approved from a tacit knowing in which the reality present is simply comprehended and experienced directly as personal knowledge (Polanyi, 1958, p. 228) The focus, then, must be upon not simply religious experience, but the varieties of experience that are comprehended as religious. It is better to think of religious experiences in light of Wittgenstein's (1945–1949/1953) notion of "family resemblance." We can identify the family resemblance among experiences we classify as religious, but not by finding a single criterion that they all must share. The characteristics making an experience religious or spiritual are clearly not the discrete, isolated components that can be identified in any experience. As Leech (1985) has argued, hardly any experience could fail to qualify as "religious" or "spiritual" under some framework. (An exception may be mysticism, as discussed in Chapter 11.)

Wildman and McNamara (2010) have demonstrated this point in research contrasting a wide range of religious and spiritual experiences with ordinary ones. The measure they used was not created from specifically religious or spiritual experiences. The Phenomenology of Consciousness Inventory (PCI) gives a quantitative profile of the contents and qualities of personal consciousness across 26 measures grouped into 12 major dimensions (Pekala, Steinberg, & Kumar, 1986). Wildman and McNamara noted that, compared to ordinary experiences, religious and spiritual experiences were recognized as altered meaningful states of consciousness that compelled attention and were accompanied by increased imagery and internal dialogue that were not simply under voluntary control. As in the drug experiences discussed later in this chapter, even negative affective aspects of religious and spiritual experiences were ultimately welcomed and experienced as positive. This is consistent with Luhrmann's (2012) study of contemporary American evangelicals who experience communication with a personal God, based partly upon their learning to respond by attentive absorption into an alternate reality whose ontological reality is acknowledged. Šhram (2017) has used similar methods to suggest that in some cultures, psychopathology and depression may be considered signs of Satanic possession.

Anomalous Experiences and Counterintuitiveness

What is "religious" or "spiritual" for some is merely "anomalous" for others. Earlier investigators identified anomalous experiences within a fiercely reductionistic frame, often attributing them to "magical" (e.g., erroneous) thinking (Zusne & Jones, 1989). The philosopher Strawson (1959) identified two characteristics that mark the metaphysics of individuals, and cognitive scientists (especially anthropologists heavily influenced by evolutionary theory) have suggested that there are two basic cognitive mechanisms related to each of the metaphysical options articulated by Strawson. One is the existence of material objects, described in Strawson's language by "M-predicates." M-predicates apply to material objects and include descriptions of their mass and volume, as well as the fact that matter occupies space. However, "P-predicates" uniquely apply to persons. They include such things as intent and purpose. Individuals or persons, in Strawson's metaphysics, can be described by both M- and P-predicates. However, some objects (e.g., statues) are purely material, and no P-predicates apply to them. In religious and spiritual traditions, the claim is that some persons (ghosts, gods) have no material bodies and are thus described in purely P-predicate terms.

Cognitive scientists have argued that persons have evolved cognitive mechanisms to identify both material and animate objects. Furthermore, the basic "default" position is that if in doubt, one assumes that an object is animate. For instance, if one is uncertain that the object is a large rock or a bear, it is safest (has survival value) to assume it is a bear until further information disconfirms it. Thus, as Guthrie (1993, 2007) notes, the tendency to anthropomorphism is part of our evolutionary makeup and is the process by which nonexistent spiritual beings are created. In this view, spiritual beings have no independent ontological status.

Perhaps the most completely reductionist theorist in this area is Boyer. Not only has he identified what he calls the "naturalness of religious ideas" (Boyer, 1994), but he has identified the cognitive mechanisms by which (to use the title of his book) he asserts that *Religion [Is] Explained* (Boyer, 2001). The basic assumption is that counterintuitiveness is what is involved in spiritual or religious experiences. There are a limited number of "supernatural templates" (Boyer, 2001, pp. 77–78) that create religious and spiritual beings and events by the application of counterintuitive properties to them. However, there are limits to the nature and type of counterintuitive properties that a person, animal, or object can have. For instance, if a ghost is to be credible, it can walk through a wall, but it must have other characteristics associated with "real" persons to be believable. Thus, what makes something counterintuitive is that one cannot infer anything further from the counterintuitive property. For instance, as Hinde (1999, p. 72) notes, no other inference follows from the claim that ghosts walk through walls. However, for real objects and persons, knowing one fact allows other inferences (e.g., "If other people can see me, I can hide from their view"). Boyer claims that the list of "spiritual templates" created by counterintuitiveness is quite limited. Table 10.1 presents this list, which, in Boyer's (2001, p. 78) view, is exhaustive.

Boyer argues that this very limited range of templates constitutes the cognitive basis for the diverse contents of mythology, science fiction, cartoons, and religious writing. Thus, as other cognitive scientists have done, Boyer "explains" religions by an evolutionary process that mixes two cognitive mechanisms selected for survival value—one to identify physical objects (M-predicates), and the other to identify animate objects that might be potential predators (P-predicates). This ultimately reductive view of religion simply asserts that persons are predisposed to postulate counterintuitive agents, especially when ambiguous stimuli are framed within cultural predispositions that support such conclusions (Atran, 2002; Bloom, 2004). The claim to have identified a basic cognitive process that creates both gods and cartoons with equal ontological status is clearly offensive to adherents of many faiths. It can be contrasted with cognitive claims to preparedness that are nonreductive, as discussed in Chapter 4. Other methodological approaches would limit the reductive claims of cognitive scientists.

Research informed by phenomenological methods keeps open the possibility of nonreductionist views of even the more extreme anomalous experiences (Porpora, 2006). Rather than simply being counterintuitive templates, superior intelligences or beings, if they exist, may be limited in the ways they can make more limited intelligences aware of them. The constraints may be gradually lifted as individuals themselves become more spiritually realized. Cardeña, Lynn, and Krippner (2000b) identify anomalous experiences as those that, though perhaps experienced by a substantial segment of the population, are nevertheless believed to deviate from ordinary experience or from the usually accepted definitions of

TABLE 10.1. Boyer's Catalogue of Supernatural Templates

Counterintuitiveness applied to:	Examples
Persons[a]	
Physical properties	Ghosts, gods with immaterial bodies
Biological properties	Gods that do not grow old or die
Psychological properties	Unblocked perception; prescience
Tools and artifacts	
Biological properties	Statues that "bleed"
Psychological properties	Statues that "hear" what you say

Note. Data from Boyer (2001, pp. 78–79).
[a]Animals can also have all these properties.

reality (Cardeña, Lynn, & Krippner, 2000a, p. 4). These experiences need not be identified as religious, but clearly many often are. This is especially the case for near-death and mystical experiences, which continue to be represented in the second edition of a handbook (Cardeña, Lynn, & Krippner, 2014) devoted to the scientific exploration of anomalous experiences. These experiences often gain added meaning when they are embedded in religious discourse that both explains and legitimates them (Taves, 2009; Streib & Hood, 2016). An even more expanded view is one in which anomalous experiences are seen as having ontological validity. In this sense, the most intriguing handbook is Miller's (2012a), which is the first major handbook devoted to psychology and spirituality that explicitly rejects secular materialism and a science framed within the ontological limits of this view (Miller, 2012b). In this sense, Miller is following the example already noted with respect to James, in which the reality of experienced religion refuses to be limited by the constraints of a too narrowly and often crudely materialistic psychology (Hood, 2012b).

This new openness on the part of some psychologists can be illustrated by shifting attitudes to hallucinatory experiences, as the recent history of modifications in the American Psychiatric Association's *Diagnostic and Statistical Manual of Mental Disorders* (DSM) shows. Despite the fact that DSM has been criticized both theoretically and scientifically (see, e.g., Kirk & Kutchins, 1992), it is in widespread normative use in at least North America. In its last several revisions, moreover, it has included cautions about identifying hallucinations and possession experiences as pathological if there is normative support for these practices. This was made especially clear in DSM-III-R:

> When an experience is entirely normative for a particular culture—e.g., the experience of hallucinating the voice of a deceased in the first few weeks of bereavement in various North American Indian groups, or trance and possession states occurring in culturally approved ritual contexts in much of the non-Western world—it should not be regarded as pathological. (American Psychiatric Association, 1987, p. xxvi)

In DSM-IV, a hallucination was defined only as "a sensory perception that has the compelling sense of reality of a true perception but that occurs without external stimulation of the relevant sensory organ" (American Psychiatric Association, 1994, p. 767); it is not automatically deemed to be an indication of mental illness. The text revision of this manual (DSM-IV-TR) simply cautioned that "a clinician who is unfamiliar with the nuances of an individual's cultural frame of reference may incorrectly judge as psychopathology those normal variations in behavior, belief, or experience that are particular to the individual's culture" (American Psychiatric Association, 2000, p. xxxiv). Finally, the most recent edition (DSM-5) identifies culture-related diagnostic issues; it notes, for example, that "An individual's cultural and religious background must be taken into account in evaluating the possible presence of delusional disorder. The content of delusions also varies across cultural contexts" (American Psychiatric Association, 2013, p. 93).

Williams and Faulconer (1994) have persuasively noted the fallacies involved in definitional efforts to determine the "pathology" of religious beliefs. The consequences are immense once one realizes that religious beliefs are less characteristic of individuals and are more cultural or subcultural ways of interpreting experiences. If so, psychological processes, even "pathological" ones, cannot be used to reductively explain away religiously interpreted phenomena. Perhaps one of the most controversial examples is illustrated by responsible investigators' refusing to dismiss reports of alien abduction experiences (hereafter abbreviated as

AAEs) out of hand. Clearly, AAEs are likely to raise problems for those who think that the umbrella of religious discourse opens too wide when it legitimates such experiences. Yet Research Box 10.1 shows how even claims to unidentified flying object (UFO) sightings and AAEs are difficult to explain exhaustively by psychological processes if one simply frames experiences in a manner suggesting that they might be true. Such experiences are gaining significant subcultural support (Appelle, Lynn, & Newman, 2000; Skal, 1998). As such, it is less profitable to ask what causes these experiences than to try to understand the experiencing of the world from within a tradition, culture, or subculture that validates and finds meaningful what others can only describe as anomalous experiences from within their own perspective.

Exhaustive efforts to classify religious experiences would not have appealed to James, who preferred to let the experiences speak for themselves, unfettered by what he would probably have seen as the tyranny of classification schemes. However, Hardy's conclusions (reached ostensibly independently of James) are interesting, as they are precisely what James concluded much earlier. Both James and Hardy affirmed the evidential value of religious experiences as at least hypotheses suggesting the existence of a transcendent reality variously experienced. As for the psychological consequences, the power of prayer is acknowledged; early childhood experiences are considered significant; and feelings of safety, security, love, and contentment are regarded as concomitants of religious experience. Few religious experiences are negative. By the very understanding of religion, at least in the West, experiences attributed to God must be ultimately positive (Spilka & McIntosh, 1995).

Other studies of voluntarily submitted reports of religious experience are not inconsistent with either James's or Hardy's claims (Ahern, 1990; Hardy, 1966; Hay, 1987, 1994; Laski, 1961; Maxwell & Tschudin, 1990). However, much of this research favors a methodology that probably biases the simple conclusion that religious experiences are resolutions of discontent. This research probably solicits reports of religious experiences congruent with a simple, if not naïve, view of religion. These reports are often evaluated by persons committed to a positive assessment of religious experience. Few negative experiences are reported, and almost none that were inconsequential or failed to produce positive fruits are volunteered. In this sense, asking persons to report religious or spiritual experiences may be tapping general cultural views (especially in cultures heavily influenced by the Judeo-Christian tradition) that religious experiences are "good" and resolve problems. For instance, Lupfer and his colleagues have demonstrated that attributions are likely to be made to God only for events with positive outcomes (Lupfer, Brock, & DePaola, 1992; Lupfer, DePaola, Brock, & Clement, 1994). Although their research applies primarily to conservative Christians, other research suggests the general tendency among all believers to attribute to God only experiences with positive outcomes (Spilka & McIntosh, 1995).

However, not all religious or quasi-religious experiences may be positive in nature, and not all may be entirely culturally determined. For instance, Hufford (1982) has extensively investigated the "Old Hag" phenomenon common to Newfoundland. According to Newfoundland folk legend, what some might be tempted to dismiss as merely a nightmare is in fact a direct supernatural encounter with the Old Hag, a being who produces night paralysis and terror. Hufford (1982, p. 245) found this experience to occur in at least 15% of the population. One succinct description of the experience was given by a 20-year-old university student Hufford interviewed: "You are dreaming and you feel if someone is holding you down. You can do nothing, only cry out. People believe that you will die if you are not awakened" (quoted in Hufford, 1982, p. 2). Hufford notes that although culture affects the way the

A controversial issue in the study of religious or spiritual experience is the persistent finding that individuals who report such various experiences also report various paranormal experiences (Zollschan, Schumaker, & Walsh, 1995). Furthermore, studies employing survey data reveal that the reports of paranormal experiences have antecedents and structures similar to those in the reports of other ecstatic experiences commonly accepted as religious or spiritual (Fox, 1992; Yamane & Polzer, 1994). Paranormal experiences are a subclass of anomalous experiences. Among those who study anomalous experiences, the perception of unidentified flying objects (UFOs) and their more recent elaboration into "alien abduction experiences" (AAEs) have begun to generate a considerable body of scientific curiosity. Jung (1958/1964), while referring to the citing of UFOs as "visionary" (p. 315) or "symbolic" (p. 387), nevertheless cautioned that psychology alone cannot exhaust the explanation for such sightings. More recently, investigators such as Strassman (2001) have suggested that certain chemicals affecting brain receptor sites for serotonin may elicit awareness of dimensions of reality in which reports of AAEs become possible as actual events. However, as with many religious or spiritual experiences, psychologists are more likely to be comfortable with explanations within the mainstream of realities that other psychologists are likely to accept. For instance, Skal (1998) has noted that the term "flying saucer" came into vogue only after newspaper headlines in June 1947, when a Boise, Idaho pilot named Kenneth Arnold described nine strange objects flying near Mount Rainier as moving "like a saucer if you skipped it across the water" (quoted in Skal, 1998, p. 204). Newspaper headlines reported "flying saucers," and quickly individuals began to reporting sighting of them. Thus cultural expectations based upon journalistic headlines that actually were in error might have played a role in shaping what have become common sightings of "UFOs." Instead of moving "like saucers," they became identified as "flying saucers."

Apparently even less plausible than the existence of UFOs are claims to AAEs, which typically include being captured and taken aboard a UFO and being subjected to physical, mental, and spiritual examinations before being returned to earth (Bullard, 1987). Other more extreme claims may include the taking of tissue samples, the implantation of objects into the body, and even the birth of alien-hybrid babies (Jacobs, 1992). As fantastic as these claims appear, explanations must accept the fact that the reports of such experiences are no more frequent among mentally ill people than among those without mental illness (Jacobson & Bruno, 1994; Parnell & Sprinkle, 1990). Among the most plausible and least controversial explanations for these reports are fantasy proneness or boundary deficits; using culturally available scenerios derived from film and other media sources; confusing subjective experiences with objectively real events; suggestibility and hypnosis (especially when such reports are "recovered" in therapeutic encounters using hypnosis); sleep disorders; and various possible psychoses in at least a minority of cases (Appelle, Lynn, & Newman, 2000). However, the fact that AAEs often contain "theophanies" (the receipt of explicit religious or spiritual messages) links them to other experiences that are more common within mainstream faith traditions. Lest skeptics too quickly consider these experiences to be simply bizarre manifestations that are exhaustively explainable by the social sciences, they might be cautioned that those who have studied these experiences in depth have found that the dismissal of their truth or reality, as with many claims to more mainstream religious experiences, is more difficult than one might at first think (Appelle, 1996; Strassman, 2001; Skal, 1998). It has been more than half a century since Jung said of UFOs (much less AAEs), "If military authorities have felt compelled to set up bureaus for collecting and evaluating UFO reports, then psychology, too, has not only the right but also the duty to do what it can to shed light on this dark problem" (1958/1964, p. 416).

experience is described, it does not determine the experience itself. The experience is likely to occur in hypnogogic sleep states and is not associated with pathology (Hufford, 1982). Table 10.2 shows that while cultural knowledge about the Old Hag is related to having the experience, people unfamiliar with the cultural knowledge about the experience nevertheless also report it. Thus cultural knowledge does not alone account for the report of this experience. After 10 years of study, Hufford concluded: "The content of the experience cannot be satisfactorily explained on the basis of current knowledge" (1982, p. 246).

Hufford's (1982) sympathetic study of the Old Hag phenomenon, as well as research on AAEs, suggests that the study of religious experiences is moving toward careful descriptions of such experiences from the perspective of those who have them—and toward the possibility that even the reality claims of seemingly bizarre experiences may have validity. For instance, Laubach (2004) has suggested "psychisms" as a descriptive term to cover a wide range of anomalous and counterintuitive experiences. From the perspective of the experiencer, such experiences are psychic intrusions into the stream of consciousness that are interpreted as not originating within the self's normal information channels (Laubach, 2004, p. 242). Persons who experience psychisms give them the same evidential force as sensory experiences and hence subjectively confirm their esoteric beliefs. That many of these are rejected by mainstream religious traditions accounts for the fact that many who are spiritual but not religious accept highly subjective experiences and beliefs that confirm them in opposition to communal practices and conformity. As with some spiritual transformations, psychisms are self-authenticating (Paloutzian, Swenson, & McNamara, 2006). However, as noted in Research Box 10.2, even psychisms can be sustained by a process of social support.

TABLE 10.2. The Old Hag Experience: The Relationship between Cultural Knowledge and Personal Reports of the Experience, and a Description of the Experience

Reporting of personal Old Hag experience as a function of accurate cultural knowledge in a sample of 93 Newfoundland students

	Reporting experience	Not reporting experience
Accurate knowledge	15.1% ($n = 14$)	24.7% ($n = 23$)
Inaccurate knowledge	7.5% ($n = 7$)	52.7% ($n = 49$)

Description of the Old Hag experience

Primary features (definitive)
1. Subjective impression of wakefulness
2. Immobility variously perceived (paralysis, restraint, fear of moving)
3. Realistic perception of actual environment
4. Fear

Secondary features (experiences contain at least one of these, often more)
1. Supine position
2. Feeling of presence
3. Feeling of pressure
4. Numinous quality
5. Fear of death

Note. Data from Hufford (1982, pp. 25, 30).

RESEARCH BOX 10.2. Accepting the Reality of Psychic Intrusions
(Romme & Escher, 1989, 1996)

A patient diagnosed with schizophrenia, who heard voices and who had read Jaynes's (1976) book postulating a "bicameral mind," was intrigued with the fact that there once was strong cultural support (as in ancient Greece) for what psychiatrists often dismiss today as mere hallucination. Appearing on Dutch television with this patient, Romme and Escher invited those who heard voices to contact them. This sampling procedure, like that of Hardy as described earlier in the text, was far from scientific. Yet it did reveal how a self-selected sample of persons (450) described coping with what some might dismiss as only auditory hallucinations, but are experienced as psychic intrusions.

Some of the people who responded to Romme and Escher's invitation were interviewed in depth concerning their process of adaptation to the voices they heard. For the approximately one-third of persons who successfully coped with voices, the general process of successful adjustment followed a clearly identified pattern that fell into three main phases:

Phase I (*startle*): Voices appear suddenly, often following stress. Persons may panic. They often feel confused and powerless. Persons struggle, try to avoid the voices, or try to make the voices disappear.

Phase II (*organization*): Persons begin to adjust to voices. There are great individual differences. Some common techniques of adjustment include ignoring negative voices or deciding to listen to them only at certain times. Positive voices are listened to more frequently, and a person may even respond to them.

Phase III (*stabilization*): Persons accept voices, and often find that they can have positive influences. Voices are integrated into an otherwise normal life.

Limits and Transcendence: The James–Boisen Formula

Before looking at particular studies of religious experience, we are going to suggest the wisdom of James's simple formula for religious experience. For while James is most often noted for his insistence on the richness and diversity of religious experience, he also suggested that a resolution of a previously experienced uneasiness is the thread from which all religious experience is woven. James is not alone in this.

Boisen (1936, 1960) noted that what distinguishes religious experience from otherwise intense, but pathological, experience is that religious experience is a resolution of what would otherwise be a devastating defeat. For Boisen as for James, it is not the nature of the experience that defines it as religious, but its results. Religious experiences, like some pathological experiences, force a confrontation with great personal disharmony. But there is a difference: the outcome. A religious experience marks the successful resolution of an inner conflict defined in transcendental terms. A limit has been reached and meaningfully transcended.

This James–Boisen formula meshes nicely with both theological and psychological perspectives in which the concepts of limits and transcendence are related (Corssan, 1975; Johnson, 1974). In the simplest sense, a total involvement and awareness of limits produce the discontent and disharmony (James's uneasiness or discontent) that creates the possibility of transcendence. It is the very confrontation with limits, however conceived, that can produce despair and the tragedy of defeat if such limits are oppressively interminable—or joy and the ecstasy of transcendence when such limits are overcome. This is the sense in which Bowker (1973) has emphasized that the psychological origin of the sense of God must be rooted not in the particulars of experience, but rather in terms of content that meaningfully points to limits to be surpassed. In this sense, God is always "beyond," and the psychology of religious experiencing is the experience of this "beyondness" through the transcendence of previously experienced limits.

We have a rather basic perspective within which to organize the empirical literature on religious experience. It can be traced back to James's notion of discontent and resolution, but only if we keep in mind the fact that both discontent and resolution are *interpretations* rooted in James's definition of religion. In a fundamental sense, religious experience is the meaningful transcendence of limits of the resolution of discontent, rooted in a sense of the divine. Not surprisingly, then, religious experience is almost infinite in its varieties. It is the *understanding in a religious vocabulary* of the process of discontent and its resolution that makes an experience religious (Taves, 1999). According to Taylor (2002), this is part of James's lasting legacy to an empirical psychology that is adequate to taking a nonreductive approach to religion.

Sundén's Role Theory

If there is a typicality to religious experience, it comes from the uniformity of interpretation found within particular traditions. Traditions define what are relevant religious experiences. The experience of being religious varies across traditions. Perhaps most compatible with this perspective is the work of the Swedish psychologist Hjalmar Sundén (see Holm, 1995; Holm & Belzen, 1995). His theory of religious experience is truly social-psychological in nature. Most important for our present purposes is Sundén's conclusion that religious traditions, particularly in the form of sacred texts, provide the templates or models that make *religious* experience possible. In other words, the interpretation or perception of events in terms modeled by stories from sacred texts is what makes experience religious. Without knowledge of a religious tradition and its sacred texts, religious experiences are not possible. For example, many would not associate the handling of serpents with religion, as noted earlier in this chapter. However, in some southern Appalachian churches, serpent handling is a religious experience perceived to be in obedience to God's will as one of the five signs specified in Mark 16:17–18. These "sign-following" churches obey what they perceive to be God's will. Signs of obedience include speaking in tongues, casting out of demons, laying hands upon the sick, handling serpents, and the drinking of poisonous substances (Brown & McDonald, 2000; Burton, 1993; Hood, 1998; Hood & Williamson, 2008a, 2008b; Kimbrough, 1995; Pelton & Carden, 1974).

Serpent Handling as a Religious Experience

In 18th-century North America, "rattlesnake gazing," or staring at snakes in the wild, was a common practice. Settlers, strongly informed by Biblical narratives, found in rattlesnake gazing a significance that attributed supernatural powers to this "agent of Satan." As one historian of popular religiosity (Lippy, 1994, p. 79) notes, "a people familiar with the biblical story of the serpent's tempting of Eve might well be predisposed to assume that the rattlesnake and other serpentine creatures did indeed possess supernatural power." However, rattlesnake gazing was never practiced as a religious ritual or acknowledged by any formal religious denominations.

At the turn of the 20th century, Holiness sects in Appalachia emphasized numerous Biblical texts (e.g., Mark 16:17–18; Luke 10:19) by which the handling of serpents gained a religious significance. In its early history, the Church of God championed serpent handling as one of the "five signs" (Williamson, 1995). In obedience to their interpretation of scripture, believers handled serpents, or (with reference to Luke 10:19) walked upon them. Serpent handling was popularized by George Hensley, who modeled the handling of serpents in churches. Later abandoned by the Church of God (whose members continue to engage in some of the signs, such as speaking in tongues), the practice persists in Holiness sects throughout Appalachia. In Sundén's role theory, both the scriptural text and the modeling of this text in actual practice permit believers to handle serpents as a religious act (Hood & Kimbrough, 1995). In addition, in terms of our notion of limits and transcendence, the actual handling of serpents in services permits a transcendence of the real possibility of death that lies at the rational basis of the fear of handling rattlesnakes and other vipers (Hood, 1998; Hood & Kimbrough, 1995; Hood & Williamson, 2008b). Whether serpent handlers are bitten or not, whether they live or die, they believe that they live and act in obedience to God's word based upon their understanding of the Bible (Hood, 1998). Research Box 10.3 presents a study that focuses upon the experience of serpent handling from the believers' own perspective.

The example of serpent handling illustrates one criticism of the study of religious experience in North American psychology. It is a criticism leveled against James and to some extent inherent in the appeal to "experience." In general, it would appear that the demand to describe "experience" is a plea to identify something unique, intense, or exceptional in one's life. "What did you experience?" is one of those questions that focus on extremes, much as the expletive "What an experience!" is likely to identify something exceptional in one's life. In one of the early critiques of James's *The Varieties of Religious Experience*, Crooks (1913) bemoaned James's fascination with the extreme and unusual in religious experience, at the expense of the more common experiences characteristic of religion. In a similar vein, Starbuck (1904) urged other psychologists of religion to avoid a focus upon the extremes in religious experience. The echoes of such criticism are still heard today, but largely fall upon deaf ears. It would appear that for many social scientists, ordinary piety and the commonplaces of religious experience are as James saw them—the duller religious habits. What fascinated James most were the more passionate expressions of the extremes of religious experience. Little has changed in this regard since *The Varieties*. The empirical literature has a Jamesian focus, if not in method, in terms of the topics that have elicited interest and study.

THE BODY IN RELIGIOUS AND SPIRITUAL EXPERIENCE

In her presidential address to the Society for the Scientific Study of Religion, Meredith McGuire (1990, p. 284) posed this interesting question: "What if people—the subjects of our research and theorizing—had material bodies?" McGuire answered her own rhetorical question by noting three broad themes in which the social sciences might better appreciate what she aptly termed the "mindful body" (p. 285): in the experience of self and others; in the production and reflection of social meanings; and in the body's significance as the subject

---

RESEARCH BOX 10.3. What Is It Like to Handle a Serpent?
(Williamson & Pollio, 1999)

Williamson and Pollio taped sermons by serpent handlers, delivered spontaneously immediately after the handling of serpents. Eighteen sermons were analyzed for their basic thematic contents. Five themes emerged, all understood within the context of a powerfully embodied experience of handling serpents in obedience to the believer's understanding of such passages in the Bible as Mark 16:17–18 and Luke 10:19.

Theme I: The experience of anointment or feeling moved by God to handle the serpent.

Theme II: The reality of being in the presence of death. A common phrase that preachers use is "There is death in these boxes" (the serpent boxes in which serpents are carried to church and contained when not being handled).

Theme III: Feeling of uniqueness and of separation between "us" (believers who handle serpents) and "them" (others who do not handle serpents or even ridicule believers who do).

Theme IV: The power of true knowing. The experience of being special, of understanding truly God's word and of living what they often identify as "the good way."

Theme V: Intense joy and affective pleasure, most typically identified as "joy unspeakable."

As Williamson and Pollio note, if one simply assumes truth to be perspectival, their phenomenological approach and the identification of meaningful themes in the experience of serpent handling allow a researcher "to see the world as the religious practitioner sees it, unaffected (as far as possible) by theories external to the practitioner's belief and experience" (1999, p. 216).

Note. Adapted from Williamson and Pollio (1999). The phenomenology of religious serpent handling: A rationale and thematic study of extemporaneous sermons. *Journal for the Scientific Study of Religion, 38,* 203–218. Copyright © 1999 Blackwell Publishing, Ltd. Adapted by permission.

---

and object of power relations. Although McGuire's concern is more sociological than psychological, her appeal to reconsider the body is useful for psychologists who tend to reduce the body to the study of physiological processes. This is a particularly pernicious tendency in the psychology of religion.

Perhaps one of the most shortsighted views of religious experience is to assume that such experiences are merely emotional. The "merely" here has a negative connotation; it suggests that since what is perceived as religiously meaningful is physiological in origin, it can be discounted. James (1902/1985) identified such disclaiming views as "medical materialism":

Medical materialism finishes up Saint Paul by calling his vision on the road to Damascus a discharging lesion of the occipital cortex, he being an epileptic. It snuffs out Saint Teresa as an hysteric, Saint Francis of Assisi as a hereditary degenerate. George Fox's discontent with the shams of his age, and his pining for spiritual veracity, it treats as a disordered colon. (p. 20)

The point, of course, is not that physiological processes may not be involved in religious experience, but that some psychologists think the identification of the physiological processes involved in religious experience "reduces it away." Yet no experience is identical to the processes involved in its occurrence. This is not to say that physiological processes such as arousal may not be involved in some aspects of religious experiencing. What is crucial is that such arousal be appropriately identified as part of a broader context, which is identified as religious because of other than merely physiological processes. The consideration becomes not simply arousal, but arousal contextualized and interpreted.

Taves (1999) has shown that from Wesley to James, North American Protestantism has struggled with evaluating the legitimacy of experiences based upon what is known about how they can be elicited. Her basic categories involve two dimensions: supernatural versus natural origins, and religious versus secular interpretations. Those who interpret experience religiously and attribute it to a supernatural origin are essentially religious apologists doing religious psychology. Those who interpret experience in secular scientific terms and attribute them only to natural causes are doing what she calls the psychology of religion. The interesting effort to interpret natural experiences in religious language is what Taves (1999, p. 348) refers to as the "mediating" tradition—an effort that can be linked to William James and the desire to establish a comparative scientific study of religion in general.

Physiological Arousal and Religious and Spiritual Experience

It has long been noted that when persons describe their experiences, there are often large physiological components to their descriptions. It appears that as embodied selves, human beings must have feelings to claim to have experienced something. Yet in a critical survey of current psychological theories of feeling, Hill (1995, p. 355) flatly states that "there are no general overarching theories of affect guiding research on religious experience." However, in the conceptual literature on religious experience, there is a broad-based theory that has generated considerable discussion. It is essentially a social-constructionist theory, which argues that there are no natural emotions. Emotions are constructed, interpreted, and recognized according to cognitive interpretations of physiological arousal. Much of this theory is based upon the psychological research of Schachter (1964, 1971) and his two-factor theory of emotion.

Within the conceptual literature on religious experience, Proudfoot (1985) has focused upon Schachter's two-factor theory of emotion as providing a conceptual critique in support of constructionist theories of religious experience. Schachter's theory essentially argues that the identification of an emotional experience requires both physiological arousal and a cognitive framework within which to identify the meaning of the arousal. Neither alone is sufficient to determine an emotional experience. In other words, persons tend to know how they feel or what they experience in terms of two quite different processes: (1) what the arousal circumstances were (external, perceptual, or cognitive factors), and (2) what internal physiological processes the persons are aware of. Hence the labeling of physiological arousal is not due just to physiological arousal per se, but to the specific circumstances in which the physiological arousal occurs. In this view, otherwise unanticipated physiological arousal may be labeled as "fear," "awe," or "anger," depending upon the circumstances in which it occurs. Proudfoot (1985) relies upon Schachter's theory to defend the thesis that experience cannot be religious until and unless it is identified and interpreted to be religious. Thus, consistent with Sundén's role theory (discussed above), without religious training and instruction to provide a context for interpretation, one cannot have a religious experience.

In a now classic study, Schachter and Singer (1962) injected a drug, epinephrine (adrenaline), into persons participating in an experiment they were told was intended to test the effects of a vitamin compound on vision. In fact, half the participants received an injection of epinephrine, which reliably produces increased respiration and heart rate, slight muscle tremors, and an "edgy" feeling. The other participants received a placebo (saline solution), which produces no physiological feelings. Hence the experimenters could be fairly assured that only the experimental group would experience physiological arousal. The participants in the experimental group were further divided into three groups: One group was told truthfully what physiological effects to anticipate; one group was misinformed and told to anticipate numbness, itching, and perhaps a headache; one group was given no information. Contextual cues were then provided for all persons in the experiment. The cues were provided by "stooges" of the experimenter, who were in the room with the real subjects, presumably as participants in the experiment. The stooges acted either euphoric or angry.

Results of the experiment were generally as predicted and support a cognition-plus-arousal theory of emotional experience. Persons who experienced no physiological arousal (the placebo [saline solution] group), or who were given correct information as to expectations, did not use environmental cues to label their emotions. On the other hand, those with incorrect information or no information tended to interpret their emotions to be congruent with the cues—as euphoric when the stooges acted euphoric, and as angry when the stooges acted angry. Both observation (through one-way mirrors) and self-report measures were used in this study. In both experimental groups, physiological arousal was generally properly identified (e.g., change in heart rate). The placebo group reported no physiological changes. Hence Schachter and Singer (1962) argued that, given a situation of unanticipated physiological arousal, external cues (in this case, the stooges' feigned emotional behavior) influence the labeling of what emotion is occurring. Whether it is labeled as angry, happy, or sad depends upon the context for unanticipated physiological arousal. Specific emotions are thus socially constructed.

Since its inception, Schachter's two-factor theory has generated much debate (see Kemper, 1978; Marlasch, 1979; Plutchik & Ax, 1967). Despite major methodological criticisms of the Schachter and Singer (1962) study, its importance for a theory of religious experience is that physiological processes per se cannot account for emotional experiences; cognitions must also occur, at least in ambiguous circumstances (Azari, 2006; Hill & Hood, 1999b).

It is important to note that Schachter's theory gives a place to both cognition and physiological arousal. More recently, theorists have begun to champion more extreme views that minimize the role of physiology in emotions. For example, the almost purely cognitive view of Lazarus (1990) is that emotions are organized psychophysiological reactions. The organization requires cognitive appraisal. Thus, without cognition or appraisal, emotions are impossible; they are merely unspecified physiological activation. However, the relevance of cognition–arousal theories such as Schachter's, and the more cognitive appraisal theories such as Lazarus's, is that the articulation of experience gains religious relevance from the tradition within which experience gains its validity. As Taves (1999) argues, language matters. How an experience is described and narrated is an integral part of what it means to have this experience, rather than some other. The more one is knowledgeable about a tradition, the more one can experience what it is the tradition defines as religious. Sundén's role theory meshes nicely with the cognitive aspect of these theories, insofar as familiarity with religious texts and traditions is the rich source for appraisals that a situation is religiously relevant. Traditions provide the relevant cognitions.

In our own view of limits and transcendence, cognition–arousal and appraisal theories suggest that physiological arousal may be a factor initiating feelings that become meaningfully religious only if other appropriate conditions are met. The relevant question is this: Under what conditions will physiological arousal be interpreted religiously? Modern research suggests what James long ago insisted: When a person interprets an experience as religious, one must in the end look at the immediate content and context of religious consciousness. However, much of the research literature on religious practices has been more concerned with aspects of arousal than with the context in which arousal is interpreted. Both prayer and meditation have been studied in terms of the state of the brain's arousal during these practices.

Meditation and Prayer

The activities of prayer and meditation have in common an effort to withdraw from normal waking consciousness and a concern with attention to another reality, often considered to be transcendent. Of course, we must be careful with language here: Prayer and meditation are affirmed by devout individuals to be meaningful confrontations with a "deeper" or "higher" reality, or perhaps, as in the case of Zen, simply a full appreciation of reality as it is. For instance, Preston (1988) has shown how converts to Zen are socialized into an interpretation of reality that is based upon nonconceptual meditative techniques, which demand attentiveness to reality presumably as it is, in and of itself.

Naranjo and Ornstein (1971) distinguish between "ideational" and "nonideational" mediation. The former encourages and utilizes imagery that is common within a tradition; the later seeks an imageless state and avoids attention to unwanted imagery that may occur during meditation. The fact that much imageless meditation is widely recognized as a spiritual practice has contributed to the psychophysiological study of meditation. Rather than assess either verbal reports or behavior, investigators have focused upon physiological measures, particularly of brain activity. This has proven a particularly useful technique for studying persons who are otherwise apparently "just sitting."

We have noted in Chapter 3 the preliminary status of any strong claim to have identified physiological determinants of religious experience. Seeking a precise physiology of either prayer or meditation may be one of those chimerical tasks that serve to satisfy those who will accept the reality of spiritual things only if they can identify their bodily correlates. Experience is no more "real" because one can identify its physiological correlates than it is the case that identical physiological correlates of meditative states mean that the experiences are necessarily the "same." The experience of mediation and prayer is more than its physiology (Azari, 2006).

Sundén thought that his role theory was particularly useful in addressing the question "How are religious experiences at all psychologically possible?" (Wikstrom, 1987, p. 390). Jan van der Lans (1985, 1987) utilized Sundén's theory in a study of students selected to participate in a 4-week training course in Zen meditation. They were told simply to concentrate on their breathing for the first 14 sessions. Then they were told to concentrate without a focus upon any object—a method called *shikantaza* in Zen. Participants were divided into those with (*n* = 14) and those without (*n* = 21) a religious frame of reference, based upon intake interviews. Instructions varied for each group: The religious group was told to anticipate experiences common in meditation within religious traditions, and the control group was told to anticipate experiences common in meditation used for therapeutic purposes.

Dependent measures included writing down every unusual experience after each daily session, and by filling out a questionnaire on the last day of training that asked participants specifically whether they had had a religious experience during meditation. The daily experiences were content-analyzed according to a list of 54 experiences categorized into five types: bodily sensations; fantasies, illusions, and imagery (hallucinations); changes in self-image; new insights; and negative feelings. Responses per category were too low for any meaningful statistical analyses. However, the number of persons reporting a religious experience during their Zen meditation varied as a function of presence or absence of a premeditative religious frame. Half of the religious participants reported a religious experience during meditation, while none of the control group (those without a premeditative religious frame) did. In addition, all participants were asked a control question at the end of the study: Had their meditations made them feel more vital and energetic? The groups did not differ on this question.

The conclusion we may draw from this research is that the actual practice of meditation elicits a specifically religious experience only for those with a religious frame of reference. If we assume equivalent meditative states in both groups (e.g., achievement of alpha states), the meaningfulness of such a state is dependent upon the interpretative frame one brings to the experience. Of course, a paradox is that within Zen, interpretative frames are minimized; hence this research employed a technique more compatible with prayer within the Christian tradition, in which interpretation plays a more significant role (Holmes, 1980). Still, it is clear that experience, meaningfully interpreted, is dependent upon whatever framework for interpretation can be brought to or derived from the experience. Sundén's role theory simply argues that familiarity with a religious tradition is the basis from which religious experiences gain their meaningfulness—and without which *religious* experiences are not possible.

Whereas Zen mediation emphasizes contemplation without an object, Deikman (1966) empirically investigated contemplative meditation, in which the emphasis is upon focused concentration upon a single object. What is important about Deikman's work is that contemplative meditation is often associated with the mystical tradition, in which the goal is a state of unity that is devoid of content or imagery. This is introvertive mysticism, as discussed in Chapter 11. However, it is also known that various experiences are likely to occur as one concentrates, including imagery of various sorts. Much of this imagery is readily understandable in the psychology of perception as afterimages, stabilized retinal images, and hypnogogic imagery. If not interpreted as meaningful, such imagery is largely irrelevant; it is left as minimal experience without meaning. However, if such experiences are specifically interpreted to be distractions and not part of one's meditative goal, such experiences have no inherent religious meaning and are only clues that one has yet to reach the desired imageless state. Furthermore, to focus upon such imagery will distract achievement of the imageless, introvertive mystical state.

Deikman's study was unusual, in that it reported the results of a prolonged series of meditative sessions derived primarily from two participants. They simply sat in comfortable chairs and for 30 minutes focused attention upon a blue vase. Contemplative meditation requires that one simply contemplate the meditative object, without attention to thoughts or peripheral sensations. In Deikman's study, no religious object was used as a meditative object; hence, in term of Sundén's theory, religious frames of reference were unlikely to be elicited. Deikman's study was thus phenomenological—that is, an effort to provide a clear description of whatever appeared to the subjects' consciousness. Wulff (1995) notes that phenomenological studies try to reclaim for psychology the preeminence of experience. Deikman's (1966) study and the Williamson and Pollio (1999) study of serpent handlers (see Research Box 10.3) are among the few studies that have attempted to reclaim experience for psychology. Each provided careful descriptions and documentation of phenomena that were not all expected by the participants or easily interpreted as *merely* subjective phenomena. These studies have left open the possibility that contemplative meditation and serpent handling allow an openness to experience that permits other aspects of reality to be revealed.

Other descriptive studies of meditation and of serpent handling likewise reveal a rich variety of experiences, many of which cannot simply be dismissed as subjective states (Goleman, 1977, 1988; Hood, 1998; Naranjo & Ornstein, 1971). It may be that phenomenological methods are the most appropriate for descriptively exploring experiences that often have religious importance (Hood, 2002b; Hood & Williamson, 2008b). As Wulff (1995, p. 197) has stated, "Indeed, systematically appropriated and developed by even a handful of investigators, phenomenological psychology could revolutionize the field."

One of the earliest topics in psychology, and one that continues to occupy the interests of psychologists of religion, is the efficacy of prayer. However, it is only recently that psychologists have become interested in empirical (much less experimental) studies of prayer, which Heiler (1932) argued to be central to religion. Since there are few firm data on which to base a theory of prayer, it is not surprising for Janssen, de Hart, and den Draak (1990) to note that "no convincing psychological theory [of prayer] exists." However, surveys of the empirical literature on prayer share a consensus that prayer is multidimensional (Spilka & Ladd, 2013). Several multidimensional models have been proposed. In their own summary of the empirical literature, Spilka and Ladd rely heavily upon a model first proposed by Foster (1992), in which the focus is upon the directionality of prayer—either outward, upward, or inward.

Part of the problem with much of the empirical research on prayer is that instead of focusing upon the content and phenomenology of prayer, researchers have focused upon its correlates. Galton (1869), one of the earliest measurement psychologists, argued persuasively on the basis of statistical analysis that prayer has no demonstrable objective benefits. However, he argued just as persuasively for the beneficial effects of prayer on subjective well-being. The shift to a focus upon subjective well-being in prayer research has been helpful for the study of religious experience in two senses. First, subjective well-being involves experience—how one feels or reacts to situations as a function of prayer. Second, few religionists or scientists would find a test derived from a participant's own wishes to be very meaningful, and thus there has been a shift away from study of the mere efficacy of prayer in objective terms. The scientists find such studies deficient because people obviously cannot wish the world to conform to their desires in any efficacious sense, and few researchers would bother to think further empirical tests of such hypotheses worthwhile. The religionists find such theorizing inadequate because mature faith in virtually every tradition is likely to be seen as shifting from requesting that a person's own will be done to asking that the divine will be done. In the latter case, apparently unanswered prayers (outcomes not corresponding to those requested) can be successfully interpreted as meaningful in terms of a more mature reflection upon the nature of faith, as emphasized by Godin (1968, 1985).

Poloma and her colleagues have made significant contributions to the contemporary empirical study of prayer (Poloma & Gallup, 1991; Poloma & Pendleton, 1989). Not only have they reliably measured several types of prayer (colloquial, meditative, petitionary, and ritualistic), but they have focused upon the more psychologically meaningful measures of (1) experiences during prayer and (2) subjective consequences of prayer. Thus much of Poloma et al.'s work is in the quality-of-life tradition, which meaningfully assesses the subjective aspects of human experience (Poloma & Pendleton, 1991).

"Quality of life" is a multidimensional construct that includes existential well-being, happiness, life satisfaction, religious satisfaction, and negative affect (reverse-scored). Prayer is also multidimensional, with various types of prayer differentially relating to experienced quality of life. For instance, meditative prayer is most closely related to religious satisfaction and existential well-being. On the other hand, only colloquial prayer predicts the absence of negative affect, whereas ritual prayer alone predicts negative affect (Poloma & Pendleton, 1989). Thus not simply frequency of prayer, but the nature and type of prayer, determine the experiential consequences of prayer.

Another contribution of Poloma and her colleagues is to focus upon the measurement of actual experiences during prayer. Poloma's prayer index is presented in Table 10.3. This index consistently correlates with quality of life, regardless of the objective status of those who pray. Thus in the specific case of variables used in religion, assessing objective outcomes may be less relevant than assessing subjective ones, as others have noted (Brown, 1966, 1994). Specifically, in research on prayer, Brown (1966, 1968) has noted that the belief in the objective efficacy of even petitionary prayer decreases with age and spiritual maturity.

This turn away from attempting to document the physical consequences of prayer makes work such as Loehr's (1959) on the efficacy of prayer on plant growth less worthy of critical methodological commentary than irrelevant. It is simply the wrong kind of issue to address. If the focus is upon the change in intentionality, consciousness, or affect of those who pray, then the focus of prayer is rightly on its subjective quality.

In this regard, both Poloma and her colleagues, and Hood and his, have derived remarkably similar factors in their multidimensional approach to the measurement of prayer. Table 10.4 presents their similar factor structures, which are remarkable for their independent derivation—one by a team of sociologists, the other by a team of psychologists. Furthermore, the high reliability of all scales suggests the robust nature of the multidimensional criteria of prayer that Poloma's and Hood's groups have both identified.

Both Poloma's and Hood's groups have noted that "contemplative" (Hood's term) or "meditative" (Poloma's term) praying—a nonpetitionary attempt merely to become aware of God—leads to unique experiences. For instance, Poloma and Pendleton (1989, p. 43)

TABLE 10.3. Poloma's Index of Prayer Experience

1. How often during the past year have you felt divinely inspired or "led by God" to perform something specific as a result of prayer?

2. How often have you received what you believed to be a deeper insight into a spiritual or Biblical truth?

3. How often have you received what you regarded as a definitive answer to a specific prayer request?

4. How often have you felt a strong sense of God during prayer?

5. How often have you experienced a deep sense of peace and well-being during prayer?

Answer options: once or twice,   monthly,   weekly,   daily.

Note. Republished with permission of Religious Research Association from Poloma and Pendleton (1989). Exploring types of prayer and quality of life research: A research note. Review of Religious Research, 31, 46–53.

TABLE 10.4. Poloma's and Hood's Prayer Factors Compared

Poloma's four factors[a]	Hood's four factors[b]
Meditative (alpha = .81)	**Contemplative (alpha = .82)**
How often do you spend time just "feeling" or being in the presence of God?	When you pray or meditate, how often do you seek to be one with God or ultimate reality?
How often do you spend time worshipping or adoring God?	When you pray or meditate, how often do you seek a perfect harmony
Ritualistic (alpha = .59)	**Liturgical (alpha = .81)**
How often do you read from a book of prayers?	When you pray or meditate, how often do you recite sacred phrases or words?
How often do you recite prayers that you have memorized?	When you pray or meditate, how often do you read from sacred texts?
Petitionary (alpha = .78)	**Petitionary (alpha = .90)**
How often do you ask God for material things you might need?	When you pray or meditate, how often do you seek blessings for others?
How often do you ask God for material things your friends or relatives may need?	When you pray or meditate, how often do you seek forgiveness for yourself?
Colloquial (alpha = .85)	**Material (alpha = .65)**
How often do you ask God to provide guidance in making decisions?	When you pray or meditate, how often do you seek material things for yourself?
How often do you talk with God in your own words?	When you pray or meditate, how often do you seek material things for others?

[a]Republished with permission of Religious Research Association from Poloma and Pendleton (1989). Exploring types of prayer and quality of life research: A research note. *Review of Religious Research, 31,* 46–53.
[b]Adapted from Hood, Morris, and Harvey (1993). Adapted by permission of the authors.

note that with the exception of life satisfaction, each of their quality-of-life measures relates to only one type of prayer. Consistent with our focus on subjective experience, meditative prayer relates most closely to an existential quality of life. Similarly, Hood and his colleagues found that contemplative (Poloma's meditative) prayer related most strongly to measures of mystical awareness (a feeling of unity), religiously interpreted for intrinsically religious individuals who prayed (Hood, Morris, & Watson, 1989). On the other hand, extrinsically religious individuals who prayed had disruptions of both religious and nonreligious imagery during contemplative prayer—suggesting the inability to quiet the mind and eliminate images. Furthermore, they did not experience a sense of unity, as intrinsic participants did. Thus it may be that different interpretations of experience reflect actual differences during experience, as well as differences in the types of prayer that intrinsically and extrinsically religious persons engage in.

Although more research is clearly needed, it is readily apparent that the shift away from the study of the efficacy of petitionary prayer is a step in the right direction. Brown (1994, pp. 45–46) has argued that if one restricts prayer to the narrow view of merely "asking for things," than prayer is perhaps more characteristic of unbelievers. Faber (2002) argues that a naturalistic understanding of prayer links it to magical behavior as understood in contemporary anthropology. Measurement-based research has clearly established the multi-dimensionality of prayer, and future research will undoubtedly contribute to a deeper understanding of the subjective experience of prayer. Although the empirical study of prayer is an established part of the psychology of religion (Francis & Astley, 2001), no generally agreed-upon theory of prayer has emerged (Gorsuch, 2008). In this sense, theories such as Sundén's role theory will become more relevant, as knowledge of traditions and texts is required to illuminate the meaningfulness of prayer within the communities of those who pray. Ladd and Spilka (2002) are developing a cognitive theory of prayer capable of empirical testing (Ladd & Spilka, 2002; Spilka & Ladd, 2013). Others are focusing on the specific process of praying. Research Box 10.4 reports one of the few empirical studies of the needs stated for prayer, the content of prayer, and its effects.

RESEARCH BOX 10.4. A Content Analysis of the Praying Practices of Dutch Youths (Janssen, de Hart, & den Draak, 1990)

In 1985, a sample of 192 Dutch high school students was asked to respond to three open-ended questions regarding prayer: (1) "What is praying to you?", (2) "At what moments do you feel the need to pray?", and (3) "How do you pray?" Using a computer technique to analyze the content of the response to these three questions, Janssen and colleagues were able to summarize prayer structure according to the following sentence: "Because of some reason, I address myself to someone in a particular way, at a particular place, at a particular time, to achieve something." They diagrammed this sentence as follows:

	2. Action (predicate)	
	3. Direction (indirect object)	
	4. Time (adverbial adjunct 1)	
1. Need	5. Place (adverbial adjunct 2)	7. Effect
(conditional adjunct)	6. Method (adverbial adjunct 3)	(direct object)

The percentages of content references to each structural category for the four most frequent citations within that category were as follows[a]:

1. *Need* (83%): personal problems (60%); sickness (23%); happiness (20%); death (16%).
2. *Action* (83%): talk/monologue (38%); talk/dialogue (36%); ask/wish (33%); meditate (22%).
3. *Direction* (60%): God/Lord (80%); Spirit/Power (13%); Someone (11%); Mary/Jesus (2%).
4. *Time* (20%): evening/night (90%); day (8%); dinner (8%); anytime (5%).
5. *Place* (34%): bed (86%); home (11%); church (11%); outside (9%).
6. *Method* (55%): alone (55%); prayer, formal (17%); low voice (19%); aloud (4%).
7. *Effect* (37%): help/support (38%); favor (34%); remission (13%); rest (10%).

[a]Percentages for the seven structural aspects are based upon $n = 192$. Percentages for content within each structure are based upon the number of participants who reported that structural aspect. See the Janssen et al. paper, p. 102, Table 1.

Bänziger, Janssen, and Scheeps (2008) have replicated the research reported in Research Box 10.4 with a large sample ($N = 1,008$) of Dutch participants. In addition, they have identified four types of prayer (meditative, religious, impulsive, and petitionary). These two studies are significant in showing that even in a highly secularized society such as the Netherlands, individuals continue to pray. However, the nature of prayer for the unchurched is different. For instance, the meditative prayer of Poloma and Hood is directed toward closeness to God, whereas Bänziger et al. (2008, p. 261) note that unchurched individuals' meditative prayer is focused upon themselves.

Altered States of Consciousness

At the other extreme from phenomenological and introspective descriptions of consciousness are studies that focus upon neurophysiological states. Part of their appeal is the obvious scientific legitimacy of "hard" data—the pure descriptive facts of identifiable physiological processes. Three areas have gained some considerable influence among those interested in the psychology of religion.

The catchall phrase "altered states of consciousness" rapidly emerged in the 1960s for what has become a loosely knit area focused upon the empirical study of experiences previously assumed to be pathological or anomalous (Berenbaum, Kerns, & Raghavan, 2000; Reed, 1974; Zusne & Jones, 1989). Included in this area are such phenomena as hypnosis, dreaming, meditation, drug experiences, and a number of other "fringe" topics (e.g., parapsychology and near-death experiences). Much of this literature is more popular than academic. Until recently, the serious academic study of such experiences has assumed that such experiences have no objective validity. However, among sympathetic researchers there has been a shift in attitude: The experiences themselves are positively valued and assumed to have ontological validity. In other words, previous efforts to provide reductive explanations of such experiences are now overshadowed by descriptive efforts to explore the experiences' meaning and validity, including their objectivity (Berenbaum et al., 2000). Much of this is incorporated into modern "transpersonal psychology"—an area yet to be clearly defined or to have general academic and research support among mainstream psychologists (Greenwood, 1995). However, it is apparent that investigators are beginning to study empirically a wide variety of experiences that are immensely relevant to religion. Much of this research promises to enliven the psychology of religion by including within the discipline phenomena that religious traditions take seriously.

Tart (1975) has been extremely influential in linking transpersonal psychology and altered states of consciousness. Basically, an altered state of consciousness is characterized by an introspective awareness of a different mode of experiencing the world. Loosely speaking, for example, everyone experiences dreaming as an altered state of consciousness relative to the normal waking state. Each altered state of consciousness has a typical pattern of functioning, recognized as such by the person. Hence things that might seem strange or bizarre are not really so when they are recognized as normal for that particular state of consciousness. Furthermore, persons move in and out of various states of consciousness. In Zinberg's (1977) view, there are alternate states of consciousness, not simply one normal and appropriate state of consciousness. Generally, it is assumed that the more open to experience one is, the more states of consciousness one can experience. More controversial is Tart's claim that knowledge is state-specific—in other words, that it is derived from, and appropriate to, a particular state of consciousness and may not be applicable to other states. Thus many religions are seen as state-specific sciences, with knowledge claims that are valid only within the parameters of the experiences and interpretations provided by these traditions. This parallels the concept of "ideological surround," discussed in Chapter 12. In a sense, new religious movements represent the sociological counterpart to the psychology of alternate states of consciousness.

Although much of transpersonal psychology (especially the claim to state-specific knowledge) is controversial, the concept of altered states of consciousness is often supported by a physiological base. Most typically, this consists of identifying alterations in neurophysiology that are assumed to be associated with such states. None of these models have achieved any degree of consensus, and most are at best speculations, in neurophysiological terms, about processes assumed to underlie various altered states of consciousness. Perhaps most often cited is Fischer's (1971, 1978) cartography of mental states linked to a continuum of arousal. This continuum ranges from hypoaroused tranquility, to normal everyday consciousness, to arousal, to hyperarousal, and finally to ecstasy. Although extensive discussion of the neurophysiology of consciousness is beyond the scope of our concerns, the important point is that neurophysiological correlates (verified or not) have given altered states of consciousness a respectability within mainstream science, especially insofar as consciousness is studied as a brain process. This respectability comes at the same time that others are affirming the much more controversial claim that the objects revealed in such altered states of consciousness cannot be dismissed as merely subjective phenomena.

As new technologies emerge to allow noninvasive neurophysiological measurement of ongoing experience, neurophysiological correlates of more typical religious experiences can be identified, as we have noted in Chapter 3. The research by Azari et al. (2001) discussed in Research Box 3.2 provides additional support for the claim that religious experience is a cognitive attributional phenomenon that often includes a causal claim as to its origins (Proudfoot & Shaver, 1975; Proudfoot, 1985). It also demonstrates that much of the speculation regarding the neurophysiological correlates of religious experiences is likely to be effectively tested in laboratory conditions with a variety of new technologies.

Speaking in Tongues (Glossolalia)

"Glossolalia," or speaking in tongues, is a universal religious phenomenon (May, 1956). Jaynes (1976) asserts that it is always a group phenomenon and that it fits well into the general bicameral paradigm, including the strong cognitive imperative of religious belief in a cohesive group, the induction procedures of prayer and ritual resulting in the narrowing of consciousness (trance), and the archaic authorization of the divine spirit in a charismatic leader. Whereas Jaynes (1976) asserts the musical and poetic nature of glossolalia, Samarin (1972) finds it to be merely a meaningless, phonologically structured human sound. Lafal, Monahan, and Richman (1974) dispute the claim that glossolalia is meaningless. Hutch (1980) claims that glossolalia aims to amalgamate the sounds of laughing and crying—signs of both the joy and pain of life. Early psychologists attributed glossolalia to mental illness, but later researchers have made a strong conceptual case for distinguishing glossolalia from what are only superficial clinical parallels (Kelsey, 1964; Kildahl, 1972). Empirically, glossolalia is normative within many religious traditions, including some Pentecostal and Holiness denominations in the contemporary United States. Thus it is not surprising that empirical studies comparing glossolalic with nonglossolalic controls have consistently failed to find any reliable psychological differences, including indices of psychopathology, between the two groups

(Goodman, 1972; Hine, 1969; Malony & Lovekin, 1985; J. T. Richardson, 1973). However, it is also true that, as Lovekin and Malony (1977) found in their study of participants in a Catholic charismatic program of spiritual renewal, glossolalia per se may not be particularly useful in fostering personality integration.

The real focus of research has been on whether or not glossolalia occurs only in a trance or altered state of consciousness. Goodman (1969), an anthropologist, has documented the cross-cultural similarity of glossolalic utterances. She attributes this similarity to the fact that glossolalia results from an induced trance. The trace state itself, for neurophysiological reasons, accounts for the cross-cultural similarity of glossolalia (Goodman, 1972). Her model of the induction of a trance state follows closely Jaynes's general bicameral paradigm (Goodman, 1988). She argues for induction techniques generated by religious rituals in believers. This trance state produces an altered perceptual state in which previous limits are transcended. One participant in her research stated the case for limits and transcendence quite succinctly: "At first you feel that you have come to a barrier, and you are afraid. All of a sudden you are beyond it and everything is different" (quoted in Goodman, 1988, p. 37). This altered perceptual state is identified by Goodman as the "sojourn." It is followed by "dissolution," or the return to ordinary perceptual states, and by the joy and euphoria of having had this sacred experience.

Samarin (1972) has challenged Goodman's cross-cultural data on the grounds that all her samples were from similar Pentecostal settings, even though the data were collected within different cultures. Samarin also points out that preaching patterns identified in typical Appalachian Mountain settings are similar to those found in glossolalia. This is the case, even though such preaching does not occur in a trance state; hence there is no reason to infer that glossolalia can only be elicited in trance states. This view is also supported by Hine (1969). More recently, however, Philipchalk and Muller (2000) demonstrated increased activation of the right hemisphere relative to the left in a small sample of participants who allowed infrared photography before and after speaking in tongues. The opposite was found before and after reading aloud. These data suggest the activation of the right hemisphere in glossolalia, and not necessarily the existence of a trance state.

Obviously, the outcome of the debate on whether or not trance states are necessary for such religious experiences as glossolalia or serpent handling is partly conceptually clouded (Hood & Williamson, 2008b, pp. 102–116). It would require a clear operational definition of glossolalia at one level and a clear operational definition of trance at another level to test whether the two covary, much less to see whether glossolalia can only be elicited in a trance state. Although such research has yet to be done, the debate has been useful as another instance of religious experience's gaining a foothold in mainstream social science by raising issues of possible physiological correlates. It is assumed that since such physiological processes can be identified in hard scientific terms, the experiences they facilitate have at least that validity. Of course, once again, for religiously committed individuals, such faint praise is less than sufficient. Experience attributed to the gods or to one's God must have more reality than the physiological conditions that facilitate them. A participant observation study of glossolalia, conducted over many years in Scandinavian countries and presented in Research Box 10.5, suggests that trance is not a necessary condition for glossolalia to occur.

The issue of whether or not trance states are required for glossolalia is paralleled in participant observation studies of serpent handlers. Williamson (1995) has emphasized that serpent handlers have historically been associated with denominations such as the Church of God, which once sanctioned *both* serpent handling and glossolalia. Based upon

RESEARCH BOX 10.5. Sundén's Role Theory and Glossolalia (Holm, 1987b)

Holm is among the foremost researchers who have focused upon the social and contextual factors that facilitate glossolalia. He collected recordings of hundreds of Pentecostal meetings in Scandinavian countries over several years. He thus studied speaking in tongues within religious contexts where it was normative. He found that there were few linguistic impediments to producing glossolalia, and thus that a trance state was not necessary for one to speak in tongues. However, he also noted that a trance state could remove social inhibitions and hence facilitate glossolalia in some Pentecostalists.

Relying heavily upon Sundén's role theory, Holm conducted in-depth interviews with 65 Pentecostalists. Glossolalia is modeled both by relevant Biblical texts regarding the Pentecost story, and by others in services who speak in tongues. Individuals must wait for this experience to occur as a true "baptism of the Holy Spirit" and not attempt to produce the experience themselves. Holm noted that approximately two-thirds of his sample first spoke in tongues at some kind of religious meeting. Other believers' speaking in tongues, combined with an initiate's readiness to have this experience as a model in text and practice, produces the "gift of tongues." The emotional excitement that accompanies this experience is a function of a true "baptism of the Holy Spirit" and a religious sense of its presence. Subsequent doubts as to whether or not the glossolalia was perhaps self-produced are allayed by church members and authorities who assure its validity. Repeated glossolalic experiences confirm and solidify what can now be routinely experienced. It is important to note that in Holm's sample, 12 persons never spoke in tongues. Personality factors such as inhibitions (and perhaps neurophysiological factors as well) suggest that even with appropriate readiness and both textual and actual modeling, the experience is not available to all.

Note. See also Holm (1991, especially pp. 142–145) and Hood (1991).

extensive participant observation on serpent handlers, Hood (1998) noted that some handlers believe that faith alone is sufficient for handling serpents, while others argue that only when "anointed" should one handle serpents. Anointing is the case that most closely parallels the claim to trance. That believers can handle serpents through either faith or anointing supports the claim that trance is not necessary for serpent handling, as it is not necessary for glossolalia. In one unique study, a serpent handler in an anointed state agreed to be videotaped and have his electroencephalogram taken. Research Box 10.6 presents the result of this study.

RELIGIOUS IMAGERY: THE RETURN OF THE OSTRACIZED

It has been well over 50 years since a distinguished psychologist prophesied the "return of the ostracized" to psychology (Holt, 1964). The "ostracized" that Holt spoke of was imagery, and its return has fostered the development of the psychology of religion in two ways. First, as Bergin (1964) has emphasized, it has helped shift the emphasis from psychology as the study of behavior to psychology as the study of inner experience. Second, it has fostered interest in religious experience, given the unquestioned centrality of imagery within the world's great faith traditions (LaBarre, 1972b). Imagery as a central fact of much human experience often gains unique relevance when interpreted religiously. The spontaneous presence or cultivated facilitation of imagery is central to many religious traditions. However, before we discuss religious imagery, we must briefly consider the issue of hallucinations.

Hallucinations

Many studies question the existence of hallucinations as a unique phenomenon. Fischer's (1969) identification of a perception–hallucination *continuum* is supported by a massive literature suggesting that hallucinations are not simply characteristic of organic deficiencies and are not necessarily psychopathological (Bentall, 1990, 2000; Hood, 2007). We have already noted the cautions by the American Psychiatric Association in successive editions of DSM that both religion and culture must be considered in discussing delusions. In many cultures, hallucinations are positively valued and are understood as meaningful confrontations with real spiritual beings. Al-Issa (1977) argues that the effort to classify experiences as "real" or "imaginary" is a preoccupation of Western psychiatrists, while Bourguignon (1970) has documented the meaningfulness of hallucinations in more than 60% of her sample of 488 societies worldwide. Thus whether or not an image is hallucinatory depends upon cultural and social factors, not simply neurophysiology.

RESEARCH BOX 10.6. Electroencephalogram of a Believer When Anointed (Woodruff, 1993)

In Holiness sects, as in many Pentecostal groups, anointment by the Holy Ghost is believed to occur when the spirit of God possesses an individual. Anna Prince, a member of a serpent-handling Holiness sect, partly defined anointing as follows: "It's a spiritual trancelike strand of power linking humans to God; it's a burst of energy that's refreshing, always brand new; it brings on good emotions. One is elated, full of joy" (quoted in Burton, 1993, p. 140). The famous serpent handler Pastor Liston Pack stated, "The anointing is hard, real hard to explain; and 'cause if I was to tell you that you had to feel just like me, I might tell you wrong, you see, but if you didn't know me, you would think I was havin' a stroke or somethin' tremendous was takin' place" (quoted in Burton, 1993, p. 140).

At researcher Thomas Burton's request, Liston Pack agreed to be videotaped and to have electroencephalographic (EEG) recordings taken while he was in an anointed state. Michael Woodruff did the recording and interpretation of the recordings. His four major conclusions were as follows: (1) Liston Pack's EEG showed no abnormal clinical signs; it was neither a self-induced epileptic seizure nor brought on by some unknown state. (2) Liston Pack had a great deal of control over his mental state, given his ability to prepare for anointment in a laboratory setting among skeptical scientists. (3) There was a sudden conversion from alpha to beta when anointment began, with beta predominant throughout the experience. The EEG was that of an aroused individual, but was accompanied by observations of an individual having a religious experience. It was *not* similar to that of a Zen monk in contemplation. (4) Overall, the EEG patterns of Liston Pack were more similar to patterns found in hypnosis than in meditation. However, Woodruff cautions that self-hypnosis is only a hypothesis worthy of further study and ought not to be confused with self-delusion.

Furthermore, hallucinations are common in normal or nonhospitalized populations. Tien (1991), using DSM-III-R criteria for the lifetime presence of hallucinations, found that between 11 and 13% of a randomly selected general population had experienced them at some point. This percentage range corresponds closely to that found in a survey done well over 100 years ago in Great Britain (Sidgewick, 1894). Thus, as critical reviews of the literature by Bentall (1990, 2000) clearly show, hallucinations are neither inherently pathological nor uninfluenced in either content or evaluation by culture. Psychologists have most typically studied auditory hallucinations, and as Research Box 10.7 notes, a consensus has been reached as to their explanation by psychologists who typically study participants in a laboratory context. The consensus reached by these psychologists largely vanishes when hallucinations are studied within their social context. We have already noted Luhrmann's (2012) study of Evangelicals who talk to God and for whom God talks back. Differences between studies are heavily influenced by whether or not the researchers are committed to the methodological exclusion of the transcendent.

Cultural and social processes facilitate the reporting of imagery, whether or not it is defined as hallucinatory (Al-Issa, 1977, 1995; Bentall, 2000; Bourguignon, 1970). One major

---

RESEARCH BOX 10.7. Are Auditory Hallucinations Misattributions of Inner Speech? (Bentall, 1990, 2000)

Bentall (2000) has summarized what he refers to as a "widespread consensus" about the nature of auditory hallucinations. Basically, auditory hallucinations are identified as misattributions of inner speech. "Inner speech" has long been identified as a normal psychological process; it refers to the internal dialogue people use to regulate or evaluate their own behavior. At about 3 years of age, children begin to regulate their behavior by talking out loud to themselves in the same fashion they have been talked to by their primary caregivers. Children then learn to talk to themselves quietly—a form of subvocalization. Subvocalization is a common part of normal development.

Bentall (1990, 2000) summarizes much physiological research indicating that the onset of self-reported auditory hallucinations corresponds to identifiable subvocalizations, regardless of whether subvocalizations are recorded by measuring muscle movements or by using sensitive electromyographic measures. Bentall summarizes other research indicating that the areas in the brain involved in speech are activated during the report of auditory hallucinations. Furthermore, the content of auditory hallucinations has been shown to match the content of actual recorded subvocalizations. Since the onset and content of auditory hallucinations correspond to those of subvocalizations, an individual who hallucinates may be making a misattribution—attributing to an external source what in fact is produced internally.

A psychologist of religion might hypothesize that religious belief influences not only the content of hallucinations, but perhaps their form as well. For instance, Catholics may be more likely to report visual hallucinations, while Protestants may be more likely to report auditory hallucinations. In any case, the study of hallucinations among religiously devout individuals within a cultural context is much needed and should help clarify the role of belief and expectations in legitimating, if not offering ontological options for, what otherwise are simply misattributions.

influence on the content of hallucinations is religion. For instance, as Kroll and Bachrach (1982) have documented, visions in the Middle Ages had almost exclusively religious content. Religions have also long been noted for their interest in fostering such activities as prayer and meditation, which either are aimed at or indirectly facilitate the elicitation of religious imagery (Clark, 1983; Larsen, 1976; Pelletier & Garfield, 1976). Similarly, apparently spontaneous experienced imagery possesses great significance when it is sanctioned as meaningful within religious traditions. For instance, Catholicism makes a distinction between a "vision" and an "apparition" that parallels psychological distinctions between "imagery" and "hallucinations." Volken (1961) notes that apparitions are perceived as "exterior" and are a special case of visions within Catholicism. A purely secular person would be tempted to call an apparition a hallucination, suggesting that it therefore has less objectivity than a "real" perception. However, social scientists have gained some insight into factors influencing the reports and sanctions of images of both Mary and Jesus, two dominant figures within the Christian tradition—whether these reports are considered apparitions, hallucinations, or simply images.

Images of Mary within the Catholic Tradition

Several investigators have focused attention upon reports of images of the Virgin Mary associated with the Roman Catholic faith tradition. We use the term "image" in a neutral sense, to cover both the possibility that such occurrences are hallucinations (nonveridical perceptions) or apparitions (veridical perceptions accepted within the Catholic tradition). In either case, social-psychological factors clearly determine the frequency of the reports of such experiences, their acceptance as authentic by the Catholic Church, and the differential appeal of the cult of the Virgin Mary. Much of the current research has been stimulated by the work of Carroll (1983, 1986).

Catholics have long accepted the worship of Mary as part of their faith tradition. Included in this worship is the recognition by the Church of apparitions of the Virgin Mary throughout history. Modern apparitions have ranged from the Miraculous Medal of the Immaculate Conception in France in 1830 to the visions at Medjugorje in the former Yugoslavia in 1981 (Perry & Echeverría, 1988). Sociological studied have focused upon the factors that influence the Catholic Church to accept only *some* reported apparitions of Mary as legitimate. For instance, Warner (1976) provides critical historical documentation in support of her claim that sanctioning apparitions of the Virgin Mary has often been linked with official support for sexual suppression. Perry and Echeverría argue that apparitions have been used both to facilitate social control on the part of the Catholic Church and to boost national prestige. Their latter claim is congruent with Carroll's (1983, 1986) claim that even when countries have similar frequencies of reports of Marian apparitions, such as Spain and Italy, social and political factors have led to differential legitimatization of the apparitions by central Church authorities.

More relevant to the empirical psychology of religion is the fact that Carroll's theoretical orientation is largely classical Freudian theory, in which it is assumed that repressed sexual desires largely account for hallucinations and fantasies. Thus Carroll treats all apparitions of the Virgin Mary as hallucinations, differentially legitimated by central Church authorities. His empirical efforts focus upon predicting characteristics of Marian apparitions from history in terms of classical Freudian theory. His thesis can be readily summarized in three major claims.

First, the Catholic doctrine of the Virgin Mary incorporates three beliefs: Mary was virginally conceived; her maidenhead (hymen) was never ruptured (*in partu* virginity); and Mary remained a lifelong virgin. Thus Mary is unique in religious mythology in that she is a perpetual virgin, totally devoid of sexuality. In Freudian theoretical terms, Mary symbolizes sexual denial.

Second, Carroll provides demographic and historical data to document that the cult of Mary is strongest in countries when the machismo complex is most common. The machismo complex essentially entails fierce sexual domination of women by men, often strongly culturally supported.

Third, Carroll provides anthropological and ethnographic data to show that in areas where the Mary cult and the machismo complex are strongest, males come from father-ineffective families. In Freudian terms, a father-ineffective family assures strong and delayed attachment to the mother on the part of her male children. Using Freudian Oedipal theory, Carroll argues that males strongly attached to their mothers have intense erotic repressions that can effectively be expressed in attraction to the cult of the Virgin Mary. The idealized Virgin Mary represents the denial of sexual attraction to one's mother; the machismo complex displaces eroticism onto other women, who are treated primarily as sex objects; guilt is assuaged by attraction to the passion of Christ, in which the male identifies with the need for punishment. Thus sexual sublimation accounts for the appeal of the cult of the Virgin Mary.

Carroll's provocative thesis is rare in the psychology of religion, as it incorporates historical, anthropological, ethnographic, and social-historical facts into a single, coherent theoretical framework. It has also led to several empirical studies. For instance, Carroll utilized Walsh's (1906) extensive identification of Marian apparitions associated with the Catholic Church that included those officially recognized by the church, as well as those not legitimated. All apparitions from the years 1100 to 1896 for which three empirical criteria could be documented resulted in a sample of 50 (see Carroll, 1986, pp. 225–226, for a list of these). The three empirical criteria were as follows: (1) The seer was in a waking state; (2) the seer both heard and saw Mary; and (3) the image of Mary was not provided by an identifiable physical stimulus. Assuming sexual sublimation to foster susceptibility to Marian hallucinations (apparitions), Carroll predicted that the seer should be unmarried (and hence likely to be celibate). Table 10.5 presents the results of Carroll's study for 45 of the 50 separate apparitions for which the celibacy status of the seer could be assumed. Inspection of this table shows that 94% of the seers could be assumed to be celibate; this supports the sublimation thesis. Of course, one cannot be assured that every unmarried seer was celibate, but the available data do suggest that married (and thus almost assuredly noncelibate) seers were unlikely to report apparitions for the years studied (1100 to 1896).

What of women seers? Freudian theory suggests that sexual sublimation applies to females as well as males. In the female case, identification with Mary on the part of females permits expression of repressed sexuality, since a daughter obtains the father by identifying with her mother. Although Freudian Oedipal theory is controversial (Shafranske, 1995), Carroll's use of this theory does lead to specific, empirically testable predictions. In this case, Carroll predicted that the gender of the seer would relate to whether or not apparitions of Mary would contain additional male figures (such as Jesus or adult male saints). He based this prediction upon the fact that males desire exclusive possession of the mother and do not want father figures present. Since females identify with the mother in order to obtain access to the father, they should want father figures present. Classifying the same 50 apparitions noted above, this time for gender of the seer, permitted Carroll to cross-tabulate this with whether or not male figures were present in the reported Mary apparitions. These results are

TABLE 10.5. Assumed Celibacy Status of Seers at Time of Their First Apparition of the Virgin Mary

Status	n	%
Assumed celibate		
Clerics	18	40
Unmarried		
Child	8	18
Adolescent	9	20
Adult	8	18
Assumed not celibate		
Married	2	4

Note. Adapted from Carroll (1983). Vision of the Virgin Mary: The effects of family structures on Marian apparitions. *Journal for the Scientific Study of Religion, 22,* 205–221. Copyright © 1983 the Society for the Scientific Study of Religion. Adapted by permission.

presented in Table 10.6 for the 47 of the 50 seers for whom the gender and adulthood of male figures appearing with Mary could be clearly identified. Inspection of this table indicates that most apparitions studied did not have adult males in them. However, a gender effect was clearly identified for males; that is, males were unlikely to report a male present in their Marian apparitions. For females, a male was as likely to be present as not to be present. Most importantly for Carroll's thesis, females were much more likely to report apparitions with males present than were males, whose Marian apparitions seldom included other adult male figures (Carroll, 1986).

If we assume Marian apparitions to be hallucinations (non-sensory-based imagery), than Carroll's theory argues that psychological factors predispose individuals to experience hallucinations that may be compatible with religious traditions legitimating such imagery in the form of apparitions. Thus religious tradition and psychological dispositions may interact to allow a powerful experience for some, which, when formally sanctioned by the authorities of the tradition, become powerful vicarious experiences for others within that tradition as well. They can believe through faith what the original seers have experienced firsthand. A test of Carroll's thesis, using a sample of Protestant males and preference for images of Mary and Christ, is presented in Research Box 10.8.

TABLE 10.6. Relationship between Sex of Seer and Likelihood of at Least One Adult Male in a Marian Apparition

	Male in Marian apparition?			
	Yes		No	
Sex of seer	n	%	n	%
Male	2	7	25	93
Female	10	50	10	50

Note. Although these data are significant according to Fisher's exact test (one-tailed), phi = .35, $p < .05$, the cases were probably not independent, since earlier apparitions probably influenced later ones. Data from Carroll (1986, p. 145).

RESEARCH BOX 10.8. An Empirical Test of Carroll's Psychoanalytic Theory
of Apparitions (Hood, Morris, & Watson, 1991)

Carroll's thesis that sexual sublimation is involved in the male attraction to the cult of the
Virgin Mary in Roman Catholicism was tested by Hood et al. in a sample of non-Catholic,
Christian males. Independent samples of raters were used to identify (1) crucifixes ranked
according to the degree of Christ's suffering they represented, and (2) artistic renderings
of the Virgin Mary ranked and rated for (a) eroticism and (b) nurturing quality. Four
crucifixes reliably varying in degree of suffering expressed (and one plain cross, as a
control) were used as stimuli. Five pictures of the Virgin Mary, reliably varying in erotic
and nurturing quality (with one identified as *equally* nurturing and erotic, as a control)
were also used. These stimuli were then rated for personal preference by 71 non-Catholic
males, all of whom either agreed or strongly agreed on a 5-point Likert scale that "My
whole approach to life is based upon my religion." These males had also taken a measure
developed by Parker (1983; Parker, Tupling, & Brown, 1979) to measure self-recalled
maternal bonding. This was used as a measure of strong attachment (ambivalently erotic
and nurturing) to one's mother.

　　Participants were taken one at a time into a room in which the crucifixes and the cross
were mounted on one wall, and the pictures of the Virgin Mary were mounted on another
wall. They were first seated in front of the wall on which the crucifixes and cross were
randomly numbered and hung, and were asked to take a moment to contemplate them.
They then answered the question "Which cross or crucifix best expresses what Christ
means to you?" followed by "Which cross or crucifix next best expresses what Christ means
to you?" This was continued until one remained, and participants were asked, "Why did
you not choose this cross/crucifix?" A similar procedure was then followed as participants
were seated in front of the wall with the five pictures of the Virgin Mary.

　　Consistent with the theory of the role of sexual sublimation in reports of Marian
apparitions, Hood et al. predicted that males strongly but ambivalently attached to their
mothers would have a preference for (1) a suffering Christ and (2) the ambivalently erotic/
nurturing Virgin Mary representation. Results supported these predictions. The more
males recalled ambivalent and strong attachments to their mothers as measured by the
bonding scales, the more likely they were to prefer a suffering Christ figure and the
ambivalent Virgin Mary figure. In terms of Freudian theory, the ambivalent attraction
to one's mother also involves the unconscious sense of guilt and the identification with
a Christ who suffers painfully. Freudian theory is often controversial and susceptible to
varying interpretations. It is best viewed as one interpretation of any set of data—even
those proposed as a test of Freudian theory, as in this study of Carroll's speculative theory.

　　Studies of hallucinations or apparitions of the Virgin Mary have important conceptual
relevance for the empirical study of religion. What is crucial is the fact that the meaningful
status of imagery varies with the context within which it is interpreted and with the nature
of the ontological status the image is given (Bettelheim, 1976; Klinger, 1971; Singer, 1966;
Watkins, 1976). Anthropological studies of apparitions have rightly cautioned against ignoring the cultural context of apparitions. Apolito (1998, p. 24) warns against Carroll's "relent-
less psychological reductionism" and states that visionary realities are complex constructions
that are more than mere "hallucinations." Yet Carroll's work remains a provocative effort to

explain apparitions within the assumption of the methodological exclusion of the transcendent.

Visions of Christ

If Marian apparitions are largely restricted to the Catholic tradition, visions of Jesus Christ occur within both Catholicism and Protestantism. Wiebe (1997, 2000) has made an extensive study of such visions reported by 30 living visionaries. Like much of the other research on visions, his sample is largely unrepresentative and certainly not an adequate scientific sample from a specified population, Yet, as with Hardy's and Hufford's work (described earlier in this chapter), the value of Wiebe's work is in his effort to provide extensive detailed descriptions of visions from the perspective of the visionaries. Although a social scientist is likely to be reluctant to claim any non-natural basis for religious imagery, it is interesting that careful phenomenological descriptions of imagery experiences—whether they are called hallucinations, apparitions, or visions—reveal that psychologists have yet to explain them fully.

Wiebe discusses efforts to explain visions of Christ in three broad areas (supernaturalistic, mentalistic, and neurophysiological). However, as Hufford (1982) concludes in regard to the Old Hag phenomenon, Wiebe (2000) concludes that "These visions elude adequate naturalistic explanation . . . and continue to provide a profound sense that a reality that does not belong to our world has been manifested" (p. 139). Lundmark (2010) has noted this in a case study of a dying woman who experienced a vision of Jesus. Thus, as in popular studies of both Marian apparitions (Garvey, 1998) and encounters with Jesus Christ (Sparrow, 1995), the belief that a reality has been encountered—that a figure has actually been seen that cannot be dismissed as merely a hallucination—is an essential part of the experience. In an innovative recent study, Silver, Olson, Larsen, and Hood (2017) had students use a computer sketch program to present how Jesus appeared in their "mind's eye," with no implication that this image had any factual ontological base.

Rodney Stark (1999) has proposed a general theory of revelations, which places the often limited psychological study of visions or hallucinations within a broader social context. His model, which is empirically testable but has been largely ignored by psychologists, is presented in Table 10.7.

The Facilitation of Religious Imagery

Religious imagery plays a role in many religious traditions and is of immense relevance to any empirical psychology of religion. Much of the more clinical and conceptual literature in the psychology of religion—for instance, the literature associated with Jungian, object relations, and transpersonal theory—explores images in depth (Beit-Hallahmi, 1995; Greenwood, 1995; Halligan, 1995). Experimental study of imagery has also been of interest in the long tradition of studies of "sensory deprivation" or isolation. As we shall see, restricting external perception enhances the probability of imagery. Not surprisingly, psychologists have sought ways to enhance both solitude and isolation to facilitate the occurrence of imagery.

Few contemporary psychologists would dispute Pylyshyn's (1973, p. 2) claim that "imagery is a pervasive form of human experience and is of utmost important to humans." Indeed, as both Shephard (1978) and Lilly (1977) have noted, situations of isolation, solitude, and focused concentration often elicit unanticipated and undesired imagery that can disrupt

TABLE 10.7. Stark's General Model of Revelations

1. Revelations will tend to occur in cultures that support communication with the divine.
2. A wide variety of mental phenomena can be interpreted as communication with the divine.
3. Most revelations are confirmatory (i.e., they support existing beliefs within the tradition).
4. There are individual differences in the ability to receive revelations.
5. Novel revelations are likely to come from devout believers who perceive shortcomings within their tradition.
6. Social crisis increases the probability of perceiving shortcomings within one's tradition.
7. During periods of social crisis, the number of persons both receiving and accepting revelations is maximized.
8. Confidence that one has received a revelation is increased to the extent that others accept the revelation.
9. Revelations are more likely to be accepted from members of intense primary groups.
10. Further revelations are likely if the recipient is reinforced.
11. Increased revelations and reinforcement increase the probability of novel or heretical revelations.
12. As religious movements become successful, they attempt to curtail novel revelations.

Note. Data from Stark (1999, p. 308).

ongoing activities. Examples of such situations include focusing upon a radar scope, attending to concerns during space travel, and surviving during prolonged periods of isolation. Thus it is not surprising that early experimental studies of isolation, using isolation tanks, often documented imagery that was disruptive and disturbing to research participants (Lilly, 1977; Zubeck, 1969). The very phrase "sensory deprivation" emphasizes the negative. However, within many religious traditions, withdrawing from "worldly" perceptions and "turning within" have long had a valuable and privileged status. For instance, some forms of both prayer and meditation involve withdrawal from external sensory attention, which may produce imagery that is religiously meaningful. LaBarre (1972a, p. 265; emphasis in original) has gone so far as to claim:

> Every religion in historic fact, began in one man's "revelation"—his dream or fugue or ecstatic trance. Indeed, the crisis cult is *characteristically* dereistic, autistic, and dreamlike precisely *because* it had its origins in the dream, trance, "spirit" possession, epileptic "seizure," REM sleep, sensory deprivation, or other visionary state of the shaman–originator. All religions are necessarily "revealed" in this sense, inasmuch as they are certainly not revealed consensually in secular experience.

Although LaBarre's position may be extreme, it does emphasize the obvious relevance of imagery to religious traditions. It is thus curious that sensory isolation research has neither focused upon the elicitation of imagery with religious samples nor concerned itself with the specific elicitation of religious imagery among samples, whether religious or not.

The exclusion of external sources of stimulation in isolation studies led early investigations to coin the term "sensory deprivation." Many assumed that the images present in such studies must be hallucinations. However, early isolation ("deprivation") studies produced exaggerated results that are now readily identifiable largely as artifacts of the experimental setting (Zubeck, 1969). In particular, the use of isolation tanks provided the means to control external sources of stimulation. A typical isolation tank is an enclosed, soundproofed, and lightproofed container filled with magnesium salt solutions, heated to external body temperature (34.1°C), and adjusted for specific gravity so that a person simply floats partly submerged. The uniqueness of the isolation tank situation, combined with excessive experimental forewarnings and precautions, elicited panic and bizarre reactions in some participants. However, as studies progressed, it was discovered that if participants were knowledgeable (i.e., were initiated into the experiences likely to be facilitated by the isolation tank), negative reactions became exceedingly uncommon. Instead, participants explored the variety of experiences common to altered-states research in an almost universally positive fashion (Lilly, 1956, 1977; Lilly & Lilly, 1976; Suedfeld, 1975). Most importantly for our interests is the imagery elicited in isolation tank experiences—imagery that is seldom appropriately identified as merely hallucinatory (Suedfeld & Vernon, 1964).

Imagery is readily elicited in isolation tanks if participants are relaxed and unfearful, and if they are given specific instructions to attend to internal states, contents, and processes. Unstructured phenomena such as focused or diffuse white light, as well as various geometric forms and colors, are common and rapidly explainable by the psychology of perception. For instance, spontaneous neural firing in the retina, a common phenomenon, is attended to in isolation studies and hence becomes a part of conscious awareness. Some of these phenomena are common in meditation and prayer, as discussed above.

More detailed instructions and time in the isolation tank can lead to more meaningful images—some similar to hypnogogic imagery, and other similar to meaningful figures not unlike those found in dreams. Both the report and content of imagery are heavily influenced by set and setting (Jackson & Kelly, 1962; Rossi, Sturrock, & Solomon, 1963). As in psychedelic research, hallucinations are rare in isolation tanks. Persons do not see images they mistakenly expect to exist in time and space, as they would see objects of everyday perception. However, with appropriate set and setting, participants do experience imagery that has ontological significance. The imagery is not simply dismissed as "subjective." In this sense, isolation tanks can facilitate genuine religious experiences. Research Box 10.9 reports one study in which set and setting were used to facilitate religious experiences under isolation tank conditions.

Other researchers have begun to explore ways to experimentally induce imagery and other forms of religious experience. Masters and Houston (1973), noted for their pioneering work on the varieties of psychedelic experience, have developed a mechanical device to induce altered states of consciousness. Essentially a suspended platform that responds to the slightest movement, the device is claimed to induce a trance state rapidly in most participants. With proper set and setting, individuals report imagery and similar experiences. Once again, the relevant point is that when investigators take a serious interest in the elicitation of experiences, participants, especially when selected for their interest and sensitivities, may report significant religious experiences. In a similar vein, Goodman (1990) claims to have discovered 30 specific body postures that can reliably elicit altered states of consciousness. These postures are derived from ancient cave drawings as well as from anthropological research. Unique in Goodman's research is her claim that these specific body postures elicit states of consciousness in which perceptions of an expanded reality are accessible. Although her thesis is controversial, it is clearly empirically testable. Again, the issue is that sympathetic researchers are taking seriously not simply the induction of altered states of consciousness,

RESEARCH BOX 10.9. Sensory Isolation and the Elicitation of Imagery
(Hood & Morris, 1981b)

Hood and Morris utilized an isolation tank to provide a setting in which the elicitation of imagery could be facilitated. The isolation tank was 7.5 feet long, 4 feet high, and 4 feet wide. The tank contained a hydrated magnesium sulfate solution with a density of 1.30 grams/cc, a depth of 10 inches, and a temperature of 34.1°C (approximate external body temperature). Participants were totally enclosed in the tank, which was also soundproofed and light-proofed. The tank itself was in a small soundproofed room. Participants were nude in the tank and floated there for 1 hour.

A person can expect a variety of imagery phenomena under isolation conditions, including geometric forms, light, and images of meaningful figures. As part of the appropriate ethical concerns in doing such research, participants were forewarned to anticipate such experiences. However, participants were also instructed to try to control their images.

In a double-blind procedure, half the participants were instructed to try to imagine religious figures, situations, and settings, while the other half were instructed to try to imagine cartoon figures, situations, and settings. Thus the researchers attempted to encourage specific imagery among religious types, for whom such imagery should be relevant. Furthermore, it was predicted that intrinsically religious persons would report more religious imagery, based upon the assumption that their participation in religion is more devoutly experientially based than that of extrinsically religious persons. Twenty intrinsically and 20 extrinsically religious participants had been selected for their extreme scores on either the Intrinsic or Extrinsic religious orientation scale.[a] Results of this study are presented in the table below.

| Reported imagery | Set condition | Religious type | | | |
| | | Intrinsic | | Extrinsic | |
		Mean	SD	Mean	SD
Religious figures	Cartoon	2.10	0.86	1.10	0.32
	Religious	3.10	0.74	1.90	0.74
Cartoon figures	Cartoon	2.30	0.95	2.50	1.27
	Religious	1.30	0.68	1.50	0.71
Meaningful figures	Cartoon	2.30	0.95	2.30	1.06
	Religious	2.00	1.16	2.50	0.97
Geometric forms	Cartoon	2.40	1.08	1.60	0.70
	Religious	2.00	1.05	2.30	0.82
Light	Cartoon	2.30	1.16	2.10	0.88
	Cartoon	2.10	0.74	2.90	0.57

Note. From Hood and Morris (1981b, p. 267). Copyright © 1981 the Society for the Scientific Study of Religion. Reprinted by permission.

(continued)

RESEARCH BOX 10.9. *(cont.)*

Statistical analyses of these data revealed that there was no overall tendency for either religious group to report more imagery when the images were those well documented to occur under isolation conditions (e.g., geometric forms, meaningful figures, light). However, under the set conditions, intrinsically religious persons reported more cued religious imagery than extrinsically religious persons did, while the groups did not differ in cartoon imagery. Thus the report of more religious imagery under cued conditions was not a function of the intrinsic participants' greater tendency to report imagery. Indeed, the intrinsic participants even reported more religious imagery under the cartoon cue than extrinsic participants reported religious imagery under the religious cue. That these results were not simply functions of demand characteristics (with intrinsic participants more sensitive to reporting more religious imagery when cued) is supported by additional work in which intrinsic participants did not report more religiously relevant imagery than extrinsic participants when asked to give religious responses to Rorschach cards.

[a]The intrinsic participant group had an Intrinsic scale mean of 38.9 (*SD* = 4.01) and an Extrinsic scale mean of 26.4 (*SD* = 5.12). The extrinsic participant group had an Extrinsic scale mean of 35.4 (*SD* = 3.93) and an Intrinsic scale mean of 20.9 (*SD* = 4.22). The Allport and Ross (1967) scales were used.

but the ontological reality of what is revealed in the experience. In this sense, the psychology of religion is forced to confront spiritual claims as it explores the reports of individuals whose experience may have evidential force.

ENTHEOGENS AND RELIGIOUS EXPERIENCE

It has long been recognized that many religions have employed various naturally occurring and synthetic substances in their religious rituals. However, until the discovery of psychedelic drugs, it was rather arrogantly assumed that concern with the facilitation of experience by drugs was the domain of anthropology and sister disciplines concerned with less "advanced" religions. In a controversial discipline with the cumbersome name "archeopsychopharmacology," researchers combine ancient texts and artifacts with contemporary cross-cultural studies of the use of naturally occurring psychedelic substances to speculate on the origins of religions. For example, Allegro (1971) contends that the origin of the Judeo-Christian tradition may have been heavily influenced by altered states facilitated by the use of naturally occurring psychedelic substances, such as the mushroom *Amanita muscaria*. So influenced, too, Wasson (1969) argues, was the sacred *Soma* of the ancient Indian text *Rig Veda†* by the use of a mushroom with psychedelic properties, the fly agaric. Merkur (2000) argues that the manna of the Old Testament was bread containing ergot, a naturally occurring psychoactive fungus. He also argues that within the Judeo-Christian tradition, Philo of Alexandra, Rabbis Moses Maimonides, and Saint Bernard of Clairvaux refer to special meditations to be practiced when taking psychoactive substances. Shanon (2008, pp. 59–63) argues that five powerful experiences in Moses's life parallel experiences known to be facilitated by naturally occurring entheogens common to the Middle East. Dannaway, Piper, and Webster (2006) have traced the use of psychoactive preparations of ergot in a variety of religious traditions, including Persian, Greek, Jewish, and Islamic sects. Beckstead (2007) and Peterson (1975) have documented the use of entheogens by Joseph Smith and his earliest Mormon converts. Indeed, Kramrisch, Otto, Ruck, and Wasson (1986) argue that *all* religions originated from the use of naturally occurring entheogens. Finally, Wasson, Hofmann, and Ruck (1978) have argued that an ergot similar to LSD was integral to the Eleusinian mystery cults of ancient Greece, and from there influenced Western philosophy. More conservatively, Fuller (2000) has carefully documented the use of drugs throughout American religious history.

There is little doubt that the facilitation of altered states of consciousness by entheogens is one of the ways in which those likely to identify themselves as spiritual can lay claim to a religious significance for the particular experiences that in Taves's (2009) terminology are deemed to be religious. Although the widely speculative theories of archeopsychopharmacology cannot be empirically confirmed, they have raised a crucial question at the center of the social-scientific study of religion and the more general study of entheogens: Can entheogens facilitate or produce religious experiences? Those who argue the case most persuasively prefer the term "entheogens" to now outdated terms such as "psychedelics" to describe plants or chemical substances that facilitate primary religious experiences (Forte, 1997). It is the term we currently prefer, especially as we focus upon the facilitation of religious experience by means of chemical substances. (The facilitation of specifically mystical experiences by entheogens is discussed in Chapter 11.)

The literature on the psychology of entheogens is immense, easily running to several thousand studies. Much of the U.S. research has been stopped by legislation against these drugs, so that Rätsch (1990, p. 2) has concluded: "Since the beginning of the 1970s, there has been little new research into psychedelic substances." While Rätsch's claim must be qualified—given both the significant current research by anthropologists and ethnobotanists with naturally occurring plants around the world, and the study of entheogens in European countries (where laws are more flexible)—the measurement-based empirical study of entheogens has clearly been drastically curtailed by U.S. drug laws. However, there nevertheless remains an extensive body of research on these drugs (Lukoff, Zanger, & Lu, 1990). Selective reviews are readily available, including the general overall review by Aarson and Osmond (1970), Dobkin de Rios's (1984) cross-cultural survey, and Barber's (1970) methodological review. Masters and Houston's (1966) review focuses upon the varieties of psychedelic experience, while Lukoff et al. (1990) focus upon religious and transpersonal states facilitated by psychedelic drugs. Roberts and Hruby (1995) have produced a useful bibliographic guide to entheogens. Most recently, Ellens (2014) has edited a two-volume summary of the history and practices associated with seeking the sacred by means of psychoactive substances.

Curiously, very few studies to date have used religious variables for directly assessing the religious importance of entheogens, despite a vast, often contentious conceptual literature on chemical substances and religion. Although the archeopsychopharmacological speculations of Wasson and his colleagues may be extreme, their basic assumption has been common within both psychological and religious studies. It has long been noted that there is an obvious similarity between various religious experiences and drug-induced experiences. Before the turn of the 20th century, in fact, Leuba (1896) argued that religious experiences in advanced traditions must be invalidated, because of their similarity to drug-induced states in less advanced traditions. The essentials of Leuba's argument have been more recently advanced by Zaehner (1972), who argues that because an experience is drug-induced, it cannot be genuinely religious. These largely conceptually based debates do little to advance a scientific understanding of the possible religious importance of entheogens. One can no more invalidate an experience because its physiology is known than one can invalidate physiology because its biochemistry has been identified. As Weil (1986) has emphasized, the similarity of psychedelic substances found within plants, animals, and the human brain suggest that any simple distinction between natural and artificially induced states is arbitrary.

Our concern is with the religious significance of chemical substances. In particular, we focus upon the question of whether or not some chemicals can induce or be used to facilitate a religious experience. We include as "entheogens" such drugs as LSD, mescaline, and psilocybin, since in both scientific studies and street use, reports indicate similar psychological experiences from these drugs (Aarson & Osmond, 1970; Stevens, 1987; Wells & Triplett, 1992). However, as Brown (1972) cautions, drugs that produce similar psychological effects need not have identical biochemical properties.

The term "psychedelic," the most common precursor to "entheogen," has a controversial history (Stevens, 1987). Debates over the common name for the class of drugs we are discussing have produced a range from "hallucinogenic" to "psychotomimetic" to "psychedelic" to "entheogen." "Hallucinogenic" is the most inadequate term, since hallucination is one of the *least* common responses to psychedelic drugs (Barber, 1970). Although these drugs do produce various visual and imagery effects, whether users' eyes are open or closed, they do not produce perceptions that have no external stimulus (hallucinations). "Psychotomimetic" was the term favored by early researchers who thought that this class of drugs produces psychoses or psychotic-like states. Given the cultural evaluation of psychoses, the negative connotations of "psychotomimetic" are obvious; however, it is well established that the ability of psychedelics to elicit sudden psychoses in otherwise normal persons is highly exaggerated (Barr, Langs, Holt, Goldberger, & Klein, 1972). "Psychedelic" was the term most favored by those who favored the "mind-manifesting" aspect of these drugs. It is the most common term today, despite its positive connotations among participants in the 1960s deviant drug culture and its still-current association with the illicit street drug culture (Stevens, 1987). As noted above, those who prefer to focus upon the religious significance of these plants and chemical substances prefer the term "entheogens."

For well-established physiological reasons, entheogens can be expected to produce reliable alterations in visual and other imagery, which to informed and stable participants are likely to be interesting objects of conscious exploration (Durr, 1970; Strassman, 2001). Meaningful images that occur under the influence of these substances, with the user's eyes closed, are not typically attributed to the object expected to exist in the world (in the sense that if the user were to open his or her eyes, the object would be in physical reality). Likewise, when the user's eyes are open, alterations in perception of objects are noted as perceptual alterations of existing objects, not changes in the actual physical objects or the perception of objects that in fact are not real. However, the user's ability to interpret perceptions in terms of a meaningful frame can transform his or her perception of the world. In Sundén's theory, a religious frame should enhance the power of entheogens to facilitate religious experiences. With an appropriate religious set and setting, entheogens can facilitate religious experiences, insofar as one under the influence of these substances may for the first time see the world in terms appropriate to a particular system of meaning. In this sense, the "other-worldly" property of entheogens is well established and provides their obvious link to religion. Religious beliefs often assert realities and possibilities of experience that are quite foreign to everyday secular experience. In addition, as noted in Chapter 9, religions often encourage such experiences in believers (or, at a minimum, urge believers to respect these experiences in others).

Masters and Houston (1966) found that under the influence of entheogens, religious imagery was quite common, even when many participants did not identify themselves as having a "religious" drug experience. For instance, religious architecture was one of the most common images reported, but Masters and Houston (1966) claim that this was more a sense of aesthetic appreciation than a genuine religious interest. Still, the commonality of religious imagery in their sample of 206 participants is impressive. Over half of these participants saw images of specific religious persons, such as Christ, Buddha, or various saints (Masters & Houston, 1966, p. 265).

The frequent report of religious imagery is likely to be a function of set and setting, long known to be major determinants of the content of imagery elicited by entheogens (Barr et al., 1972; Barber, 1970). In light of Sundén's role theory, we would expect that if individuals were given the appropriate familiarity with religious frames, many substance-facilitated experiences would be experienced as religious. It would be naive to claim that religious experiences are substance-specific effects. Rather, the power of entheogens to facilitate religious experience lies in the extent to which states of consciousness, altered by chemical substances, are seen as relevant in religious terms. Within U.S. culture, the ironic fact is that mainstream religions sends mixed signals relative to religious experience—often encouraging and validating experiences when interpreted as originating in God, but discouraging and invalidating experiences that are known to be chemically facilitated. The fact that many participants in studies using entheogens experience religious imagery and use religious language to describe otherwise secular imagery (e.g., cosmological events) is difficult to assess. Masters and Houston (1966) noted that the use of sacramental or religious metaphors was a common practice for their participants, even though genuine religious experiences may have been rare. Here the problem is how to judge the genuineness of any experience; obviously verbal reports of religious imagery and religious language are, even in Sundén's theory, necessary but not sufficient criteria for religious experience.

Grof (1980) has argued that the therapeutic use of entheogens often provides a set and setting that encourage the report of religious and transpersonal experiences. Many of these experiences are interpreted in terms of Jungian theory, which is particularly favorable to describing religious imagery. Thus we would expect religious imagery in LSD psychotherapy sessions to be common and to increase if the set and setting are made even more explicitly religious—for instance, by having religious symbols in the therapeutic room. Leary (1964) compared the reported LSD experiences of clients of two different therapists—one who used an explicitly religious context for therapy, and one who did not. These data are presented in Table 10.8. Inspection of this table indicates that the evaluation of the LSD experience as the greatest personal experience was a function of religious context; in addition, whether an experience was interpreted as religious or not was clearly affected by the religious context of the therapy. Although these results confound possible differences in therapists with set/setting differences, if we assume that therapists in religious contexts are global contextual factors, having a religious context clearly facilitates a religious experience.

Research Box 10.10 presents a study in which autobiographical accounts of various experiences, including hallucinogenic drug experiences, were shown to differ reliably in the way they were described. The use of linguistic analysis is innovative in the psychology of religion. For instance, Altmeyer et al. (2015) have used linguistic analytical techniques to show how in both Germany and America, religion is seen as related to beliefs and rules endorsed by

TABLE 10.8. LSD Therapy Experience as a Function of Religious Set/Setting

	Percentage of clients saying yes	
	Therapist A, using no religious context (n = 74)	Therapist B, using religious context (n = 96)
Felt LSD was greatest personal experience	49	85
Felt LSD was a religious experience	32	83
Felt a greater awareness of God, higher power, or ultimate reality	40	90

Note. Data from Leary (1964, p. 327).

groups, while spirituality is more associated with feelings and a sense of interconnectedness. As we shall see in Chapter 11, other forms of linguistic analysis have been used to suggest differences between "genuine" and "false" mystics. Thus it is important not to lose sight of innovative techniques such as those reported in Research Box 10.10, because they remain useful and can be modified with new technologies.

Although the hostility of mainstream religion to the use of entheogens is well documented, the irony is that entheogens have relevance to the range of experiences typically called "religious." It is a mistake not to acknowledge the possibility that chemically facilitated

---

**RESEARCH BOX 10.10. The Language of Altered States
(Oxman, Rosenberg, Schnurr, Tucker, & Gala, 1988)**

Oxman and his colleagues collected 94 autobiographical accounts of personal experiences. The texts were divided into four categories: schizophrenic experiences; drug-induced hallucinogenic experiences; mystical/ecstatic experiences; and autobiographical controls (identified as personally important experiences). The texts were coded into 83 lexical categories by means of standardized computer programs.[a] The four groups were significantly different in word frequencies in 49 of the 83 lexical categories. Using lexical content to classify the three altered states of consciousness and the control experiences indicated that the altered states of consciousness were more different from one another than similar. Schizophrenic experiences were characterized by an abnormal illness experience associated with a negative self-evaluation. Drug-induced hallucinogenic experiences were characterized by positively aesthetically experienced visual and auditory phenomena. Mystical/ecstatic experiences were characterized by life-altering encounters with God, associated with a sense of power and certitude. When discriminant-function analysis was employed, 84% of the experiences could be correctly identified by their word frequencies. The authors assumed that the actual experiences were different, given that different words were used to describe the experiences.

[a]These were the General Inquirer Computer Content Analysis Program and the Harvard-111 Psychosociological Dictionary (see Stone, Dunphy, Smith, & Ogilvie, 1966).

states of consciousness may have ontological validity. Indeed, identifying them as religious both contextualizes them and gives them such validity. However, the mere elicitation of a single experience, however "religious," probably lacks sustained life-transforming power if it is not contextualized within some tradition. Roszak (1975, p. 50; emphasis in original) has argued that the focus upon specific behaviors or experiences elicited as "religious" can be distorting:

> The temptation, then, is to believe that the behavior which has thus been objectively veri-fied is what religious experience is *really* all about, and—further—that it can be appropri-ated as an end in itself, plucked like a rare flower from the soil that feeds it. The result is a narrow emphasis on special effects and sensations: "peak experiences," "highs," "flashes" and such. Yet even if one wishes to regard ecstasy as the "peak" of religious experience, that summit does not float in midair. It rests upon tradition and a way of life; one ascends such heights and appreciates their grandeur by a process of initiation that demands learning, commitment, devotion, service, sacrifice. To approach it in any hasty way is like "scaling" Mount Everest by being landed on its top from a helicopter.

Stevens (1987) has documented the history of the original "psychedelic movement" and its failure to have mind-altering substances accepted for sacramental use within a reli-gious frame. In this sense, the "psychedelic movement" must be judged in terms of the cul-tic and sectarian movements discussed in Chapter 10. However, exceptions include some Native American religions, whose long history of sacramental use of peyote demonstrates that entheogens can be incorporated into religious frameworks and used to facilitate experi-ences whose meaning is truly religious (Bergman, 1971; LaBarre, 1969). It is also possible that entheogens are prime triggers of mystical experiences under appropriate set and setting conditions, as discussed in Chapter 11.

The cultural bias against entheogens has not only affected the serious study of these chemicals, but made it difficult to take a balanced view of the range of their effects (Forte, 1997; Walsh, 1982). Furthermore, several reviewers have argued that typical double-blind studies are particularly inappropriate ways to investigate entheogens, especially since participants who are assigned to the control conditions are likely to be immediately aware of this fact (Bakalar & Grinspoon, 1989; Yensen, 1990). Many researchers have supported the view that ingestion of psychedelic substances on the part of researchers is a valid (and, some claim, necessary) method of study. Such self-involvement has plagued the history of the "psychedelic movement" in the United States and promises to fuel future controversies in which research on entheogens and religion takes on many of the characteristics of religious movements, as discussed in Chapter 9.

OVERVIEW

Religious experiences are as varied as the interpretations individuals can bring to their lives. It is less relevant to seek the common elements of religious experiences than to find higher-order abstractions for identifying a class of varied phenomena. The James–Boisen formula that religious experience is a successful resolution of discontent is basic to most faith traditions. However, few studies have placed religious experience within a context to determine its functionality over time. Methodological considerations still loom large in the evaluation of empirical research. Although few researchers are now satisfied with correlation studies, debates that have dominated the empirical psychology of religion continue between those who favor the rigor and control provided by laboratory research (Saroglou, 2014b) and those who seek to place the study of religion within a cultural and historical perspective (Belzen & Hood, 2006). Others have provided examples of multi-disciplinary research using both qualitative and quantitative methods and both idiothetic and nomothetic methods, without privileging any one method over all others (Streib & Hood, 2016). The particulars of discontents and resolutions are provided by Sundén's role theory, which not only allows tradition, text, and practice to model appropriate perceptions and interpretations that facilitate religious experiences within a faith tradition, but permits longitudinal studies needed for true tests of the James–Boisen formula.

Common religious practices, such as prayer and meditation, have been studied in terms of the physiological correlates and subjective contents of these experiences. As we shall see in Chapter 11, more and more true experimental methods are applied to areas in which experimentation was long thought difficult if not impossible. Some have, as it were, facilitated a sense of divine presence not in the church, synagogue, or mosque, but in the laboratory. Speculations about the neurophysiology of dramatic religious experiences, such as glossolalia and hallucinations, demand additional empirical investigation with new neurophysiological techniques that continue to be developed. Dynamic theories illuminating the processes involved in determining the content of hallucinations have been tested and promise to foster both controversy and additional research.

Imagery has returned as a focus of research, as methodological behaviorism has been seen as too limited in scope for any deep study of religion, and metaphysical behaviorism has been found no more philosophically adequate than is the methodological exclusion of the transcendent from a field in which transcendence may be an essential defining characteristic. Entheogens remain of interest, despite legal impediments in the United States to research. The fact that religious imagery can be facilitated by entheogens, in the appropriate set and setting, assures the continued relevance for the psychology of religion of techniques to alter states of consciousness—not simply out of curiosity, but as a response to realities that remain ontologically relevant to any nonreductive psychological exploration of religion or spirituality.

CHAPTER 11

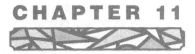

Mysticism

In Hinduism, in Neoplatonism, in Sufism, in Christian mysticism, in Whitmanism, we find the same recurring note, so that there is about mystical utterances an eternal unanimity which ought to make a critic stop and think and which brings it about that the mystical classics have, as has been said, neither birthday nor native land.

How can an individual human claim union with God without compromising divine transcendence and elevating the creature beyond its proper status? Are not claims to union inherently blasphemous?

According to our yogic traditions, *samadhi* means complete awareness of God, or to put it in less religious terms, *samadhi* means that your mind and the mind of the universe are, for a time, merged in an absolute ecstatic union.

The fascination of the subject of mysticism is not, I suggest, simply a fascination with some intense psychological experiences for their own sake, but rather because the answers to each of these questions are also ways of defining or delimiting authority.

The breadth and intensity of the interest in mysticism during the last half of the twentieth century have given rise to many different interpretations of mysticism and many conflicting theories about it.

This problem of the secularized interpretation of amorphous mystical experiences has been raised repeatedly since the Enlightenment.[1]

The focus upon mysticism in this chapter highlights the central role that mystical experi-ence has occupied in conceptual discussions of religion for over a century. The claims of mystics dominate contemporary discussions concerned with the evidential value of religious experience. "Evidential force" and "evidential value" are the phrases most linked to debates as to whether or not religious experiences such as mysticism provide sufficient grounds for asserting the truth of various religious beliefs (Clark, 1984; Davis, 1989; Swinburne, 1981). For some, mystical experience cannot support a belief that one has united with God or expe-rienced ultimate reality. For others, mysticism is an experience that provides sufficient war-rant for belief in God or ultimate reality—or, in Hick's (1989, 2010) term, "the Real." As Katz

---

[1] These quotations come, respectively, from the following sources: James (1902/1985, p. 324); McGinn (1989, p. vii); Lenz (1995, p. 215); Jantzen (1995, p. 1); Ruffing (2001, p. 1); and Scholem (1969, p. 16).

(1977) notes, those who assert the evidential force of mystical experience provide an ecumenical umbrella under which diverse religious claims can be sheltered as simply different expressions of one fundamental truth. This avoids the embarrassing particulars of religious experiences, which, like the particulars of religious belief expressed in dogmatic terms, tend to separate one faith from another as discussed in Chapter 10 (Schuon, 1975). Although as social scientists we need not address theological or philosophical debates directly, our methods and analyses cannot avoid philosophical and religious implications. As both Jones (1994) and Miles (2007) have noted, science and religion are not identical, but neither can they be categorically separated or viewed as mutually exclusive orientations. At a minimum, mysticism is the best candidate for a distinct, *sui generis* experience that has been recognized across diverse traditions and cultures (Jones, 2016; Otto, 1917/1923). It also is the best candidate to refute the common assertion by empirical psychologists that there are no specifically religious emotions (e.g., Saroglou, 2014a, p. 366).

CONCEPTUAL ISSUES IN THE STUDY OF MYSTICISM

The theological and philosophical literature on mysticism is extensive (see Hood, 2005b, 2006; McGinn, 1991). Our concerns as social scientists are restricted to the aspects of these literatures that have direct relevance for empirical research. Of immediate concern is the clarification of the nature of mystical experience, as well as of its relationships to other forms of religious experience.

According to Thorner (1966), mystics claim that the perceptual referent in religious experience is a unity within the world. This unity is not linked to any one perceptual object; instead, all objects are unified into a perception of totality or oneness. However, the mystical experience of a unity within the world emphasized by Thorner is only one form of mysticism. Following Stace (1960), we refer to this as "extrovertive mysticism." We contrast extrovertive mysticism with another form of mysticism, "introvertive mysticism." This is an experience of unity devoid of perceptual objects; it is literally an experience of "no-thing-ness." Perceptual objects disappear, and a pure consciousness devoid of content is reported. Forman (1990a) has referred to this as "pure consciousness experience." What is important for now is that only extrovertive mysticism has as its perceptual referent a unity that transcends individual, discrete objects of perception. There are discrete objects of perception, but they are all seen unified in their particularity as nevertheless one. The unity in extrovertive mysticism is with the totality of objects of perception; the unity in introvertive mysticism is with a pure consciousness, devoid of objects of perception. Stace (1960, p. 131) has suggested that extrovertive mysticism is a less developed form, perhaps preparatory to introvertive mysticism. Forman (1990a) argues that extrovertive mysticism is a higher form of mysticism to which introvertive mysticism is only preparatory. Hood (1989) has argued that extrovertive mysticism is likely to follow upon introvertive mystical experience, but he does not claim it to be a "higher" experience. These conceptual arguments have been given renewed consideration by Marshall (2005) and Jones (2016), with substantial agreement that the experiences reported are in some fundamental sense real.

In this chapter, we focus upon mysticism in empirical terms. As we shall see, if introversive and extrovertive mysticism can be measured, the relationship between the two can be studied as an empirical issue. Yet, whether the experience of unity is introversive or extrovertive, it is this experience that by scholarly consensus uniquely characterizes mysticism

(Hood, 2006; Jones, 2016). Although social scientists cannot confirm any ontological claims based upon mystical experience, they can construct theories compatible with claims to the existence of such realities. Hodges (1974) and Porpora (2006) have argued that the scientific taboo against the supernatural can be broken, as long as hypotheses about the supernatural can be shown to have empirical consequences. Likewise, Hood (2012b, 2014a) has argued for a methodological agnosticism in which one cannot a priori rule out the ontological possibilities inherent in mystical experience. In Garrett's (1974) phrase, "troublesome transcendence" must be confronted by social scientists as much as by theologians and philosophers. There is no reason why scientists cannot include specific hypotheses derived from views about the nature of transcendent reality in empirical studies of religious experience, as long as specific empirical predictions can be made. The source of the predictions may reference even the unobservable and the intangible. All that is required is that there be identifiable empirical consequences. Jones (1986) has stated the case as follows:

> Invoking Occam's Razor [i.e., the philosophical principle that the best explanation of an event is the simplest one] to disallow reference to factors other than sensory observable ones is question begging in favor of one metaphysics building up an ontology with material objects as basic. (p. 225)

Jones echoes the classic claim of William James that mystics base their experience upon the same sort of processes that all empiricists do—direct experience. James would restrict the authoritative value of mystical experience to the person who had the experience, but would view it as a hypothesis for the social scientist to investigate (Hood, 1992a, 1995c). However, mystics are united in the belief that such experiences are real, and many nonmystics are convinced of the reality of the experience even if they personally have not had it. Thus, as Swinburne (1981) argues, mystical experience is also authoritative for others:

> . . . if it seems to me I have a glimpse of Nirvana, or a vision of God, that is good grounds for me to suppose that I do. And, more generally, the occurrence of religious experience is prima facie reason for all to believe in that of which the experience was purportedly an experience. (p. 190)

Social scientists are often too quick to boast that their own limited empirical data undermine ontological claims. Religious traditions cannot be adequately understood without the assumption that transcendent objects of experience are believed to be real and foundational to those who experience them (Hood, 1995a). It is also possible that they not only are believed to be real, but are in fact real as well. Furthermore, their reality may be revealed in experience. Carmody and Carmody (1996, p. 10) define "mysticism" as "a direct experience of ultimate reality." This definition remains a hypothesis capable of empirical investigation. To presuppose otherwise is less persuasive than once thought. Bowker (1973), after critically reviewing social-scientific theories of the sense of God, has noted that it is an empirical option to conclude that at least part of the sense of God might come from God. In our terms, religious views of the nature of the Real suggest ways in which it can be expressed in human experience. This can work in two directions, both deductively and inductively. Deductively, one can note that if the Real is conceived in a particular way, then certain experiences of the Real can be expected to follow. Thus we can anticipate that expectations play a significant role in religious experience, often confirming the foundational realities of one's faith tradition. Inductively, we can infer that if particular experiences occur, then the possibility that the Real exists is a reasonable inference—a position forcefully argued by Berger (1979). Thus we can anticipate that experiences, some unanticipated, may lead some to seek religions for their illumination. O'Brien (1965) has gone so far as to include in his criteria for a mystical experience that it be unexpected. Religious traditions adopt both options in confronting mystical and numinous experiences. In this sense, a rigorous methodological atheism that Flournoy (1903) raised to a methodological postulate is unwarranted in the study of religious and mystical experiences (Hood, 2012b; James, 1902/1985; Porpora, 2006).

Not surprisingly, then, mystical experiences have long been the focus of empirical research and provocative theorizing among both sociologists and psychologists. We first explore classic efforts to confront these experiences. These classic views are of more than historical interest, as they set the range of conceptual issues that continue to plague the contemporary empirical study of mysticism. Our focus upon classic views is not exhaustive. We focus upon representatives of three major social-scientific views regarding mystical experience: as erroneous attribution, as a heightened state of awareness, and as evolved consciousness.

REPRESENTATIVE CLASSICAL VIEWS OF MYSTICISM

Mysticism as Erroneous Attribution

Preus (1987) has emphasized that the classical social-scientific theorists of religion, with only a few exceptions, had little doubt that they could provide genuine reductive explanations of religion. Such explanations purported to replace religious attributions with purely secular claims to processes involved in mystical experience as illuminated by science. Furthermore, it was commonly assumed that once the social sciences illuminated the true nature of religious experience, then religious claims based upon such experiences would lose much of their persuasive force.

The early psychologists of religion could not help confronting mysticism in light of this assumption. The mystical claim to have experienced God could not be uncritically accepted by psychologists. Much of the scientific validity of psychology was seen to rest upon its ability to provide scientific explanations for spiritual and religious claims. Thus, despite the fact that in the popular mind psychology was seen as a spiritual discipline, most psychologists saw the public interest in spiritual matters as a way to help develop the science of psychology, if psychology could explain the spiritual in natural-scientific terms (Coon, 1992; Taves, 1999). In *The Psychology of Religious Mysticism*, Leuba (1925) provided one of the earliest physiological theories of mysticism. Considerably less sympathetic to religion than William James was, Leuba insisted that mystical experience could be explained in physiological terms. He also insisted that no transcendental object is necessary for mystical experience, and that only physiological processes and a natural-scientific framework can illuminate these experiences. He was one of the first psychologists to argue forcefully that mystical experience provides no evidential force for religious beliefs. Mystics do not encounter God in their experience, Leuba claimed; rather, mystics use their beliefs to interpret their experience, ultimately erroneously. His now-classic study of mysticism was echoed in the general French tradition of the emerging discipline of psychiatry, in which mental states—including many religious ones interpreted by those who experienced them—were understood in terms of their origins in physiological and psychological processes that were often deemed pathological. At one time, the American Psychiatric Association produced a widely accepted declaration announcing that mystical experience is erroneous pathological attribution. However, empirical scholars quickly refuted this claim, as we discuss in this chapter.

Reductive sociologist Emile Durkheim (1915) argued for mystical experience as the apprehension of individuals' dependence upon a transcendent object; however, this object is society, not a divine being or reality. The genuine experience of being part of a larger unity is correct, but a misattribution applies this to God instead of its real origin, society. Thus any theory that claims to explain experiences of union with the Real in terms of processes that can be identified as purely physiological, psychological, or social must claim to interpret mysticism by misattribution. A corollary is that when individuals realize the true source of their experience of union, the religious quality (in terms of transcendent claims) will disappear. In the social sciences, William James in psychology and Petrim Sorokin in sociology refused to stand as the best representatives of accepting mystical experiences as veridical of realities ignored by most social scientists (Hood, 2014b).

Mysticism as Heightened Awareness

Although most early social scientists reveled in the apparent power of psychology to explain religion in general and mystical experiences in particular, William James best represented the paradoxical position of the emerging science of psychology. Hood (1992a, 1995c) has traced the efforts of James to avoid religious concepts, such as the soul, in developing psychology as a natural science. In *The Principles of Psychology* (1890/1950), James saw no need for the concept of a soul or for any transcendent dimension to human consciousness; however, in *The Varieties of Religious Experience* (1902/1985), he noted that the facts of mystical experience require a wider dimension to human consciousness. He favored Myers's (1903/1961) notion of a subconscious, in which James argued that a wider self may emerge. Furthermore, he argued that this natural process may be one in which the human self merges with God. Thus, although the empirical facts cannot prove the existence of a God, mystical experience provides the basic experiential fact from which God as a genuine "overbelief" to explain the process is a viable hypothesis. Mystical experiences thus have reasonable evidential force, in James's view (Hood, 2000a, 2002a). More recently, empirical psychologists have reintroduced Myers to a new generation of scholars who have succumbed to reductive materialism, in opposition to what is referred to as an irreducible mind that cannot be explained in terms of a building-block approach (Kelly et al., 2007; Marshall, 2015).

James's views created much controversy among early psychologists, who were anxious to separate psychology from religious views. But James's insistence that mystical experiences are valid forms of human experience—incapable of being reductionistically explained by either physiological or psychological processes—provided a counter to the emerging natural-scientific possibility that religious experiences may have a truly transcendent dimension (Hood, 2002a; Taves, 1999). James's view was simply that one may encounter God in mystical experiences, regardless of the processes identified by the scientists that are operating during the experience. Taylor (2002) argues that this is one of James's lasting contributions to psychology, relevant to those who would assume that "The believer is thought to have invented the delusion that beguiles him [or her]" (p. 55).

In terms used previously, science cannot rule out that a mystical experience is an experience of the Real or of a foundational reality that may be necessary for the experience to occur. At a minimum, the *belief* in the reality must be there. As James stated in his notes for his Gifford Lectures on mysticism, "Remember, the whole point lies in really believing that through a certain point or part in you, you coalesce and are identical with the Eternal" (quoted in Perry, 1935, Vol. 2, p. 331).

Mysticism as Evolved Consciousness

Evolutionary theory has been a continuous influence on psychology since its inception, and, as we have done in several chapters, we once again propose it as a major paradigm for the psychology of religion (Kirkpatrick, 2005). Mysticism has been proposed by some as a form of consciousness that is evolving, much as consciousness has evolved from the nonreflective consciousness that characterizes animals to the reflective consciousness that characterizes people. Not only are persons aware, but they are aware that they are aware; that is, they can reflect upon their awareness. Bucke (1901/1961) is most closely identified with the theory that following upon reflexive awareness in the evolution of consciousness is a cosmic consciousness or mystical state of awareness of unity with the cosmos. He documented the increased presence of individuals over time whom he saw as examples of persons expressing this cosmic consciousness. Basic to his theory is the notion that cosmic consciousness is evolving in the human species, becoming more frequent (even though by citing as exemplars of mystics such persons as Buddha and Christ, Bucke made the absolute frequency of mystical experience quite rare in any population). Nevertheless, as opposed to theorists who described mysticism as pathological or as a union with a religiously defined transcendent object, Bucke saw cosmic consciousness as the natural, advanced form of consciousness toward which the human species is evolving. As consciousness evolves, it evolves into a mystical consciousness.

The philosopher Bergson (1911) gave the major impetus to evolutionary theories of mysticism by identifying mystical experience with the direct awareness of the evolutionary process itself (*élan vital*), which he saw as the basis of all life. Kolakowski (1985) has argued that sociological studies of mysticism both support and are compatible with Bergson's linking of mystical experience and his *élan vital*—a point worth emphasizing in terms of the tendency of many psychologists of religion to provide reductive evolutionary views of religious and mystical experience. Another mystical evolutionary view that is consistent with a nonreductive religious view is found in the work of de Chardin (1959).

Alister Hardy (1965, 1966) proposed that a cosmic consciousness is gradually emerging within the human species as a whole. His theory provides a thoroughly naturalistic basis for mystical experiences as evolved forms of consciousness. Unlike Bucke, Hardy assumed that mystical states are common. Late in his life, after his retirement from a career in zoology, he began soliciting reports of religious experiences and initiated efforts to provide a classification system of them. We have mentioned his empirical work in Chapters 8 and 10, and we discuss it further in the section on survey research below.

Our task in the remainder of this chapter is to focus on the empirical literature. As we shall see, many of the issues raised in the classical and conceptual literatures on mysticism are paralleled in the empirical literature (Hood, 2012b). By interrelating these two, we hope to contribute to what McGinn (1991, p. 343) has termed the "unrealized conversation" between social-scientific investigators and those involved in the history and theory of mystical traditions.

THE EMPIRICAL STUDY OF MYSTICISM

Central to any empirical study of mysticism is measurement based upon operationalized terms. There are almost as many definitions of "mysticism" as there are theorists. Well over 100 years ago, Inge (1899) evaluated at least 26 definitions of it and concluded that no word in the English language had been employed more loosely. Not surprisingly, much of the current conceptual literature on mysticism debates various definitions and classifications of mysticism—often, obviously, on the basis of prior theological or religious commitments. For instance, Zaehner (1957) argued for a clear distinction between "theistic mysticism" and other forms of mysticism, primarily on theological grounds. Likewise, in an often-cited example, the renowned Jewish scholar of mysticism Buber (1965) referred to his own experience of an "undivided unity," which he had thought to be union with God, but later felt to be an inappropriate interpretation. In a similar vein, James (1902/1985) refused to give serious consideration the considerably refined classification systems of mystical states associated with the Catholic mystical tradition, believing them to be primarily driven by theological considerations unrelated to actual experience. The Protestant theologian Ritschl claimed that neo-Platonism had so influenced the history of mysticism that it had become the theoretical norm for mystical experience, and that the universal being viewed as God by mystics is a "cheat" (quoted in McGinn, 1991, pp. 267–268). Finally, feminist theorists have accused both authorities within mysticism and scholars who study mysticism of falsely universalizing perspectives that, when deconstructed, can be seen as efforts to silence women—including accepting "ineffability" as a criterion of mysticism precisely so that women can say nothing of their experience (Jantzen, 1995).

From this sampling of views, it is clear that any definition of mysticism is likely to encounter conceptual criticism. However, at the empirical level, it is clear that the distinction between experience and its interpretation and/or evaluation carries some weight. Thus, even in the case of Buber cited above, an experience of unity can be identified, regardless of how it is interpreted. The measurement of mysticism is possible once some operational indicator is identified. A considerable consensus exists that an experience of unity is central to mystical experience. Indeed, debates on mysticism often center on precisely how this unity is to be interpreted. Accordingly, measurements of mysticism identifying an experience of unity that is variously interpreted are quite congruent with the conceptual literature. They can also provide empirical tests of some of the issues central to that literature.

There are three major ways in which mysticism has been operationalized and measured in empirical research:

1. Open-ended responses to specific questions intuitively assumed to tap mystical or numinous experiences. These responses may then be variously coded or categorized.
2. Questions devised for use in survey research. Of necessity, these questions are brief, limited in number, and worded in language easily understandable for use in surveys of the general population. However, they are relevant as indicators of both a numinous sense of presence and an experience of unity.
3. Specific scales to measure mysticism.

As we shall see, how mysticism is operationalized and measured is related to the kinds of data provided to answer the various questions about mysticism. Accordingly, we discuss empirical studies in terms of the predominant operational and measurement strategies employed.

Studies Using Open-Ended Responses to Assess Mystical Experiences

Laski's Research

One of the more curious mainstream references in the empirical study of mysticism is Laski's (1961) research on ecstasy—curious, because of its severe methodological inadequacies. Laski, a novelist untrained in the social sciences, became interested in whether or not the experience of ecstasy she had written about in a novel was experienced in modern life. Initially using a convenience sample of friends and acquaintances sampled over a period of 3 years, she essentially asked persons to respond in an interview to the primary question: "Do you know a sensation of transcendent ecstasy?" (Laski, 1961, p. 9). If she was asked to explain what was meant by "transcendent ecstasy," she told her respondents to "Take it to mean what you think it means" (Laski, 1961, p. 9). It only took 63 persons to produce 60 affirmative responses, perhaps because of the highly educated and literary nature of Laski's friends (20 of the 63 identified themselves as writers). Laski's own belief was that the transcendent ecstasy is most likely to be related to a family of terms that includes "mysticism," "oceanic feeling," and "cosmic consciousness" (1961, p. 5). However, an attempt to replicate her interview results with a sample distributed through mailboxes to 100 homes in a working-class area of London resulted in only 11 returns, with only 1 of these responses answering affirmatively the reworded question: "Have you ever had a feeling of unearthly ecstasy?" (Laski, 1961, pp. 526–533). We need only note here that different methods with different samples radically alter the nature of the data one may collect!

Thus Laski's 1961 text primarily analyzed responses obtained from her 60 interviews and from comparisons to 27 literary and 24 religious excerpts from published texts (selected for their intuitive demonstration of ecstatic experiences similar to those reported by the interview group). Her work is an extensive discussion of various means of classifying and identifying the nature of these experiences, primarily in terms of the language used to describe them. Laski's own limited data-analyzing skills were balanced by her perceptive analysis of language. The citations of the primary texts and interviews make it easy for the reader to judge the value of Laski's own analyses. Her conclusions raise several issues that have been the focus of more rigorous studies, including those with children and adolescents discussed in Chapters 4 and 5.

Among Laski's conclusions is that transcendent ecstasy is a subset of mystical experience, defined and demarcated by the language used to describe it. It can be of three subtypes: experience of (1) knowledge, (2) union, or (3) purification and renewal. It is transient, and is triggered or elicited by a wide variety of circumstances and contexts. Generally, it is pleasurable and has beneficial consequences. However, it need not have unique religious value or provide evidential force for the validity of religious beliefs. Laski's own preference was to interpret transcendent ecstasy as a purely human capacity to experience joy in one's own creativity. She concluded that in both the past and the present, those who believe that they have experienced God are indeed mistaken; they have made a misattribution (Laski, 1961, pp. 369–374).

Social scientists continue to cite Laski's work, less for its methodological rigor than for its powerful description and analysis of instances of mystical experience. The assumption of many that mysticism is a rare phenomenon, characteristic of only a few, is belied by Laski's work. Her examples ring true to many persons' experiences, as we shall see. Furthermore, her interview procedures and her willingness to use the participants' own terms and language to analyze experiences have parallels in modern phenomenological research (Wulff, 1995).

Hood's Research

Open-ended responses to specific questions such as the ones we have been discussing can yield massive amounts of material, difficult to summarize. Statistical rigor and classification often yield to a rich descriptive presentation. However, such studies can be used to test empirical hypotheses as well. Hood (1973b) selected two extreme groups from a sample of 123 college students who responded to Allport's Intrinsic and Extrinsic religious orientation scales. The 25 highest-scoring subjects on each scale (Intrinsic mean = 41.8, SD = 2.9; Extrinsic mean = 49.2, SD = 3.7) were invited to participate in interviews regarding their "most significant personal experience." The 41 participants (20 "intrinsic subjects" and 21 "extrinsic subjects") described a wide variety of experiences, few of which were explicitly identified as religious. However, coding experiences for their mystical quality on five criteria revealed that, as predicted, intrinsic subjects' most significant personal experiences were reliably coded as mystical more frequently than were extrinsic subjects' most significant personal experiences (see Table 11.1). This held not only for the total, global assessment of mysticism, but for each of the five criteria used to identify mysticism. Despite the wide diversity of actual experiences (from childbirth to drug experiences), these could be coded as mystical more often for intrinsic subjects than for extrinsic subjects. It is important to note that few participants spontaneously described any experience as mystical; coders using theory-derived criteria categorized experiences as mystical or not. The role of language in defining experience from both first- and third-person perspectives is complex and is a topic of intense conceptual debate (Hood, 2006; Jantzen, 1995; Katz, 1992; Scharfstein, 1993). Yet at the purely empirical level, Hood's study indicates that experiences can be reliably coded as mystical by independent raters using theory-based criteria, even if the respondents themselves do not identify their experiences as mystical.

Research by Thomas and Cooper and by the Hardy Centre

However, if individuals affirmatively respond to an item measuring mysticism, does it mean that their experience was mystical as judged by others? Thomas and Cooper suggest that it may not be so. In two studies (Thomas & Cooper, 1978, 1980), they had persons from colleges, religious groups, and civic organizations respond to one of the items most frequently used in survey research (to be discussed below) to assess mystical experience. The item was "Have you ever had the feeling of being close to a powerful spiritual force that seemed to lift you out of yourself" (Thomas & Cooper, 1978, p. 434). Research Box 11.1 discusses these two studies in greater detail.

The findings of Thomas and Cooper are supported by classifications of the religious experiences solicited from and sent in to the Alister Hardy Religious Experience Research Centre, as described in Chapter 10. Much as Alister Hardy collected and classified samples

TABLE 11.1. Most Significant Personal Experiences Coded for Mystical Criteria in Intrinsic and Extrinsic Persons

Mystical criteria	Intrinsic ($n = 20$)	Extrinsic ($n = 21$)	Chi-square	Contingency coefficient[a]
Total				
Mystical	15	3		
Nonmystical	5	18	13.0***	.49
Loss of self				
Yes	14	3		
No	6	18	10.9***	.46
Noetic				
Yes	17	3		
No	3	13	7.6**	.39
Ineffable				
Yes	19	4		
No	1	17	21.0**	.58
Positive				
Yes	19	12		
No	1	9	6.0*	.36
Sacred				
Yes	18	6		
No	2	15	13.8***	.56

Note. Adapted from Hood (1973b). Religious orientation and the experience of transcendance. *Journal of the Scientific Study of Religion, 12*, 441–448. Copyright © 1973 the Society for the Scientific Study of Religion. Adapted by permission.
[a]Upper limit of contingency coefficient = .71.
*$p < .02$. **$p < .01$. ***$p < .001$.

of plankton during his career as a zoologist, numerous samplings from over 5,000 reports of religious experience at the Hardy Centre have been collected and variously classified. The most extensive classification is based upon the initial 3,000 cases Hardy collected. Variations occurred in the wording of the appeal for reports of such experiences, depending on the source of publication. In some cases, brief descriptions from literature were given to illustrate the type of experience in which the researchers were interested (Hardy, 1979, p. 18). Most common was this one in a pamphlet widely circulated in the United Kingdom:

> All those who feel they have been conscious of, and perhaps influenced by, some Power, whether called God or not, which may either appear to be beyond their individual selves or partly, or even entirely, within their being, are asked to write a simple account of their feelings and their effects. (Hardy, 1979, p. 20)

Not surprisingly, Hardy and his colleagues found that the reports of the materials submitted defied easy classification: "So many of them were a mixture of widely different items" (Hardy, 1979, p. 23). Hardy's own elaborate classification system, composed of 12

RESEARCH BOX 11.1. Measurement and Rates of Mystical Experiences
(Thomas & Cooper, 1978 [Study 1], 1980 [Study 2])

In Thomas and Cooper's first study, only young adults ages 17–29 were used (44 males, 258 females). In the second study, 305 persons representing three different age groups—17–29 years ($n = 120$), 30–59 years ($n = 110$), and 60 years and older ($n = 75$)—responded to the same survey question. In each study, those who answered "yes" went on to describe their experience in open-ended fashion, and raters coded the responses to place them in one of the categories described below. The percentage who answered "yes" was identical in both studies and is typical for survey research (34%). However, when the open-ended descriptions were analyzed for frequency and type of experience reported, all experiences were reliably placed into one of four response categories derived from a portion of the initial sample.

The frequencies and types of experiences reported, based upon open-ended descriptions to "yes" responses to the question "Have you ever had the feeling of being close to a powerful spiritual force that seemed to lift you out of yourself?", were as follows. (Note that these percentages are based on n's of 302 for Study 1 and 304 for Study 2; coder agreement was 94% overall for both studies.)

Type 0: No experience (Study 1, 66%; Study 2, 66%). Respondents answered "no" to question.

Type 1: Uncodable (Study 1, 8%; Study 2, 10%). Respondents answered "yes," but responses were irrelevant or could not be reliably coded.

Type 2: Mystical (Study 1, 2%; Study 2, 1%). Responses included expressions of such things as awesome emotions; a sense of the ineffable; or a feeling of oneness with God, nature, or the universe.

Type 3: Psychic (Study 1, 12%; Study 2, 8%). Responses included expressions of extraordinary or supernatural phenomena, including extrasensory perception, telepathy, out-of-body experience, or contact with spiritual beings.

Type 4: Faith and consolation (Study 1, 2%; Study 2, 16%). Responses included religious or spiritual phenomena, but without indications of either extraordinary or supernatural elements.

Despite minor variations in frequencies of experience categories between these two studies (perhaps because of the larger age range in Study 2), there is remarkable agreement not only in the identical percentage of affirmative responses in both studies, but also in the fact that the *least* frequent content category for the open-ended responses was mystical.

The importance of these two studies is that if affirmative responses in a single-item survey question are accepted at face value, many diverse experiences may be clustered together. In terms of our specific concern with mystical experiences, no more than 2% of the 34% who responded to the survey question presumed to be a measure of mysticism actually described mystical experiences in open-ended descriptions. The criteria for mysticism compatible with those typically cited in the conceptual literature—such as an ineffable sense of union with God (personal) or the universe (impersonal)—were not evident. Thus survey items to assess mysticism may do so poorly according to more rigorous criteria, and may overestimate the actual rates of reported mystical experience in samples.

major categories (most with numerous subclassifications), yielded a total of 92 classifications. Some of these referred to the development and consequences of the experience, and did not describe the experience proper. Each experience was rated for the presence or absence of any classification category. Most relevant to our concerns in this chapter are those experiences that were coded in terms of mystical or numinous criteria. Few of these were: The most specific mystical category, "Feeling of unity with surroundings and/or with people," characterized only 168 of the initial 3,000 experiences coded, or 5.6% (Hardy, 1979, p. 26). The most numinous classification, "Sense of presence (not human)," characterized 369 or 12.3% of these 3,000 reports (Hardy, 1979, p. 27). Thus, despite the fact that Hardy felt his appeal would yield reports of evidential value—akin to spiritual reports in the Bible and accounts by mystics—only a small minority of the experiences were either mystical or numinous when coded for relevant criteria by independent raters. For instance, Hay (1994) has identified six major types of religious experiences in the Hardy archives, only one of which is "experiencing in an extraordinary way that all things are One" (pp. 21–22).

Hay's Research

Hay and Morisy (1985, p. 14) asked a random sample of 266 residents of Nottingham, England, a version of the Hardy appeal: "Have you ever been aware or influenced by a presence or power, whether you call it God or not, which is different from your everyday self?" Of the 172 who consented to be interviewed, 72% (124) answered "yes." Eliminating 17 of these (who apparently misunderstood the question or who could not describe the experience) left 107 persons who were able to describe in detail the experience (or the most important experience, if they had more than one). Using the respondents' own language, the researchers classified the experiences into one of seven categories as follows: presence of or help from God (28%), assistance via prayer (9%), intervention by presence not identified as God (13%), presence or help from deceased (22%), premonitions (10%), meaningful patterning of events (10%), and miscellaneous (8%) (Hay & Morisy, 1985, p. 217). Although these categories were purely provisional, once again it is evident that persons who were responding to particular questions were in fact reporting a wide range and type of experiences. This was true even though the specific wording of the Hardy appeal used in this study was field-tested and assumed to draw out both the mystical and numinous qualities of religious experience. Yet no mystical experiences could be coded (except perhaps if included under "miscellaneous"), and only 28% were explicitly numinous in terms of a sense of presence identified with the holy (God).

In a similar study, Hay (1979, p. 165) found a high (65%) affirmative response rate to whether an individual could ever remember "being aware of or influenced by a presence or a power, whether you call it God or not, which is different from your everyday self." Respondents were 100 randomly selected students in a postgraduate teacher certificate course at Nottingham University, England. Despite the fact that the question was worded to cover mystical or numinous experiences—by focusing upon whether the experience was of a personal ("presence") or impersonal ("power") nature—classification of extended interviews in which affirmative respondents described their experience yielded only 32 of 109 (29.4%) experiences that were clearly either mystical or numinous. These were 10 (9.2%) experiences of unity (mystical experience), and 22 (20.2%) experiences of an awareness of God (numinous experience). Consistent with the work of Vernon (1968) cited below, Hay (1987) also found that 24% of the atheists or agnostics responded affirmatively to this question, compared with 36% of the population as a whole.

Summary of Studies Using Open-Ended Responses

Overall, we can conclude that open-ended responses to specific questions presumed to elicit reports of mystical experiences reveal little of scientific value, beyond the fact that individuals (from children through senior citizens) readily report such experiences. The richness of their reports varies with their linguistic capacities. They cannot be taken as uncritical evidential value for the realities they describe, and they may be highly influenced by personal concerns of those making such reports. Finally, depending on investigators' own classification interests, such reports can be almost interminably classified and cross-referenced. This means that first-person descriptions of experience are unlikely to correspond closely to third-person classifications of these same experiences However, this research tradition does remind us that responses to such questions, even if reliably quantified, mask a rich subjective variation of immense importance to those whose experiences are studied.

Survey Research

Emerging simultaneously with, and influenced by, open-ended reports of mystical experience are survey studies. As noted earlier, such studies use a few specific questions, often answered simply "yes" or "no." What survey studies lose in terms of the range and depth of description of experiences, they gain in terms of identifying the frequency and reporting of such experiences in the general population. Their results are also easily quantified and allow correlations with a wide variety of demographic and other variables to provide a distinctive empirical base that complements merely conceptual discussions of these experiences. We focus here on the body of survey research that has asked questions intended by the researchers to be direct measures of mystical experiences. Fortunately, several surveys have used identical questions over several years and even within different cultures, so some comparisons over time and cultures can also be made, at least at the descriptive level.

One caution must be noted before we begin, however. Intercorrelations among different items to measure mystical experiences across different surveys are not available. Although we can anticipate positive correlations, it is not clear that this will always be the case; nor can we be certain of the magnitude of such correlations. Hence each item must be judged in itself as an operational measure of the experience in question. Four major questions have dominated the majority of surveys covering since 1960. Accordingly, we summarize these data in terms of the survey questions used, each identified by the name most closely associated with the formulation of the initial question.

The Stark Question

In their sampling of churches in the greater San Francisco area in 1963, Glock and Stark (1965) asked, "Have you ever as an adult had the feeling that you were somehow in the presence of God?" (p. 157, Table 8-1). With a sample size just under 3,000 respondents (2,871), 72% answered "yes." Because the question specifically emphasized a *feeling* of God's presence, it was presumed to tap religious experience rather than belief. Not surprisingly, the majority of religiously committed, institutionally involved persons answered "yes." Only 20% of all Protestants sampled ($n = 2,326$) and 25% of all Catholics sampled ($n = 545$) answered "no."

Vernon (1968) isolated a small sample of 85 persons who indicated "none" when asked about religious commitment. In this sample of "religious nones," 25% nevertheless answered the Stark question affirmatively. Thus, even among those with no institutional religious commitment, a significant minority of adults reported experiencing a sense of God's presence.

The Bourque Question

In a series of surveys, Bourque and her colleagues utilized the following question to assess religious experience: "Would you say that you have ever had a 'religious or mystical experience'—that is, a moment of sudden religious awakening or insight?" (Back & Bourque, 1970, p. 489). They also cited results from three Associated Press surveys using this question; these surveys were conducted in 1962, 1966, and 1967 in the United States. Over time, the percentage of persons answering "yes" increased from 21% in 1962 ($n = 3,232$) to 32% in 1966 ($n = 3,518$) to 41% in 1967 ($n = 3,168$). Gallup (1978) used this item in a U.S. national survey in 1976 and found that 31% answered affirmatively in a sample of 1,500. More recently, Yamane and Polzer (1994) reported the results of two Gallup surveys in 1990—one in June and one in September, each using a sample of 1,236—and found a stable affirmative response frequency of 53%.

Thus, over a period exceeding a quarter of a century, representative samples of persons in the United States reported having a religious or mystical experience, defined as a moment of sudden religious awakening or insight. The range of affirmative responses was large (21–53%), but lower than the typical affirmative response to the Stark question.

Bourque (1969; Bourque & Back, 1971) also created an index of religious experience composed of three questions—the Stark and Bourque questions already noted, plus a third: "Have you ever had a feeling of being saved in Christ?" In a sample of 3,168, a total of 990 (31%) answered affirmatively to all three questions; 794 (25%) to any two; and 566 (18%) to at least one (Bourque & Back, 1971, p. 10).

The Greeley Question

Another question widely used in survey research and accepted as an operational measure of reported mystical question is associated with the work of Greeley (1974). The question most typically used is "Have you ever felt as though you were close to a powerful spiritual force that seemed to lift you out of yourself?" It has been administered as part of the General Social Survey (GSS) of the National Opinion Research Center. The GSS, mentioned in earlier chapters, is a series of independent cross-sectional probability samples of persons living in noninstitutional homes in the continental United States, who are at least 18 years of age and English-speaking. It was found that overall, in a GSS sample of 1,468, 35% of the respondents answered "yes" to this question (Davis & Smith, 1994).

Hay and Morisy (1978) administered a similar question to a sample of 1,865 in Great Britain and found that 36% answered in the affirmative. In the two studies by Thomas and Cooper (1978, 1980) discussed above, the 34% affirmative responses revealed few responses that were truly mystical when independently coded for criteria of mysticism. On the other hand, Greeley (1975, p. 65) found that a very high percentage (29%) of those who positively answered his question agreed with "a sense of unity and my own part in it" as a descriptor of their experience. Thus most of the 34% answering "yes" to the Greeley question also appeared to accept a mystical description of unity as applying to the experience. It may be that, methodologically, checking descriptors of experience increases the positive rate of mystical experiences over spontaneous descriptions of the experiences in open-ended interviews.

In a survey of 339 persons, McClenon (1984) found the lowest affirmative response rate to the Greeley question (20%). A decade later, Yamane and Polzer (1994) analyzed all affirmative responses from the GSS to the Greeley question in the years 1983, 1984, 1988, and 1989. A total of 5,420 individuals were included in their review. Using an ordinal scale where respondents who answered affirmatively could select from three options—"once or twice," "several times," or "often"—yielded a range from 0 (negative response) to 3 (often). Using this 4-point range across all individuals who responded to the Greeley question yielded a mean score of 0.79 (SD = 0.89). Converting these to a percentage of "yes" as a nominal category, regardless of frequency, yielded 2,183 affirmative responses, or an overall affirmative response rate of 40% of the total sample who reported ever having had the experience. Independent assessment of affirmative responses for each year suggested a slight but steady decline. The figures were 39% for 1983–1984 combined (n = 3,072), 31% for 1988 (n = 1,481), and 31% for 1989 (n = 936).

The Hardy Question

As noted above, Alister Hardy's interest in religious experience focused methodologically on soliciting open-ended responses from persons to both literary examples and descriptions of religious experiences. The most common description used by Hardy (noted above) was slightly modified by Hay and Morisy and used in several survey studies.

The precise wording of the Hay and Morisy question was "Have you ever been aware of or influenced by a presence or power, whether you call it God or not, which is different from your everyday self?" (1978, p. 207). Their survey was conducted in Great Britain. Respondents were chosen from a two-stage stratified sample: names randomly drawn from the electoral register, supplemented with randomly drawn names of nonelectors from the households of the selected electors. In their sample of 1,865, 36% answered affirmatively to the question. In the more restricted sample of 172 homes in an industrial area of England (described earlier), Hay and Morisy (1985) found the high affirmative response rate of 72%. The high rates were probably a function of face-to-face interviews, which have been shown to increase the number of affirmative responses to survey questions dealing with religious experience. However, Hay (1994) also found a 65% affirmative response rate to his version of the Hardy question in a random sample of postgraduate students at Nottingham University, England. He extensively interviewed respondents regarding their experiences, but the actual affirmation of the experiences occurred before the interview. It may be that anticipating a discussion of reports of religious experience increases the rate of such reports. Hay (1994, p. 8, Table 3) also cites a study by Lewis, in which a high affirmative response rate to the Hardy question was obtained in a British sample of 108 nurses from two different hospitals in Leeds. Again, face-to-face interviews may have been a factor increasing response rates.

In a Gallup sample of 985 British citizens, Hay and Heald (1987) found a rate more typical of other general surveys using the Hardy question: 48% of their sample responded affirmatively to the question. This closely matches the 44% rate found in previously unpublished data based upon an Australian sample of 1,228 by Morgan Research (the Australian affiliate of the Gallup Poll organization) and cited by Hay (1994, p. 7). A survey in the United States of 3,000 sampled produced a 31% affirmative response rate, closely matching the 35% response rate produced in a sample of 3,062 from the Princeton Research Center (1978, cited by Hay, 1994) a few years earlier. Hay (1994, p. 7, Table 1) also cites two unpublished Gallup Polls commissioned by the Hardy Centre in 1985, indicating a 33% affirmative response to the Hardy question in a sample of 1,030 in Britain, and a 10% higher rate (43%) for a similar sample of 1,525 in the United States. Finally, Back and Bourque (1970) reported three different Gallup surveys done in the United States, with affirmative response rates to the Hardy question of 21% in 1962 ($n = 3,232$), 32% in 1966 ($n = 3,518$), and 41% in 1967 ($n = 3,168$).

Thus surveys from 1962 through 1987 in the United States, Britain, and Australia suggest a fairly wide range (21–72%) of affirmative responses to the Hardy question. However, when the higher rates obtained from anticipated in-depth interviews are ignored, the affirmative response rates average in the 35–40% range for the Hardy question—paralleling fairly closely those for the Greeley and Bourque questions, and for the Stark question when the respondents are not restricted to church or synagogue members. Thus, overall, it appears that 35% of persons sampled affirm some intense spiritual experience, felt by the researchers to measure mystical and/or numinous experience. At a minimum, then, the reports of such experiences have been clearly and conclusively established by survey studies to be statistically quite common among normal samples. What are we to make of these reports?

Most survey studies have included additional questions and demographic characteristics that can be correlated with the reports of religious experience. No simple pattern has emerged from the studies mentioned above, and unfortunately each study must be considered in terms of its sampling and the statistical models used. The range of data analysis is large, from naïve to state-of-the-art sophistication. The major consistent findings are easily summarized: Women report more such experiences than men; the experiences tend to be age-related, increasing with age; they are characteristic of educated and affluent people; and they are more likely to be associated with indices of psychological health and well-being than with those of pathology or social dysfunction. Thus Scharfstein's (1973) "everyday mysticism" is supported by survey research in affirming the commonalty of mysticism among both institutionally and noninstitutionally committed religious persons within the United States, the United Kingdom, and Australia.

Several studies have focused upon the communication patterns of persons who have such experiences, noting that these persons do *not* talk about their experiences with others. Even Tamminen (1991, p. 62) noted this among his Scandinavian sample; the failure to communicate such experiences starts in childhood, as we have discussed in Chapter 4. This may well account for the persistence of the belief that such experiences are uncommon. The irony is that at least one-third of the population claims to have such experiences, but few people talk about them publicly. This hidden dimension of religious experience is well documented and can be clarified by other studies, to be discussed below. However, before we discuss these studies, one cautionary note is needed—one that confronts the issue of the language and experience central to much of the conceptual and empirical literature on mysticism.

A Cautionary Note: Mysticism and the Paranormal

Since its inception, North American psychology has been linked in the popular mind with psychic phenomena. As Coon (1992) has documented, many founding North American psychologists fought hard to separate the emerging science of psychology from "spiritualism" and "psychic," to which it was connected in the popular mind. Few psychologists, then or now, believe in the reality of parapsychological phenomena. Hood (1994, 2000a) has identified religion and parapsychology as perhaps the most controversial research area in the psychology of religion.

Yet within research on mysticism, several empirical facts emerge that are problematic. First, several of the key theoreticians and empirical researchers have explicitly linked mysticism to parapsychology, with varying degrees of sympathy to both. These include such major figures as Greeley (1975), Hardy (1965, 1966), and Hood (1989, 2008a). Historians have also documented the relationship of paranormal phenomena to the history of religious experience in North American Protestantism (Coon, 1992; Taves, 1999). Second, in classifications of open-ended responses to single-item questions to measure mysticism, one of the most common code categories is "paranormal." Thus many persons who affirm what the researcher assumes to be a mystical or numinous item are in fact reporting paranormal experiences, such as telepathy, clairvoyance, or contact with the dead. Third, survey studies of mysticism commonly include items to assess paranormal experiences. For instance, paranormal experiences are included in the 1984, 1988, and 1989 GSS data. In virtually every survey, paranormal and mystical experiences are positively correlated: Persons who report paranormal experiences often report mystical experiences as well, and vice versa. Seldom is only one type of experience reported. Further support for this claim is that factor analysis of survey items including mysticism and paranormal experience indicate that extrasensory perception, clairvoyance, contact with the dead, and mysticism form a single factor; this means that these are empirically measuring one thing in the popular mind. Thalbourne and his colleagues propose the term "transliminality" to account for the common factor underlying all these experiences (Thalbourne, Bartemucci, Delin, Fox, & Nofi, 1997; Thalbourne & Delin, 1999). If we exclude *déjà vu* experiences, which are also included in survey studies but neither conceptually nor empirically linked to paranormal experiences, the pattern of affirmative responses is as high as or higher than the range of affirmative responses to religious items. As an example, Table 11.2 compares the distribution of affirmative responses to three items assessing paranormal experiences with the distribution of such responses to the Greeley question about mysticism.

TABLE 11.2. Comparison of Affirmative Responses to Four Questions about Mystical or Paranormal Experiences in 3 Years of the GSS

Year	Extrasensory perception	Clairvoyance	Contact with the dead	Mysticism
1984	$n = 1,439$ 67%	$n = 1,434$ 30%	$n = 1,445$ 42%	$n = 1,442$ 41%
1988	$n = 1,456$ 64%	$n = 1,440$ 28%	$n = 1,459$ 40%	$n = 1,451$ 32%
1989	$n = 922$ 58%	$n = 983$ 23%	$n = 991$ 35%	$n = 988$ 30%

Note. The four questions asked were as follows:

> *Mysticism*: Have you ever felt as though you were close to a powerful spiritual force that seemed to lift you out of yourself?
> *Extrasensory perception*: Have you ever felt as though you were in touch with someone when they were far away from you?
> *Clairvoyance*: Have you ever seen events that were happening at a great distance as they were happening?
> *Contact with the dead*: Have you ever felt as though you were in touch with someone who had died?

Based on Fox (1992, p. 422).

Clearly, Table 11.2 reveals that reports of parapsychological experiences are at least as common as those of mystical experiences. This fact, combined with the strong intercorrelation among parapsychological and religious items that in a general sample often yield a single factor, suggests that what is being tapped in these surveys is some assertion of experiencing a reality different from that postulated by mainstream science (Targ, Schlitz, & Irwin, 2000; Thalbourne et al., 1997; Thalbourne & Delin, 1999). However, the nature of that reality is open to serious question. We have seen that open-ended responses to survey questions yield a wide range of experiences. It is likely that some respondents simply want to affirm experiences that offer evidential support not only for alternative beliefs, but also for their own self-importance. Furthermore, it is likely that to tease out separate reports of such experiences as mystical and numinous experiences would require studies of sophisticated populations for whom such distinctions can be made, in terms of both conceptualizations and actual experience. However, it would seem that sampling from religiously committed persons would best allow distinctions between the religious and parapsychological experiences often associated with religion but perhaps best independently identified. For instance, the conceptual literature on mysticism clearly separates paranormal experiences from mystical ones. Measurement studies that find a common factor such as the one noted above may need more sophisticated samples to separate responses to parapsychological and mystical items. Moreover, many religious traditions carefully dissociate themselves from what they would term "occult" practices.

Some empirical evidence for this view is that when samples are carefully selected for their religious identification, paranormal experiences are infrequently cited (if at all) as instances of religious experiences. For instance, Margolis and Elifson (1979) carefully solicited a sample of persons who were willing to affirm that they had had a religious experience that the researchers accepted as indicating some personal relationship to ultimate reality. Forty-five respondents were then carefully interviewed about their experiences; to avoid interviewer bias, a structured format was employed. The 69 experiences described were content-analyzed, yielding 20 themes. These were then factor-analyzed, yielding four factors—the major one of which was a mystical factor "very similar to the classical mystical experience described by Stace and others" (Margolis & Elifson, 1979, p. 62). Two of the other three factors (a life change experience factor and a visionary factor) were clearly religious experiences. One factor, vertigo experience, was a loss of control experienced negatively, often triggered by drugs or music. No paranormal experiences were reported. Thus it is likely that survey questions worded to avoid religious language probably elicit a variety of experiences, including paranormal ones, that otherwise would not be identified as religious by the respondents.

However, in a survey study in the San Francisco Bay Area, Wuthnow (1978) found not only that the majority of all respondents claimed to have experienced paranormal phenomena, but that those affirming that they had "ever been in close contact with the sacred or holy" were the most likely to report paranormal experiences. The conceptual literature on mysticism is replete with discussion of traditions that warn against confounding paranormal and mystical experiences, even though they are often related both empirically and historically (Coon, 1992; Hood, 2000a; Taves, 1999; Zollschan, Schumaker, & Walsh, 1995). It is unlikely that members of the general population make such distinctions, because they usually lack either the experiential base or the conceptual sophistication to make such distinctions. As Yamane and Polzer (1994) have argued, religiously committed persons may be quite adept at distinguishing religious experiences from other types of intense or anomalous experiences.

Of course, some people outside mainstream religious traditions may define paranormal experiences as "religious," or more likely by the more general term "spiritual" (Streib & Hood, 2016). It is likely that the specific presence or absence of the term "God" in survey items produces different results, in that persons committed to a mainstream religion are most likely to respond to religious language and to make distinctions among various experiences based upon religious knowledge.

For instance, Orenstein (2002) used data from Project Canada, which polls a representative sample of Canadians every 5 years. Using 1995 data based upon 1,765 cases, he found that persons who reported conventional religious beliefs were *more* likely to report paranormal beliefs. He concluded that some amount of religious belief is a necessary condition for belief in the paranormal. However, religious belief should not be equated with religious participation: Orenstein found that among those who were religious (church, etc.) attenders, there was a decreased belief in the paranormal. Thus it was among religious believers who were not religious attenders that belief in the paranormal was strongest. He suggests that this finding is characteristic of a postmodern spiritual journey (Orenstein, 2002, p. 310)— something that we discuss in more depth below when we confront the issue of distinctions between "religion" and "spirituality."

Clearly, avoiding religious language in survey questions encourages the reporting of a wider range of experiences. Likewise, it is important to distinguish between religious belief and nonreligious attendance. Many religious believers are not religious attenders and are more likely to identify themselves as "spiritual but not religious," as we discuss more fully later in this chapter. Teasing out reports of experiences from a whole host of complex factors affecting their reporting requires more complex techniques than the methodology of survey research permits. Some of these issues have been explored in more measurement-based studies, many of which are correctional. However, there are also more laboratory-based and quasi-experimental studies. These permit even more precise identification of determinants of the reports of mystical experience.

Measurement Studies

The academic psychology of religion remains heavily committed to what Gorsuch (1984) has called the "measurement paradigm." It continues to influence the new multilevel interdisciplinary paradigm proposed for the psychology of religion (Emmons & Paloutzian, 2003). However, it has also taken an experimental turn, especially among personality and social psychologists, for which measurement and experiment are the gold standard for an empirical psychology first seriously championed by Batson and Ventis (1982) in their now-classic text.

One goal of measurement is to create reliable scales from clearly operationalized concepts. Many have thought that religious experiences, particularly the mystical varieties, cannot be reliably measured. However, two approaches to their measurement have been reasonably successful and have been used in several studies.

The Religious Experience Episodes Measure: The Influence of James

One approach to measurement of mystical experiences has been to operationalize and quantify what might be called the "literary exemplar approach" of many of the more open-ended studies discussed above. Laski and Hardy gave particular examples of experiences and asked respondents whether they had ever had an experience like the one described. Hood (1970) essentially systematized this procedure in constructing the Religious Experience Episodes Measure (REEM). He selected 15 experiences from James's *The Varieties of Religious Experience*, presented them in booklet form, and had respondents rate on a 5-point scale the degree to which they had ever had an experience like each of these. Hood's approach standardized the experiences presented to research participants, and allowed a quantification of the report of religious experience by summing the degree of similarity of one's own experiences to those described in the REEM. Rosegrant (1976) modified the REEM by rephrasing "the elegant 19th century English" (p. 306) and reducing the number of items from 15 to 10. Examples of REEM items as modified by Rosegrant are presented in Table 11.3.

Both Hood's initial version and Rosegrant's modified version of the REEM have high internal consistencies, suggesting that the experiences described cluster together. Unpublished factor analysis of the REEM also yields a single factor. Overall, the use of explicit or implicit religious language suggests that the REEM is best used with religiously committed samples. It also reflects religious experience perhaps most common in North American Protestant experience—a common criticism leveled against James's classic text, from which items for the REEM were selected. Holm (1982) found it difficult to make a meaningful translation of the REEM into Swedish, and had to create a version of the REEM appropriate to Swedish culture by selecting Nordic tales.

TABLE 11.3. Items from the Modified REEM

To what extent have you ever had an experience like this?

God is more real to me than any thought or person. I feel his presence, and I feel it more as I live in closer harmony with his laws. I feel him in the sunshine, or rain, and my feelings are best described as awe mixed with delirious restfulness.

Or like this?

I would suddenly feel the mood coming when I was at church, or with people reading, but only when my muscles were relaxed. It would irresistibly take over my mind and will, last what seemed like forever, and disappear in a way that resembled waking from anesthesia. One reason I think that I dislike this kind of trance was that I could not describe it to myself; even now I can't find the right words. It involved the disappearance of space, time, feeling, and the things I call my self. As ordinary consciousness disappeared, the sense of underlying essential consciousness grew stronger. At last nothing remained but a pure, abstract, self.

Or like this?

Once, a few weeks after I came to the woods, I thought perhaps it was necessary to be near other people for a happy and healthy life. To be alone was somewhat unpleasant. But during a gentle rain, while I had these thoughts, I was suddenly aware of such good society in nature, in the pattern of drops and every sight and sound around my house, that the fancy advantages of being near people seemed insignificant, and I haven't thought about them since. Every little pine needle expanded with sympathy and befriended me. I was so definitely aware of something akin to me that I thought no place could ever be strange.

Note. From Rosegrant (1976). The imact of set and setting on religious experience in nature. *Journal of the Scientific Study of Religion, 15*, 301–310. Adapted from Hood (1970). (Also see Hill & Hood, 1999a, pp. 222–224.) Copyright ©1976 the Society for the Scientific Study of Religion. Reprinted by permission.

Hood (1970) initially created the REEM to test the hypothesis that intrinsically religious persons would score higher on such a measure than extrinsically religious persons would. In a sample of college students, this hypothesis was supported, with intrinsic persons scoring significantly higher on the REEM than extrinsic persons. These findings are compatible with the survey research described above, in which religiously committed persons are often identified to have high rates of reported mystical experiences. It further suggests, however, that among religiously committed individuals, intrinsic persons have higher scores (and hence perhaps report more experiences) than extrinsic persons. Using Allport's Intrinsic and Extrinsic scales to create a fourfold typology, based upon median splits on the Intrinsic and Extrinsic scales, indicated that "indiscriminately pro" (IP) persons (with high Extrinsic/high Intrinsic scores) could not be distinguished from intrinsic persons on the basis of their REEM scores. Likewise, "indiscriminately anti" (IA) persons (with low Extrinsic/low Intrinsic scores) could not be distinguished from extrinsic persons on the basis of their REEM scores. Survey researchers have often worried about "false positives" and "false negatives" in their surveys. How do we know that persons who report experiences are telling the truth? Some might not have had the experiences they report (false positives). On the other hand, how do we know that persons denying these experiences are telling the truth? Some may refuse to admit experiences they have had (false negatives).

In this study, Hood (1970) linked the methodological problem of distinguishing between intrinsic and IP persons and between extrinsic and IA persons with the possibility that IP persons often represent false positives and IA persons represent false negatives with respect to reports of mystical experience. The basis for this hypothesis is that Allport believed the indiscriminate types to be motivated by conflicting stances with respect to religion: IA persons may deny religious impulses they may in fact feel, while IP persons may feign religious impulses they may not actually experience. It is this sort of dynamic and conflictual process that Allport and Ross (1967, p. 442) felt would make the indiscriminate categories potentially of significant research interest and of "central significance" for Allport's theory.

In a second study, Hood (1978b) replicated the relationship between Allport's fourfold typology and REEM scores. This time, using Rosegrant's modification of the REEM and categorizing persons according to their religious type produced similar high REEM scores for intrinsic and IP persons and similar low scores for extrinsic and IA persons, as indicated in Table 11.4.

TABLE 11.4. REEM Scores According to Religious Type

Religious type	Score
Intrinsic ($n = 31$)	Mean = 48.81, SD = 12.21
IP ($n = 46$)	Mean = 50.89, SD = 14.79
Extrinsic ($n = 39$)	Mean = 39.51, SD = 17.07
IA ($n = 31$)	Mean = 39.13, SD = 18.8

Note. $F (1, 143) = 15.69$, $p < .05$; post hoc comparisons grouped according to significant differences *between* clustered categories, at least $p < .05$. Categories *within* parentheses did not differ: (IP, I); (IA, E). Adapted from Hood (1978b). The usefulness of the indiscriminately pro and anti categories of religious orientation. *Journal for the Scientific Study of Religion, 17,* 419–431. Copyright © 1978 the Society for the Scientific Study of Religion. Adapted by permission.

In order to directly test the possibility that the indiscriminate categories might represent false positives (in the case of IP persons) and false negatives (in the case of IA persons), Hood had interviewers in a double-blind condition conduct a bogus interview that included nearly 40 personal and religious questions. These served as baseline data and also served to mask the key final question, which was prefaced by the comment that many of the preceding questions were designed to tap whether or not one had ever had a mystical experience. Persons were then asked whether they had in fact ever had such an experience. The answer to this key question, whether "yes" or "no," was then analyzed with a "Stress Analyzer," a device that measures stress by means of detecting small voice tremors. Each participant's stress level was measured by comparing the affirmation or denial of mystical experience to the baseline levels of stress in response to the bogus inventory. The numbers of persons affirming and denying mystical experiences, and the numbers showing stress when responding, are reported in Table 11.5 according to religious type.

As predicted, the proportions of persons affirming mystical experiences were similar in the intrinsic and IP groups, as were the proportions denying mystical experiences in the extrinsic and IA groups. However, intrinsic persons as a group expressed little stress when affirming mystical experiences, while IP persons showed much stress. The case was less clear for extrinsic persons. Still, more than half the IA persons exhibited stress, and while many did so when reporting mystical experiences, it may be that indiscriminate persons (whether pro or anti) indicate stress when talking about their religion (or lack of it), due to their conflictual stance with respect to religion. In any case, the large number of IP persons affirming mystical experiences with great stress is consistent with the possibility that they are "false positives," attempting to appear religious by reporting experiences they believe they should have had but perhaps have not had.

However, it is also possible that as Rosegrant (1976, p. 307) found, stress is often associated with the report of mystical experience; this was indicated by a .29 ($p < .05$) correlation between REEM scores and a measure of stress in a nature setting with 51 students. Although Rosegrant did not measure religious orientation in his study, it may be that the *lack* of correlation between mysticism and a measure of meaningfulness used in his study indicates that mystical experiences are experienced as stressful only when participants are asked for a

TABLE 11.5. Affirmation and Denial of Mystical Experience and Associated Stress by Religious Type

Religious type	Mystical experience		Stress level	
	Affirming	Denying	High	Low
Intrinsic ($n = 46$)	28	3	3	28
IP ($n = 31$)	40	6	31	15
Extrinsic ($n = 39$)	3	36	8	31
IA ($n = 31$)	12	19	18	13

Note. There was an error in the original article: The numbers for mystical experience for the extrinsic group were reversed. All differences were significant at least at $p < .05$ for all groups except the IA group for both mystical experience and stress. Adapted from Hood (1978b). The usefulness of the indiscriminately pro and anti categories of religious orientation. *Journal for the Scientific Study of Religion, 17,* 419–431. Copyright © 1978 the Society for the Scientific Study of Religion. Adapted by permission.

meaningful religious framework for interpretation. Consistent with this claim is that mystical experience as measured by the REEM is not only higher among intrinsically oriented persons, but also among religious denominations with strong norms for eliciting and interpreting mystical experiences.

Rosegrant's finding that mystical experiences as measured by the REEM were associated with stress experiences in a solitary nature setting may be misleading. It is unlikely that stress per se should serve to elicit mystical experience. Rather, the incongruity between anticipatory stress and setting stress is postulated to be a likely trigger of mysticism. In a study to test this hypothesis specifically in a nature setting, Hood (1978a) administered Rosegrant's modification of the REEM to 93 males who, as part of the requirements for graduation from a private high school, participated in a week-long outdoors program. One portion of this program entailed having students "solo." Each student was taken alone by Hood into a wilderness area; was issued minimal equipment (a tarp, water, and a mixture of nuts and candy for food); and was then left to spend the night in solitude. Various students were taken out over a five-night period, regardless of weather conditions. As some indication of the power of this experience, 29 of the 93 participants "broke solo," meaning that they returned to camp before dawn. Before each outing, anticipatory stress was measured by having the students fill out a measure of subjective stress. In addition, setting stress was fortuitously varied by the fact that some students soloed on nights when there were strong rain and thunderstorms. Table 11.6 presents the means on the REEM for participants in this exercise, according to anticipatory stress and setting stress conditions. Appropriate statistical tests indicated not only that set–setting incongruity elicited higher REEM scores, but that it made no difference whether the incongruity was between high anticipatory stress and low setting stress or low anticipatory stress and high setting stress. Either incongruity would work.

Several investigators have postulated that mystical and other intense religious experiences are related to and perhaps often elicited by hypnotic trance states. For instance, Gibbons and Jarnette (1972) suggest that at least some religious experiences may be trance states induced by stimuli outside awareness. Both historians (Taves, 1999) and anthropologists (Lewis, 1971) have long argued for the similarity between hypnotic and religious ecstatic states. Hood (1973a) found a correlation between the original form of the REEM and the Harvard Group Scale of Hypnotic Susceptibility (Shor & Orne, 1962) of .36 ($p < .01$) in a

TABLE 11.6. Mean REEM Scores for Participants under High- and Low-Stress Nature Solo Conditions, According to Anticipatory Stress Levels

Anticipatory stress	Setting stress	
	High	Low
High	32.44 ($SD = 12.75$) ($n = 16$)	52.83 ($SD = 14.72$) ($n = 12$)
Low	51.43 ($SD = 9.37$) ($n = 21$)	42.07 ($SD = 4.95$) ($n = 15$)

Note. Adapted from Hood (1978a). Anticipatory set and setting: Stress incongruity as elicitors of mystical experience in solitary nature situations. *Journal for the Scientific Study of Religion, 17*, 278–287. Copyright © 1978 the Society for the Scientific Study of Religion. Adapted by permission.

sample of 81 fundamentalist Protestants willing to be hypnotized. This is consistent with the finding that fundamentalist Protestants who report significant conversion experiences are also hypnotically suggestible (Gibbons & Jarnette, 1962), and with the historical linkage of hypnosis with Protestant conversion experiences in North America (Taves, 1999). Perhaps the loss of sense of self reported in mystical experience parallels the loss of self in hypnotic states. However, we must be careful *not* to equate mysticism and hypnosis on the basis of similar processes that might operate in both.

It is also worth hypothesizing that the wide diversity of triggers or conditions facilitating mystical experiences (as noted in survey and other studies) may have in common the fact that an individual fascinated by any given trigger experiences a momentary loss of sense of self, being "absorbed" or "fascinated" by his or her object of perception. Tellegen and Atkinson (1974) have proposed "absorption," or openness to absorbing and self-altering states, to be a trait related to hypnosis. The only empirical study using both their measure of absorption and a measure of mysticism is a study by Mathes (1982) relating mysticism, absorption, and romantic love. Unfortunately, Mathes did not report the correlation between mysticism and absorption. However, in his study, a measure of romantic love (Rubin, 1970) was correlated with mysticism for both males and females. This is consistent with being fascinated or "absorbed" by the object of interest in both experiences. It is also consistent with the fact that both love and sexuality are frequently cited as triggers of mysticism in open-ended questionnaire and survey studies.

The relationship between mysticism and hypnosis has been negatively interpreted, particularly by psychodynamically oriented investigators. Both hypnotic susceptibility and intense religious experiences, especially mystical ones, are interpreted either as regressions to early states of ego development or as signs of weak adult ego development (Allison, 1961; Owens, 1972). Both Hood (1985) and Parsons (1999) have noted that claims to a relationship between weak ego development and religious experience are derived from primarily a priori theoretical commitments of dynamic theorists that not only are conceptually unwarranted, but lack empirical support. In the only direct empirical test of a relationship between weak ego development and intense religious experience, both the conceptual and empirical inadequacies of this hypothesized relationship were demonstrated.

Hood (1974) administered the most psychometrically sophisticated measure of ego strength (Barron's [1953] ego strength scale) to a sample of 82 college students who also took the initial 15-item version of the REEM. Overall, there was a significant negative correlation ($r = -.31$) between the REEM and Barron's scale, appearing to support the claim that intense experience is related to weak ego strength. However, part of the problem is conceptual, in that Barron's scale contains several religiously worded items; these religiously worded items are scored so that agreement indicates weak ego strength. This suggests a conceptual bias against religious experience, so that one can simply assume that many religious beliefs reflect poor ego development and then use them as a measure of weak ego strength. Hood separated Barron's scale into two parts: the religiously worded items and the residual, nonreligiously worded items. Correlating these with the REEM yielded markedly different results, as noted in Table 11.7.

Inspection of this table is instructive in two senses. First, negative correlations, supposedly indicating weak ego strength among persons reporting mystical experiences, were found with religiously worded items scored to indicate weak ego strength! This link reveals the conceptual basis of these items, and confounds many supposedly empirical findings. Removing the religious items removed any significant relationship between weak ego strength and

TABLE 11.7. Correlations between the REEM and Barron's Total Ego Strength Scale, Religiously Worded Items, and Residual Items

	Nonreligiously worded items	Religiously worded items	REEM
Total ego strength scale	.47*	.93*	−.31*
Religiously worded items		−.46*	−.55*
Nonreligiously worded items			−.16

Note. Adapted from Hood (1974). Psychological strength and the report of intense religious experience. *Journal for the Scientific Study of Religion, 13*, 65–71. Copyright © 1974 the Society for the Scientific Study of Religion. Adapted by permission.
*p < .01.

religious experience. Furthermore, a nondynamically oriented measure developed for use in survey research revealed that among a sample of 114 college students, those with higher adequacy in psychological functioning as measured by this index had significantly higher REEM scores than those with lower adequacy as measured by this index.

Thus not only is there little conceptual or empirical support for the claim that weak ego strength must characterize persons who have intense religious experiences; such persons may be *more* psychologically adequate than those who do not report such experiences. This latter claim is consistent with the normality of the report of mystical and numinous experiences noted in survey studies, and also with theories that are more sympathetic to religion. For instance, Maslow's (1964) popular theory of self-actualization postulates that more actualized persons are most likely to have and report "peak experiences" (Maslow's term for mystical and other related experiences). Although his theory has generated little rigorous empirical research to support this claim, it serves as a useful conceptual counter to dynamic theories that postulate a relationship between regression and religious experience, for which there is also little rigorous empirical support.

The Mysticism Scale (M Scale): The Influence of Stace

James was the source for the range of experiences, both numinous and mystical, selected for the REEM. One criticism of the REEM is that while it does contain both numinous and mystical experiences according to the criteria discussed earlier, it is not particularly theory-driven. However, this is not the case with the Mysticism Scale (M Scale; Hood, 1975). It was developed as a specific operationalization of Stace's (1960) phenomenological work, in which he identified both introvertive and extrovertive mysticism and their common core. It is commonly employed as the most widely used empirical measure of mysticism (Lukoff & Lu, 1988).

Prior to the development of the M Scale, Stace's criteria for mysticism had influenced assessments in psychedelic research seeking to document the ontological validity of experiences elicited under drugs. Stace's criteria were developed under the assumption of causal indifference. That is, the examples used by Stace were accepted as mystical, whether elicited under drug conditions or not (Stace, 1960, pp. 29–31). Research Box 11.2 presents a summary of, and follow-up data from, what is perhaps the most famous study in the psychology of religion—Pahnke's (1966) "Good Friday" experiment.

RESEARCH BOX 11.2. Drugs and Mysticism:
Pahnke's "Good Friday" Experiment (Pahnke, 1966; Doblin, 1991)

In the psychology of religion's most famous and controversial study, Pahnke, as part of his doctoral dissertation, administered the drug psilocybin or a placebo in a double-blind study of 20 volunteers, all graduate students at Andover–Newton Theological Seminary. The subjects met to hear a broadcast of a Good Friday service after they had been given either psilocybin (experimental group) or nicotinic acid (placebo group). Participants met in groups of four, each consisting of two experimental subjects and two controls matched for compatibility. Each group had two leaders assigned, one of whom had been given psilocybin. Immediately after the service and then 6 months later, participants were administered a questionnaire, part of which consisted of Stace's specific common-core criteria of mysticism.

Nearly a quarter of a century later, from November 1986 to October 1989, Doblin contacted the original participants in the experiment. By either phone or personal contact, he was able to interview nine of the control participants and seven of the experimental participants from the original study. In addition, he was able to administer Pahnke's questionnaire to them. Thus we have the responses on Stace's criteria of mysticism immediately after the service, then 6 months later, and finally nearly 25 years later. Assigning each score as the percentage of the possible maximum for that criteria, according to Pahnke's original procedure, yields the following results.

	Original Pahnke study				Doblin follow-up study (nearly 25 years later)	
	Immediate		6 months later			
Stace category	Exptls. ($n = 10$)	Controls ($n = 10$)	Exptls. ($n = 10$)	Controls ($n = 10$)	Exptls. ($n = 7$)	Controls ($n = 9$)
1. Unity:						
a. Internal	70%	8%	60%	5%	77%	5%
b. External	38%	2%	39%	1%	51%	6%
2. Transcendence of space/time	84%	6%	78%	7%	73%	9%
3. Positive affect	57%	23%	54%	23%	56%	21%
4. Sacredness	53%	28%	58%	25%	68%	29%
5. Noetic quality	63%	18%	71%	18%	82%	24%
6. Paradoxicality	61%	13%	34%	3%	48%	4%
7. Ineffability	66%	18%	77%	15%	71%	3%
8. Transience	79%	8%	76%	9%	75%	9%

Note. Our table has been constructed to allow direct comparison between Doblin's percentages and Pahnke's. Terms have been altered to correspond more closely to M Scale terminology where relevant. Pahnke's criteria were not employed by Stace (e.g., transience), and some of Stace's criteria were not employed by Pahnke (e.g., inner subjectivity). Paradoxicality is not assessed by the M Scale. Smith (2000, pp. 99–105) has revealed that in the original study, one experimental subject had a disruptive psychological experience that had to be handled by administration of thorazine—a fact unfortunately not reported in the original description of the study. Exptls., experimental participants.

STUDIES AT JOHN HOPKINS AND RELATED RESEARCH

Griffiths, Richards, McCann, and Jesse (2006) sought to advance the Good Friday study. This benchmark study was a significant advance over Pahnke's (1966) study for several reasons. First, it was a highly sophisticated (double-blind, between-groups, crossover) design conducted at a major American university, Johns Hopkins. Thirty entheogen-naïve volunteers received psilocybin and methylphenidate (Ritalin) in counterbalanced order over two sessions. Methylphenidate was chosen as an active placebo control, because it and psilocybin have similar time course effects on blood pressure. An additional 6 randomly assigned volunteers received methylphenidate on the first two sessions and unblinded psilocybin on the third session. The purpose of this condition was to obscure the study design to both participants and guides. This was successful. Despite the use of an experienced entheogenic guide (who was drug-free when guiding) and additional knowledgeable monitors, almost one-quarter of sessions were misclassified, with methylphenidate identified as psilocybin or psilocybin identified as some other drug. Thus, unlike Pahnke's original study, this study was successful in its double-blinding.

The 36 participants (20 females) were volunteers with some religious and/or spiritual interests. They were all medically and psychologically healthy, without histories of prior entheogen use. Ages ranged from 24 to 64 (mean age was 46). Most were college graduates, and half had postgraduate degrees. Thirty participants were told that they would receive psilocybin and also that various other drugs might be administered (double-blind conditions), while 6 participants who received methylphenidate in the first two sessions were told that in the third session they would receive psilocybin. All participants met with the primary monitor over four sessions (for 8 hours total) and on four occasions (for 4 hours total) after each session. The primary purpose was to develop rapport and trust and to minimize any negative reactions.

This study was and is a longitudinal study, in that participants will be followed up and assessed on a wide variety of measures at various intervals. For our present purposes, we focus only upon the assessment of mysticism in this study. The assessment occurred in several ways. Before and 2 months after the study, participants took the M Scale. Seven hours after drug ingestion, participants took a modified version of Pahnke's questionnaire to assess mysticism. Thus both measures of mystical experience were directly related to Stace's phenomenologically identified "common core" (see below).

Results of the study indicated that 7 hours after drug ingestion, participants in the experimental group had significantly higher scores on the modified Pahnke questionnaire than the controls receiving methylphenidate had. Likewise, 2 months after the experiment, psilocybin participants had higher scores on the Hood M Scale than the methylphenidate controls had. Scores on the Hood M Scale *after* psilocybin predicted the spiritual significance of the experience ($r = .77$) in a 12- to 14-month follow-up (Griffiths, Richards, Johnson, McCann, & Jesse, 2008). Scores on all three factors of the M Scale (Interpretation, Introvertive Mysticism, and Extrovertive Mysticism; see below) were significantly greater than the initial screening scores at both the 2-month and 12- to 14-month follow-ups for those receiving psilocybin. The majority of psilocybin participants rated their experience in the study as one of the five most spiritually significant in their lives at both follow-ups.

Pahnke's (1966) original study, Doblin's (1991) long-term follow-up, and the studies by Griffiths et al. (2006, 2008) are important in demonstrating the effect of set and setting on drug-facilitated mystical experiences, using Stace's explicit criteria. The general discussion of entheogens and religious/spiritual experience in Chapter 10 obviously applies to this experiment. Yet in terms of this chapter, Pahnke was the first investigator to attempt explicitly to operationalize Stace's criteria of mysticism. His original questionnaire has been variously modified through the years, with many additional, nonmystical items added. However, the basic items relating to Stace's core criteria of mystical experience have remained virtually unchanged, and this allows direct comparisons among Pahnke's original study, Doblin's follow-up study, and the studies by Griffiths and his colleagues. The most recent, expanded versions of Pahnke's questionnaire include items relevant to peak experiences. It is clear that the concept of "peak experiences" has been broadened to include a wide variety of experiences, only some of which are mystical in Stace's sense of the term. Fortunately, the studies by Griffiths and his colleagues employed the M Scale. The M Scale is explicitly designed to measure Stace's criteria of mysticism—distinct from a wide range of other experiences, including peak experiences. Thus this research can be seen as facilitating mystical experiences in solitary settings as verified by a widely used measure of mysticism. It also provides support for the common-core thesis (discussed below)—something the experienced guide in these studies strongly supports, based upon his own extensive experience with entheogens (Richards, 2008, 2016).

The use of empirical measures is one way in which the "genuineness" of chemically facilitated reports of mystical experiences can be judged. Insofar as experiences reported under diverse sets and setting yield the same scores, then claims that chemically facilitated experiences are not genuine lack merit (Hood, 2014a). In the John Hopkins research, the experiences reported had high mysticism scores, comparable to those reported in other studies without the use of entheogens. Further evidence of "genuineness" comes from the construction of a measure similar to the M Scale, the Mystical Experience Questionnaire (MEQ; MacLean, Leoutsakos, Johnson, & Griffiths, 2012). The researchers used a self-report sample of 1,602 participants who responded to an Internet survey of psilocybin use. Exploratory factor analysis of items selected from both the original Good Friday measures and the M Scale yielded a four-factor solution: Mysticism (including unity, noetic, and sacred items), Positive Mood (including a sense of awe), Transcendence of Space and Time, and Final Ineffability. A final 30-item MEQ was constructed by a confirmatory factor analysis of a separate sample of 440 participants for whom both M Scale and MEQ scores were obtained. Samples were largely white and well educated, and 50% of respondents were female. Not surprisingly, given the admitted psilocybin use, the vast majority of participants identified themselves as spiritual but not religious (70%). The remaining identified as spiritual and religious (13.5%) or neither religious nor spiritual (16%). Given the overlap in items, it is not surprising that the total scores on the M Scale and the MEQ were highly correlated ($r = .81$). Correlations between the total score on the M Scale and subscales of the MEQ varied from .79 for Mysticism to .47 for Final Ineffability. The issue of how individual facets of the M Scale (and MEQ?) can shift is addressed later, but here it is important to note the continuity in studies documenting that entheogens do provide one means of experimentally facilitating experiences that, if not deemed religious, clearly are deemed spiritual. However, for now, it is worthy to note that among those reporting having a chemically facilitated mystical experience ($n = 1,410$) and those reporting having had no mystical experience ($n = 192$) on all factors of both the M Scale and the MEQ, there were significant differences, with those reporting the experience having the highest factor scores.

Hood and Morris (1981a) took virtually all items used in previous (pre-1980) empirical assessments of mysticism and factor-analyzed them into scales, all with adequate reliability.

These were then administered to a sample of respondents who rated the items for their applicability to defining mysticism as they understood it. Next, they rated each item as to whether or not they had ever had experienced it. The respondents did not differ in knowledge about mysticism, including whether or not they personally identified themselves as having had a mystical experience. However, persons denying having a mystical experience did not mark items they knew to define mysticism as experiences they had had, whereas those affirming a mystical experience did. Thus persons who were equally knowledgeable about mystical experiences differed in whether nor not they marked an item as being experienced as a function of having a mystical experience. This suggests that persons can know what mysticism is and yet not have an experience of it. This further suggests, despite the possibility that both demand characteristics and the abstract nature of many items assessing mysticism may contribute to "false positives" in studies of mysticism (Wulff, 2000), that respondents can be knowledgeable about mysticism and still deny that they have had the experience. Perhaps Scharfstein (1973) is correct in warning that mysticism may be more common than social scientists have heretofore thought. Certainly his claim to an "everyday mysticism" is supported by survey research and by measurement-based studies involving reported experiences with psilocybin and other entheogens (Hood, 2014b).

While the MEQ focuses upon the report of a single mystical experience triggered by psilocybin, as opposed to the M Scale's focus upon any lifetime mystical experience (however triggered), Sears (2015) has proposed a hypothesis of continuity between waking states and dreaming states. Historically, it is well established that mystical experiences across traditions and cultures have been associated with dreams (Goll & Goll, 2006). Sears (2015) initially constructed a dream-specific scale called the Spiritual Dreams Scale (SDS), using Hood's M Scale and language specific to the American evangelical sample he studied. Like many researchers using the M Scale, Sears found a three-factor solution; he identified these factors as Mystical Psychology (Passivity), Perceived Alternate Reality (Ineffability), and Noesis. Sears's study with evangelicals is not inconsistent with similar three-factor solutions for versions of the M Scale that use language compatible with evangelical Christian views (Hood & Williamson, 2000).

In a follow-up study, Sears and Hood (2016) modified the SDS to use more neutral language, not favoring any single faith tradition. Translated into Nepalese, this scale was administered to self-identified Hindus (largely higher-caste) and Christian Nepalese (largely middle- or lower-caste), and the results were analyzed via appropriate statistical techniques. The structure of the resulting 24-item Dreaming Mysticism Scale (DSM) that emerged from this study bears a marked resemblance to the results of prior M Scale analyses involving American Christians, Iranian Muslims, and Chinese Christians and non-Christians (cf. Hood, Morris, & Watson, 1993; Hood et al., 2001; Chen et al., 2012). With their various three-factor solutions for lifetime reports of mystical experience in a wide diversity of samples from diverse cultures, these studies differ from the MEQ in adopting an interpretation–extroversion–introversion typology, according to which (1) interpretation is framed by positive/religious affect and noesis; (2) extroversion comprises unity and inner subjectivity; and (3) introversion consists of ego loss, ineffability, and timelessness/spacelessness. This particular arrangement of facets has come to be known as the "Hood factor solution" (see Chen et al., 2012). Apart from a stray ego loss item and the splitting of timelessness/spacelessness items among all factors, the breakdown of the DMS with Nepali Christians and Hindus matches the Hood solution.

COMMON-CORE THEORISTS VERSUS DIVERSITY THEORISTS

Given that the M Scale is based upon Stace's demarcation of the phenomenological properties of mysticism, it is also of necessity driven by some of Stace's theoretical concerns.
Most central is the fact that Stace has become the central figure in the debate between
what we call the "common-core theorists" and the "diversity theorists." Common-core theorists assume that people can differentiate experience from interpretation, such that different
interpretations may be applied to otherwise identical experiences. This theory is often characterized by its opponents as if it claims that there is an absolute, unmediated experience.
In fact, Stace (1960) and other common-core theorists simply distinguish between degrees
of interpretation, arguing that at some level, different descriptions can mask quite similar if
not identical experiences.

Diversity theorists—led by Katz (1977), who edited an entire volume in response to
Stace's work—argue that no unmediated experience is possible, and that in the extreme, language is not simply used to interpret experience but in fact constitutes experience. Proudfoot
(1985) is among the contemporary theorists (heavily influenced by psychology) who argue for
the role of language in the constitution of, and not simply in the interpretation of, experience.

Just as Katz marshaled a series of scholars in opposition to Stace's common-core thesis,
Forman has marshaled others in opposition to the diversity position of Katz. In two edited
works (Forman, 1990b, 1998), scholars associated with Forman have argued that at least with
respect to introvertive mysticism, the diversity thesis fails. The basic argument is that since
introvertive mysticism is an experience devoid of content, it cannot be qualified by various
descriptors; nor can language play a role in its construction. Hence introvertive experience
(identified as "pure conscious experience" by Forman, 1990a) may be variously interpreted
after the fact, but as experience it lacks content. It thus is legitimately as Stace conceptualized it—a common core to mysticism, independent of both culture and person—and has
become the basis for constructing what Forman (1998) refers to as a "perennial psychology."
Parsons (1999) has also championed this phrase.

Studies in the Good Friday tradition clearly establish that when entheogens are ingested
under appropriate set and setting conditions, they can facilitate mystical experiences, in both
group (Pahnke, 1966) and individual (Griffiths et al., 2006) sessions. The consistent use of
measures derived from Stace's common core indicates that these facilitated experiences are
indistinguishable from mystical experiences that occur "spontaneously" or by other facilitated
means, such as prayer or meditation (Nichols & Chemel, 2006). Thus psilocybin and even
methylphenidate (Ditman et al., 1969) can serve as psychoactive sacramental substances.
Further research indicates that psilocybin is a more effective facilitator than methylphenidate, but even the latter can facilitate the reporting of mystical experience (Hood, 2014a).
Experiments in the Good Friday tradition can be interpreted to support the common-core
thesis, in that both "spontaneous" and facilitated mystical experiences are indistinguishable
as measured by the M Scale (Hood, 2012a) or the MEQ (MacLean et al., 2012).

Although we cannot further engage this rich conceptual literature here, we should
emphasize that three fundamental assumptions are implicit in Stace's work and in that of the
common-core psychologists. First, the mystical experience is itself a universal experience
that is essentially identical in phenomenological terms, despite wide variations in ideological
interpretation of the experience (the common-core assumption). Second, the core categories
of mystical experience are not all definitionally essential to any particular mystical experience, since there are always borderline cases, based upon fulfillment of only some of the

criteria. Third, the introvertive and extrovertive forms of mysticism are conceptually distinct: The former is an experience of unity devoid of content (pure consciousness), and the latter is an experience of unity in diversity, with content. However, these are not two distinct experiences of unity, but are intimately intertwined in ways yet to be empirically clarified. The psychometric properties of the M Scale should reflect these assumptions, and insofar as they do, they are adequate operationalizations of Stace's criteria. The question for now is this: Does empirical research support a common-core conceptualization of mysticism and its interpretation?

FACTOR-ANALYTIC TESTS OF THE COMMON-CORE CLAIM

The M Scale consists of 32 items (16 positively worded and 16 negatively worded items), covering all but one (paradoxicality) of the original common-core criteria of mysticism proposed by Stace. Independent investigators (Caird, 1988; Reinert & Stifler, 1993) have supported Hood's original work indicating that the M Scale contains two factors. For our purposes, it is important to note that Factor I consists of items assessing an experience of unity (introvertive or extrovertive), while Factor II consists of items referring both to religious and knowledge claims. This is compatible with Stace's claim that a common experience (mystical experience of unity) may be variously interpreted. The factor analysis by Caird (1988) supported the original two-factor solution to the M Scale. Reinert and Stifler (1993) also supported a two-factor solution, but suggested the possibility that religious items and knowledge items might emerge as separate factors. This would split the interpretative factor into religious and other modes of interpretation, which would not be inconsistent with Stace's theory. This would allow for an even greater range of interpretation of experience—a claim to knowledge that can be either religiously or nonreligiously based. This is consistent with the distinction between spirituality and religion, to be discussed later in this chapter. However, the factor-analytic studies cited above were far from definitive; notably, they suffered from adequate participant-to-items ratios. Overall, however, they consistently demonstrated two stable factors—one an experience factor associated with minimal interpretation; the other an interpretative factor, probably heavily religiously influenced.

Hood, Morris, and Watson (1993) proposed a three-factor solution to the M Scale, based upon a more adequate sample size. This three-factor solution fitted Stace's phenomenology of mysticism quite nicely, in that both introvertive and extrovertive mysticism emerged as separate factors, along with a third interpretative factor. Hood and his colleagues then undertook to directly test Stace's common-core theory of mysticism with both exploratory and confirmatory factor-analytic procedures.

A persistent problem with the M Scale is that it attempts to be neutral with respect to religious language. For instance, the scale refers to experience with ultimate reality, not to experience of union with God. However, the language of neutrality is perplexing, as emphasized by the diversity theorists: How do we know that union with God is the same experience as union with ultimate reality? Two issues are empirically relevant.

First, no language is neutral. Hence, to attempt to speak of union with "God" or "Christ" in language that references only "ultimate reality" suggests to some conservative religionists a "New Age" connotation. Likewise, to reference "God" or "Christ" is itself problematic for secularists. Although the distinction between experience and interpretation acknowledges that language is an important interpretative issue, it also forces us to focus upon the experiential basis from which genuine differences in interpretation can arise. Like texts, measurement scales use particular language and thus confound the distinction between interpretation and experience. However, empirical methods are available to suggest how this confound can be clarified. One method is to show similar factor structures despite different language.

Second, individuals demand that profound experiences be interpreted. In Barnard's (1997) extended treatment of James's theory of mysticism, a mystical experience is defined as one that is necessarily "transformative" with respect to contact with some transpersonal reality. Although we do not accept this definition of mysticism as properly Jamesian, it does indicate that intense transformative experiences will be acknowledged in some language that identifies, defines, and expresses what the experienced transpersonal reality is. In Jamesian terms, this language is less constructionist of the experience than descriptive of it. Therefore, those who have experienced "ultimate reality" may not wish to claim it as "God." Even more, Christians may want that reality to be identified as "Christ"—something that non-Christian mystics may eschew. Thus the claim of what is experienced is important as part of the "social construction" of the expression of experience. However, differently expressed experiences may have similar structures if we can avoid confounds with language issues.

Hood and Williamson (2000) created two additional versions of the M Scale. Each paralleled the original M Scale, but, where appropriate, made references either to God or to Christ. Both the original M Scale and either the God-language version or the Christ-language version were given to relevant Christian-committed samples. The scales were then factor-analyzed to see whether similar structures would emerge. Basically, whether the M Scale items were phrased in terms of God, Christ, or more "neutral" words, the structures were identical. The structures for all three versions matched Stace's phenomenologically derived model quite well. For all versions of the scale, clear introvertive, extrovertive, and interpretative factors emerged. The exception was that, as Hood and Williamson (2000) anticipated, ineffability emerged as part of the introvertive factor in all samples, and not as part of the interpretative factor (as suggested by Stace). However, as Hood and Williamson note, an experience devoid of content is inherently "ineffable," as there is no content to describe.

In additional research, Hood et al. (2001) translated the M Scale into Persian and administered this scale to a sample of Iranian Muslims. The scale in its original English version was also administered to a U.S. sample. Confirmatory factor analysis was then used to directly compare Hood's model of mysticism in both samples (with ineffability as part of introvertive mysticism) to other possible models, including Stace's (where ineffability is part of the interpretative factor). The overall results showed that both Stace's and Hood's models were better than any other models, and that Hood's model of mysticism was better than Stace's. Thus, empirically, there is strong support to claim that as operationalized from Stace's criteria, mystical experience is identical as measured across diverse samples, whether expressed in "neutral language" or with either "God" or "Christ" references. Both Stace's and Hood's versions of the basic structure of mysticism emerging from this research are presented in Table 11.8.

Three-factor solutions to the M Scale clearly provide the most adequate overall measures of mysticism in terms of compatibility with Stace's theory. Furthermore, Hood's three-factor solution with ineffability as part of introvertive mysticism is clearly the most psychometrically adequate. It is preferred for future research. However, for now it seems fair to conclude that the common-core view has strong empirical support, insofar as regardless of the language used in the M Scale, the basic structure of the experience remains constant across diverse samples and cultures. This is a way of stating the common-core thesis in measurement-based terms.

TABLE 11.8. Conceptual (Stace's) and Empirical (Hood's) Models of Mystical Experience: The Perennialist View

The Stace model of mystical experience—phenomenologically derived

Introvertive Mysticism	Extrovertive Mysticism
a. Contentless Unity	a. Unity in Diversity
b. Timeless/Spaceless	b. Inner Subjectivity

Interpretation
a. Noetic
b. Religious
c. Positive Affect
d. Paradoxicality (not measured in M Scale)
e. Ineffability (alleged)

The Hood model of mystical experience—empirically derived

Introvertive Mysticism (12 items)	Extrovertive Mysticism (8 items)
a. Contentless Unity items	a. Unity in Diversity items
b. Time/Space items	b. Inner Subjectivity items
c. Ineffability items	

Interpretation (12 items)
a. Noetic items
b. Religious items
c. Positive Affect items

Correlational and Empirical Research with the M Scale and Other Measures

Most empirical research with the M Scale to date has used the two-factor solution initially reported by Hood (1975), in which introvertive and extrovertive mysticism are not independently measured, forming as they do part of the minimal phenomenological factor (Factor I). Thus the majority of studies of mysticism to date using two-factor solutions do not separately identify differential predictions for introvertive and extrovertive mysticism, but rather merge these two as a single factor expressing experiences of unity (see Hood, 2002b). As noted above, the MEQ does not separate these.

CROSS-CULTURAL VARIATIONS

Researchers in the fairly new area of positive psychology are making significant contributions to the psychology of religion by focusing upon virtues common across great cultures. For instance, Dahlsgaard, Peterson, and Seligman (2005) noted that of seven virtues identified across eight traditions, transcendence of self (mysticism) is explicitly mentioned in the Abrahamic faith traditions of the West (Christianity, Islam, Judaism) and in the two explicit faith traditions of the East (Hinduism, Buddhism). Empirical studies have demonstrated similar factor structures for the M Scale among adherents of the three Abrahamic faiths for which explicit references to transcendence are well documented: Israeli Jews (Lazar & Kravetz, 2005), Iranian Muslims (Hood et al., 2001), and American Christians (Hood & Williamson, 2000). Similar results have been obtained among adherents of the two Eastern traditions in which such explicit references are well documented: Tibetan Buddhists (Chen, Hood, Yang, & Watson, 2011) and Hindus in India (Anthony, Hermans, & Sterkens, 2010).

However, Dahlsgaard et al. (2005) argue that transcendence is also implicit in the two indigenous faith traditions of China, Confucianism and Taoism (as well as Athenian philosophy) —traditions not associated with claims to the existence of God or gods. No studies to date have used the M Scale with either Confucianists or Taoists. However, as we note below, this is a fruitful area for research. A useful distinction here from the psychology of religion is that transcendence, as Streib and Hood (2016) note, can be "vertical" (and hence religious) or "horizontal" (and hence spiritual). Horizontal transcendence need not involve any ontological claims about God, but may include a sense of union with humankind, a oneness with the cosmos, or a sense of oneness with nature (Anthony et al., 2010; Streib & Hood, 2011). Thus scholars using Stace's common-core thesis have applied it to the remaining traditions identified by Dahlsgaard and colleagues (King, 1990; Roth, 1995, 1999).

Thus, beginning with Holm's (1982) research in Sweden (see below), the cross-cultural usefulness of the M Scale has been well established, supporting the report of mystical experience in cultures that hold transcendence as a virtue. However, as MacLean et al. (2012) have noted with respect to the M Scale, each criterion in Stace's common-core model is measured by four facets, two positively and two negatively worded. These facets may operate differently in various cultures, likely due to issues of interpretation. For instance, although several studies have provided strong support for a three-factor structure of mystical experience, results from recent studies suggest a lack of cross-cultural reliability in the composition and number of factors. For example, studies of the M Scale using confirmatory factor analysis have indicated alternative factor structures for Christians, Muslims, and Hindus in India (Anthony et al., 2010), Tibetan Buddhists (Chen, Hood, et al., 2011), and Chinese Buddhist monks and nuns (Chen, Qi, Hood, & Watson, 2011). In these studies, the alternate models outperformed the Hood and Stace models and required modifications of factor number (e.g., a single factor that subsumed unity, noetic quality, and ineffability; Anthony et al., 2010) and factor composition (e.g., noetic quality loading on the extrovertive factor and positive mood loading on the introvertive factor; Chen, Hood, et al., 2011), Although such variations are methodologically problematic (rather than refuting the common-core thesis altogether), they suggest how mixed methods can adjust the overall model to reflect genuine experiences of transcendence as understood within a particular culture. For instance, Tibetan Buddhists wanted to indicate clearly that they did not want to endorse an experience of greater unity viewed in Western terms as substantial and suggestive of a permanence (Chen, Qi, et al., 2011). In areas as sensitive as mysticism, mixed methods are essential (Streib & Hood, 2016).

One of the earliest translations of the M Scale was that prepared by Holm (1982). Unlike the REEM, the M Scale could be meaningfully translated into Swedish and could be studied similarly to the way it was investigated in North America. Holm not only confirmed a two-factor solution closely paralleling Hood's initial mysticism and interpretation factors, but also found that in correlating the M Scale with ratings of a person's most significant personal experiences, Factor I correlated best with experiences reported by individuals *without* a Christian profile, while Factor II best related to more traditional Christian experiences. The revised Swedish version of the REEM, using Nordic accounts of intense experiences appropriate to Finnish–Swedish culture, also showed similar patterns to Hood's research with the REEM in North America. Holm (1982) stated:

> We also discovered one factor which could be called a general mysticism factor and another where the experience was interpreted on a religious/Christian basis. The "religious interpretation factor" had strong correspondences with religious quality in the interviews and with the background variables of prayer frequency, Bible study, church attendance and attitude

towards Christianity. This factor thus covered experiences with an expressly Christian profile. It showed high correlations with the intrinsic scale, with the expressively Christian
narratives on the REEM and with the religious quality on the interviews. Thus, overall,
in a Finnish–Swedish culture the M Scale and REEM functioned very closely to how they
function in American culture. (p. 273)

Interestingly, Holm also noted that the distinction between a general mysticism factor
(or impersonal mysticism) and a religious factor (or personal mysticism) has parallels with
early research on mysticism in Sweden by Söderblom (1963), who identified these as "infinity
mysticism" and "personality mysticism," respectively (see Holm, 1982, pp. 275–276). More
recently, Holm (2008) has summarized his research on mysticism by noting that mysticism
can occur both within and outside religious traditions. The latter is simply a generalized
mysticism without need of specific religious interpretation. This insight has proven to be substantially supported by empirical research discussed below. However, it raises the question
of whether or not the report of mystical experience is genuine.

GENUINENESS OF MYSTICISM

If one takes seriously the reports of mystical experience as possibly being veridical, or something "Real," then one can address the genuineness of any report. Sundararajan and her colleagues have employed innovative methods using computer-based programs that assess how
people describe their experiences. Guided by Otto's (1917/1923) classic analysis of mystical
experience as an ineffable response to the numinous or transcendent, Hopkins and Sundararajan (2015) compared two German mystics—one (Johannes Tauler) widely acknowledged as
genuine, and the other (Thomas Müntzer) often seen as a revolutionary who used language
suggesting mystical experiences that many thought he did not have. Using two different word
count programs, Hopkins and Sundararajan found that Tauler used words suggestive of experience as affectively "near," while Müntzer's words were suggestive of reflective cognition
that was affectively "distant." In another innovative study, Sundararajan and Kim (2014) compared Mother Teresa's writings to both Tauler's and Müntzer's; they found her confessional
writings to be suggestive of genuine experiences of what has long been identified as the "dark
night of the soul," associated with a sense of abandonment by God and most explicitly articulated by a Spanish mystic, Saint John of the Cross. The results suggested that reflections on
spiritual suffering, which loom large in both medieval German mysticism and Mother Teresa's writings, constitute an adaptive approach to negative emotions. The results also seemed
supportive of Fowler's (1994, 2001) assertion that Mother Teresa was perhaps a candidate for
the highest stage of faith development, which few ever attain. Her being recognized as a saint
in 2016 by Pope Francis suggests that Fowler's view may indeed have merit. Although this
work has not gone without historically based criticism (Friedman, 2015), Sundararajan and
her colleagues have shown how innovative methodologies can be used empirically to address
issues of interest in the psychology of religion—in this case, to understand how believers
experience sacred realities.

Triggers of Mystical Experience

Accepting that mystical experience is normal has led some to search for personal and cultural factors that affect what might be appropriate "triggers" for mystical experiences.

Survey research has long established that a variety of triggers can elicit mystical experiences. Although some triggers are consistently reported—prayer; church attendance; significant life events, such as births and deaths; and experiences associated with music, sex, and entheogens—one seeks in vain for a common characteristic shared by such diverse triggers. Empirically, it is more useful to focus upon what triggers function to elicit mystical experience in different persons. Research Box 11.3 presents the results of a study in which the evaluation of experience was shown to be a function (1) of the normative legitimacy of the trigger, (2) of the experience, and (3) of the alleged open-mindedness of respondents.

RESEARCH BOX 11.3. Differential Evaluation of Experiences and Triggers by High- and Low-Dogmatism Persons (Hood, 1980)

Hood was interested in how the evaluation of intense experiences would vary as a function of the identification of triggers among open- and closed-minded persons. From published sources, he selected one true report each of an aesthetic, a mystical, and a religious experience, independently operationalized for equal intensity. These unlabeled experiences were then presented in a booklet along with Rokeach's (1968) Dogmatism scale, claimed to be a measure of "open-mindedness." Three versions of the booklet were constructed, so that the experiences described could be described as a result of drugs, prayer, or unspecified factors. The experiences were rated on an evaluative semantic differential scale, with higher scores indicating a more positive evaluation. This part of the study clearly showed that the more normative the experience, the more positively it was viewed, so that religious experiences were evaluated more positively overall. Aesthetic and mystical experiences were evaluated less positively overall than religious ones, but did not differ from each other in valence of evaluation. In addition, as predicted, the more normative the trigger, the more positively it affected the evaluation of the experience. Experiences triggered by prayer were more positively evaluated than those with unspecified triggers. Drug triggers lowered the evaluation of all experiences. These effects were most pronounced for the high-dogmatism persons. The actual mean evaluations for each experience coded by trigger for high- and low-dogmatism groups were as follows. (This table is based upon 93 low- and 93 high-dogmatism subjects; 31 subjects in each group rated the three experiences as triggered by drugs, 31 as triggered by prayer, and 31 as triggered by unspecified factors [none].)

Subjects		Aesthetic experience triggered by			Religious experience triggered by			Mystical experience triggered by		
		Drugs	Prayer	None	Drugs	Prayer	None	Drugs	Prayer	None
High-dogmatism	Mean	53.16	62.65	59.94	55.97	66.68	60.03	47.87	59.87	54.00
	SD	9.4	4.1	8.3	9.6	8.9	9.3	12.3	9.5	10.7
Low-dogmatism	Mean	51.988	61.32	57.86	54.50	62.10	59.61	48.02	57.45	53.65
	SD	9.9	7.3	9.0	8.7	8.1	8.6	11.4	9.7	10.7

Note. Republished with permission of Religious Research Association. From Hood (1989). Social legitimacy, dogmatism, and the evaluation of intense experiences. *Review of Religious Research, 21,* 184–194. Permission conveyed through Copyright Clearance Center, Inc.

Sex and eroticism are often cited as triggers of mystical experience. Consistent with the vast conceptual literature relating mysticism and eroticism (Kripal, 2001), Hood and Hall (1980) hypothesized that individuals would use similar gender-based descriptions to describe both mystical and erotic experiences. Open-ended descriptions of mystical and erotic experiences by both males and females were coded for the use of active, agentive language or receptive language. As predicted, females used receptive terms to describe both their erotic and mystical experiences. However, while males used agentive language to describe their sexual experiences, they did not describe their mystical experiences in such terms. Rating their mystical and erotic experiences on words independently established to be either agentive or receptive also showed that females described both erotic and mystical experiences in receptive terms, but that males described only their sexual experiences in agentive terms. The researchers suggested that the compatibility of erotic and mystical experiences for females is aided by the masculine imagery common in the Christian tradition, which facilities congruent expression of eroticism and mysticism for females but inhibits it for males. Consistent with this claim is a study by Mercer and Durham (1999), who found scores on the M Scale to be significantly correlated with scores on a measure of gender orientation. Specifically, persons with feminine and androgynous orientations had higher M Scale scores than persons with masculine orientations. Mercer and Durham suggest that persons scoring high on the M Scale are those who have developed a feminine self-schema (cognitive structure), through which they process data in a way that facilitates the unity of reality and facilitation of mystical experiences. Similar arguments have been made within the conceptual literature on mysticism (Kripal, 2001).

Rather than focusing upon particular concrete triggers, Hood has argued that more abstract conceptualization may permit a more empirically adequate investigation of conditions and circumstances that trigger mystical experience. In particular, theological and philosophical interest in the concept of "limits" is useful (Grossman, 1975). At the conceptual level, the idea of limits entails transcendence; in fact, awareness of limits makes the experience of transcendence possible. Perhaps the sudden contrast that occurs when a limit is suddenly transcended yields a contrast effect similar to a figure–ground reversal, in which what was previously unnoticed is thrown into stark relief. Hood (1977) has noted that such sudden contrasts are common in nature settings, particularly those in which stress is involved. The fact that nature is a common trigger of mystical experiences is well documented in survey studies, and often such experiences are associated with stress, which is itself sometimes cited as a trigger. In one study described earlier, the set–setting incongruity hypothesis was supported when the REEM was used as a measure. It has also been supported in research using the M Scale.

Hood (1977) took advantage of a week-long outdoors program at a private all-male high school. In this week-long program, graduating seniors took a trip in which they engaged in a variety of outdoor activities varying in degree of stress. Three particularly stressful activities were examined: rock climbing and rappelling (for the first time, for many students); whitewater rafting (down a river rated as difficult); and the experience (described earlier in this chapter) of staying alone in the woods at night with minimal equipment. A nonstressful activity (canoeing a calm river) was selected as a control. Just prior to participating in each activity, participants were administered a measure of subjective anticipatory stress for that activity. Immediately after each activity, the participants completed the M Scale to assess mystical experience. The comparisons between set and setting stress for each high-stress activity supported the hypothesis that the interaction between these two types of stress would elicit reports of mystical experience. It is important to note that anticipatory stress varied across situations, such that whether or not a particular person anticipated a given situation as stressful was not simply a function of its independently assessed situation stress. Second, in stressful situations, those anticipating low stress scored higher on mysticism than those anticipating high stress. Thus set–setting stress incongruity elicited reports of mystical experience—not simply stress per se, either anticipatory or situational. Additional support for this hypothesis was found by using the canoe activity as a control; no student anticipated this activity to be stressful. Given the congruity between anticipated stress and setting stress (both low), low M Scale scores resulted, as predicted. However, in high-stress activities anticipated as high in stress, low M Scale scores were also hypothesized and obtained. Only the incongruity between setting and anticipatory stress produced high M Scale scores. Furthermore, with only one exception, these results held for both Factor I and Factor II scores; this suggested not only that the minimal phenomenological properties of mysticism were elicited, but also that they were seen as religiously relevant in the broad sense of this term. This replicates the findings discussed above with solo experiences in a nature setting when the REEM was used as a measure.

Mystical experiences are common in nature and meditative prayer, both of which are often solitary conditions. Hence factors that meaningfully enhance solitude may facilitate the report of mystical experience. Experimentally, it is possible to enhance solitude through the use of an isolation tank. If a religious set is given in an isolation tank, would the combination of set and enhanced isolation facilitate the report of mystical experience? Research Box 11.4 reports a study in which Hood and his colleagues explored this question.

Overall, then, studies (mostly employing the M Scale) have been successful in correlating mysticism with predicted variables of theoretical significance. Quasi-experimental studies involving efforts to elicit mystical experience have also produced useful results. It is simply not true that mystical experiences cannot be elicited under experimental or quasi-experimental conditions. Of course, we make no claim that investigators have caused such experiences—only that they have produced conditions under which such experiences are likely to occur.

Additional Measures of Mysticism

Although Hood's M Scale has been most commonly used in studies of mysticism, additional measures are associated with the work of Leslie Francis and his colleagues, and of Michael Thalbourne and his colleagues.

THE FRANCIS–LOUDEN MYSTICAL ORIENTATION MEASURES

Similar to Hood's use of Stace's common-core criteria to develop the M Scale, Francis and Louden (2000a) drew upon Happold's (1991) seven criteria for mysticism to develop two useful measures of mysticism. As Hood and his colleagues have done, Francis and his colleagues have used phenomenology and measurement to complement one another in the best spirit of the call for a new multilevel interdisciplinary paradigm. The Francis–Louden measures operationalized Happold's seven criteria for mysticism: ineffability, noesis, transiency, passivity, oneness, timelessness, and true ego. Factor analyses confirmed the psychometric validity of the classifications and produced a long and a short measure; there is both a 21-item Index of Mystical Orientation (Francis & Louden, 2000a) and a 9-item Short Index

RESEARCH BOX 11.4. The Differential Elicitation of Mystical Experience in an Isolation Tank (Hood, Morris, & Watson, 1990)

Solitude is often cited as one trigger of religious and mystical experiences. Hood and his colleagues placed individuals in a sensory isolation tank to maximize solitude. The tank was approximately 7.5 feet in diameter and 4 feet high. It contained a hydrated magnesium sulfate solution with a density of 1.30 grams/cc, a constant temperature of 34.1°C, and a depth of 10 inches. The tank was totally enclosed, lightproof, and soundproof. It was equipped with an intercom system so that a participant could communicate with an experimenter in another room.

Each participant in the study was placed in the isolation tank after being told about the typical images likely to occur under these conditions. In addition, participants were given a specific religious set (in boldface) or nonreligious control set (italics) as follows:

> I am now going to invite you to keep silent for a period of ten minutes. First you will try to attain silence, as total silence as possible of heart and mind. Having attained it, you will expose yourself to whatever (**religious revelation**/*insight*) it brings.[a]

Participants had previously taken the Allport and Ross (1967) religious orientation scales and could be classified as intrinsic, extrinsic, and "indiscriminately pro" (IP) individuals. A modified version of the M Scale was used that allowed a simple "yes" or "no " response to each item, so that the participants could respond over the intercom while still in the isolation tank. Results were as predicted: Under the religious set, both intrinsic and IP participants reported more religious interpretation of their experiences (higher Factor II scores) than extrinsic participants. However, the IP participants reported less minimal phenomenological properties of mysticism (lower Factor I scores) than either the intrinsic or the extrinsic participants. This suggests that IP participants wished to "appear" religious by affirming religious experiences they did not actually have. Extrinsic participants had these experiences, as indicated by their Factor I scores, but did not describe them in religious language. Intrinsic participants both had the experiences and described them in religious language.

Further support for these views was evident in the control conditions. When participants were not presented with a religious set, none of the groups differed in the minimal phenomenological properties of mysticism (Factor I). However, intrinsic persons still interpreted their experiences in religious terms (Factor II), whereas neither extrinsic nor IP persons described their experiences in religious language in the control condition. Thus the isolation tank elicited similar experiences in subjects of all religious types. The difference in Factor II under set conditions for the types suggests that intrinsic persons consistently interpreted their tank experiences as religious; extrinsic persons consistently interpreted their tank experiences as less religious; and IP persons only interpreted their tank experiences as religious when given an explicit religious set.

---

[a]These instructions were adapted from those used by de Mello (1984) in his study of prayer.

of Mystical Orientation (Francis & Louden, 2004). Given Francis's established interest in Eysenck's (1981) personality theory, he and his colleagues used these measures to demonstrate that mysticism was related to extroversion, but unrelated to neuroticism and psychoticism, in a large sample of Roman Catholic priests (Francis & Louden, 2000b). This replicated earlier research with a sample of over 200 male clergy that found the same results (Francis & Thomas, 1996), as well as research by Argyle and Hills (2000) using an independently constructed measure of mysticism. However, in a study relevant to our discussion in Chapter 10 of Eastern and Western forms of meditation, Kaldor, Francis, and Fisher (2002) found a difference between a sample of Eastern meditators and a sample of Christians who prayed: Christian prayer was associated with low psychoticism scores, but Eastern meditation was associated with high psychoticism scores, as measured by a Revised Eysenck Personality Questionnaire.

In two earlier studies, Francis and his colleague attempted to test Ross's hypothesis that in terms of Jungian theory as operationalized in the Myers–Briggs scale, the perceiving function is crucial for individual differences in religious expression (Ross, Weiss, & Jackson, 1996). Using the Short Index of Mystical Orientation, both Francis (2002) and Francis and Louden (2000b) failed to find support for Ross's hypothesis. However, in a sample of over 300 individuals who stayed at a retreat house associated with Ampleforth Abbey, Francis, Village, Robbins, and Ineson (2007) found clear support for Ross's hypothesis, using the full 21-item Index of Mystical Orientation.

Edwards and Lowis (2008b) have proposed a measure of attitudes to mysticism, as distinguished from reported mystical experience. This promising measure has been used in one study, suggesting that attitudes toward mysticism and mystical experience as measured by the long version of the Francis–Louden Index of Mystical Orientation may relate differently to personality traits such as psychoticism (Edwards & Lowis, 2008a). Research on attitudes toward mysticism and the three factors of Hood's M Scale is needed, especially since attitudes toward mysticism may be more influenced by interpretive factors than reports of mystical experience may be (Edwards & Lowis, 2008a, p. 156).

THALBOURNE'S MEASURE OF TRANSLIMINALITY

Hood (2008c) has argued that scholars have overemphasized James's commitment to a uniform treatment of mysticism. Barnard (1997, p. 63) has noted that ultimately James equates mystical experience with any submarginal or subliminal state, including a wide variety of experiences that defy easy classification. Among these submarginal experiences is James's "diabolical mysticism," a "sort of religious mysticism turned upside down" (James, 1902/1985, p. 337). In this sense, the measure of transliminality developed by Thalbourne (1998) is the most nearly Jamesian measure of mysticism we have. It is a single-factor scale measuring essentially subliminal states of consciousness. Thalbourne and Delin (1994, p. 25) have coined the term "transliminal" to refer to a common underlying factor that is largely an involuntary susceptibility to inwardly generated psychological phenomena of an ideational and affective kind. However, transliminality is also related to a hypersensitivity to external stimulation (Thalbourne, 1998, p. 403); as such, transliminality becomes a Jamesian measure of the submarginal region, where "'seraph and snake' abide there side by side" (James, 1902/1985, p. 338).

Lange and Thalbourne (2007) have also developed a single-factor measure of mysticism that is more restricted than the transliminal domain, but is similar to James's treatment of mysticism in *The Varieties*, as it allows for interval scaling of intensity of experiences (as an empirical "mystical ladder" of sorts). However, at the empirical level, the single-factor measure of transliminality links such phenomena as schizotypy, magical ideation, creativity, and paranormal experiences as interrelated. This is different from Hood's conceptualization of mysticism based upon Stace's criteria, in which relationships between mystical experience and other states are treated as independent empirical hypotheses. For instance, using the earlier two-factor solution of Hood's M Scale, Byrom (2009) has noted that the experiential component has a stronger relationship with a measure of magical ideation than the interpretative component does. Thalbourne's measure of transliminality would suggest this, as both magical ideation and mysticism are components of the underlying single factor of transliminality. Masterful studies using mixed methods by Kohls and his colleagues (Kohls & Walach, 2006, 2007) are beginning to document the role of actual spiritual practices (as opposed to mere beliefs) in separating out positive experiences of ego loss (mysticism) from negative ones (psychoses). It appears that spiritual practices buffer otherwise negative effects that might occur due to transliminality (Kohls, Hack, & Walach, 2008; Kohls, Walach, & Wirtz, 2009).

MYSTICISM AND PSYCHOPATHOLOGY

In this chapter, we have presented considerable support for the commonality of reports of mystical experience among normal persons. However, despite the fact that such reports are firmly established as normal phenomena among healthy individuals, it remains true that there has been a considerable bias against mystical experience among many clinically oriented specialists. For instance, the Group for the Advancement of Psychiatry (GAP) answered its own question, *Mysticism: Spiritual Quest or Psychic Disorder?*, in favor of the latter (GAP, 1976). This view is based largely upon well-established similarities between mysticism and madness at the purely experiential level (Boisen, 1936).

The most reasonable position is that both normal and psychotic individuals can have mystical experiences. Empirical support for this fact is provided by Stifler, Greer, Sneck, and Dovenmuehle (1993), who administered Hood's M Scale along with other measures to three relevant samples (*n* = 30 each): psychiatric inpatients who met formal diagnostic criteria for psychotic disorders, and who also displayed "notable religiously oriented symptoms" (p. 368); senior members of various contemplative/mystical groups; and hospital staff members (as "normal" controls). Stifler et al. found that the psychotic and contemplative groups could not be distinguished from one another on their mysticism scores, but that both differed from the hospital staff controls. Thus both psychotic and contemplative individuals reported mystical experiences more often than controls. Although these data are correlational, it is reasonable to assume that mysticism neither causes nor is produced by psychoses. Rather, psychotic individuals, like contemplative persons, can have or report such experiences. What distinguished the psychotic from the normal mystics in Stifler et al.'s study was not mystical experience, but rather dimensions of personality structure. The psychotic mystics exhibited resistance and rigidity, as opposed to the normal mystics, who exhibited openness and fluidity. Thus it was not simply mystical experience, but the reactions to the experience, that distinguished psychotic from normal mystics. This finding is supported by research using mixed methods (qualitative and quantitative). For instance, Kohls et al. (2008) have demonstrated that among persons who have mystical experiences, those who are adept at spiritual practices are more prone to experience these states as positive. Thus not simply belief, but actual spiritual practice, is a necessary component of a positive mystical experience. As we note elsewhere in this chapter, those who have meaningful religious frames to interpret their mystical experiences are unlikely to have psychotic reactions to them (Hood & Byrom, 2010).

Consistent with research affirming that mysticism might be pathological is work on temporal lobe epilepsy, commonly assumed to be associated with reports of mystical and other religious experiences (see Chapter 3). For instance, Persinger (1987) has argued that what he terms the "God experience" is an artifact of changes in temporal lobe activity. He has been able to elicit a sensed presence of God in laboratory studies, using weak complex magnetic fields to stimulate the frontal lobes (Persinger, 2002; Hill & Persinger, 2003). However, Granqvist et al. (2005) have demonstrated that the sensed presence of God in temporal lobe stimulation studies is due to suggestibility and not to the application of complex magnetic fields. Likewise, in a study of 46 outpatients in the Maudsley Epilepsy Clinic, Sensky (1983) found that patients with this type of epilepsy did not have a higher rate of mystical experiences (or general religious experiences) than a control population. By contrast, a study by Persinger and Makarec (1987) found positive correlations between scores on their measure of complex epileptic signs and the reports of paranormal and mystical experiences in a sample of 414 university students. Overall, temporal lobe studies suggest that even if mystical experience is commonly associated with temporal lobe activity, it is no more common in actual patients with such epilepsy than in control populations with normal temporal lobe activity. Hence there is no firm empirical basis from which to assume neurophysiological deficiencies in those reporting mystical experiences.

On the contrary, as noted in Chapter 3, the biological basis of religious experience in general and mysticism in particular suggests that, if anything, such experiences are normal. They can occur in persons with neurophysiological or psychiatric disorders, but this does not make mystical experience itself psychopathological. Even if mysticism and madness are viewed as different aspects of the same experience (Heriot-Maitland, 2008), how one interprets or frames the experience is the crucial determinant of whether the experience is positive or negative (Granqvist & Larsson, 2006; Hood & Byrom, 2010). It is also worth emphasizing that despite the identification of neurophysiological processes that facilitate mystical experiences, the neurophysiology does not rule out the possibility that such experiences have a basis in reality (Azari, 2006; d'Aquili & Newberg, 1993, 1999). As Deikman (1966) has said, the unity revealed in mysticism may be the unity of reality.

TOWARD A THEORY OF MYSTICISM: RELIGIOUS AND SPIRITUAL

The rather substantial body of conceptual and empirical literature on mysticism has not yielded any coherent theory that has been accepted by more than a few investigators. Perhaps consistent with Chapter 3, as suggested just above, are neurophysiological theories of mysticism. As Wulff (2000) concludes, his own survey of research on mysticism suggests that some fundamental internal mechanism is operating. Yet Wulff also notes the methodological issue raised by the fact that it is not uncommon for investigators who were originally neutral about mysticism to become convinced of its reality as other than a merely subjective state, and to seek out explanations compatible with the ontological assertions of the experience. William James followed this path (Hood, 2000a, 2002b), and insofar as mystical experiences are noetic, perhaps so should we. Thus we end this chapter with a theory of mysticism that is not linked to proposed internal mechanisms, but to Deikman's (1966) claim noted above that the unity of the mystical experience may in fact be a unity that is objectively real. However, our theory, rooted in the pioneering but neglected work of Troeltsch's (1931) description of two types of mysticism, remains neutral with respect to theological or cosmological claims to the reality experienced as unity. Nevertheless, it is rooted in historical processes that facilitated the emergence of mystics as independent types, and is consistent with the empirical data on mysticism, religion, and spirituality.

Mysticism within and outside Religious Traditions: The Emergence of "Mystics"

Both Bouyer (1980) and Smith (1977) note that the word "mysticism" comes from the Greek and derives its meaning from the verb "to close." Applied initially to the very specific Greek mystery rites whose rituals were secret or "closed" to outsiders, the term gradually evolved to refer simply to any knowledge that is enigmatic (Bouyer, 1980, p. 44). The term has a distinct history within Christianity, emerging in three distinct transformative stages. Bouyer identifies these stages as "Biblical," "liturgical," and "spiritual."

Only later in its history has the term come to mean a particular experience—what Bouyer has described as an "ineffable mode of experimental knowledge of divine things" (1980, p. 51). It is important to note that "mystical experience" was formerly not thought to be psychologically illuminated by a mere subjectivity, but was viewed as an experience grounded in what is ontologically "real" in terms of the objective description of Biblical truth that also inspired all Christian liturgy. Smith (1977) suggests that the derivation from the pagan rites came to mean the closing of the mind to all external things (i.e., all things not of divine illumination). The crucial point for our empirical concerns is that whatever the focus upon mystical experience may have been, it was contextually dependent upon claims for it as the objective realization of a truth less ineffable than that contained in sacred texts and expressed in sacred liturgy. Thus, as Katz (1983) has argued, mysticism is often conservative—expressing itself within a tradition, not standing outside and opposed to it. Furthermore, empirical studies suggest that mystical experiences interpreted within a tradition have the most meaning and transformative power (Deikman, 1966; Hood, 2008b; Ruffing, 2001; Wittberg, 1996).

As McGinn (1991) has noted, self-identified "mystics" are a more recent historical phenomenon. It thus behooves social scientists to develop a theory of how mysticism became divorced from specific faith traditions. The separation, while never complete, suggests a tension that mystics in the third ("spiritual") sense of Bouyer's classification have always faced within their traditions. It also serves as an umbrella that can meaningfully cover the contemporary debate over religion and spirituality.

The Religion–Spirituality Debate in Relation to Mysticism

As we have discussed in earlier chapters, this tension has been best captured in the social-scientific literature by the comparison and contrast between two terms—"religion" and "spirituality" (Pargament, 1999). For some, "religion" has become a term that identifies institutional aspects of a faith tradition. This includes beliefs and rituals adhered to and practiced, but seen by some people as devoid of an "inner, experiential dimension." For these people, the preferred term is "spirituality." Wulff (1997) claims that the "new spirituality" employs an emergent model of a journey or quest whose goal is the realization of some innate capacity, variously conceived. He rightly notes that this model has deep roots in historical faith traditions. He states with reference to the Christian tradition, "Indeed, the classic Christian mystics would find every element in the model familiar" (Wulff, 1997, p. 7). He further notes that the shift from "religious" to "spiritual" is simply the focus upon inner processes emphasized by the latter rather than the former term. He goes on to assert that what is "conspicuously new" in contemporary spirituality is the lack of an explicit transcendent object outside the self (Wulff, 1997, p. 7). Here, of course, are serious ontological issues not to be avoided (Deikman, 1966; Hood, 2002b; Parsons, 1999; Porpora, 2006). However, our focus here is upon a theory to account for the emergence of spirituality within the framework of a larger theory of mysticism. Pargament (1999, p. 7) has argued that discussions and studies of spirituality lack theoretical grounding—something that is desperately needed. Although there are some interesting efforts to develop theoretically grounded views of spirituality (e.g., Helminiak, 1998), our intent is to develop a theory that is grounded in historical facts and can frame the empirical data.

Troeltsch's Model: Church, Sect, and Two Types of Mysticism

Troeltsch's theory, as developed in *The Social Teaching of the Christian Churches* (1931), has been explored in Chapter 9 in terms of the distinction between church and sect. However, Troeltsch was clearly using an expanded typology derived from Weber, in which, besides church and sect as forms of religious organization, he identified a third type—mysticism. Ironically, Troeltsch was popularized among North American scholars by H. R. Niebuhr, especially in his *The Social Sources of Denominationalism* (first published in 1929 and thus antedating the English translation of Troeltsch's text by 2 years). Niebuhr dropped Troeltsch's third type, mysticism, so that subsequent theorizing and empirical research on church–sect theory has largely ignored mysticism. The reasons for this are in dispute, but it is clear that neither Niebuhr nor Troeltsch thought highly of mysticism, and that neither saw it as characteristic of the North American religious landscape (Garrett, 1975; Steeman, 1975). Whatever the reason, as Garrett (1975, p. 205) has noted, mysticism has experienced "wholehearted neglect" at the hands of sociological investigators. Among psychologists, the wholehearted neglect is of a historically grounded theory. Thus, if sociologists have a relevant theory, psychologists have the relevant data (many of which have been presented above). In the remainder of this chapter, we develop a general theory of mysticism that incorporates two mysticisms—that of the church and of what Parsons (1999, p. 141) has called "unchurched mysticism."

According to both Bouyer (1980) and Troeltsch (1931), one form of mysticism is an inherent tendency to seek personal piety and an emotional realization of a faith within the individual; it serves simply to intensify commitment to a tradition. Only when mysticism emerges as an independent religious principle—as a reaction to the church and the sect form—does it become a new social force and seek an independent philosophical (today, psychological!) justification. These two forms of mysticism must be clearly distinguished—something social scientists have failed to do even when acknowledging Troeltsch's mysticism. Garrett (1975, pp. 214–215) simply identifies these two forms as M_1 and M_2.

In the widest sense, mysticism is simply a demand for an inward appropriation of a direct inward and present religious experience (Troeltsch, 1931, p. 730). It takes the objective characteristics of its tradition for granted, and either supplements them with a profound inwardness or reacts against them as it demands to bring them back "into the living process" (Troeltsch, 1931, p. 731). This is Garrett's M_1 or Troeltsch's "wider mysticism." We identify this as "religious mysticism" for two reasons. It is a mysticism that, according to both Troeltsch (1931, p. 732) and Bouyer (1980, p. 51), is found within all religious systems as a universal phenomenon. Thus, as an empirical fact, it entered Christianity partly from *within* (insofar as Christianity entails the same logical form as all traditions relative to this type) and partly from *without* (from other sources that were "eagerly accepted" by Christianity) (Troeltsch, 1931). Concentrating among the purely interior and emotional side of religious experience, it creates a "spiritual" interpretation of every objective aspects of religion, so that mystics typically stay within their tradition (Katz, 1983).

However, Troeltsch also identifies a "narrower, technically concentrated sense" of mysticism (1931, p. 734). This is Garrett's M_2. It is a mysticism that has become independent in principle from, and is contrasted with, religion. It gives rise to "spiritual religion." It claims to be the true inner principle of all religious faith. This we refer to as "spiritual mysticism," but the term "spiritual" is redundant. This type of mysticism breaks away from religion, which it disdains. It accepts no constraint or community other than ones that are self-selected and self-realized. It is a "spiritual religion," with the term "religion" as redundant here as "spiritual" is above (Hood, 2006). It is the basis of what Forman (1998) and Parsons (1999) identify as a "perennial psychology" rooted in mysticism, which now allows one to be identified as a mystic, rather than as a Buddhist, Catholic, or Jew. It is what many today profess to be "spirituality" as opposed to "religion."

Research on Distinctions between Religiousness and Spirituality

Kenneth Pargament and his students have taken the lead in descriptive and correlational work identifying distinctions between religious and spiritual self-identification (Zinnbauer et al., 1997; Zinnbauer & Pargament, 2005). One motivation for Zinnbauer et al.'s (1997) study, to borrow part of the title of the article in which these data are presented, was to "unfuzzy the fuzzy" (a phrase first coined by Spilka).

Data were solicited from 11 different small convenience samples, ranging from "conservative Christian college students" to "New Age groups." Most of the 364 participants were either college students or members of some religious group. Exceptions included a small sample of residents of a nursing home ($n = 20$) and another one of mental health workers ($n = 27$). Overall, 78% of participants identified themselves as "religious," while 93% identified themselves as "spiritual." It is worth noting that in both Roof's (1993, 1999) research on "baby boomers" (see Research Box 11.5, below) and the Zinnbauer et al. (1997) study, most religious persons considered themselves to be spiritual (74% in the latter study). Overall, few of Zinnbauer et al.'s participants thought religiousness and spirituality to be identical concepts (2.6%) or entirely nonoverlapping concepts (6.7%). Thus, for most, religiousness and spirituality were somehow and variously intertwined. Nearly identical percentages identified themselves as religious but not spiritual (4%) or as neither (3%); all we need to note is that very few people considered themselves religious but not spiritual. Hence, for most participants, religion was inherently involved with spirituality.

Content analysis of participants' descriptions of religion and spirituality in the Zinnbauer et al. (1997) study revealed what sociological studies have also confirmed: The most common categories for spirituality were experiential, while those for religion were belief-based. This is consistent with Day's (1994) distinction, found in his interview with "Sandy" and with other Sierra Project participants (see Research Box 11.6, below). Not surprisingly, the greatest differences between self-ratings were found among participants who were members of religious groups distant from traditional expressions of faith, such as "New Age groups" and Unitarians. Although members of more traditional faiths might differ in levels of self-rated religiousness and spirituality, within specific groups such as Roman Catholics there was no significant difference, whereas among "New Age groups" self-rated spirituality greatly exceeded self-rated religiousness. Furthermore, consistent with Roof's (1993, 1999) perceptive observation, more conservative religious groups made less distinction between spirituality and religiousness (Zinnbauer et al., 1997).

These data are also congruent with previous empirical work. In particular, the finding that mental health workers are more "spiritual" than "religious" replicates previous work on mental health professionals. Shafranske (1996a) has reviewed the empirical research on the religious beliefs, associations, and practices of such professionals. Focusing primarily on samples of clinical and counseling psychologists who are members of the American Psychological Association, Shafranske notes that psychologists are less likely to believe in a personal God, or to affiliate with religious groups, than other professionals or the general population. In addition, while the *majority* of psychologists report that spirituality is important to them, a *minority* report that religion is important to them (Shafranske, 1996a, p. 153). Shafranske summarizes his own data and the work of others to emphasize that psychologists are more like the general population than was previously assumed. However, Shafranske (1996a, p. 154) lumps together various indices as the "religious dimension," and this is very misleading. In fact, psychologists neither believe, practice, nor associate with the institutional aspects of faith ("religion") as much as they endorse what Shafranske properly notes are "noninstitutional forms of spirituality" (1996a, p. 154). One could predict that in forced-choice contexts they would be most likely to be "spiritual but not religious." Empirically, three facts about religious and spiritual self-identification ought to be kept quite clear.

First, most persons identify themselves as *both* religious and spiritual. These are largely persons sampled from within faith traditions, for whom it is reasonable to assume that spirituality is at least one expression of and motivation for their religion (e.g., institutional participation). Hence many measures of spirituality simply operate like measures of religion (Gorsuch & Miller, 1999).

Second, a significant minority of individuals use spirituality as a means of at least partly refuting or even ridiculing religion. This is particularly obvious in qualitative studies, where individuals identify their spirituality in defiant opposition to religion. They actually oppose various aspects of institutional religion, such as its authority, its more specific ("closed") articulation of beliefs ("dogma"), and its practices ("ritual"); they seek to move away from religion in order to become "more developed" spiritually. The move is from belief to experience, as Day (1994) perceptively notes. This is consistent with the research on deconversion discussed in Chapter 8.

Third, religiousness and spirituality overlap considerably, at least in North American populations. The majority of the U.S. population in particular is religious *and* spiritual, in terms of both self-identification and self-representations. Exceptions are easy to identify, but we ought not to lose sight of the fact that they are *exceptions*. Significantly, they include not only scientists in general, but psychologists in particular (Beit-Hallahmi, 1977; Shafranske, 1996a). Among these people, a hostility to religion as thwarting or even falsifying spirituality is evident. This hostility is readily revealed in qualitative studies in which there is some degree of rapport between interviewer and respondents. One sociological study—Roof's research on baby boomers, which has already been discussed to some extent in Chapters 6 and 8—is presented in Research Box 11.5.

RESEARCH BOX 11.5. Qualitative Sociological Study of Religion
versus Spirituality (Roof, 1993, 1999)

Roof (1993) has characterized the 76 million U.S. adults born in the two decades after World War II as a "generation of seekers" who are either "loyalists" (those who have stayed with their religious tradition), "returnees" (those who experimented with options before returning to their religious tradition), or "dropouts" (those who have left their tradition). Roof (1993) noted that a distinguishing feature among the "highly active seekers" he interviewed was a preference to identify themselves as "spiritual" rather than "religious." Twenty-four percent of these had no religious affiliation. Such highly active seekers were but a minority (9%) of all Roof's participants, but they seem to have captured the interest of researchers in what we might identify as the "spiritual turn" in the scientific study of religion. Roof's (1999) follow-up text reveals similar findings regarding self-identification. Asking, "Do you consider yourself religious?" and "Do you consider yourself spiritual?" in nonconsecutive places in open-ended interviews (but always in that order) revealed an overall weak association between the two identifications (gamma = .291). However, the association was higher among "strong believers" (gamma = .439) than among "highly active seekers" (gamma = .196). Other data, including the question "Which is best: to follow the teachings of a church, synagogue or temple, or to think for oneself in matters of religion and trust more one's own experience?" (Roof, 1999, pp. 320–321), suggested that those identified as seekers were least likely to rely upon institutional authority or to think that such authority should overrule their own conscience. An Asian American participant who was no longer active in the Methodist Church captured well what we are suggesting: "You can be spiritual without being religious. I think religious ... would be more specific. The faith is more specific, certain doctrines. Spiritual would be general, wider. I think that's how you can be spiritual without being religious. Maybe even religious without being spiritual. Show up for church and go through the motions" (Roof, 1993, p. 78).

The emergence of the discussion of spirituality among psychologists of religion parallels sociological concern with a vocal minority of highly active seekers whose spirituality is most typically identified as mystical (Bellah, Marsden, Sullivan, Swidler, & Tipton, 1996; Roof, 1993, 1999). It also characterizes much of the empirical literature on deconversion and spiritual transformation discussed in Chapter 8. A qualitative psychological study is presented in Research Box 11.6.

Empirical support for qualitative studies that have identified a minority of persons intensely opposed to religion while identifying themselves as spiritual is readily available. For instance, Zinnbauer et al. (1997, p. 553) used a modified form of Hood's M Scale (unity items only) and found that in their overall sample, self-rated religiousness did not correlate with mystical experience ($r = -.04$), but self-rated spirituality did ($r = .27$, $p < .001$). Furthermore, there was a significant difference between the mean mysticism scores for the "equally spiritual and religious" group and the "spiritual but not religious" group, with the latter scoring significantly higher. The percentages of self-identification into groups ("neither religious nor spiritual," "religious but not spiritual," "spiritual but not religious," and "equally religious and spiritual") in Hood's data reasonably parallel Zinnbauer et al.'s (1997) data for mainstream college students. The scores on the M Scale, as well as the group comparisons, are also consistent with Zinnbauer et al.'s data.

Use of the complete M Scale provides further clarification. As in Zinnbauer et al.'s data, the means for the two experiential factors were greater for the "spiritual but not religious" group than for the "equally spiritual and religious" group. However, the difference was not significant for the Introversive Mysticism factor (one that is quite compatible with classical Christianity), but it was significant for the Extroversive Mysticism factor (an experience less traditional within Christianity) (see Hood, 1985). The truly significant difference lay between the "spiritual but not religious" and "equally spiritual and religious" groups on the one hand, and the "religious but not spiritual" and "neither" groups on the other. A crucial point, consistent with previous research, was that both "spiritual-only" and "equally religious and spiritual" persons reported mystical experience more often than "religious-only" or "nonreligious" persons. Also important was that on the Interpretation factor, the "equally religious and spiritual" group scored higher than the "spiritual but not religious" group; again, however, the real difference was between these two groups and the "religious but not spiritual" and the "neither" groups.

Thus we can summarize these data by stating that mystical experience ("spirituality") is commonly reported by individuals who identify themselves as spiritual rather than religious,

---

RESEARCH BOX 11.6. A Qualitative Psychological Study of Religion versus Spirituality (Day, 1994)

The Sierra Project, which was specifically designed to increase knowledge about students' stages of moral development, began with the 1979 class at the University of California–Irvine. A crucial aspect of this study (and its continuation since 1987 by researchers associated with Boston University) is the use of both traditional empirical and narrative-based qualitative methodologies (see Day, 1991, 1994; Whiteley & Loxley, 1980). Day (1994) reported the results of in-depth interviews with three Sierra participants chosen by the Boston research team after listening to hundreds of hours of audiotaped interviews. Day wrote up the results of an interview with one participant, "Sandy," in an idiothetic presentation rare in psychology.

The interview probed Sandy's views on both religion and spirituality—a tactic based upon researchers' belated recognition that earlier Sierra participants might have purposefully avoided discussion of religion, especially religious beliefs (Day, 1994, p. 160). Thus questions on religion and spirituality were strategically placed within the schedule on subsequent interviews.

Sandy took great care to distinguish religion from spirituality. In her words, "Religion is organized, dogmatic, and social. Spiritual is individual, intimate, personal. Religion tells you what is good or true and tells you who is favored and who is not. It operates in fixed categories. Spirituality is developed. You have to work hard at it and to be conscious about it and take time for it. Sometimes, in order to grow spiritually, you have to go beyond or even against religious doctrine" (Day, 1994, p. 163). Sandy's concern with doctrine was important. Day noted that she would probably protest if identified as a "believer." She neither identified herself nor wanted others to label her as "religious" (Day, 1994, p. 165).

and by those who identify themselves as equally religious and spiritual. In other words, there is a mysticism ("spirituality") both within and outside of religious traditions. The mysticism outside religion is what Holm (2008) has referred to as "generalized mysticism." This ought not to surprise us. As noted earlier, Katz (1983) reminds us that most mystics, even when struggling against their faith tradition, stay within it. Religious mysticism is inherently conservative in this limited sense. For most religious people, belief adequately expresses their mystical experiences, and their religious rituals facilitate them (Hood, 1995a). But for some "independent" mystics, spirituality is only constrained and choked by belief. These independent mystics are those who consider themselves spiritual but not religious.

Hood (2003, 2005b, 2006) has reviewed several empirical studies using various indices of mysticism. Overall, a clear pattern emerges: Spirituality is more closely identified with mystical experience, whereas religion is more closely identified with a specific religious interpretation of this experience. Thus the current debate on religiousness and spirituality is really neither new nor theoretically unexpected. It has now been 50 years since Vernon (1968) noted that those who answered "none" to questions of religious preference were ignored in the scientific study of religion. He argued that perhaps a parallel could be drawn to those in political surveys who identify themselves as "independents." Such persons, he noted, are not without political convictions (1968, p. 223). "Spiritual but not religious" persons, or "nones," are perhaps religious independents, paralleling political independents. In response to the question "Have you ever had a feeling that you were somehow in the presence of God?", Vernon found that some of those who rejected membership in formal religious groups (the "nones") answered either "I am sure" (5.9%) or "I think so" (20%). Thus 26% of the "nones" nevertheless thought or were sure they had had an experience of God. This percentage closely matches survey reports of mystical experience across a wide range of populations, religious and otherwise, as discussed above. They are also congruent with psychological research indicating that "nones" often score higher on measures of the minimal phenomenological properties of the experience than on the religious interpretation of the experience (Hood & Morris, 1981b). Vernon also noted the problem that his religious "nones" had with using religious language to describe mystical experiences. So there is not simply the finding of spirituality emerging in opposition to religion, but the persistent failure by social scientists of religion to study the experiences of those who do not primarily identify themselves as religious. If these people are more willing to identify themselves as "spiritual" than as "religious," it has been a social-scientific oversight to think that they have nothing to do with "religion" (Streib & Hood, 2011).

In a major effort to clarify the semantics and psychology of spirituality, Streib and Hood (2016) concluded that the M Scale serves well to identify what many people today understand as "spiritual." An advantage is that this measure is well grounded theoretically and is an excellent predictor of both self-rated spirituality and spiritual self-identification. Streib and Hood (2016, Chs. 11 and 27) suggested then that the usefulness of the M Scale for the "spiritual but not religious" and for those "both spiritual and religious" is due to the widespread notion that spirituality is an experience-oriented approach to unite with some kind of transcendence. This fact, combined with the fact that transcendence can be vertical (religious), horizontal (spiritual), or both, is more than justification for the fact that the present book remains titled *The Psychology of Religion*, whether religion is explicit or implicit.

OVERVIEW

Clearly, mystical experience remains a central concern for those who would link the conceptual and empirical literatures on religious/spiritual experience. The mystical and the numinous remain contenders for the unique in religion and spirituality. They also provide an experiential basis that may require serious attention to the ontological claims of those who have such experiences. McClenon (1990) has argued that the uniformity in the reporting of a wide range of anomalous experiences suggests that cultural determination of these interpretations may account for less variance than many suppose. We have discussed many examples of such experiences in Chapter 10. Similar arguments apply to numinous and mystical experiences. Although social scientists may not offer "proofs" for such claims, neither can they without hubris deny the possibility that religion contains truths. Indeed, such truths may be as necessary for the experience as the more restricted claim that the *belief* in such truths is necessary. Few persons have such experiences without believing in their possibility in advance or becoming converted to their truth after the fact.

Research on mystical experiences is best approached in terms of what each methodology can contribute. The descriptive material of open-ended and qualitative studies enhances the narrowness and precision of survey research. Yet both methods have revealed similar triggers and consequences of these experiences, and both methods have confirmed the normality of their occurrence. Survey research provides correlations and patterns suggestive for laboratory and quasi-experimental studies, which in turn have shown that mystical experience can be facilitated and follows patterns compatible with the results from open-ended and survey research. All these are then given various conceptual alternatives by the theological, philosophical, and historical literatures.

If there is any picture to be suggested at this point, it must be sketched in broad lines. Yet even this picture is helpful. Mysticism is a normal phenomenon, reported by healthy and functioning persons who struggle to find a meaningful framework within which to live out this experience as foundational—as at least what is real for them, if not in some sense as the ultimate "Real." Mysticism, real or Real, has proven itself susceptible to empirical investigation. As noted above, we now have several useful measures of mysticism. Clearly, however, much remains to be done. Future progress will surely be in the spirit of the call for a new interdisciplinary multilevel paradigm for the psychology of religion. Even if McGinn (1991, p. 343) is correct in his fear that an empirical reading of mystical texts from a psychological perspective has only an "ambiguous contribution" to make, he is correct in noting that psychological investigators and those involved in studying the history and theory of mysticism must cooperate in what to date is an "unrealized conversation."

CHAPTER 12

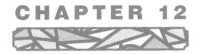

Religion, Morality, and Prejudice

[Religion] makes prejudice and it unmakes prejudice. . . . Some people say the only cure for prejudice is more religion; some say the only cure is to abolish religion.

NO to condom distribution in the schools, NO to taxpayer funding of abortion, NO to sex-education classes in the public schools that promote promiscuity, NO to homosexual adoptions and government-sanctioned gay marriages.

. . . being helpful is a scriptural criterion of true religion (James 1:27), and humans will ultimately be judged on their efforts on behalf of those in need of aid or comfort (Matthew 25:31–46).

Religious involvement is an especially strong predictor of volunteering and philanthropy.

. . . terrorism is religious because religion provides the moral justification for killing and the images of cosmic warfare that impact a heady illusion of power. . . . every major religious tradition has served as a resource for violent actors.[1]

Religion has much to say about morality. Christians, Jews, Buddhists, Muslims, and Hindus may not agree on the nature of God, or on religious rituals and teachings, but they do tend to agree about moral issues. In fact, when it comes to ethics, major world religions are amazingly consistent in their teachings about right and wrong, especially concerning murder, stealing, and adultery. In Christianity and Judaism, this distilled essence of morality is captured by the Ten Commandments. And all major world religions seem to teach some version of "Do unto others what you would have them do unto you."

Persons with a proreligious orientation would be inclined to argue that religion has tremendous potential to improve our world by teaching an ethical system that would benefit all of us. In fact, the theologies of such diverse religious bodies as Buddhists, Christians, and Jews have claimed that faith and morality are inseparable (Spilka, Hood, & Gorsuch, 1985). In contrast, some people are not convinced that religion holds the key to morality in the world, and they may argue that it can actually cause intolerance and suffering. Some of

---

[1]These quotations come, respectively, from the following sources: Allport (1954, p. 444); a fund-raising letter distributed in March 1995 by the Christian Coalition, quoted in Birnbaum (1995, p. 22); Ritzema (1979, p. 105); Putnam (2000, p. 67); and Juergensmeyer (2000, p. xi).

these individuals, such as Richard Dawkins and Sam Harris, have become rather prominent in popular culture (see the discussion of the anti-theist movement in Chapter 9).

We can all think of examples in which religion has apparently resulted in tolerance, helpfulness, and personal and interpersonal integrity. Mother Teresa spent her life in appalling conditions in order to help the poor, the sick, and the downtrodden in the cause of Christian charity. Martin Luther King, Jr. faced considerable danger, and was eventually assassinated, in his religiously based fight for equal rights and self-respect for black Americans. Churches, mosques, and synagogues provide money, housing, and social support for homeless persons and for refugees from other lands. Soup kitchens and halfway houses are sponsored by religious organizations. The list could go on and on.

On the other hand, many examples can be cited where religion has seemed to have no impact at all in encouraging positive behavior, or where it may even have contributed to dishonesty, intolerance, physical violence, and prejudice. The Christian-based Ku Klux Klan, still in existence in much of the United States, spreads hatred of blacks, Jews, and Catholics. Terrorist activities throughout the world are often conducted in the name of religion. Many wars and other violent conflicts in today's world are religiously based: Shiites and Sunnis battle in the Middle East; Catholics and Protestants still sporadically clash in Northern Ireland; Sikhs and Hindus die in violent conflicts in India; ethnic and religious "cleansing" occurred in Bosnia (of Muslims by Christians) and continues in Sudan (of Christians by Muslims); the Taliban in Afghanistan has taken away women's rights and has also attacked Western aid workers for being open about their Christian beliefs; extremist Palestinian Muslim groups send suicide bombers to kill Israeli civilians; and Israeli Jews respond with military violence against Palestinians. Again, the list could go on and on.

Religious faith is complex, and it would therefore be a mistake to oversimplify the relationship between religion and morality—especially in light of the many unique religious groups, orientations, and dimensions that may have different understandings of "right and wrong." Furthermore, we should not assume that religion has an impact on ethics through the process of "moral development" in childhood and adolescence. We have shown in Chapter 4 that Kohlberg and other researchers on moral development see religion as quite distinct from moral reasoning and the emergence of morality in general.

It has been pointed out that different religious groups may have different ways of thinking about moral issues, possibly because of religious identification and the beliefs associated with that identification (see Seybold, 2016, Chs. 6 and 7, for an excellent discussion). Cohen and Rozin (2001) found that Protestants, partly because they were more likely to believe that mental states are controllable and likely to lead to action, rated a target person with "inappropriate mental states" (p. 697—e.g., not honoring one's parents, or thinking about having a sexual affair) more negatively than did Jews. As a result, Cohen and Hill (2007) have argued that Allport's conceptualization of Intrinsic and Extrinsic (abbreviated throughout this chapter as I and E) religious orientations—with an emphasis on beliefs and other cognitive activities for I, and an emphasis on personal and (particularly) social benefits for E—may have a Protestant bias. For example, from a Jewish perspective (which places a much greater emphasis on community and ritual), the E items "One reason for my being a church member is that such membership helps to establish a person in the community" and "I pray chiefly because I have been taught to pray" may contain quite a different meaning from Allport's notion of E as flagrantly utilitarian. Indeed, Cohen and Hill (2007) found that Jews (in comparison to Protestants and Catholics) stress values of community and descent in their understanding of religion. Furthermore, important life experiences were more likely to include a social component for Jews, as opposed to a more guided focus on God and personal beliefs among Protestants (Catholics were between the two). As a result, Jews were found to be the least I and the most E; Protestants were just the opposite by being the most I and the least E (again, Catholics were between the two on both measures). Thus defining "mature" religion as I and "immature" religion as E may, these authors have speculated, reflect a Protestant bias (Allport was an Episcopalian). To be sure, religious traditions to some extent lead people to think about moral issues differently, and also to judge others differently, depending on the others' expressed thoughts about moral issues. However, evidence suggests that the ways in which people *reason* about religious and moral conflicts are quite similar (Cobb, Ong, & Tate, 2001).

Quite apart from formal moral development in Kohlbergian or other terms, and the ways in which people think about morality, it has been claimed that religiousness is associated with being a "better person" in numerous ways. In addition to broad moral imperatives such as "love thy neighbor," many religions have specific things to say about various personal issues: honesty and cheating; substance use and abuse; sexual behavior; criminal behavior and delinquency; domestic abuse; helping others; and prejudice and discrimination. After a brief discussion of moral attitudes and religion, we explore each of these areas in turn, attempting to determine whether religion and morality are associated.

MORAL ATTITUDES

It is not surprising that religion is related to people's attitudes on a host of morality-related issues. Typically, people who are religious (as measured in many different ways) are more "conservative" in their attitudes. In general, those who are more religious show more opposition to abortion (Bryan & Freed, 1993; Strickler & Danigelis, 2002), AIDS education (Ford, Zimmerman, Anderman, & Brown-Wright, 2001), divorce (Hayes & Hornsby-Smith, 1994), pornography (Lottes, Weinberg, & Weller, 1993), contraception (Krishnan, 1993), premarital sexuality (Bibby, 2001; Barkan, 2006), homosexuality (Rowatt, Tsang, et al., 2006), feminism (Wilcox & Jelen, 1991), nudity in advertising (Alexander & Judd, 1986), suicide (Domino & Miller, 1992), euthanasia (Shuman, Fournet, Zelhart, Roland, & Estes, 1992), amniocentesis (Seals, Ekwo, Williamson, & Hanson, 1985), heavy metal and rap music (Lynxwiler & Gay, 2000), and women going topless on beaches (Herold, Corbesi, & Collins, 1994). Highly religious individuals are also more likely to support marriage (Hayes & Hornsby-Smith, 1994), capital punishment (Bibby, 1987), vengeance (Cota-McKinley, Woody, & Bell, 2001), traditional sex roles (Larsen & Long, 1988), conservative political parties (Bibby, 1987), more severe criminal sentences (Altemeyer & Hunsberger, 1992), and censorship of sex and violence in the mass media (Fisher, Cook, & Shirkey, 1994). These lists surely just scratch the surface of such relationships, but they should give the reader an idea of the many diverse links between religion and moral attitudes. However, it should also be noted that the relationship between religion and moral issues does not necessarily remain constant. For example, Strickler and Danigelis (2002) found that general religiosity had become less powerful as a predictor of abortion attitudes in 1996 than in 1977, though religious fundamentalism in particular had become a stronger predictor of opposition to abortion during the same time period.

Perhaps no morally related social topic has generated as much recent controversy as sexual orientation, with religiousness as a primary factor. Not surprisingly, there appears to be a relationship between theologically conservative religion and negative attitudes toward homosexuality (Herek, 1987, 1994; Rowatt, Tsang, et al., 2006; Wilkinson, 2004). Religion has been found to be one of the major predictors of opposing views on social and political issues related to sexual orientation. One study (Olson, Cadge, & Harrison, 2006), consisting of a nationally representative survey of over 1,600 respondents, found sexual orientation to be the most prominent issue in "moral values" discourse in American politics at that time. Over a decade later, it appears that the prominence of this issue has not abated. Olson et al. also found that religion, more than any other demographic variable, predicted attitudes about same-sex unions, with conservatives (especially Protestant conservatives) more likely to oppose such unions. Of interest, however, was their finding that religiousness was less capable of predicting support for a constitutional amendment to prevent same-sex marriage than in predicting general attitudes about the topic. Research by Mavor and Gallois (2008) found a two-factor model that maps attitudes toward moral issues on two separate dimensions: group attitudes and moral orientation attitudes. This is useful in that the researchers distinguished between an external behavioral model (i.e., believing in civil rights for homosexual individuals while also believing that the behavior is immoral) from an internal ideology (believing that the behavior is immoral). This model may help clarify the Olson et al. (2006) findings.

Sexual orientation issues (e.g., same-sex marriage and other civil rights for gays and lesbians, as well as bisexual and transgender individuals) have been increasingly raised for consideration at both the federal and state levels. At this writing, 37 states and the District of Columbia have legalized same-sex marriage, and the U.S. Supreme Court legalized such marriages nationwide on June 26, 2015. The very fact that these issues are being considered by courts and legislators probably heightens the fervency of different views, especially among those holding traditional views, who often find the consideration of such issues threatening. One study (Oldmixon & Calfano, 2007) found that although decision making pertaining to gay/lesbian issues was primarily a function of legislators' partisanship and ideology (both of which correlate with religiosity), members of the U.S. Congress show a high degree of responsiveness to religious groups, especially conservative Protestants. We return to the topic of religion and views of homosexuality later in this chapter.

It is one thing to oppose, for example, premarital sex or alcohol use on the basis of religion, and quite another to act consistently with this attitude when the opportunity presents itself. Furthermore, it is possible that one's personal position on ethical issues may differ from one's public stance. For example, it has been found that people who personally oppose abortion on moral or religious grounds may actually *favor* legal abortion (Scott, 1989). And 70% of a sample of Seventh-Day Adventist young people endorsed their church's prohibition of premarital sex, but 54% of the sample reported that they had engaged in premarital sex (Ali & Naidoo, 1999). Thus, although associations between faith and moral attitudes are informative, they do not always accurately predict how religion will relate to moral *behavior*. So we now survey several areas of behavior with strong ethical implications, in order to assess the role of religion in people's actions. However, as we shall see, beliefs and behavior are often intertwined in the research literature; it is therefore sometimes necessary to focus on attitudes generally in order to gain insights into moral behavior, despite the problems in doing so.

MORAL BEHAVIOR

Honesty and Cheating

Research suggests that academic dishonesty in high school and university settings is quite common, even among religious college students. One investigation (Spilka & Loffredo, 1982) reported that 72% of a group of religious college students admitted that they had cheated on examinations. Another study (Cochran, Chamlin, Wood, & Sellers, 1999) found that 83% of college students admitted to at least one act of academic dishonesty (e.g., plagiarism on an essay, cheating on an examination). Bruggeman and Hart (1996) noted that when given incentives to lie and cheat, their sample of both religious and secular high school students revealed "surprisingly high levels of dishonest behavior" (p. 340). Even among Mormons, a group known for a conservative and strict approach to moral issues, 70% of a sample of more than 2,000 adolescents admitted that they had cheated on tests at school (Chadwick & Top, 1993). Apparently cheating is quite widespread among high school and college students, even among students who consider themselves religious.

Does Religion Make Any Difference?

Does religion make any difference at all? The results are mixed. Overall, research results over several decades suggest that if religion does have an influence, it is a small influence at best. Early studies (Hartshorne & May, 1928, 1929; Hartshorne, May, & Shuttleworth, 1930; Hightower, 1930) investigated a possible link between religiousness and cheating in their massive studies involving some 11,000 school children in the 1920s. These researchers devised ingenious tests for cheating—for example, by measuring peeking during "eyes-closed" tests, and by checking whether students had changed their original answers when allowed to grade their own exams. In the end, they found essentially no relationship between religion and honesty or cheating. Later research, involving behavioral measures and diverse samples, has confirmed that religion does not decrease cheating behavior. Guttman (1984) investigated sixth graders from religious schools in Israel and discovered that religious children indicated some resistance to temptation on a paper-and-pencil test, but were actually more inclined to cheat on a behavioral measure. Smith, Wheeler, and Diener (1975) studied undergraduate college students, categorizing them as involved in the "Jesus movement" or as being otherwise religious, nonreligious, or atheistic; no differences emerged with respect to their tendency to cheat on a class examination when the opportunity was available. More recently, however, Huelsman, Piroch, and Wasieleski (2006) found that religiousness was related to less academic dishonesty, but only in women.

Perrin (2000), using a behavioral measure, did find that religious college students cheated less. Because such behavioral investigations of cheating are rare, this study is highlighted in Research Box 12.1. Unfortunately, the cheating in this research was necessarily quite mild, involving 1 point on a single weekly quiz, and only four of seven measures of religion (all single-item measures) achieved statistical significance. In another behaviorally based study of cheating on a computerized version of the Graduate Record Examination, Williamson and Assadi (2005) found that religious orientation was unrelated to cheating. In their study, induced low self-esteem was the major predictor of cheating. However, behavioral studies investigating the effect of religious priming on cheating, have found that individuals engaged in less cheating when primed with religious words, regardless of religious beliefs or commitment (Randolph-Seng & Nielsen, 2007; Shariff & Norenzayan, 2007). Therefore, the results

RESEARCH BOX 12.1. Religiosity and Honesty (Perrin, 2000)

Perrin carried out this study in an attempt to address problems in the literature, including the paucity of studies on religion and honesty; measurement problems, such as the tendency for dependent measures to rely on self-reports rather than behavior; and inconsistencies in the results of relevant investigations.

Perrin's own study had two main components. First, students in a large lecture course at a university in the western United States completed a survey that included seven items on religiosity. These items were intended to tap frequency of church attendance, participation in religious activities (such as Bible study), frequency of prayer, belief in life after death, whether respondents considered themselves to be "born again" and to be "strong Christians," and the frequency with which they had had religious experiences (i.e., being "very close to a powerful, spiritual force that seemed to lift you out of yourself" [p. 539]). We are not told what else was on the questionnaire, or what the reliability of the seven religiosity items might be.

Second, there was a simple but effective measure of honesty. In one of the weekly quizzes in this class, the teaching assistant intentionally graded them incorrectly, so that *everyone* received 1 additional point on that quiz. Students were then informed that an error might have been made in grading. They were to regrade their own quizzes and write, at the top of an unrelated assignment that they were handing in, one of three phrases: "I owe you a point," "Quiz graded correctly," or "You owe me a point."

Results indicated that, first, honesty was hard to come by in this investigation, as had been found in previous research. Of the 130 students included in the analyses, just 32% honestly admitted receiving an extra point on the quiz. Fifty-two percent said that the quiz was graded correctly, and 16% actually tried to get another point in addition to the point they received from the teaching assistant's "mistake." More important, however, were the comparisons of honesty across the religion item responses. For all seven items, the results were in the expected direction, such that more honesty was apparent for more religious responders. However, the results achieved significance for just four of the seven items (church attendance, frequency of other religious activities, belief in life after death, and born-again status). The most dramatic difference in scores seems to have been for church attendance: 45% of weekly (or more frequent) attenders, but just 13% of those who attended once a year or less, honestly reported the 1-point error on their quiz.

Finally, the results do confirm a stark reality for "religious people." Even among the most highly religious people in this study, as defined by seven quite different items, the majority of students apparently lied about the results of their quiz. It would seem that truly high percentages of honesty are difficult to find in groups of religious or nonreligious persons.

Unfortunately, this study had a relatively small sample about which we know little (e.g., age, percentage of men and women, race/ethnicity, religious affiliation, extent of personal religiosity), as well as only a brief measure of religiosity without established reliability and validity. Results are reported only in percentages of some rather unique combinations of response categories, and so on. For these reasons, it would be helpful to see the results replicated, with more standard measures and more information about samples and analyses. At the same time, this study is one of very few that has attempted to use a behavioral measure of honesty, and we hope that it will stimulate additional and much-needed investigations in this area.

of these studies cannot be seen as representing a major shift in findings when behavioral measures are used. However, behavioral measures of cheating deserve further attention and follow-up research.

Those studies that have found a negative link between religiousness and cheating have usually involved self-reports rather than actual behavioral measures. Of course, self-reports are subject to bias, either intentionally or unintentionally. Grasmick and his colleagues (Grasmick, Bursik, & Cochran, 1991; Grasmick, Kinsey, & Cochran, 1991) have investigated the relationship between religion and self-reported admission of how likely respondents would be to cheat on their income taxes (and, in one study, to commit theft and to engage in littering) in the future. There was some tendency for more religious persons to indicate that they were less likely to cheat on their taxes (and less likely to litter, but there was no significant relationship for theft). Similarly, a nationwide Dutch survey (ter Voert, Felling, & Peters, 1994) found that "strong Christian believers" reported holding a stricter moral code with respect to "self-interest morality" (different forms of cheating). And Storch and Storch (2001) found that higher I religious scores were negatively related to reported rates of academic dishonesty.

These findings suggest that as researchers probe deeper into the religious variable and consider such things as degree of religious commitment or religious orientation, the "no relationship found" conclusion may be an oversimplification. For example, in a study using a behavioral measure of cheating, Shariff and Norenzayan (2011) found that whether or not participants cheated depended on their view of God. Specifically, they found that only participants who viewed God as punishing or unloving were less likely to cheat.

It is often the case that when only self-report measures are used, "lie scales" (i.e., scales assessing the tendency to present oneself in a socially desirable manner) are included in the research instrument to determine whether respondents are prone to provide inaccurate data, whether intentionally or not. Francis and Johnson (1999) found no relationship between scores on a lie scale and either church attendance or personal prayer among primary school teachers (see also Francis & Katz, 1992; Gillings & Joseph, 1996; Lewis & Joseph, 1994). However, in other studies, religiosity has been linked with *higher* lie scale scores (e.g., Francis, Pearson, & Kay, 1983; Lewis & Maltby, 1995), indicating a possible bias among religious respondents. We must therefore be careful with such self-report findings, regardless of what the results suggest; what people say they will do is not always consistent with their actual behavior.

Religion and Honesty: Summary

In the end, the results are mixed. Although religious people say that they are more honest than less religious persons, such findings seem to be contradicted by other research showing no relationship, or even a positive relationship, between lie scale scores and religiosity. In addition, the evidence from studies of actual behavior to support the position that religious people are somehow more honest, or less likely to lie or cheat, than are their less religious or nonreligious peers is at best weak. In view of the clear teachings of most faiths on such issues, we are left to ponder why religion does not have a more significant impact in reducing cheating *behavior*.

Substance Use and Abuse

Religious teachings across diverse groups typically oppose the abuse of such substances as alcohol and illicit drugs. One might expect, therefore, that faith would be associated with decreased substance use/abuse. And, in fact, the related literature generally does confirm the tendency for more religious persons (as defined in many different ways) to be less likely to use and abuse alcohol and drugs. The range of studies in this area is impressive, focusing variously on alcohol, tobacco, and illicit drugs used for nonmedical purposes (e.g., cocaine, heroin, amphetamines, barbiturates, and psychedelic substances). Some studies focus on either alcohol *or* "drugs," but many investigate the impact of religion on both. Here we consider the findings of the various studies together, because their results are so similar.

The Negative Relationship between Religion and Substance Use/Abuse

Research since the mid-1970s continues to show, as it has for decades, that religion is an important negative predictor of alcohol and substance use (Ford & Hill, 2012; Gorsuch, 1995; Hill & McCullough, 2008; Michalak, Trocki, & Bond, 2007). Religiousness—especially being actively involved in one's religion (attending services, engaging in scriptural study, etc.)—predicts lower levels of alcohol abuse among college students, even after researchers control for such related variables as grade point average, ethnicity, and social support (Dulin, Hill, & Ellington, 2006). Religious participation seems to be a key in religiousness as a predictor. For example, in a Canadian inpatient population, those who participate in more frequent worship reported lower levels of current and past alcohol abuse (Baetz, Larson, Marcoux, Bowen, & Griffin, 2002). Similarly, Bazargan, Sherkat, and Bazargan (2004) found that religious participation had a significant negative relationship with alcohol use 6 hours prior to seeking emergency care. Dunn (2005) found that the importance of religion was a predictor of less initiation of alcohol use, less current alcohol use, and less likelihood of having tried binge drinking among high school seniors. Similar findings have been documented for tobacco use (Nonnemaker, McNeely, & Blum, 2006).

Studies document what many large-scale surveys (sometimes involving samples of 5,000 people or more) have found—namely, that people who are religious are less likely to abuse alcohol and other drugs (Ford & Kadushin, 2002; Hill & McCullough, 2008; Johnson, Sheets, & Kristeller, 2008; Park, Bauer, & Oescher, 2001; Sutherland & Shepherd, 2001). Furthermore, these findings tend to hold regardless of age or gender and, with few exceptions, across cultures. Consistent findings have been obtained in countries and regions as disparate as Central America (Kliewer & Murrelle, 2007), Canada (Hundleby, 1987), Nigeria (Adelekan, Abiodun, Imouokhome-Obayan, Oni, & Ogunremi, 1993), Scotland (Engs & Mullen, 1999), the Netherlands (Mullen & Francis, 1995), Sweden (Pettersson, 1991), Israel (Kandel & Sudit, 1982), Australia (Najman, Williams, Keeping, Morrison, & Anderson, 1988), Thailand (Assanangkornchai, Conigrave, & Saunders, 2002), Spain (Grana Gomes & Munoz-Rivas, 2000), Saudi Arabia (Qureshi & Al-Habeeb, 2000), and China (Wu, Detels, Zhang, & Duan, 1996). The relationship has been demonstrated among Filipino Americans (Gong, Takeuchi, Agbayani-Siewert, & Tacata, 2003) and Mexican American youths (Marsiglia, Kulis, Nieri, & Parsai, 2005), in addition to the U.S. ethnic groups usually studied (European Americans and African Americans). This effect has even been found among the children of individuals addicted to opium (Miller, Weissman, Gur, & Adams, 2001). *Parental* religiosity is also apparently linked with less substance abuse among children (Foshee & Hollinger, 1996; Merrill, Salazar, & Gardner, 2001).

THE MAGNITUDE AND GENERALITY OF THE RELATIONSHIP

The size of the relationships between religiosity and substance use noted above varies from study to study. Research shows that on average, negative correlations with alcohol, tobacco, and marijuana use are in the −.15 to −.20 range—small to moderate correlations, in other words (Benson, 1992b; Yeung, Chan, & Lee, 2009). These results usually remain significant even after the effects of age, gender, race, region, education, income, and other variables are controlled for.

However, we should not assume that other variables are inconsequential. Mason and Windle (2002), in a 1-year longitudinal study, found that religious attendance initially seemed to predict fewer subsequent alcohol problems. But when peer, family, and school influences were statistically controlled for, the relationship disappeared. A Finnish study of adolescents (Winter, Karvonen, & Rose, 2002) showed a negative correlation between religiousness and alcohol use only for a rural sample; there was no relationship for an urban sample. There are also suggestions that gender is important, with stronger relationships for women than for men (e.g., Templin & Martin, 1999). A study by Corwyn and Benda (2000) is highlighted in Research Box 12.2, to give the reader a better appreciation for the complexities of "controlling for other variables" and ways in which the relationship between religion and substance use can be further specified.

RESEARCH BOX 12.2. Religiosity and Church Attendance:
The Effects on Use of "Hard Drugs" after Sociodemographic and Theoretical
Factors Were Controlled For (Corwyn & Benda, 2000)

This questionnaire study involved 532 students in grades 9–12 from three inner-city public high schools in a metropolitan area on the U.S. East Coast. The authors pointed out that "church attendance" has been a favorite measure of religion in studies of religion and substance use, but because this measure is confounded by other variables, they suspected that personal religiosity might be a more appropriate measure. The authors also wondered about the extent to which the relationship between religion and substance abuse might be mediated by other variables. That is, there has been some question about whether religion is related to substance abuse simply because of its relation to other relevant variables, or whether religion makes some unique contribution to the relationship that cannot be "explained" by resorting to those other variables. Also, relatively few studies have investigated the use of "hard drugs" (e.g., cocaine, heroin) in relation to religiosity.

The results of this study led the authors to conclude that "church attendance, like attendance in a college classroom, is at best a vicarious indicator of commitment and a poor measure of performance" (p. 253). Indeed, church attendance did not show a negative association with hard drug use, but personal religiosity (e.g., private prayer, Bible study) did show the expected negative association. Indeed, the results indicated that personal religiosity was negatively correlated with self-reported hard drug use even after other strong predictors found in the literature were statistically controlled for.

This investigation is of course limited by the nature of the sample (inner-city high school students) and the measures (relatively few single items were used to generate measures of church attendance and personal religiosity), as well as the use of self-reports for all dependent variable information. However, this investigation did consider a variety of other potentially influential variables, without assuming that the initial correlations themselves justified the conclusion that religion is negatively related to hard drug use.

NEW RELIGIONS

The negative association between religion and substance use/abuse is not limited to traditional religious groups. Although there is evidence that individuals who become members of cults often have a history of greater drug and alcohol utilization before joining (Rochford, Purvis, & NeMar, 1989), research suggests that their subsequent use of these substances often declines, sometimes dramatically (Galanter & Buckley, 1978; Richardson, 1995). In fact, these sorts of findings led Latkin (1995) to suggest that "The study of new religions may provide insights into methods of improving drug treatment programs" (p. 179). On the other hand, new or alternative religions sometimes also encourage substance use. For example, some cults from the 1960s and 1970s openly advocated LSD use (Gorsuch, 1995).

WHY DOES THIS RELATIONSHIP EXIST?

It is one thing to find an association between variables, and quite another to explain *why* that relationship exists. There are probably many factors involved in the inverse correlation between religion and substance use/abuse, and various theories have been proposed to explain the association (see DeWall et al., 2014; Ford & Kadushin, 2002; Gorsuch, 1995). Benson's (1992b) review of the related empirical literature led him to infer:

> Nearly all of these efforts appeal to the social control function of religion, in which religious institutions and traditions maintain the social order by discouraging deviance, delinquency, and self-destructive behavior. Religion, then, prevents use through a system of norms and values that favor personal restraint. (p. 216)

Gorsuch (1995) has pointed out two mechanisms that may be operating here. First, as clearly noted in the quotation above, socialization processes may decrease substance use through the internalization of (religious) antiabuse norms. Drawing on a distinction made by the classical social theorist Emile Durkheim (1915), we call this the "normative" function of religion—the notion that religion provides a reference group that prescribes what one's attitude and behavior toward alcohol and other substances should be. Thus affiliation with conservative reference groups (e.g., churches that teach against substance use) should negatively predict substance use. Second, Gorsuch maintained that religion may serve as an alternative (i.e., to drugs or alcohol) means of meeting basic needs, such as the need to relieve mental anguish or social anxiety, or as an alternative to a sense of meaninglessness and alienation. We refer to this second mechanism, again following Durkheim's lead, as the "integrative" function of religion—the notion that the religious group provides an individual with a sense of acceptance, and that such social support lessens reliance on other anxiety-reducing mechanisms, such as the use of alcohol or drugs.

Consider, for example, research showing that the negative relationship between religion and substance use is stronger for white than for black adolescents in the United States (Amey, Albrecht, & Miller, 1996). Furthermore, different aspects of religiosity are better predictors for blacks than for whites. A study of adolescents (mostly 14- and 15-year-olds) in Ohio and Kentucky found that church attendance was a better negative predictor of alcohol use among blacks, but that fundamentalism was the better negative predictor for whites (T. L. Brown, Parks, Zimmerman, & Phillips, 2001). Though it is not precisely clear what these findings mean, Ford and Kadushin (2002) have offered an explanation along the lines of the distinction between the normative and integrative functions of religion. Their study of over 18,000 individuals found that though the normative dimension of religion was important for both races, it had much greater power in predicting alcohol use among whites. In contrast, the integrative dimension seemed to have greater predictive power among blacks. Ford and Kadushin suggest that the influence of the organizational church, especially in the black community, should be understood in terms of not just its doctrinal teachings, but also its position as a provider of social support and its ability to meet basic psychological needs. In a similar vein, Wallace, Brown, Bachman, and Laviest (2003) found that religion operated as a protective factor for white youths at an individual level, whereas for black youths the influence of religion seemed greater at a group level.

Benson (1992b) has argued that in addition to social control mechanisms, religion decreases alcohol and drug use/abuse indirectly by "promoting environmental and psychological assets that constrain risk-taking" (p. 218). He is referring here to religion's attempts to encourage positive behaviors through promoting family harmony and parental support, as well as through sponsoring prosocial values and social competence. Others have similarly concluded that religious young people are generally less likely to engage in health-compromising behaviors and more likely to engage in health-enhancing behaviors (Wallace & Forman, 1998). Research is needed to assess the extent to which such indirect mechanisms are effective deterrents to drug and alcohol use/abuse.

There are interesting variations in the relationship between religion and substance use/abuse across faith groups. Cochran (1993), for example, found that in the case of alcohol consumption, this association was strongest for religious bodies that condemn alcohol, perhaps reflecting the normative function of religion. However, faiths that are silent regarding alcohol revealed little influence of religiousness. Similarly, research (Chawla, Neighbors, Lewis, Lee, & Larimer, 2007; Walker, Ainette, Wills, & Mendoza, 2007) has further documented that the negative linkage between religion and substance use may reflect the perceived perception of others, such that less substance use is found among those who associate with less tolerant groups. Individuals apparently find that their ability to refuse drugs or alcohol is enhanced by both private and public religiosity, as one study among African American adolescents and young adults found (Nasim, Utsey, Corona, & Belgrave, 2006).

Of course, the association of religiousness and substance use may reflect other, more personal characteristics as well. Perhaps the most pervasive line of research suggests that self-control, often a virtue stressed in religious traditions, may help explain the rather consistent findings that link religion to better health, including lower substance use and abuse (e.g., DeWall et al., 2014; McCullough & Willoughby, 2009; Desmond, Ulmer, & Bader, 2013; Kim-Spoon, Farley, Holmes, Longo, & McCullough, 2014; Kim-Spoon, McCullough, Bickel, Farley, & Longo, 2014; Walker et al., 2007). Several researchers suggest that the effect of religiousness on substance use is mediated through personal self-control and less personal tolerance for deviance. The study by Walker and associates also found that parental support and less parent–child conflict were associated with decreased substance use. Other research findings have identified the importance of belief in high God control in addition to (not replacing) internal control (Goggin, Murray, Malcarne, Brown, & Wallston, 2007), and a combination of the I and Quest religious orientations (Jankowski et al., 2015), as predictive factors in lower alcohol use.

The Role of Religion in Prevention and Treatment of Substance Abuse

Some of religion's role in inhibiting substance abuse may derive from its role in preventing abuse before it begins. For example, Stewart (2001) found that religious beliefs seemed to act as a buffer for university students, deterring them from making an initial decision to use alcohol or drugs. In this sense, religion may play a role in prevention.

It is likely that some prevention, treatment, and support programs could benefit from the aspects of religion that combat substance abuse, though research is needed to clarify what those specific elements are. Regarding prevention, there are now several studies showing that religion is a protective factor in the development of alcohol or drug dependence (e.g., Borders, Curran, Mattox, & Booth, 2010; Button, Hewitt, Rhee, Corley, & Stallings, 2010; Haber et al., 2013; Mason, Schmidt, & Mennis, 2012). However, one study (Webster, 2015) showed no relationship between level of spirituality and substance use. Another study (Burris, Sauer, & Carlson, 2011) found that religious commitment, but not a measure of spiritual transcendence, predicted lower underage alcohol use, suggesting that perhaps measures of spirituality are tapping something different regarding substance use than are measures of religious commitment. Supporting this notion, Mason et al. (2012) found that social religiousness and religious support, but not private religiousness, were protective factors among adolescents for marijuana and tobacco use. It may be that the social indicators of religiousness better reflect the values of religious teachings about substance use than do measures of private religious or spirituality.

Regarding treatment, Gorsuch (1995) and Benson (1992b) suggested over two decades ago that religion may be especially effective for religious people who want their beliefs to be considered in a nurturing and supportive treatment context for substance abuse. The majority of empirical studies suggest that spirituality or religiousness is a facilitative factor in substance abuse recovery—often because those who report high religiousness or spirituality also show positive mental health characteristics, such as increased coping and optimism, greater perceived social support, and so on (Arnold, Avants, Margolin, & Marcotte, 2002; Collins, 2007; Martin, Ellingsen, Tzilos, & Rohsenow, 2015; Robinson, Cranford, & Webb, 2007; Shields, Broome, Delany, Fletcher, & Flynn, 2007; Sterling et al., 2006, 2007). Several of these studies include behavioral components. For example, those who report being more religious are abstinent from illicit drugs significantly longer during the first 6 months of a treatment program (Avants, Warburton, & Margolin, 2001) and are more successful in recovering from addiction (Jarusiewicz, 2000). One large-scale study (Shields et al., 2007), based on a national sample of over 10,000 individuals in 70 different drug treatment programs, concluded that a religious or spiritual emphasis in treatment programs was moderately positively related to treatment outcomes, though the researchers admitted difficulty in assessing the specific contribution of religion as compared to these treatment programs' other features. Sterling et al. (2006) also found that a spiritual treatment component was helpful, but only to clients who desired such a component. This team of researchers (Sterling et al., 2007) also found that clients reported spiritual growth during substance abuse treatment that had a spiritual emphasis; such treatment provides a sense of meaning and hope, which in turn may have an impact on treatment outcome.

Probably the most well-known treatment approach that includes a religious element is that of Alcoholics Anonymous (AA). Though the organization has had some success in treating alcoholism over the years (Oakes, Allen, & Ciarrocchi, 2000), some authors would argue that AA's success, especially as portrayed in the mass media, is overrated (see, e.g., Bufe, 1991). AA is essentially a secular organization, but it has incorporated aspects of religious experience and practices into its treatment approach, especially a reliance on a higher power (God) as the source of rehabilitation (Morreim, 1991). Tonigan, Miller, and Schermer (2002) found that belief in God appears not to be necessary in deriving AA-related benefits; however, they discovered that relative to spiritual and religious clients, atheists and agnostics were less likely to initiate and sustain AA attendance. Also, in another study, theists were more likely to maintain sobriety longer than agnostics or atheists (Zemore & Kaskutas, 2004).

Caveats

One drawback of the many studies on religion and substance use/abuse is that they typically rely on self-reports—a recurring theme throughout this text. If, as Batson, Schoenrade, and Ventis (1993) have suggested, religious persons (especially those with an I orientation) have an inclination toward socially desirable responses, it is possible that they are reporting a kind of ideal image of themselves, rather than an accurate assessment of actual substance use and abuse.

In addition, most of the studies in this area, particularly those conducted prior to the 1990s, have examined religiousness in a very general sense, relying on such measures as church attendance and affiliation. Though church attendance does seem to be an important variable with regard to substance use, these measures are probably overly simplistic. Some of the more recent studies have used more sophisticated scales of personal religiosity and religious orientation. There is evidence that in some specific contexts, the usual negative relationship between religion and substance use/abuse may disappear, or may even be reversed. For example, some studies of adolescents have revealed the usual negative relationship with substance use, but have also found a *positive* relationship between some aspects of religion (e.g., proscriptiveness) and binge or problem drinking (e.g., Kutter & McDermott, 1997), or between early (teen) religiosity and increased adult alcohol use (Galaif & Newcomb, 1999).

The results of relevant studies are correlational, leading to some difficulties in interpretation. The most obvious cause-and-effect interpretation seems to be that greater religiosity somehow protects individuals from substance use and abuse. However, it is conceivable that substance use decreases religiosity. For example, adolescents who experiment with alcohol or drugs may find less room for religion in their lives, and the "hassles" of religious proscriptions for substance use may make religious teachings seem less relevant to their lives and therefore less important. At the least, there may be a reciprocal causal relationship between religiosity and substance use (e.g., Benda, 1997; Benda & Corwyn, 2000; Corwyn, Benda, & Ballard, 1997). However, the development and increased use of more sophisticated statistical procedures are helpful, though not conclusive, in suggesting the more likely causal directions.

Furthermore, in spite of repeated findings of low to moderate negative correlations between religion and substance use/abuse, there are exceptions. Some "failures" to find the expected association may reflect unique cultural or religious situations. For example, studies carried out in Iran (Spencer & Agahi, 1982), in Colombia (Marin, 1976), and among Chinese students in Singapore (Isralowitz & Ong, 1990) have shown no link between religion and alcohol or drug use. Other "failures" may simply be related to the generally weak nature of the relationships; slightly weaker correlations in some samples, or small sample sizes, might also result in "no relationship" results. In addition, as noted above, there have been reports of a positive relationship between religion and *problem* drinking (e.g., Alem, Kebede, & Kullgren, 1999).

Finally, we must remember that the "substances" considered in this section sometimes play a part in religious ceremonies or rituals for specific faith groups, and that within this context their use may actually be increased by religious involvement. For example, religious ceremonial use was one justification for drinking alcohol in Nigerian (Oshodin, 1983) and in Mexican and Honduran (Natera, Renconco, Alemendares, Rosowsky, & Alemendares, 1983) samples. In the 1960s, as noted earlier, some new religious groups encouraged the use of LSD, and Clark (1969) and Siegel (1977) have argued that psychedelic drugs may contribute to religious experiences and behaviors. In a different vein, Westermeyer and Walzer (1975) have even suggested that drug use among young people may occur in part because it generates personal and social benefits that would formerly have been derived from religious practice. It has also been noted that traditional religious-based festivals may serve as a vehicle for binge drinking, as well as violence against women (Perez, 2000).

Religion and Substance Use/Abuse: Summary

The vast majority of studies in this area reveal a negative link between religion and substance use/abuse. The relationship is typically rather weak; there are also confounds to consider, as well as occasional failures to replicate the effect. But, all in all, it is impressive how general and consistent the association is across diverse samples and studies. Until the 1990s, the overall literature on substance use/abuse made only token acknowledgment of religion as an important explanatory variable, and then only as one of many possible cultural influences (see, e.g., Gorsuch, 1995; Petraitis, Flay, & Miller, 1995). However, as more and more studies are being published, it is likely that religion will be increasingly recognized as an important predictor variable.

Sexual Behavior

Traditionally, religion has acknowledged the proper role of sexuality as being for procreative purposes within a marital relationship. Consequently, virtually any sort of sexual expression outside heterosexual marriage has been considered inappropriate and sinful. These norms have been both strong and stable across the centuries, but societal changes regarding these standards, particularly in Europe and North America, may have an impact on the attitudes and behavior of religious individuals and groups. The population at large and some religious groups are currently showing an increased tolerance of premarital sex, same-sex behavior, and even some extramarital sexual behavior. As far back as 1991, Cochran and Beeghley pointed out that

> some churches have addressed the problem by adjusting and softening their stand, while others have steadfastly avoided such secularization. As a result, there are significant differences in the official stands taken toward nonmarital, particularly premarital sex, among mainstream religious bodies in America. (p. 46)

Religion and Sex outside Marriage

Not surprisingly, among Christians the conservative Protestant churches have most resisted a softening of attitudes toward nonmarital sex. Petersen and Donnenwerth (1997) examined more than 14,000 cases from longitudinal data obtained from 1972 to 1993. Their results showed that, across the years, mainline Protestants and Catholics were more willing to alter their traditional beliefs about sex before marriage; however, conservative Protestants showed no such willingness. Cochran and Beeghley (1991) examined cumulative data from the National Opinion Research Center's General Social Survey (GSS) series conducted in the United States between 1972 and 1989, involving almost 15,000 people. Though they found an overall tendency for religious persons to disapprove more strongly of premarital sexuality, extramarital sexuality, and homosexuality than did the less religious respondents, there were notable variations across different religious groups (see Table 12.1), apparently indicative of the official doctrines of U.S. churches. The more strongly one's (religious) reference group condemns and prohibits various sexual acts, the more likely one is to disapprove of such practices. This is found across most major religious traditions. Muslims, in particular, are less likely to report premarital and extramarital sexuality (Adamczyk & Hayes, 2012).

RELIGION AND PREMARITAL SEX

In spite of differences between religious traditions, including denominations within Protestantism, research has generally found that stronger religious beliefs and involvement are associated with self-reported decreased nonmarital sexual activity, especially premarital and extramarital sexual intercourse. A considerable research literature supports this conclusion. For example, a longitudinal New Zealand investigation revealed that for both men and women, being involved in religious activities (as measured at both age 11 and age 21) predicted abstinence from sexual intercourse until at least age 21 (Paul, Fitzjohn, Eberhart-Phillips,

TABLE 12.1. Attitudes toward Nonmarital Sexuality: Percentages Saying Specific Behaviors Are "Almost Always Wrong" or "Always Wrong" among Different Religious Groups

Religious group	Attitude toward . . .		
	Premarital sexuality	Extramarital sexuality	Homosexuality
Nonaffiliated	10	66	49
Jewish	18	75	43
Catholic	36	87	77
Episcopalian	25	85	66
Presbyterian	36	89	76
Lutheran	40	90	81
Methodist	43	91	84
Baptist	49	90	89
Other Protestant	55	93	86
Total sample	40	88	79

Note. Based on Cochran and Beeghley (1991).

Herbison, & Dickson, 2000). Other studies have also shown that various measures of religiosity are related to decreased premarital sexual activity (e.g., Barry, Willoughby, & Clayton, 2015; Holder et al., 2000; Lammers, Ireland, Resnick, & Blum, 2000; Zaleski & Schiaffino, 2000), though at least one study suggests only a weak relationship (Cochran, Chamlin, Beeghley, & Fenwick, 2004). Most of this research involves adolescents, and the findings hold true with emerging adults (Barry et al., 2015). Barkan (2006) has found that the general pattern of results discovered with adolescents applies to adults as well: The number of premarital sexual partners is fewer among the religious (partly because of moral disapproval of premarital sex), and the association of religiousness and premarital sexuality is stronger for European Americans than for African Americans.

However, Barkan's finding that the relationship of religiousness with premarital sexuality activity is about the same for men as it is for women has not been consistently reported. Sometimes religion has been shown to be a stronger predictor of more conservative attitudes and behavior for women than for men (e.g., McFarland, Uecker, & Regnerus, 2011), while other studies have suggested that the effects of religion on sexual behaviors are stronger for men (e.g., Luquis, Brelsford, & Rojas-Guyler, 2012). Further research is needed to unpack these findings.

RELIGION AND MARITAL INFIDELITY

High religiousness has also been linked to lower levels of marital infidelity. Atkins, Baucom, and Jacobson (2001) found that frequent churchgoers reported less extramarital sexual activity than did nonattenders. However, this difference was moderated by marital satisfaction; that is, the difference between church attenders and nonattenders was largest among those who were in "very happy" marriages. In marriages described as "pretty happy" or "not too happy," not only was more extramarital sexual activity reported, but the differences based on church attendance were eliminated, suggesting that marital discontent may be a stronger predictor of extramarital sexual activity than religiosity may be. In subsequent work, Atkins and Kessel (2008) found that religious attendance, but not strength of faith, perceived nearness to God, or prayer, was a predictor of past infidelity. In fact, people who reported high religious importance but infrequent religious attendance were *more* likely to have had a past affair.

In general, though, the degree of religious affiliation (at least for Christians), in terms of both attendance at religious services and acceptance of biblical beliefs, predicts less self-reported marital infidelity (Burdette, Ellison, Sherkat, & Gore, 2007). One question that can be asked is whether the negative association between religion and extramarital sexuality is due to religious proscriptions or due to a higher level of marital satisfaction, including sexual satisfaction, among religious married couples. McFarland et al. (2011) found that among married older adults, religiousness was unrelated to sexual satisfaction and frequency. However, they also found a small positive relationship between the degree to which daily life was infused with religion and sexual pleasure. Similarly, Hernandez, Mahoney, and Pargament (2011) found that when sexuality in a marriage relationship was viewed as sacred, married individuals reported greater marital and sexual satisfaction.

QUALIFICATIONS

As is the case with research on religion and substance use/abuse, the research here is almost entirely correlational, so we must resist the temptation to draw causal inferences prematurely.

The bulk of the literature appears to assume that the causal direction is from religion to sexuality; given religious teachings about sexual morality, this assumption is not so much unreasonable as it is perhaps premature. We should entertain the possibility that sexual beliefs and practices may influence religious commitment. Vasilenko and Lefkowitz (2014) found, for example, that individuals may become less religious following initial sexual intercourse, perhaps to address intrapersonal tension due to dissonant cognitions. Furthermore, since many decisions about both religion and sexuality often occur at about the same time, some third variable may influence both religious and sexual decisions.

Another problem is that the literature is not consistent in its measures of religiousness or spirituality. Though researchers often bemoan church attendance as a measure of religiousness, research indicates that in the case of sexuality, frequency of religious attendance is sometimes more important than religious beliefs or attitudes. For example, in a study of Australian adults, the frequency of attendance at religious services was the key finding; infrequent attenders held relatively liberal sexual attitudes and behavior patterns, more similar to those of nonreligious peers than to those of regular attenders (de Visser, Smith, Richters, & Rissel, 2007; see also Atkins & Kessel, 2008; Landor & Simons, 2014; Murray, Ciarrocchi, & Murray-Swank, 2007). This is not to say that religious beliefs and attitudes are unimportant predictors of sexuality, for, indeed, they are; however, it does suggest that those who are more immersed in ongoing socialization with like-minded others through attendance at religious services and events are more likely to adhere to religious teachings regarding sexuality.

That said, it is unfortunate that there has not been more research interest in the relationship of specific religious *orientations* to nonmarital sexual attitudes and behavior. Haerich (1992) investigated the role of the I and E religious orientations in the sexual attitudes of about 200 undergraduate psychology students. Consistent with other research, Haerich found that lower church attendance and religiousness were (by self-report) weakly but significantly associated with more permissive attitudes toward nonmarital sexuality, as measured by a sexual permissiveness scale. Furthermore, permissive attitudes were negatively linked to I scale scores and positively associated with E scale scores, usually in the moderate .20 to .30 range. This is consistent with Woodroof's (1985) finding that extrinsically religious persons were more likely to be nonvirgins and to have had more sexual experience than intrinsically religious persons. Haerich interpreted these findings as indicating that greater commitment to religious institutions (high I scores) is associated with decreasing permissiveness, whereas people with a religious orientation that focuses on personal comfort and security (high E scores) will, in a similar manner, use sexual intimacy to contribute to their personal comfort and security. However, this interpretation must be considered speculative, pending further research. One study, for example, found that *both* I and E scores were linked with decreased sexual activity (Zaleski & Schiaffino, 2000).

Finally, it should be noted that more religious young people tend to be less knowledgeable about sexual issues. For example, adolescents reporting no religious affiliation were found to have the fewest misconceptions about condom use (Crosby & Yarber, 2001). Furthermore, women who are religious are less likely to use sexual and reproductive health services (Hall, Moreau, & Trussell, 2012). We need more research on how such misconceptions and/or lack of knowledge about sexuality may affect premarital sexual activity and the likelihood of premarital pregnancy or sexually transmitted diseases. Some authors (Zaleski & Schiaffino, 2000) have speculated that although religion helps to protect adolescents from initiating sexual activity, it does not seem to have a protective effect against practicing unsafe sex, at least among those who are already sexually active. Possibly this failure of religion to protect against unsafe sex is related to a fear among conservatives that education about safe sex implicitly communicates an endorsement of sexual activity outside the marriage relationship. It may also be that in some religious circles, sexuality is a taboo subject matter beyond the message of abstinence, even in families.

RELIGION AND NONMARITAL SEX: SUMMARY

There is little dispute about the consistent tendency for religion to be negatively related, albeit sometimes weakly, to nonmarital sexual attitudes and behaviors. However, it is also evident that the relationship is not as simple as was once thought, and future research needs to consider various issues: denominational differences in sexual standards and behavior; the importance of religious attendance; religious orientation; knowledge and misconceptions about sexuality; and gender.

Clergy Sexual Abuse

Clergy sexual abuse, especially in the Roman Catholic Church, has been a problem for centuries (Isley, 1997). In light of intense media coverage of the sexual abuse of children by priests, one might suspect that there is an abusing priest lurking in every parish. However, Sipe (1990, 1995) has estimated that just 2% of priests are pedophiles, and that possibly 4% would be classified as "ephebophiles" (those who reveal sexual attraction and behavior toward adolescents). Also, as these figures suggest, postpubescent adolescents are more likely to be abused than are prepubescent children (see Plante, 1999). Of course, even these small percentages translate into substantial numbers of abusing priests in the United States.

RESEARCH ON CLERGY ABUSE

The situation is too complicated to be explained by simple reference to mental disturbance or to a pattern of egocentric, immature, and narcissistic personality traits. For example, it has been pointed out that the clerical profession exposes clergy to sexual temptation—women or men who "fall in love" with their pastors, or parishioners who bare their most intimate problems to ministers, rabbis, or priests. Such actions make both the clergy and those who seek their help vulnerable to exploitation. Given such encounters, it may not come as a surprise that one study of 1,500 Catholic priests over a 25-year period indicated that about half had violated their celibacy vows (Schaffer, 1990). Other work reports that between 42 and 77% of women clergy claim that they have been sexually harassed or abused (see Culver, 1994; Fortune & Poling, 1994; Simpkinson, 1996). Though some estimates suggest that up to one-third of U.S. ministers admit to having engaged in sexual misconduct (Fortune & Poling, 1994), most work indicates that about 25% of pastors have had some kind of sexual involvement with a parishioner (Culver, 1994; Lebacqz & Barton, 1991). Actual intercourse rates between 10 and 15% have been reported (Culver, 1994). In the 1983–1993 decade, one concerned organization documented over 1,150 such incidents (Fortune & Poling, 1994).

Of course, in terms of the number of parishioners directly affected by clergy sexual advances, the percentages are much lower. According to the 2008 GSS (a survey with a nationally representative sample), 3.1% of women who attended religious services at least monthly reported a sexual advance by a clergy member since they turned 18 (Chaves & Garland, 2009).

It should be noted, however, that the considerable amount of unflattering attention given in recent years to the sexual misconduct of Roman Catholic clergy has led many to overestimate the pervasiveness of the problem. For example, the John Jay Report (John Jay College of Criminal Justice, 2004) has estimated that 4% of priests have sexually abused minors, and that this percentage is approximately the same as that found among clergy of other religious traditions and among others with unsupervised positions with children (e.g., coaches, Scout leaders, teachers). It is also slightly lower than that found among the general male population in the United States as a whole (Plante & Aldridge, 2004). Furthermore, despite what appears to be reported by the media, the victims of priest sexual abuse are not exclusively male. In fact, research suggests that female victims were purposefully targeted by priests at about the same rate as male victims (Terry & Frielich, 2012). Holt and Massey (2012) suggest that clergy abuse, Catholic or otherwise, appears to be more a function of opportunity than of targeting one gender or the other.

Efforts at psychologically characterizing clergy who perpetrate abuse have met with limited success, in part because of the variety of such abuse. These episodes can involve heterosexual or homosexual behavior and the mistreatment of children or adults. Among other possibilities, one scheme identifies what might be termed "passive/neurotic" perpetrators and "angry/impulsive" perpetrators (Camargo & Loftus, 1993). Another framework distinguishes six different types (Hands, 1992). Yet another attempt was based on the statistical technique of cluster analysis, and focused on Roman Catholic priests and brothers who had been identified as child sexual offenders (Falkenheim, Duckro, Hughes, Rosetti, & Gfeller, 1999). This investigation identified four clusters of abusers, which were labeled as follows by the authors: Sexually and Emotionally Underdeveloped; Significantly Psychiatrically Disturbed; Undefended Characterological; and Defended Characterological. Unfortunately, we still do not know how to recognize any of these types of clerics before they do damage.

The application of psychological and psychiatric labels to clergy sexual abuse has not proven particularly useful, for although such behavior is unacceptable, individual cases often involve many unique, sometimes tragic circumstances that would also influence average people. Furthermore, especially in cases involving abuse of children, many years may pass before complaints are lodged or legal action is taken. In such cases, issues of memory accuracy and the legitimacy of so-called "repressed memory" become important (see, e.g., Loftus & Guyer, 2002; Qin, Goodman, Bottoms, & Shaver, 1998).

CLERGY SEXUAL ABUSE: SUMMARY

In any profession, perfection is an unrealizable ideal. However, people frequently look to the clergy as ideal role models, forgetting that they are subject to the same stresses, problems, motives, and shortcomings as are parishioners and congregants themselves. Clergy, especially when celibacy is expected as part of their role, may experience considerable conflict over personal sexuality (Fones, Levine, Althof, & Risen, 1999). Perhaps better procedures are needed to select those who enter the religious professions; however, screening processes will undoubtedly contain a fair amount of error for some time to come. Psychological and character disorders will therefore persist in religious institutions. Little, however, can be done about such difficulties until they become evident, and the tragedy is that when they do come to light, there will be victims—clerics and laypersons alike.

Criminal Behavior and Delinquency

The literature on religion and crime rates is ambiguous and even somewhat contradictory; this is hardly surprising, once we consider a few points of clarification. Besides the complex issue of how religiousness or spirituality is defined and operationalized, there are equal ambiguities in defining and measuring criminal behavior. The term "criminal and delinquent behavior" covers considerable territory, some of which is discussed elsewhere in this chapter (such as clergy sexual abuse, serious cases of cheating/dishonesty, or illicit drug use). Also, there is sometimes confusion regarding where to draw a line between mental disorder and criminal behavior. Furthermore, crime statistics themselves may be unreliable. Definitions of crimes may vary from one jurisdiction to the next; some governments and police agencies may be more zealous in enforcing laws; and much crime surely goes unreported. Also, the methodological and statistical challenges in teasing out religion–delinquency relationships are considerable. In light of such problems, conflicting findings should be taken in stride.

Common-sense reasoning suggests that religious ties should be linked to decreased crime rates. Theoretical underpinnings of this expected inverse relationship can be traced back to Durkheim's (1915) emphasis on the social roots of religion, and particularly his social integration theory of religion's place in society. Durkheim felt that religion is integrally tied to the social order, playing an important role in legitimizing and reinforcing society's values and norms. Deviance may then stem from a breakdown in the church's role in this regard. Although the preponderance of studies do show a negative relationship, it tends to be weak to moderate and inconsistent. A review and meta-analysis of 60 investigations published from 1967 to 1998 led to the conclusion that in general, religious beliefs and behaviors were moderately negatively related to individuals' criminal behavior (Baier & Wright, 2001). However, it was noted that results varied, depending on the conceptual and methodological approaches in individual studies. This is an important point; operational definitions of crime and religion vary substantially across studies, as do samples, data collection techniques, statistical analyses, and controls for potentially confounding factors. It is not surprising that studies in this area generate conflicting results, given the tendency for "apples and oranges" to be thrown into the same bowl as if they are identical (see also Benda & Corwyn, 1997).

Furthermore, like the research on other moral issues discussed in this chapter, virtually all of the published studies on crime and religion are correlational, though it appears that many researchers assume (sometimes even slipping into causal language) that religion somehow prevents or reduces crime. However, it might also be true that those predisposed toward criminal behavior may be less inclined to attend church or see religion as important. Furthermore, much of this association may be attributable to social-environmental factors, such as a stable family environment or closeness to parents, rather than to religion itself (Benson, Donahue, & Erickson, 1989; Petts, 2009). Thus, even if the negative relationship between religion and criminal behavior is mediated by self-control, as has been shown to be the case (Pirutinsky, 2014), we cannot be sure that religiousness is the cause of less criminal behavior. In fact, higher self-control may be an important operating factor that leads to both higher religiousness and less offending (Pirutinsky, 2014).

In general, the negative relationship seems most likely to appear for "victimless activities" (e.g., the use/abuse of alcohol and drugs, fighting, consensual premarital sexual activity), rather than other delinquent behavior (Chadwick & Top, 1993), though some studies have also found religion to be related to a decreased likelihood of theft (Salas-Wright, Vaughn,

Hodge, & Perron, 2012) and violent attacks (Salas-Wright, Vaughn, & Maynard, 2014). People who are religious are also less likely to view white-collar crime as morally acceptable (Corcoran, Pettinicchio, & Robbins, 2012). Also, one study found that emerging adults who claimed to be "spiritual but not religious" were more likely to commit property crimes than those who were "religious," suggesting that the social control function of religion may play an important role (Jang & Franzen, 2013). Curiously, however, this research also found that the "spiritual but not religious" participants were also more likely to commit property crimes than those who were "neither religious nor spiritual."

It is important to go beyond simple correlational relationships, as indicated in research carried out by Peek, Curry, and Chalfant (1985). They found evidence that over time, higher delinquency rates appeared among students who declined in religiousness, compared to those who were low in religiousness throughout the same period. Such longitudinal trends may provide the basis for future investigations of adolescent delinquency.

We focus in the next section on one particular type of criminal behavior: domestic abuse.

Domestic Abuse

There has been increasing concern with the issue of domestic violence toward both spouses/partners and children. Some studies have focused on partner or child abuse that is apparently related to religious beliefs. Similar violence related to religion has been documented across cultures and through time, so we are not witnessing a phenomenon indigenous to our own time and social order (Girard, 1977). In the past, like clergy abuse, domestic abuse was often "hushed up"; people seemed to prefer to believe that it did not exist. Even today, because virtually all of the research is based on self-report that is subject to bias for many reasons (e.g., reluctance to admit to abuse, having heard overly positive or negative stories about one's childhood from parents or others, the power of suggestion), we cannot be sure how widespread the phenomenon is. Furthermore, exploratory research has even indicated that the *belief* that one was abused may be more important than *actual* abuse history in predicting some effects of abuse (Webb & Otto Whitmer, 2001).

Religious "Justification" for Abuse

Apparently religion may be seen by some people as "justifying" child or partner abuse, in the sense that it may encourage physical punishment of children or violence against one's partner (Capps, 1992, 1995; de Jonge, 1995; Greven, 1991; Kroeger & Beck, 1996; Volcano Press, 1995). These authors point to numerous Biblical passages, as well as books and articles written by religious authors that may be interpreted as encouraging the use of physical force, especially in disciplining children. It is argued that this could serve as a justification for various forms of abuse (e.g., "It is for the child's own good," "The man is the head of the household"). It should also be noted that these findings are not limited to Christianity. Similar patterns of scriptural interpretations or cultural norms have been pointed out in Islam (Ibrahim & Abdalla, 2010) and Judaism (Cares & Cusick, 2012). Furthermore, Bottoms, Shaver, Goodman, and Qin (1995) have suggested that religious beliefs can threaten the welfare of children in various ways, including the withholding of medical care and attempts to rid children of evil, as well as direct physical and psychological abuse that adults see as religiously justified. At the same time, religious institutions have usually taken strong positions against domestic abuse (Volcano Press, 1995), and current research suggests that religion is overall more of a protective factor against marital violence and child physical abuse than a factor facilitating such violence/abuse (Mahoney & Tarakeshwar, 2005).

Research on Religion and Domestic Abuse

Research in this area has generated unclear results because of such influencing factors as education, denial that abuse has taken place, reluctance to admit to having endured or perpetrated abuse, and differing definitions of abuse. For example, we might be tempted to conceive of domestic violence as only physical or sexual. But the Volcano Press (1995), for instance, has listed 98 forms of domestic abuse, including 29 that are considered physical, 16 sexual, 17 financial, 16 verbal, and 20 emotional. The research that has been carried out on this topic, however, has generally been confined to more straightforward operational definitions of "domestic abuse."

One summary of this literature indicated that those who attended church frequently were half as likely as infrequent attenders to experience physical violence themselves, or to use physical aggression against their partners (Mahoney, Pargament, Tarakeshwar, & Swank, 2001). Similarly, Ellison and Anderson (2001) found a negative relationship between church attendance and domestic violence (see also Ellison, Bartkowski, & Anderson, 1999; Wang, Horne, Levitt, & Klesges, 2009), and Lown and Vega (2001) reported that regular church attendance was associated with decreased physical abuse by a partner for Mexican American women. Brown, Cohen, Johnson, and Salzinger (1998), in a 17-year longitudinal study, found that children of regular church attenders were less than half as likely to suffer from physical abuse as were children of parents who rarely or never attended church. In a somewhat different vein, Makepeace (1987) found religion to be negatively associated with courtship violence among college students. A Canadian investigation of more than 1,000 adults reported that more frequent church attenders were the least violent (Brinkerhoff, Grandin, & Lupri, 1992). Initially, then, the research evidence seems to show a link between higher religiosity (generally speaking) and reduced domestic abuse or child physical abuse.

There have been suggestions that family abuse, generally speaking, has roots in the strong patriarchal family structure espoused by some conservative religions (Brinkerhoff et al., 1992). This patriarchal system is sometimes interpreted as justifying the subordination of women, particularly in terms of their subjection to powerful male authority (Clarke, 1986; Pagelow & Johnson, 1988), though some women may turn to religion as a source of personal empowerment in other ways (Ozorak, 1996; Wang et al., 2009). The problem may be confounded by some clergy, who counsel women to remain with abusive husbands because it is their religious duty and responsibility to stay with and obey their spouses (Alsdurf & Alsdurf, 1988); indeed, there is evidence that religious beliefs among evangelical Christian women may make them more reluctant to leave physically abusive husbands (Nason-Clark, 1997). Also, women from such patriarchal environments whose intimate partners have sexually abused their children may experience intense value conflict over the need to preserve the family, as well as their loyalty to both their abusive partners and their victimized children (Alaggia, 2001). This patriarchal issue may cross cultural boundaries. Higher levels of religiosity among Arab women in Israel were associated with the attitude that abused women should assume more personal responsibility for their husbands' violent behavior (Haj-Yahia, 2002).

Brinkerhoff et al. (1992) found that their hypothesis that more fundamentalist, conservative Protestants would be more abusive "because of the stereotypes surrounding their value of patriarchy" (p. 28) received mixed support. Conservative Protestant women, but not men, reported the highest rates of violence (37.8%), compared to mainline Protestants (28.1%), Catholics (23.9%), and nonaffiliated respondents (30.8%). It may be that a greater differential understanding or definition of abuse between the genders exists among conservative Protestants. Of course, such research is also subject to the biases already mentioned that are associated with self-reports. For example, gender differences might represent a self-serving bias or a reluctance to admit to abuse.

Consequences for the Victims of Abuse

Studies have shown that child sexual abuse has both religious and nonreligious consequences for those who are abused. Doxey, Jensen, and Jensen (1997) investigated more than 5,000 women, including more than 600 who reported being sexually abused when they were growing up. Those reporting abuse also reported higher rates of emotional and psychological problems (e.g., depression, lower self-esteem), as well as lower levels of religiousness. Bottoms, Nilesen, Murray, and Filipas (2003) found that although religion-related physical abuse is similar to non-religion-related physical abuse, abuse in the name of religion has significantly more negative implications for long-term psychological well-being. Pritt (1998) looked at the effects of sexual abuse on Mormon women and noted that it was spiritually disruptive. Among other things, such abuse created alienation from self and God, resulting in a sense of powerlessness and meaninglessness in a woman's life. The effects of domestic violence on children and women, especially when religiously justified, are profound and long-lasting (Volcano Press, 1995). A study of 1,207 male veterans reported that those who had a history of sexual abuse did report greater spiritual injury, but abuse was not related to an overall measure of current religious behavior (Lawson, Drebing, Berg, Vincellette, & Penk, 1998).

However, there are also indications that religion can help people to deal with the effects of domestic abuse, possibly through a mechanism such as social support (Coker et al., 2002; Wang et al., 2009). Elliott (1994) investigated child sexual abuse among almost 3,000 professional women. She could find no evidence that its prevalence was related to family religious affiliation, but there was a tendency for adult religious practices to mediate the severity of symptoms for those victimized as children. Similarly, Reinert and Smith (1997) found that their sample of women who had been sexually abused as children often looked to faith for support. Another investigation compared about 1,000 female teenagers who had been sexually abused to a sample of 1,000 female teenagers who had not been abused (Chandy, Blum, & Resnick, 1996). Results indicated that greater religiosity seemed to act as a protective factor against a variety of adverse outcomes. And Giesbrecht and Sevcik (2000) found that abused women from a conservative evangelical background could allow their faith either to engender shame and guilt or to provide a vehicle for hope and change. Studies such as this underline the potential of religion to help some adult survivors to cope with their earlier abuse.

Perceptions of Abuse

One's religious orientation is apparently linked to how one views partner abuse in others. Burris and Jackson (1999) experimentally varied scenarios depicting a woman who was abused by her boyfriend. They found that their undergraduate students' ratings of the abused woman and her abuser changed, depending on whether the woman was depicted as upholding or as violating religious values (see Research Box 12.3).

RESEARCH BOX 12.3. Hate the Sin/Love the Sinner, or Love the Hater?:
Intrinsic Religion and Responses to Partner Abuse (Burris & Jackson, 1999)

The authors of this study began by noting inconsistencies in the little research that exists on the relationship between religion and partner abuse. Past research, they pointed out, was limited by a possible social desirability bias (intrinsically religious people may be more prone to this bias and attempt to present themselves in a more positive light), crude measures of religiosity, and a failure to take contextual influences into account. They attempted to deal with all of these problems in their investigation of how an I religious orientation would be associated with reactions to the perpetrator and the victim of abuse, under different conditions.

Ninety undergraduate volunteers responded to the Allport–Ross I and E religious orientation scales, and were then randomly assigned to one of three conditions in which they read a vignette about a woman who was abused by her partner. The vignettes were mostly the same for all conditions, describing a situation where, after dating for 9 months, Rob asked Cheryl to marry him. She asked for a week to think about his proposal, after which they had dinner together at a restaurant. The vignettes diverged at this point. In one condition ("value-affirming"), Cheryl told Rob that their religious differences were too great; she "would not feel right about marrying outside of my faith" (p. 165), and therefore regretfully said no to his marriage proposal. In a second ("value-neutral") condition, Cheryl admitted that she did not think that she was in love with Rob, and therefore could not accept his proposal. In the final condition ("value-violating"), Cheryl said that the reason she could not marry Rob was that she needed time to resolve issues about her sexual orientation, especially her concern that she might be a lesbian. All vignettes ended with Rob throwing a glass of ice water in Cheryl's face and storming out of the restaurant, leaving Cheryl alone and crying.

Participants indicated their liking for both Cheryl and Rob on a 9-point response format, from "not at all" (1) to "very much" (9). A check indicated that after reading the vignette, all respondents did remember Cheryl's reason for turning down Rob's marriage proposal.

As expected, people with higher I scale scores tended to like the victim more when she based her decision to decline the marriage proposal on her religious values. However, when the victim (Cheryl) based her decision on value-violating concerns (that she might be a lesbian), those with higher I scores actually liked the abuse perpetrator (Rob) more. These relationships are especially interesting, because the perpetrator's behavior was identical in all conditions; the victim suffered precisely the same abuse in all conditions; and these two correlations were not found for any of the other conditions.

The authors reasoned that Cheryl's rationale for saying no to the marriage proposal gave more intrinsically religious persons a sort of contextual justification to express what otherwise would probably have been socially undesirable responses, in actually expressing liking for an abusive person. This rather subtle shift from loving the person who was abused to expressing more positive attitudes toward the abuser is disturbing, since it seems to fly in the face of intrinsically oriented individuals' "claim to endorse positive attitudes toward women and to reject many patriarchal beliefs.... The present research suggests that the commitment underlying their profession may be tenuous and undercut by other value commitments (e.g., 'family values'), however" (p. 171). The findings of this study are especially relevant to our discussion of partner abuse, because they might help to explain why victims of abuse do not always receive the expected love and sympathy from their religious group, and why sympathy for the perpetrator can sometimes override concern for the victim among religious persons.

Religion and Domestic Abuse: Summary

This is another area where it is difficult to come to firm conclusions, based on the relevant research. It is challenging to carry out research on domestic abuse for many reasons, such as potentially biased self-reports from respondents, difficulties in operationalizing concepts, lack of agreement regarding measures to be used, differential value systems in defining abuse, and so on. In spite of these problems, the most common finding has been a negative relationship between measures of religion and domestic violence. There is also some support for the claim that some domestic violence may seem to be justified by the patriarchal family structure found most often in fundamentalist or conservative religious groups. Also, victims of abuse can potentially suffer serious adverse effects for many years. Often victims become less religious, but there is evidence that religion can serve as a positive resource as well in their coping with abuse. Finally, some perpetrators of abuse may be viewed sympathetically, especially if "value violation" might have contributed to the abuse. In spite of these findings, this area of study is still in its infancy, with many research contradictions and anomalies to be resolved.

HELPING BEHAVIOR

"Help those in need." "Love one another." "Treat others as you would have them treat you." These are simple yet powerful imperatives, and similar themes are espoused by all of the world's major religions (Coward, 1986). Religion has been identified with humanity and community through such terms as "love," "justice," "compassion," "mercy," "grace," and "charity." The scriptural writings of most religions provide many examples of religious persons' being kind to and helping others in need; the New Testament story of the "good Samaritan" is a classic example. And even in contemporary society, religious organizations and individuals sometimes stand out in their efforts to assist others. Churches become involved in relief efforts to ease the effects of famines, earthquakes, wars, and other disasters. Religious groups organize and fund soup kitchens in cities large and small; they help refugees to escape from unbelievable horrors and to become established in a new land; they become actively involved as peacemakers in the world's "hot spots." Interviews with hundreds of people who rescued Jews in Nazi Europe revealed some who attributed their behavior to their religious values (Oliner & Oliner, 1988). The list of such religiously sponsored helping efforts is a long one.

Yet for many, "religion" apparently has little or nothing to do with their goodwill; present-day society offers unlimited opportunities to aid others in a secular context, and many people accept this challenge. Of course, this is why anecdotes are of little use in clarifying our understanding of the relationship between religion and helping behavior. Examples can be marshaled to show that both religious and nonreligious individuals and organizations assist others, and that they can also act with callous neglect when people cry out for assistance. Our challenge is to move beyond rhetoric and anecdotal material—to examine more general links between religion and helping, as revealed in the empirical literature.

For example, after an extensive review of the literature on prosociality, Norenzyan (2014) has concluded that religion does in fact influence moral behavior, largely due to perceptions of supernatural monitoring. He qualifies this finding, however, by pointing out that religion's connection with morality is culturally variable, and that prosociality evolved in various cultures independent of religion; hence he suggests that religion is not necessary for morality. Secular institutions, he argues, can serve the social monitoring functions of religion and thereby influence moral behavior. Still, however, whether religion is necessary or not, Norenzyan surmises that religion does a good job fulfilling this function. A growing body of research continues to suggest a complex connection between religion and helping behavior. Some would argue that the assumption of many that the more religious a person is, the more helpful he or she is toward others is at best only partially and indirectly supported—to the extent that the assumption itself is of little utility and should be disregarded (e.g., Galen, 2012). Others, however, contend that such conclusions are excessive and not well justified (Saroglou, 2012).

Research Findings

By now, as readers might guess, psychometric, methodological, and definitional issues are important in the study of helping behavior, just as they are in most areas of psychology. Norms for helping can differ across cultural or religious groups (e.g., Kanekar & Merchant, 2001). Also, in keeping with many psychological studies of religion generally, much research in this area relies on questionnaires, asking for self-reports of religiousness and helping behavior. This raises concerns about "self-presentation" issues. For example, religious persons may be concerned that they should appear to be good representatives of their faith, and therefore may be inclined to exaggerate the extent to which they help others. Fortunately, there are also some studies in this area that utilize behavioral measures, and these serve as an important counterbalance to the many questionnaire studies on helping.

Early Studies

Early survey studies in this area tended to rely on measures of frequency of church attendance as the primary measure of religiousness, with occasional forays into measures of such factors as belief in God, affiliation, or religious involvement. Assessment of "helping" typically involved self-reports (and occasionally others' reports) of one's inclination to assist others. These studies were fairly "primitive," in the sense that the measures of both religion and helping were quite simple and basic, and investigators merely looked for correlations between such general measures. These studies typically reported low to moderate positive correlations between religiousness and helping (Hunsberger & Platonow, 1986; Langford & Langford, 1974; Nelson & Dynes, 1976; Rokeach, 1969).

In contrast, early studies that incorporated actual behavioral measures found only limited evidence that religious people were necessarily more helpful than less religious or nonreligious people. In fact, Batson et al.'s (1993) review of six early studies employing behavioral measures (i.e., creatively putting people in a behavioral situation, not just asking them how they would hypothetically behave; examples included taking lost addressed letters to a mailbox, calling a garage for a stranded woman motorist without any money, and making a financial contribution to help a needy family) showed that five of the six found no evidence that more religious individuals were more helpful. Only one study showed any inclination for more religious individuals to be more likely to help than their less religious counterparts, and even this finding held only when the request came from a religious person. After reviewing these six studies, Batson et al. (1993) concluded that "this evidence strongly suggests that the more religious show no more active concern for others in need than do the less religious. The more religious only present themselves as more concerned" (p. 342).

More Recent Research

More recent research seems to confirm many of the early research findings, but also provides some new insights. Much of the newer research has looked at the broader construct of "prosocial character," which involves far more than just helping behavior; it has found clear associations between self-reported measures of religiousness and such prosocial characteristics as forgiveness (McCullough, Bono, & Root, 2005; Worthington, 2005), benevolence (Saroglou, Delpierre, & Dernelle, 2004), and agreeableness (Saroglou, 2002b). A meta-analysis (Saroglou et al., 2004) found that although the relationship between religiousness and prosocial personality traits and values is somewhat modest, it seems to exist across religions and cultures.

Once again, the vast majority of these studies rely on self-reports, which may be biased. However, one set of studies (Saroglou, Pichon, Trompette, Verschueren, & Dernelle, 2005) utilizing behavioral measures found that religiousness was indeed associated with prosociality, but with certain qualifications. These researchers conducted four studies and found that religiousness was accompanied by prosocial tendencies, including not engaging in indirect aggression in response to hypothetical daily hassles (Study 1) and being willing to help people who are known and close to them (Study 2). Studies 3 and 4 suggested that any self-reported altruistic behavior and empathy were not delusional, since peers also validated those self-reports. These results were found after the researchers controlled for such other possibilities that might explain the relationship, such as gender, honesty, social desirability bias, and attachment security; hence the relationship between religion and prosociality did not reflect these variables. However, the researchers pointed out that perhaps there are limits to the amount of prosociality (i.e., low-cost actions) related to religiousness, and that such tendencies are not necessarily extended to all people (especially if the people are not personally known).

Some early research suggested that the greater likelihood of helping among those more religious was limited to religion-related contexts (Nelson & Dynes, 1976). However, more recent investigations concluded that conservative Christians were more likely to report volunteering and giving in both religious and secular realms (Lam, 2002; Regnerus, Smith, & Sikkink, 1998; Uslaner, 2002). Furthermore, laboratory research involving economic games found that religiousness predicted cooperative behaviors in several cultures, including kibbutz members in Israel (Ruffle & Sosis, 2007), Christians in the United States (Anderson & Mellor, 2009), and Muslim students in India (Ahmed, 2009).

Dimensions of Religion and Helping

Most of the research discussed above did not take into account possible differences in helping tendencies associated with varying religious *orientations*. The reader is again reminded of Gordon Allport's two dimensions and accompanying measures of I and E religious orientations, introduced in Chapter 2 and mentioned earlier in this chapter. Briefly, the I orientation is intended to reflect what Allport (1950) called a "mature" religious sentiment—a motivation that arises from the goals set forth by the religious tradition itself. Religion is thus regarded as a *master motive* that overrides other needs, as compelling as they may be. In contrast, the E religious orientation is characterized by a utilitarian approach to religion—where religious beliefs, attitudes, and actions are endorsed to the extent that they aid in achieving other, less ultimate goals (both personal and social). One would expect that persons with an I orientation should be more helpful, since they tend to "live" their religion, and that persons with an E orientation should be less helpful, because their religion derives from self-interest. And, indeed, many investigations involving self-reports have revealed positive correlations between I scores and either helping others or professing values consistent with helping others (Benson et al., 1980; Bernt, 1989; Chau, Johnson, Bowers, Darvill, & Danko, 1990; Tate & Miller, 1971; Watson, Hood, Morris, & Hall, 1984; Watson, Hood, & Morris, 1985). Likewise, most of these studies found either negative or, more commonly, no correlations between E scores and helping-related values.

The evidence presented above suggests that more religious persons, especially more intrinsically religious individuals, tend to help others through their religious organizations in a variety of ways. Also, it would appear that I religiosity is positively but weakly related to an inclination to say that one helps others, and possibly the tendency actually to volunteer in a charitable context. There is some evidence that social desirability does not explain this relationship, though the relevant studies have relied to a large extent on self-reports. The situation is certainly not clear-cut, since the associations that have appeared tend to be weak, and they are not entirely consistent from one study to the next.

Quest as an Alternative Orientation

Batson and his colleagues have suggested that I religiousness relates positively only to the *appearance* of being more helpful (Batson, 1976, 1990; Batson, Floyd, Meyer, & Winner, 1999; Batson, Schoenrade, & Pych, 1985; Batson et al., 1993; Batson, Eidelman, Higley, & Russell, 2001), since that is what virtually all religious traditions teach. They proposed that a measure of the Quest (Q) dimension—a flexible, questioning approach to religion—might be the most direct predictor of actual helping behavior. Defined as "the degree to which an individual's religion involves an open-ended, responsive dialogue with existential question raised by the contradictions and tragedies of life" (Batson et al., 1993, p. 169), Batson developed the notion of Q from those neglected elements of Allport's (1950) original conceptualization of the mature religious sentiment. It frequently happens, when a researcher is attempting to construct a measure of a complex concept, that certain dimensions or elements of the concept are lost. This, Batson and colleagues argued, is precisely what happened when religious maturity became operationalized for measurement purposes into the I scale. The neglected elements included the recognition, and even appreciation, of the complexity of issues involved; openness to the possibility of change in religious beliefs; and ascription of a positive role to doubt.

As we know from Chapter 2, for the Q dimension to be scientifically studied, it was necessary to develop a reliable and valid measure. An early version of a Q Scale was criticized on psychometric grounds (see, e.g., Altemeyer, 1996). Batson and Schoenrade (1991a, 1991b) subsequently developed a 12-item revised Q Scale that addressed the earlier problems, and that generated Cronbach's alphas of .81 and .75 (reasonably acceptable internal-consistency scores indicating adequate reliability of the measure) in two samples. Other Q measures have also been developed (e.g., Altemeyer & Hunsberger, 1992; alpha = .88). We must be careful, however, in comparing such measures; there is little item overlap, and it is not clear to what extent different scales might tap different conceptualizations of Q. Batson's 12-item revised Q Scale has become the instrument of choice in much related research.

We spend some time here looking at Batson's research program, which stresses behavioral measures of helping rather than self-report measures. However, it should be noted that questions about the conceptual and methodological underpinnings of Q have been raised (e.g., Donahue, 1985), and that some of Batson's interpretations of results of the relationship of religious orientations to helping behavior and to prejudice (which we review later in this chapter) have been challenged.

Altruism or Egoism?

An early behavioral study in this area attempted to place the parable of the good Samaritan in an experimental context (Darley & Batson, 1973; see Research Box 12.4). Essentially, this experiment revealed no tendency for scores on religion as a *means* (similar to E), religion as an *end* (similar to I), or Q to be related to helping behavior. Darley and Batson (1973) concluded that among those who did not offer to help, the more orthodox intrinsically oriented persons might be helping for their own reasons, instead of being sensitive to those needing aid. Additional studies conducted by Batson and his colleagues (Batson et al., 1989; Batson & Gray, 1981; Batson & Flory, 1990) have pursued the "altruism versus egoism" issue concerning underlying motivation for helping by people with different religious orientations. The findings of these studies provide further support that for those who score high on Q, providing assistance is generated a concern for the victim's welfare. Those with an I orientation seem motivated primarily by a personal need to appear helpful.

This interpretation has been challenged (Gorsuch, 1988; Watson, 1993; Watson et al., 1985). Possibly those with higher Q scores helped "tentatively" because they really weren't very committed to helping in the first place, and the more assertive assistance of those with higher I scores reflected more genuine caring and concern on their part. Furthermore, we may wonder about the generalizability of findings from the relatively homogeneous and religious sample of seminary students.

Intrinsic and Quest Religion as a Source of Universal Compassion?

There is considerable discussion in the research literature about the extent to which the association of religion with prosociality is limited to like-minded individuals (e.g., other people of the same religion). Such findings may reflect a human tendency, whether religious or not, to favor those who are like us rather than different from us. For example, Ruffle and Sosis (2006) found that members of an Israeli kibbutz were more likely to cooperate with other kibbutz members than with city residents. There are also research findings that suggest that when primed with religious words or when studied in a religious context, people engage in more prosocial behaviors, such as being more generous (Ahmed & Salas, 2011; Pichon & Saroglou, 2009), more willing to volunteer (Pichon, Boccato, & Saroglou, 2007), more willing to help an ailing person (K. A. Johnson, Memon, Alladin, Cohen, & Okun, 2015), and more willing to forgive (Saroglou, Corneille, & Van Cappellen, 2009). However, some research suggests that the connection between religion and prosocial behaviors appears stronger when the beneficiaries are members of ingroups (such as others of the same faith tradition) rather than various outgroups (M. K. Johnson, Rowatt, & LaBouff, 2012; LaBouff, Rowatt, Johnson, & Finkle, 2012; Pichon & Saroglou, 2009; Saroglou, 2013), though other studies (e.g., K. A. Johnson, Memon, et al., 2015) have not found this distinction. One study (Preston & Ritter, 2013) discovered that the words that are used to prime religious thoughts matter. They found that the word "religion" primed prosociality to ingroups, while the word "God" primed prosociality to outgroups as well.

RESEARCH BOX 12.4. Situational and Dispositional Variables in Helping Behavior
(Darley & Batson, 1973)

In the parable of the good Samaritan, Jesus described a man who was robbed, beaten, and left for dead at the side of the road. Two "religious" individuals, a priest and a Levite, passed by but did not stop to help. However, a Samaritan (a religious outcast), at some cost to himself, gave the robbery victim the help he needed. Jesus apparently wanted to make the point that people should model their behavior after the Samaritan, not after "religious" people who may be so caught up in their thoughts that they do not see the needs of people around them.

Would the results differ if this situation were to occur in contemporary society? Darley and Batson attempted to construct a similar "help-needed" situation at Princeton University. Sixty-seven seminary students first completed questionnaires to assess their religious orientation, among other things. Then, one at a time, 40 of them showed up for a follow-up experimental session. They were asked to prepare a short talk based on either (1) the parable of the good Samaritan, or (2) jobs that seminary students might pursue. After having a few minutes to prepare for their forthcoming talk, participants were given a map to show them how to get to a room in another building where they would give their talk. Half of the participants were told that they would need to hurry, since they were late for their appointment.

As these students passed down an alley, they met a man who clearly seemed to be in need of help. A confederate of the experimenters was slumped in a doorway, head down, eyes closed, not moving. As each seminarian passed, the victim coughed and groaned; given the geographical setting, it was virtually impossible to miss him. The key dependent measure in this study was whether or not the students stopped to offer any kind of help. In fact, just 16 of the 40 seminarians (40%) offered assistance. And religious orientation scores—Means (similar to E), End (similar to I), or Q—did not predict who would stop to offer aid.

However, among those who did stop, an interesting finding emerged. When a seminarian offered help, the victim indicated that he had just taken his medication, he would be fine if he just rested a few minutes, and he would like to be left alone. Some of the "good Samaritans" were quite insistent, however. In spite of the victim's objections, some participants insisted on taking him into a nearby building and pouring some coffee and/or religion into him. Among only those who did stop to help, scores on the I measure correlated positively with this "I know what is best for you" helping style ($r = .43$), but scores on the Q measure were negatively associated with such insistent aid ($r = -.54$). Darley and Batson concluded that the more I-oriented seminarians seemed to be guided by a "preprogrammed" helping response, which was not affected by the expressed needs of the victim. It was almost as if the "super helpers" were satisfying their own internal need to help, rather than meeting the needs of the victim. However, those with a Q orientation had a more tentative helping style, sensitive to the person needing help, since they tended to accept the victim's statement that he really just wanted to be left alone and everything would be fine.

Before we leave our consideration of this study, there are some loose ends to tie up. Contrary to expectations, it did not make any difference whether the participant was preparing to give a speech on the parable of the good Samaritan or on jobs for seminary graduates. Apparently, thinking about helping in a Biblical context did not make participants more likely to offer aid in a similar situation. Finally, those participants in the "hurry up, you're late" condition were significantly less likely to stop and offer any kind of help than were those with no "hurry up" instructions. Apparently, the most powerful variable in determining helping behavior overall in this study was a nonreligious one—whether or not the participant was in a hurry.

Let's explore this tendency to favor religious ingroups more by considering the role of religious orientation. Batson et al. (1999, 2001) carried out two studies to investigate more thoroughly the role of the I and Q religious orientations in helping behavior—specifically, when a target person's behavior violated or threatened one's values (e.g., the person was a homosexual). These studies suggested that a high Q orientation—but not a high I orientation—was associated with broadly based compassion. Their investigations overlap two foci of this chapter (helping and prejudice) and are included here because they speak directly to the underlying motivation of religious people's helping behavior. Specifically, these authors investigated people's inclination to help, depending on the extent to which helping might violate their values. An I orientation was found to be associated with *less* help being offered for people who violated values. That is, intrinsically religious people's antipathy was not limited to value violators' (sinful) behavior, but was apparently directed at the value-violating person as well (i.e., the sinner). High Q scores, on the other hand, were associated with less help being offered to aid value-violating behavior, but there was not greater antipathy toward the value-violating person (the sinner).

Findings from a subsequent study (Mak & Tsang, 2008) were inconsistent with those found by Batson and his colleagues. They found in a behavioral study (i.e., not relying exclusively on self-reports) of 100 females at a religiously based university that those with high I scores were just as likely to help a self-disclosed gay person as much as they would help a straight person. However, regardless of the target person's sexual orientation (gay or straight), the high-I participants were less likely to help if the person was sexually promiscuous (a value-violating behavior). The authors concluded: "High intrinsic scores seemed to be related to antipathy toward the value-violation, but not toward the gay person as an individual" (p. 379). We return to this issue later in this chapter.

Furthermore, Goldfried and Miner (2002) attempted to replicate and extend Batson et al.'s (2001) work, but were led to a rather different conclusion. The "target" for helping/prejudice in Goldfried and Miner's study was a "religious fundamentalist" rather than the "gay person" targeted by Batson et al. (2001). Goldfried and Miner concluded that the Q orientation is not indicative of a universally compassionate religious style. Rather, even those with a Q orientation demonstrated discrimination against (i.e., a lesser tendency to help) someone with a different value system (here, a "religious fundamentalist"). Of particular interest is the fact that the questers' self-reports did not reflect negative opinions of the fundamentalists. Hence, even questers may demonstrate the desire to *appear* to adhere to their set of values (e.g., "open-minded") more than they actually do, similar to what Batson and his colleagues documented among intrinsically religious persons.

However, Batson, Denton, and Vollmecke (2008) replicated the Goldfried and Miner study with some important methodological differences: They restricted their study to U.S. Christians with at least a moderate interest in religion (Goldfried and Miner studied Australian students and did not limit their sample by religion or interest level) and used what they argued to be a better Q measure. They found that those Christians scoring high on Q helped someone who endorsed fundamentalist beliefs (again, the "target" person was a religious fundamentalist) as much as a nonfundamentalist, unless such help would promote closed-minded fundamentalist religion. Thus the researchers concluded that questers do extend compassion to those who violate their own values of religious open-mindedness, but not to the point that it might help promote a violation of dearly held values.

Jackson and Esses (1997) also investigated the extent to which religious orientation was related to helping behavior under different value-threatening circumstances, but focused on religious fundamentalism (abbreviated from here on in this chapter as RF)—defined as an inflexible belief that one's religious beliefs represent absolute truth that must be followed—rather than the I, E, and Q religious orientations. They found that when someone needed help and that person was a "moral violator" (e.g., a homosexual), religious fundamentalists advocated personal change rather than other forms of helping. When the persons seeking help did not violate their value system (e.g., Native Canadians, single mothers, students), the high-RF respondents were just likely to give direct help or to do what they could to empower the individuals to help themselves as to provide advice. Whether this tendency is unique to fundamentalists awaits additional research.

Religion and Helping Behavior: Summary

The study of religion and helping behavior is especially interesting because of the availability of both self-report questionnaires and investigations of actual and anticipated behavior. Furthermore, few areas have seen extensive use of theory accompanied by a systematic research program, such as that provided by Batson and his coworkers. Not all research supports Batson et al.'s conclusions that I religion is related to the *appearance* of helping, and that the assistance provided by such individuals is likely to be a preprogrammed, self-serving type of aid (Mak & Tsang, 2008; Saroglou et al., 2005). Nor is there complete support of the finding that the Q orientation is a good predictor of *actual* (behavioral) helping, and that Q-based assistance is motivated by the needs of others—a source of universal compassion (Goldfried & Miner, 2002; see also Gorsuch, 1988; Watson et al., 1984)—though Batson et al. (2008) have attempted to provide additional support. Also, Jackson and Esses (1997) have given us much to think about in their unique investigations of religion and helping. Apparently RF scores predict a tendency to attribute personal causes for need, at least to value-threatening groups. Perhaps all people, whether their orientation is I, E, Q, RF, or nonreligious, are subject to biases as defined by their own value systems—a general human tendency well documented by social psychologists.

We might also wonder whether their religious values could be used in a more positive way. Values not only serve as a potential source of threat; they may also provide a means of increasing helping behavior for religious persons. Could a direct appeal to religious values increase helping behavior—for example, by increasing perceived personal moral obligation to help among religious persons? One study suggests that such an approach might be productive, at least in the context of blood donations as helping behavior (Ortberg, Gorsuch, & Kim, 2001).

PREJUDICE, DISCRIMINATION, AND STEREOTYPING

Since most world religions espouse a common theme of "love one another," it might be expected that this teaching would have a powerful effect in reducing prejudice among the members of these religions. But research has not always supported this generalization. In fact, there is a considerable amount of research showing that as a broad generalization, the more religious an individual is, the more prejudiced that person is (Batson et al., 1993; Dittes, 1969; Gorsuch & Aleshire, 1974; Meadow & Kahoe, 1984; Myers & Spencer, 2001; Paloutzian, 1996; Spilka, Hood, & Gorsuch, 1985). However, the generalization that religion is positively correlated with prejudice is more complex than it might first appear. In fact, there are important qualifiers that must be considered—such that any broad conclusive statement about the relationship between religion and prejudice is an oversimplification, and therefore not particularly helpful.

The religion–prejudice link has a long history. It dates at least to the late 1940s, when Adorno, Frenkel-Brunswik, Levinson, and Sanford's (1950) famous studies of the authoritarian personality disclosed a positive association between religion and prejudice. In reviewing the work on religion and prejudice, we do not offer an exhaustive review of the vast literature that has accumulated in the area. Rather, we attempt to summarize different stages in the development of our understanding of the religion–prejudice relationship. We ultimately focus on promising developments that have occurred in the past few decades, involving the RF and Q orientations, right-wing authoritarianism (RWA), and intergroup conflict perspectives.

Does Religious Orientation Make a Difference?

Much of the research, especially the early research on religion and prejudice, did not take religious *orientation* into account. Some of the initial work was conducted before the conceptualization and measurement of various personal religious orientations began in the mid-1960s and later. Allport and Ross (1967) addressed this issue head-on when they published their famous article outlining the formulation of the I and E religious orientations, as well as the scales developed to measure the concepts, since this work was done in the context of their study of prejudice. Ultimately, Allport and Ross concluded that persons with an I orientation were, as expected, less prejudiced than those with an E orientation, who in turn were less prejudiced than those with an "indiscriminately pro" (IP) orientation (i.e., those who scored high on both the I and E scales). This finding concerning prejudice levels (i.e., I < E < IP) has become firmly embedded in the literature (see, e.g., Gorsuch, 1988; Hunsberger & Jackson, 2005). However, as several researchers (e.g., Donahue, 1985; Kirkpatrick & Hood, 1990; Laythe, Finkel, & Kirkpatrick, 2001) have pointed out, there were numerous problems with the original I and E concepts and scales as presented by Allport and Ross (1967).

Furthermore, just as we have discussed in the section on helping behavior, high-I persons may only *appear* to be less prejudiced. Batson et al. (1993) suggested that a measure of social desirability and the I orientation were positively correlated, making it difficult to assess the real relationship between I and prejudice. Batson, Naifeh, and Pate (1978) reported a correlation in one study between I scores and social desirability (.36), whereas other authors have been unable to find a significant relationship in this regard (e.g., Hunsberger & Platonow, 1986; Spilka, Kojetin, & McIntosh, 1985) or have reported a significant but very low correlation (.12; Duck & Hunsberger, 1999). Batson, Flink, Schoenrade, Fultz, and Pych (1986) and Batson et al. (1978) reported that I scores were negatively correlated with overt prejudice, but this relationship was not apparent when the effects of social desirability were controlled for, or when a covert behavioral measure of prejudice was used. E scores were unrelated to all measures of prejudice.

However, two other studies (Duck & Hunsberger, 1999; Morris, Hood, & Watson, 1989) found that controlling for social desirability did not change prejudice–religion relationships. Furthermore, it has been argued (Watson, Morris, Foster, & Hood, 1986) that weak positive correlations between I scores (or scores on a similar religiousness dimension) and social desirability are unique to the Crowne–Marlowe Social Desirability Scale (Crowne & Marlowe, 1964—the measure used by Batson et al., 1978, and Duck & Hunsberger, 1999). That is, such correlations are not a result of social desirability, but appear because the Crowne–Marlowe Social Desirability Scale "has a substantial number of items confounded by a religious relevance dimension" (Watson et al., 1986, p. 230). However, Leak and Fish (1989) have challenged Watson et al.'s conclusions in this regard. The reader will understand why these discrepancies make it difficult to come to firm conclusions regarding the role of social desirability in the relationship between I religiousness and prejudice.

Measures of the Q orientation have been found to correlate significantly with measures of prejudice. Batson et al. (1993) cited five studies that revealed significant negative relationships between Q scores and prejudice (Batson et al., 1978, 1986; McFarland, 1989, 1990; Snook & Gorsuch, 1985). Two other studies (Griffin, Gorsuch, & Davis, 1987; Ponton & Gorsuch, 1988) did not replicate this negative association. However, all of these studies apparently used the earlier, psychometrically weaker version of Batson's Q Scale (Batson & Ventis, 1982).

Subsequent research using Batson and Schoenrade's (1991a, 1991b) revised Q Scale have sometimes replicated the significant negative associations between Q and intolerance (Duck & Hunsberger, 1999), as did research by Altemeyer and Hunsberger (1992) with their own Q measure. Similarly, the research on helping (Batson et al., 1999, 2001) discussed earlier in this chapter seems to support the link between Q and tolerance. However, still other investigations (often with different Q measures) have obtained rather mixed results (Fisher, Derison, Polley, Cadman, & Johnston, 1994; Fulton, Gorsuch, & Maynard, 1999; Jackson & Hunsberger, 1999; Kirkpatrick, 1993).

The relationship between prejudice and the I–E dichotomy as well as Q is at best tenuous and difficult to interpret. At times it seems that the I–E distinction, which was intended to help us understand Allport's paradoxical assertion that religion both makes (the E religious orientation) and unmakes (the I religious orientation) prejudice, has instead led us into a psychometric and empirical morass of confusion. Certainly, not all authors agree with this rather bleak assessment of the research on I–E religiosity and prejudice, and some see more potential for these concepts in the future. Studies focusing on the I–E orientations continue to appear regularly in the literature, and many other I–E scales have been developed that are improvements on the original Allport and Ross (1967) scales (see Hill & Hood, 1999a). However, other approaches to religious orientation may offer more promise in explaining the religion–prejudice connection.

Values and Prejudice: Attitudes toward Homosexuality

It seems logical that for religious people, the stand of their church on issues of prejudice would have some effect on their own attitudes and behavior. However, it has been noted that the existing research on religion and prejudice rarely considers the potential impact of the formal or informal stance of one's religious group on such issues (Batson & Burris, 1994; Hood, Hill, & Williamson, 2005; Rosik, 2007a, 2007b; Watson, 1993). There may be situations in which a religious group does not attempt to negate prejudice, especially if the objects of prejudice are people who represent a threat to religious values; this is sometimes referred to as "nonproscribed prejudice." For example, a growing body of research (e.g., Cragun, Kosmin, Keysar, Hammer, & Nielsen, 2012: Gervais, Shariff, & Norenzayan, 2011) suggests that atheists are often objects of prejudice. In such cases, the same religious (e.g., high-I) persons will be likely to admit to their prejudice because it is sanctioned by their religion. To discuss the distinction between "proscribed" (forbidden) and "nonproscribed" (not forbidden) prejudice further, we focus on the topic of attitudes toward homosexuality.

Factors Associated with Prejudice against Homosexuals

Numerous authors have suggested that racial prejudice is now generally proscribed by main-line North American Christian churches, but that prejudice against homosexuals (at least among religious conservatives) is not forbidden. Certainly the link between religion and negative attitudes toward homosexuality is well established (e.g., Finlay & Walther, 2003; Fisher, Derison, et al., 1994; Gentry, 1987; Herek, 1988; Kunkel & Temple, 1992; Marsiglio, 1993; VanderStoep & Green, 1988; Whitley, 2009). Unfortunately, until fairly recently, few studies on religion and homosexuality have attempted to assess the proscribed–nonproscribed distinction. Duck and Hunsberger (1999) examined this issue by asking undergraduate students directly about church teachings related to prejudice. Their results indicated that, as predicted by Batson and his colleagues, racial prejudice was typically proscribed by students' religious groups, but intolerance toward gay men and lesbians was generally not proscribed. Furthermore, they found that I scores were negatively related to proscribed prejudice (racism), but positively associated with nonproscribed prejudice (negative attitudes toward homosexuals), in two separate studies. Also, as predicted, Q scores were negatively correlated with both proscribed and nonproscribed prejudice (although one of the four correlations was not statistically significant).

Other studies (Finlay & Walther, 2003; Fisher, Derison, et al., 1994) have documented that more frequent church attenders, as well as those who belong to more conservative denominations, are more likely to report prejudice against homosexual individuals. Within a pluralistic society, fundamentalists maintain their sectarian nature by deliberately utilizing both religious and sectarian means to maintain the boundaries of their beliefs that are functional for their way of life (Hood et al., 2005). For instance, several studies have shown that fundamentalists vote as a meaningful bloc only when candidates take significantly different stands on issues crucial to fundamentalists' beliefs. In these instances, fundamentalists vote in a manner congruent with what has been called "boundary maintenance" (Hood, Morris, & Watson, 1985, 1986). Thus fundamentalists within Protestantism attempt to maintain a tradition in the face of broader cultural changes that threaten their beliefs. In this sense, proscribed beliefs are integral to maintaining the boundaries of the faith. Proscribed behaviors and boundary maintenance among fundamentalists are widely recognized in other traditions, including Islam, despite their originally being described as North American phenomena (Marty & Appleby, 1991).

Further support for the connection between religion and nonproscribed sexual prejudice, especially among people with an I religious orientation, is found in recent research on sexual prejudice as an implicit attitude. As a reminder from material covered in Chapter 2, implicit attitudes are automatic, unconscious evaluations that have influence on thoughts, feelings, and behaviors (Greenwald & Banaji, 1995; Greenwald, McGhee, & Schwartz, 1998). Tsang and Rowatt (2007; see also Rowatt, Tsang, et al., 2006) used the most common measure of implicit attitudes, the Implicit Association Test (IAT), as a measure of sexual prejudice; they found that an I (but not E or Q) religious orientation among college students at a religious university was positively associated with implicit sexual prejudice, even when RWA was controlled for. In contrast, another study of students at the same university (again using the IAT) found that Christian orthodoxy was negatively related to implicit racism (Rowatt & Franklin, 2004). However, religious orientation (I, E, Q) was not related to implicit racism. Also, Rowatt, Franklin, and Cotton (2005) found that Christian orthodoxy and self-reported positive attitudes toward Christianity, but not religious orientation (I, E, Q) or other personality variables such as RF or RWA, predicted implicit preference for Christians over Muslims. This line of research suggests that a nonproscribed attitude, such as that toward homosexuality, is an internalized implicit component in I religion—something not found in proscribed attitudes, even when measured implicitly, such as racism or religious identity.

The studies just described all involved measures of implicit prejudice in relation to self-reports of religiousness or spirituality. However, LaBouff et al. (2010) have carried this line of research one step further by developing a validated implicit measure of religiousness or spirituality. They found that their measure was able to predict self-reported attitudes toward gay men and lesbians over and above self-reported measures of RF and RWA (two important characteristics in relation to prejudice that we discuss more fully later).

Distinguishing between the Behavior and the Person ("Sin" and "Sinner")

With regard to sexual orientation, it is common among some religious people to claim that they make a distinction between homosexual behavior ("sin") and homosexual individuals ("sinners"). In so doing, they claim that they disapprove of the behavior only, and not of the individuals who engage in the behavior. Fulton et al. (1999) reported some support for the distinction between sin and sinner from an investigation of students at a conservative Christian college with a Seventh-Day Adventist affiliation. The researchers attempted to categorize negative attitudes toward gays and lesbians into morally rationalized (sin) and nonmorally rationalized (sinner) groups. Examples of items representing these two categories are "Homosexuality is a perversion," and "A person's homosexuality should not be a cause for job discrimination," respectively (Fulton et al., 1999, p. 17). The authors found that the I orientation in particular was correlated with morally rationalized but not nonmorally rationalized antipathy: The researchers concluded that "Intrinsics appear to be relatively accepting of homosexual people, but not of homosexual behavior" (p. 19). It should be noted that this study was limited by the unique and homogeneous nature of the sample, and the use of an unpublished measure of religiousness (thus we do not know how it compares to other measures of this concept).

Other studies that speak to this issue have provided mixed results. Altemeyer and Hunsberger (1993) pointed out that religiousness was associated with condemnation of both sin and sinner on an item-by-item basis in their study of attitudes toward gay persons. Research by Batson et al. (1999, 2001), discussed earlier in this chapter in the "Helping Behavior" section, led to the conclusion that high-I individuals do *not* distinguish between sin and sinner. Batson et al. (1999) conducted a behavioral study and found that religiously devout (high-I) university students were less willing to offer a monetary prize to a homosexual person (relative to a heterosexual person), regardless of how the prize money would be used (to visit grandparents or to attend a gay pride rally). The researchers concluded that those with an I religious orientation had a general antipathy toward gays and lesbians, regardless of behavior.

However, to date, more studies appear to support the conclusion drawn by Fulton et al. (1999). Bassett et al. (2000, 2002) have provided evidence from samples of Christian college students that the distinction between homosexual persons and behavior is made by high-I individuals. The 2002 study is particularly noteworthy, in that it was a conceptual (and with some exceptions, a methodological) replication of the Batson et al. (1999) study. This team of researchers found that high-I individuals (defined by using the same cutoff on the I scale as that used by Batson et al.) made a value distinction between behavior and persons. In a later study (Bassett, van Nikkelen-Kuyper, et al., 2005), Christian college students who were either uniformly accepting or rejecting of both homosexual persons and homosexual behavior were exposed to psychological and spiritual interventions that purposed to help students more clearly value homosexual persons. The researchers found that the intervention improved attitudes toward homosexual persons and, for the uniformly negative students (i.e., those with negative attitudes toward both the gay persons and gay behavior), to homosexual behavior as well. Ironically, the intervention diminished the acceptance of homosexual behavior among those students who were initially accepting. The fact that the Bassett et al. studies involved rather homogeneous samples of Christian college students (though, again, in the one replication study, they used the same cutoff values on their measure of religious orientations as did the Batson et al. study being replicated) may have influenced the results.

Finally, the reader is reminded of the Mak and Tsang (2008) study reviewed earlier (again, see the "Helping Behavior" section), which showed that high-I participants would help a self-disclosed gay person as much as a straight person, but not when the targeted person (whether gay or straight) revealed that she was also sexually promiscuous. Again, this suggests that intrinsically religious persons make the distinction between value-violating behavior and the person who engages in that behavior.

Researchers are beginning to unpack the sin–sinner issue. What appeared to be a major predictor is less so: the distinction among the traditional I, E, and Q religious orientations. Perhaps there are other ways of assessing religious orientation that are more productive in explaining religion's link with prejudice. Of particular interest is the concept of RF.

Religious Fundamentalism and Prejudice

Early in the 20th century, William James (1902/1985) anticipated the importance of going beyond the content or orthodoxy of a person's beliefs. He argued that a rigid, dogmatic style of religious belief might be associated with bigotry and prejudice. Over the years, some investigators have used the term "religious fundamentalism" (RF) to capture this rigid, dogmatic way of being religious. However, the definition of this term was quite variable, and often did not correspond to *religious* use of the word. In fact, early researchers often used the term interchangeably with "orthodoxy of belief," "intense interest in religion," or "considerable religious involvement." Today, some researchers (but, unfortunately, not all) try to distinguish RF from other forms of religiousness.

Not surprisingly, a positive relationship between RF and prejudice has been documented in a number of studies (e.g., Altemeyer, 2003; Fulton et al., 1999; Hunsberger, Owusu, & Duck, 1999; Jackson & Esses, 1997; M. K. Johnson, Rowatt, LaBouff, Patock-Peckham, & Carlisle, 2012; Kirkpatrick, 1993; Laythe et al., 2001; Rowatt, LaBouff, Johnson, Froese, & Tsang, 2009). There has now been enough research on RF and prejudice that meta-analyses have now been conducted with regard to racism (Hall, Matz, & Wood, 2010); homosexuality (Whitley, 2009); and a number of psychological characteristics, such as authoritarianism, ethnocentrism, and various forms of prejudice (including racism and homosexuality) (McCleary, Quillivan, Foster, & Williams, 2011). The general conclusion that can be drawn from these meta-analyses is that the association of RF with racial prejudice is positive, but small (Rowatt, Shen, LaBouff, & Gonzalez, 2013). The relationship between RF and negative attitudes toward gay men and lesbians found by Whitley (2009) appears stronger (see Rowatt et al., 2013, for a more detailed description of these meta-analytic studies). As we note shortly, these findings must take into account the relationship of RF with RWA. Much of this research has utilized a scale developed by Altemeyer and Hunsberger (1992; see Research Box 12.5). To unpack this relationship further, we must consider how RF is conceptualized.

RESEARCH BOX 12.5. Authoritarianism, Religious Fundamentalism, Quest, and Prejudice (Altemeyer & Hunsberger, 1992)

Based on their conceptualization of RF (see the text), the authors developed a 20-item RF Scale, including items such as "God will punish most severely those who abandon his true religion." They developed this measure, as well as a 16-item Q measure, in several studies of university students in Manitoba and Ontario. Satisfied that their new measures were reliable and interrelated as expected among students, the authors then carried out an investigation of 491 Canadian parents of university students.

In addition to the RF and Q instruments, these adults completed a 12-item Attitudes Toward Homosexuals scale (e.g., "In many ways, the AIDS disease currently killing homosexuals is just what they deserve"); a 20-item Prejudice scale (e.g., "It is a waste of time to train certain races for good jobs; they simply don't have the drive and determination it takes to learn a complicated skill"); the RWA measure; and two additional measures of prejudice—a Posse–Radicals survey (in which participants indicated the extent to which they would pursue radicals outlawed by the government), and a Trials measure (in which respondents "passed sentence" in three court cases involving a dope pusher, a pornographer, and someone who spit on a Canadian provincial premier). The resulting web of relatively strong and significant correlations led these authors to conclude the following about the answer to the question "Are religious persons usually good persons?":

> [It] appears to be "no," if one means by "religious" a fundamentalist, nonquesting religious orientation, and by "good" the kind of nonprejudiced, compassionate, accepting attitudes espoused in the Gospels and other writings. But the answer is "yes" if one means by "religious" the nonfundamentalist, questing orientation found most often in persons belonging to no religion. Which irony gives one pause. (pp. 125–126)

The authors cautioned against overgeneralizing these findings, since there were inevitably exceptions to the rule—people scoring high on RF and low on Q who showed nonprejudiced, accepting attitudes; or people scoring low on RF and high on Q who were bigoted. But the correlations that emerged were quite strong and clear-cut. Apparently individuals who scored high on RF and low on Q, as defined here, tended to be prejudiced in a variety of ways. The authors speculated that fundamentalist beliefs can be linked to some of the psychological sources of authoritarian aggression (e.g., fear of a dangerous world and self-righteousness), as well as the tendency for high-RWA individuals to reduce guilt over their own misdeeds through their religion.

Defining Fundamentalism

RIGID DOGMATISM

Consider the following definition of RF offered by Altemeyer and Hunsberger (1992):

> the belief that there is one set of religious teachings that clearly contains the fundamental, basic, intrinsic, essential, inerrant truth about humanity and deity; that this essential truth is fundamentally opposed by forces of evil which must be vigorously fought; that this truth must be followed today according to the fundamental, unchangeable practices of the past; and that those who believe and follow these fundamental teachings have a special relationship with the deity. (p. 118)

One of the key features of this definition is the emphasis on a rigid dogmatism in the manner in which religious beliefs are held. To this extent, this definition is getting at a religious orientation that is distinct from other ways of being religious. However, there is still considerable overlap with orthodoxy (particularly Christian orthodoxy), especially if major religious sources (e.g., sacred writings) teach that there is but one set of truths about humanity and deity. Thus, when it comes to measuring RF, a person who holds orthodox views can easily be (mis)identified as a fundamentalist. To say, therefore, that this conceptualization is free of doctrinal content, as Altemeyer and Hunsberger (1992, 2005) have done, is perhaps not entirely warranted.

Nevertheless, the Altemeyer and Hunsberger (1992) definition is consistent with other theoretical work on RF (e.g., Kirkpatrick, Hood, & Hartz, 1991) and is potentially applicable to most major world religions—unlike much previous work on RF. Also, the reader will recognize that we might expect this conceptualization to be negatively related to Batson et al.'s (1993) Q orientation, which involves a questioning approach to religion; openness and flexibility; and a resistance to clear-cut, pat answers. Altemeyer and Hunsberger (1992) developed a 20-item RF Scale to measure their conceptualization, and later (2004) developed a shortened 12-item version. Both scales were balanced against response sets and generated Cronbach's alphas of .91 to .95 in different studies.

LINKS AMONG FUNDAMENTALISM, QUEST, PREJUDICE, AND RIGHT-WING AUTHORITARIANISM

Almost 70 years ago, Adorno et al. (1950) noted that religiousness was related to RWA, (as measured by the California F scale, an instrument developed by these researchers). For example, it was rare for religious people also to score low on RWA. However, Adorno et al.'s work has received considerable criticism on methodological and conceptual grounds (see, e.g., Altemeyer, 1981), and the research utilized unsophisticated measures of religion (e.g., frequency of church attendance, a single item on the importance of religion). Work by Altemeyer (1981, 1988, 1996) has confirmed that RWA may help us to understand the relatively high levels of prejudice found among religious persons scoring high on RF and low on Q. Altemeyer's reconceptualization of RWA focuses on three attitudinal clusters: authoritarian submission, authoritarian aggression, and conventionalism.

Altemeyer and Hunsberger (1992) conducted a study to assess the links among RF, Q, prejudice, and RWA (see Research Box 12.5). They found that people who scored high on their RWA measure tended also to score high on RF ($r = .68$), as well as to be prejudiced in a variety of ways (r's $= .33$ to .64). This is not to imply that all high-RWA individuals are high on RF, or the reverse. However, "off-quadrant" cases (i.e., those scoring high on RWA and low on RF, or vice versa) were quite rare, and Altemeyer (1988) concluded that RF and RWA do seem to "feed" each other. That is, they both encourage obedience to authority, conventionalism, self-righteousness, and feelings of superiority. Unfortunately, one of the problems with the RWA scale is that it includes a number of religious items, which may help contribute to the high correlation between the RF and RWA measures. Altemeyer and Hunsberger (2005) have contended that this is not a problem, since the nonreligious items on the RWA measure tend to correlate just as strongly as the religious items with the RF scores. However, even many of the items judged to be nonreligious (e.g., questions about the morality of homosexuality and the role of women) may be viewed as part of the religious meaning system by fundamentalists (see Hood at al., 2005).

DIFFERING PERSPECTIVES

The findings described above have not gone without comment in the psychology-of-religion literature; for example, Gorsuch (1993) questioned several aspects of the Altemeyer and Hunsberger (1992) study, as noted earlier. Leak and Randall (1995) have suggested that RWA's positive association with religion is limited to measures of "less mature faith development" (p. 245). They found that such measures of "less mature" religion (e.g., a scale assessing Christian orthodoxy, measures of Fowler's second and third stages of faith development [see Chapter 4], and church attendance) were positively related to RWA scores, but that measures of "more mature" religion (e.g., Batson's Q Scale, measures of Fowler's fourth and fifth faith stages, and a Global Faith Development Scale) were negatively correlated with RWA scores.

The real issue here may be semantics. Just what *is* "mature faith"? Leak and Randall have chosen to regard a Q sort of orientation as "mature" (see also Kristensen, Pedersen, & Williams, 2001). Their Global Faith Development Scale included items such as "It is very important for me to critically examine my religious beliefs and values" (p. 248), and in this respect it bears some resemblance to Q measures. It is not surprising that such measures have a negative association with RWA, as previously reported by Altemeyer and Hunsberger (1992). However, it seems a moot point to define, for example, global faith development and a Q orientation as "mature," and religious orthodoxy and RF as "less mature." Religiously orthodox persons and those with an RF orientation may feel that *their* religion is the mature one, and that Q is immature. Of course, Gordon Allport considered an I orientation to be mature and an E orientation to be immature (Allport, 1954; Allport & Ross, 1967). In any case, we would suggest that Leak and Randall's findings, aside from the maturity issue, are consistent with earlier findings of relationships among RF, Q, RWA, and prejudice.

An Alternative View of Fundamentalism: Intratextuality

Hood et al. (2005) offer an alternative perspective on RF. Though they agree that some fundamentalists are characterized by the rigid dogmatism described earlier, they suggest that to fully understand why fundamentalists so strongly adhere to their belief system, one must approach the subject matter on fundamentalists' terms (a "hermeneutical" approach, as described in Chapter 2). Much in line with the theoretical framework introduced in Chapter 1, they contend that religion provides a convincing system of meaning to fundamentalists by keeping its sacred text (which is usually written, but may be an oral text as well) as the sole source of meaning. This is not to imply that nonfundamentalists who are highly religious fail to recognize and appreciate the value of sacred writings such as the Bible. The difference is that the fundamentalist sees the sacred text as the single authoritative base to which all other elements of human experience are subordinated; such subordination to a supreme authoritative text is, according to these authors, the hallmark of RF. No sources outside the text are necessary for an understanding of absolute truth. This principle of "intratextuality" is tautologically reinforced, in that it specifies not only what truths are absolute, but also what text is sacred. Though the text requires an interpretive process, the absolute truths are not relative to human understanding and impose themselves on the reader. Furthermore, the absolute truths of the sacred text inform and regulate all peripheral belief systems (i.e., beliefs that are not specifically and directly addressed by the text itself). So, for example, fundamentalists' approach to the value of the field of psychology will be determined by their understanding of what the sacred text reveals about it. Furthermore, the text is protected from outside influences; if other beliefs or knowledge question the content of the authoritative text, they are rejected.

In contrast, the religious *non*fundamentalist utilizes the principle of "intertextuality," whereby no single text speaks authoritatively in isolation from other texts. It is the interrelationship between texts that is consulted in the process of deriving truth; this process is much more in accordance with modernistic thinking. Thus, there may be, for example, knowledge from science that may help interpret and even alter one's understanding of the text (e.g., scientific findings that might influence one's perspective on the Biblical creation account). Furthermore, peripheral beliefs may also exert influence on the interpretive process.

The Hood et al. (2005) alternative has yet to generate much empirical attention. However, research reported by Blogowska and Saroglou (2013) has demonstrated the importance of the Biblical text as religious authority in predicting attitudes, as they say "for better or worse," toward outgroups. Their research also supports the notion that RF, as defined by the nature of the authoritative texts, is distinct from general religiousness and the personality trait of authoritarianism.

What about Non-Christian Religions and Samples outside North America?

Finally, it is worth noting that the relationships described here are not unique to the specific measures and North American samples reported above. Researchers from Europe, using very different measures of religiousness, RWA, and prejudice, have found links among these measures that are quite consistent with the findings reported above (e.g., Billiet, 1995; Eisinga, Konig, & Scheepers, 1995). Apparently the findings on religion, prejudice, and RWA cut across differing variables and cultural contexts, at least within Christianity.

Hunsberger (1996) assessed RF–RWA–prejudice relationships in small samples of people from non-Christian religions in Canada. The strength of these relationships is similar to those found in samples of mostly Christian adults and university students in Canada (Altemeyer & Hunsberger, 1992) and college students in the United States (Laythe et al., 2001). These associations have also been essentially replicated with Muslim and Christian university students in Ghana (Hunsberger et al., 1999). These results seem to confirm the links among RF, RWA, and prejudice across various religious groups in North America and elsewhere. However, further research is needed to assess the relationships in larger samples, and particularly for non-Christian groups outside North America.

A series of investigations has been carried out in Belgium and the Netherlands by a group of European researchers, focusing on religious beliefs, RWA, and prejudice (Billiet, 1995; Duriez & Hutsebaut, 2000; Eisenga, Billiet, & Felling, 1999; Eisenga et al., 1990), although they did not include the same religious orientation measures described in this chapter (e.g., the I, E, Q, or RF measures). These investigations have typically revealed little or no relationship between ethnic prejudice and measures of Christian belief or attendance, although there are occasional exceptions of positive (e.g., Duriez & Hutsebat, 2000) or negative (e.g., Billiet, 1995) relationships.

Outside Europe and North America, several relevant investigations have been reported. Griffin et al. (1987) found that on the Caribbean island of St. Croix, members' commitment to the Seventh-Day Adventist Church and their I orientation were positively correlated with prejudice (e.g., withholding human rights from Rastafarians). However, the authors pointed out that church members perceived the church itself to be relatively prejudiced in this regard; therefore, this could be an instance of a positive link between an I orientation and prejudice when such prejudice is nonproscribed by one's church. In Venezuela, Ponton and Gorsuch (1988) reported a negative link between I religiousness and (ethnic) prejudice, as well as a positive association for E religiousness. The Q orientation was uncorrelated with prejudice. Of course, the proscription of specific prejudice may be specific to cultural, religious, and temporal context. For example, Lafferty (1990) argued that in South Africa racial prejudice was (until the abolition of apartheid) religiously nonproscribed, but others have pointed out that it is proscribed in North America (e.g., Batson et al., 1993; Duck & Hunsberger, 1999).

A study at a university in northern India showed a "reverse prejudice" (Murphy-Berman, Berman, Pachauri, & Kumar, 1985, p. 33), in that Hindu students allocated more money to Muslim (than to Hindu) targets in a hypothetical situation. The authors speculated that a social desirability effect might have influenced the results. Hassan and Khalique (1987) reported a tendency for Muslim college students to be more prejudiced than Hindus. In Bangladesh, Hewstone, Islam, and Judd (1993) had Muslims (the majority group) and Hindus (the minority group) evaluate targets of different religion (Muslim or Hindu) and nationality (Bangladeshi or Indian). They concluded that religion and nationality were both important predictors of outgroup discrimination.

Such studies are important in broadening the investigation of religion and prejudice to different cultural and religious groups in the world. However, these studies often do not include comparison groups; their measures and samples vary considerably; results are sometimes seemingly contradictory; and it is therefore very difficult to compare their results and make sense of them in a systematic way. Comprehensive cross-cultural research is needed— especially investigations that compare the same measures and similar samples across cultures and religious groups, while controlling for other important variables such as proscription status, demographic aspects of the sample, and the cultural context of the research (e.g., majority vs. minority status of participants).

Is Cognitive Style Relevant?

Since religions offer people a particular view of the world, potentially giving meaning to their existence and offering answers to questions about the universe and the world around them, one might wonder whether religions influence people to think in similar ways (see Hunsberger & Jackson, 2005). Some evidence does point in this direction. For example, RF is apparently related to complexity of thought about existential issues (e.g., Hunsberger, Alisat, Pancer, & Pratt, 1996; Hunsberger, Pratt, & Pancer, 1994). "High and low fundamentalists may actually perceive and deal with their own (and others') religious experiences in different ways" (Hunsberger et al., 1996, p. 218); that is, high-RF persons may tend to incorporate new information into an existing religious schema, whereas low-RF persons may be more likely to adapt their religious beliefs to accommodate religious doubts or new information. Also, the Q orientation has been associated with increased complexity of thought (Batson & Raynor-Prince, 1983) and openness to different perspectives (McFarland & Warren, 1992).

It has been suggested that such unique cognitive styles, associated with religious orientation, might help us to understand the religion–prejudice connection (Hunsberger & Jackson, 2005). Specifically, those high in RF may tend to cling to existing stereotypes, rather than changing their views in light of new information. Conversely, those with a Q orientation may be inclined to think more complexly about both religion and, for example, cultural diversity, contributing to greater tolerance of such diversity. Similarly, these individuals' tendency toward greater cognitive complexity may incline them to be less influenced by

group or social norms that tolerate prejudice. However, these possibilities are only speculative at this point.

Beyond Personal Religion to Group Effects

Several researchers have argued that research on religion and prejudice needs to expand to
focus more on intergroup issues (Altemeyer, 2003; Hunsberger & Jackson, 2005; Jackson &
Hunsberger, 1999). Historically, research on religion and prejudice has been dominated by
work involving an individual-difference perspective (especially that of religious orientation),
as reflected in much of our discussion so far in this chapter. However, it has been argued that
a group perspective could help us to understand religion–prejudice relationships.

Some theories of intergroup relations suggest that group members are susceptible to prejudice against outgroup members. For example, social identity theory (e.g., Tajfel & Turner,
1986) posits that personal self-esteem may be bolstered when group members compare themselves with other groups. In terms of religious groups, if individuals believe that their religion
is the source of absolute truth, this could enhance their self-esteem (and ingroup attachment);
it could also serve as a source of prejudice against members of other religions, who are seen
as belonging to inferior groups. In general, it could seemingly justify intolerance of people
who do not adhere to divinely revealed morality (Hunsberger & Jackson, 2005).

Similarly, realistic group conflict theory (e.g., Sherif, 1966) argues that the perception
of being in competition with other groups for valued resources can exacerbate intergroup
tension and prejudice. Perceived threat to values can apparently engender greater discrimination against disadvantaged groups by some religious people (Jackson & Esses, 1997). So,
for example, the perception that immigrants compete for jobs with established members of a
society can foster prejudice against those immigrants' religion in particular (Jackson, 2001),
even if the original perceptions of job competition are incorrect. In a similar vein, Struch and
Schwartz (1989) reported that perceived conflict of interest among different Jewish groups in
Israel was associated with intergroup negativity and endorsement of antagonistic behaviors
toward outgroups. In this context, it has been argued that stronger religious group identification is characteristic of especially devout persons—for example, those who score high on
measures of I, orthodoxy, or RF (Hunsberger & Jackson, 2005). Indeed, I scores have been
found to be strongly correlated (+.70) with religious group identification (Burris & Jackson,
2000), as have RF scores (+.46) and scores on a measure of Christian orthodoxy (+.51) (Jackson & Hunsberger, 1999).

Jackson and Hunsberger (1999) reported two studies that investigated these intergroup
conflict proposals in a religious context. Both studies reported by these authors involved
Christian and religiously nonaffiliated undergraduate students who were asked to complete
measures of their religious orientation, as well as their attitudes toward various religious outgroups. Using an "evaluation thermometer" with labels describing every 10-degree change,
participants indicated their evaluation of various groups: 0 degrees indicated "extremely
unfavorable," 50 degrees was "neither favorable nor unfavorable," and 100 degrees was
"extremely favorable." This measure has been used successfully in other research on intergroup attitudes and relations (see Haddock, Zanna, & Esses, 1993). Results suggested that
measures of RF, orthodoxy, I, E, and Q were *all* associated with more favorable attitudes
toward ingroup members (Christians, "believers") and greater intolerance of religious outgroups (atheists, "nonbelievers"). It is particularly interesting that all religious orientation
measures were associated with negativity toward outgroups, when it has been argued in the

past that the I and particularly Q orientations should be associated with tolerance of others (see the discussion earlier in this chapter). Jackson and Hunsberger (1999) concluded that "prejudice against religious outgroups is pervasive . . . religious intergroup relations are no different from any other form of intergroup relation, and . . . for a variety of reasons, group identifications can generate intergroup antagonism" (p. 521). Interestingly, people who identified themselves as atheists or nonbelievers did not show the same degree or pervasiveness of outgroup negativity toward religious groups (i.e., believers and Christians—"religious outgroups," from their perspective).

Similarly, Altemeyer (2003) found that both RF and emphasis on religious identity in childhood were associated with a "religious exclusiveness," a kind of religious ethnocentrism involving a tendency to reject atheists as well as persons of other faiths (including faiths with rather similar beliefs to their own). These studies provide evidence that religious group membership per se can contribute to intergroup prejudice, especially intolerance of religious outgroup members.

We have looked at the association between religion and prejudice through the eyes of science. However, the discussion of morality and, specifically, prejudice against gay men and lesbians forces us to revisit an issue raised in the first chapter: Namely, it is beyond the domain of science to verify or challenge the truth claims of any religious tradition. So what scientists have identified with the pejorative term "prejudice" may for religious persons simply be upholding a religiously moral standard. Before we conclude this section on religion and prejudice, we wish to discuss this particular issue in more depth in terms of what has been called an "ideological surround."

The Ideological Surround Model

In recent decades, researchers employing the ideological surround model (ISM) have examined what "objectivity" might mean in the social-scientific study of religion (Watson, 1993, 2011). The ISM most basically assumes that religions and the social sciences operate as social rationalities. Social rationalities organize community life around a shared ultimate standard (C. Taylor, 2007). For theistic religions, the standard will be some vision of God. For the social sciences, the standard will instead be some reading of nature. Both communities approach greater rationality through improvements in the organization of their communal life relative to their standards and through the development of deeper insights into their standards. In other words, religion and the social sciences have their own "objectivities."

Inferences based upon supernatural religious and natural social-scientific rationalities will not always be incompatible, but they will always be incommensurable (i.e., they do not have a common factor). Incommensurability occurs when no common metric of evaluation for comparisons can be found (MacIntyre, 1988). Ultimate standards are by definition "ultimate," and thus they cannot be judged by some shared, indisputable, "more ultimate" standard. This absence of higher standards for judging ultimate standards means that religious and social-scientific rationalities necessarily function within a surround of incommensurable ideological assumptions. Explanations of religious rationality based upon social-scientific rationality, and vice versa, cannot rest upon a universal objectivity that commands assent across communities.

Incommensurability and the problem of relativism that it helps engender, therefore, represent a challenge in efforts to understand religion and psychology. According to the ISM, this challenge requires adoption of what Nietzsche (1887/1967) once called "future objectivity."

To strive toward such objectivity, the psychology of religion in the future will need to avoid exclusive conformity with ultimate standards of either the naturalistic social sciences or any particular supernatural religion. This is so because incommensurable rationalities constitute an undeniable empirical reality that no true objectivity can ignore. Future objectivity will, therefore, require a balanced rationality that brings incommensurable rationalities into dialogue through three broad types of research programs (Ghorbani, Watson, Tavakoli, & Chen, 2016). First, proponents of naturalistic social-scientific rationalities will need to continue making critical contributions to the study of religion. In addition, however, proponents of the supernatural rationalities of religions should adopt empirical methods to analyze not only religions, but the social sciences as well (Johnson & Watson, 2012). Finally, future objectivity will call for methods that bring incommensurable religious and social-scientific rationalities into formal and empirically useful dialogue. The development of such dialogical methods has been a central objective of ISM advocates (Watson, 2011).

One implication of the ISM is that the psychology of religion can at least sometimes reflect sociological influences associated with the problem of incommensurability (Watson, Chen, Ghorbani, & Vartanian, 2015). The ISM illustrates that possibility in its analysis of the idea that conservative religiosity predicts narrow-mindedness and other psychological dysfunctions (Batson et al., 1993). Support for that claim appears in findings that scores on the RF Scale display clear linkages with closed-mindedness and psychological maladjustment (Altemeyer & Hunsberger, 1992). Also relevant are studies using a Religious Reflection Scale that was originally developed for Muslims, but that can be adapted for use with other religious traditions (Dover, Miner, & Dowson, 2007). A study examining American Christians, for example, uncovered two factors for the latter scale (Watson, Chen, & Hood, 2011). Faith Oriented Reflection (FOR) appeared in such self-reports as "Faith in Christ is what nourishes the intellect and makes the intellectual life prosperous and productive." Intellect Oriented Reflection (IOR) instead included such claims as "I believe as humans we should use our minds to explore all fields of thought from science to metaphysics." In this American sample, these two forms of reflection correlated negatively, and the RF Scale correlated negatively with IOR and positively with FOR. Such results seemed to provide clear support for the claim that conservative religious commitments promote narrow-mindedness.

Further analysis using ISM methods, nevertheless, uncovered complexities. Creation of the RF Scale occurred within a social-scientific ideological surround that sometimes describes the relationship between conservative religiosity and the wider society as a "culture war" (Hunter, 1991). That this scale presupposes a "culture war" in fact appears in its definition of fundamentalism as, in part, a faith in the "essential truth . . . opposed by forces of evil which must be vigorously fought" (Altemeyer & Hunsberger, 1992, p. 118). Dialogical ISM procedures translated the RF Scale into a less war-like Biblical Foundationalism (BF) Scale (Watson et al., 2003). Scores on the RF and BF Scales reflected different (albeit highly correlated) Christian ideological surrounds, but statistical procedures examining one while controlling for the other made it possible to examine more ideologically differentiated measures. For example, after RF was controlled for, BF predicted higher (not lower) IOR as well as FOR, and the two Religious Reflection Scale factors correlated positively rather than negatively (Watson, Chen, Ghorbani, & Vartanian, 2015). Conservative Christian commitments, therefore, were not exclusively narrow-minded, but had more open intellectual potentials that became obvious when procedures remained sensitive to nuances in Christian social rationalities.

Cross-cultural investigations further confirmed the potential openness of traditional religions. Because Iran is a theocracy, no culture war and no incommensurability exist between religion and the wider society. As might be expected, therefore, IOR and FOR were correlated positively, not negatively, among Iranian Muslims; and both broadly predicted openness and other forms of adjustment (Ghorbani, Watson, Chen, & Dover, 2013). These data paralleled earlier findings that an empirical marker of RF also predicted openness and adjustment in Iran (Ghorbani, Watson, Shamohammadi, & Cunningham, 2009). The two types of reflection were also correlated positively and predicted greater openness in Muslims in Malaysia and Hindus in India (Kamble, Watson, Marigoudar, & Chen, 2014; Tekke, Watson, İsmail, & Chen, 2015).

Correlations between IOR and FOR that are negative in the United States but positive in Iran, Malaysia, and India support the idea that sociological factors associated with incommensurability have an influence on the psychology of religion. An alternative explanation, however, might be that these cross-cultural differences merely reflect contrasts between Christians on the one hand and Muslims and Hindus on the other. Elimination of that possibility, nevertheless, appeared in a demonstration that IOR and FOR correlated positively rather than negatively in Christians living in Iran (Watson, Ghorbani, Vartanian, & Chen, 2015). Muslims and Christians will, of course, follow social rationalities based on different visions of God; but in Iran, both communities live in a theocracy where the presumption is that intellect and faith are compatible. The possible conflict between IOR and FOR in American Christians, therefore, does not appear in Iranian Christians. The deciding influence on IOR is not Christianity, but rather the ideological context in which Christianity is practiced.

Further confirmation of the potentials for religious openness appears in studies using the Religious Schema Scale (Streib, Hood, & Klein, 2010). Within this instrument, a Truth of Texts and Teachings Scale essentially assesses fundamentalism, and a Xenosophia Scale reflects an open-minded willingness to engage in dialogue with other religious traditions based upon a belief that wisdom (*sophia*) is to be found in the perspective of outsiders (*xeno*). These two scales correlate negatively in the United States and Germany (Streib et al., 2010), once again pointing toward the narrow-mindedness of conservative Christians in the West. Truth of Texts and Teachings, nevertheless, correlates positively rather than negatively with Xenosophia in Hindus in India (Kamble et al., 2014) and Muslims in Malaysia (Tekke et al., 2015) and in Iran (Ghorbani, Watson, Amirbeigi, & Chen, 2016). In addition, statistical procedures controlling for the RF Scale in the United States demonstrate that Truth of Texts and Teachings can correlate positively with Xenosophia in the West, and that the BF Scale predicts higher levels of Xenosophia and not just of Truth of Texts and Teachings (Watson, Chen, & Morris, 2014; Watson, Chen, Morris, & Stephenson, 2015).

Importantly, a study in the United States used a Defense against Secularism Scale to more directly analyze the possible influence of a "culture war" on the American religious social rationality. Defense against Secularism included such assertions as "Reason is a weapon that the culture uses to destroy faith" and "Secularist beliefs urge the use of reason and open-mindedness in political life because the real motive is to destroy our religious beliefs." This measure wholly or partially explained inverse linkages of FOR, RF, and Truth of Texts and Teachings with IOR (Watson, Chen, Morris, & Stephenson, 2015). These data, therefore, supported the notion that belief in a "culture war" against "forces of evil" that must be "vigorously fought" at least partly explains an incompatibility between American intellect and faith.

Examination of the Religious Reflection and Religious Schema Scales in Malaysia also illustrated another important element of the ISM (Tekke et al., 2015). Again, the ISM assumes that a balanced future objectivity should include research programs in which religions adopt empirical methods to describe the objectivity of their own incommensurable rationalities. An example is the Ummatic Personality Inventory, which records personality adjustment for the Muslim community or *ummah* (Othman, 2011). Within this inventory, an Ilm measure records the Muslim belief that each person is "given an intellect (*aql*) to enable him to seek knowledge (*ilm*) and to put this knowledge into practice to benefit mankind" (Othman, 2011, p. 38). As Rahman (1988) points out, "Ilm . . . is a key concept in the Quran and the second most used word after Allah" (p. 167). Especially noteworthy in the Malaysian data were findings that Ilm correlated positively not only with FOR and Truth of Texts and Teachings, but also with IOR and Xenosophia. The broader implication, therefore, is that Islam and perhaps other religious traditions may have internal ideological resources for promoting open-mindedness. Exploration of such possibilities will require empirical analyses framed within the ideological assumptions of the religious rationalities themselves.

This research into religious openness illustrates only some ISM findings that suggest the potentials of a social-scientific sensitivity to incommensurable rationalities. By empirically constructing a balanced rationality, the ISM seeks to promote development of a more expansive perspective that in the future can even more objectively understand the influences of the standards defining religion and psychology, and thus can promote the dialogue that needs to exist between them.

Now let's return to the topic of prejudice against gay men and lesbians, and consider it in terms of the ISM. This is precisely what Rosik has done (Rosik, 2007a, 2007b; Rosik, Griffith, & Cruz, 2007; see also Bassett, Smith, et al., 2005) in exploring the relationship between conservative religion and homophobia as defined by Herek's (1998) Attitudes Toward Lesbians and Gay Men Scale—Revised (ATLG-R). Rosik (2007a) found that among a sample of students from a small conservative Christian liberal arts college, 4 items of the ATLG-R were viewed as ideologically balanced (e.g., "Female homosexuality is a threat to many of our basic social institutions"), 4 items were viewed as proreligious (e.g., "A woman's homosexuality should not be a cause for job discrimination in any situation"), and 12 items were viewed as antireligious (e.g., "Sex between two men is just plain wrong"). Of particular interest is the fact that of the 12 items judged to be antireligious by the Rosik sample, all but one of the items entirely constitute what has repeatedly been found in a number of studies as the single dominant factor (called Condemnation–Tolerance) of Herek's conceptualization of homophobia—what Rosik has identified as the "moral" factor. Only one perceived antireligious item was found among the other three factors (Social Cohesion, Social Concern, and Right to Privacy). Further research by Rosik (2007b) found that the relationship between religiousness and negative attitudes toward homosexuality was entirely a function of the single moral Condemnation–Tolerance factor and its perceived antireligious items, forcing Rosik to conclude:

> Thus, homophobia as defined by the ATLG-R appeared largely explicable in terms of traditional religious moral sentiment rather than pathological adjustment that inevitably leads to negative affects toward or the suppression of certain basic civil rights for gay men and lesbians. To the extent that other scales of homophobia have similar factor structures and ideological surrounds fundamentally experienced by religious conservatives as antireligious, they may share in the need for interpretive sensitivity. (2007b, p. 151)

It is clear from much research that religious conservatives, including those with an I religious orientation, hold more negative attitudes toward homosexuality. However, simply and pejoratively labeling such attitudes as sexual prejudice or homophobia may overlook the "undisclosed but inherent ideological collision among competing visions of sexual morality" (Rosik, 2007a, p. 141). The bottom line, Rosik maintained, is that some measures of homophobia, such as Herek's (1998) ATLG-R measure, fail to consider the normative beliefs of a religiously oriented value framework. In terms of the ISM, the metrics of the social rationalities used by social scientists such as Herek and by the religious community are simply incommensurable. Rosik further suggested that successful efforts in educating and reducing homophobia in the conservative religious community will require sensitivity to their belief systems. One such normative belief, supported in yet another study (Rosik et al., 2007), is the previously discussed distinction between homosexual behavior and homosexual persons.

Religion and Prejudice: Summary

Clearly, the religion–prejudice link is far more complicated than the initial suggestion of a linear relationship between church attendance and prejudiced attitudes indicated. Indeed, recent research demonstrates that we still have much to learn about this area. Some research suggests that high RF and low Q scores are apparently linked to prejudice and discrimination; there is also some evidence that it is not RF per se that causes prejudice, but rather the tendency for those high in RF to be high in RWA as well. These conclusions, however, are not airtight and should command further investigation, given some recent contradictory empirical findings as well as theoretical and methodological challenges. Nevertheless, work from the past several decades has provided valuable insight into the religion–prejudice relationship. Perhaps a lesson learned from the ISM is that to understand why an individual holds beliefs or attitudes, whether they be prejudicial or not, the researcher must take into account the context from which such beliefs and attitudes are held.

POSITIVE PSYCHOLOGY AND RELIGION

To some, religion seems only to emphasize the darker side of human nature. To such individuals, for example, the beginning chapters of Genesis tell less of a story about creation than one about the fall of humanity. The story of Adam and Eve stresses condemnation for eating a forbidden fruit—and, more importantly, for the human frailty of giving in to temptation even when one knows that it is wrong. Similarly, Saint Augustine's *Confessions* contain a lucid account of his own spiritual struggles with lust, and Saint Thomas Aquinas's writing in *Summa Theologiae* systematically identifies and discusses the seven deadly sins. Lamenting that contemporary psychological discourse has thoroughly disregarded the wisdom of the past and is therefore "seriously deficient in addressing problems associated with impulse control, selfishness, existential meaning, moral conflict, and ethical values that were so prominent in earlier psychological reflection" (p. 5), Schimmel (1997) argued that psychology, particularly psychotherapy, should incorporate ethical and spiritual values if it is to effectively address contemporary emotional and social issues.

It is therefore perhaps not surprising that research in the psychology of religion has tended to emphasize ethical and moral guidelines as proscriptions that prohibit certain behaviors or even thoughts, as indicated by the topics thus far discussed in this chapter (with the exception of helping behavior). In the religious literature, probably the foremost examples are the Ten Commandments found in the Old Testament. Most (but not all) of these commandments warn us about our human tendency to succumb to that which is not good for us—whether it be worshipping false gods, committing adultery, or coveting another person's possessions. Sometimes, however, these guidelines are in the form of prescriptions that tell us about our potential as human beings to cultivate those characteristics deemed good.

Students of psychology may notice that one of the more substantial changes in psychology over the past few decades is the development of a new focus area called simply "positive psychology." Psychologists everywhere, so it appears, seem eager to accept the challenge of former American Psychological Association President Martin Seligman (1999; Seligman & Csikszentmihalyi, 2000) to take seriously a view of human nature that considers such strengths and virtues as compassion, empathy, persistence, gratitude, and honesty as authentic rather than derivative human experiences. Positive psychology's mission is the scientific study of the "good life"[2]—that is, what is right about human nature, what works, what is improving, what its capacities are, what makes people authentically happy. If psychology can begin to answer these questions, then our ability to handle the big questions often facing the ordinary person, such as "What makes live worth living?" or "How can life can be more fulfilling?", will be enhanced. In short, according to Sheldon and King (2001), positive psychology is "nothing more than the scientific study of ordinary human strengths and virtues" (p. 216). An obvious question for our consideration here is the extent to which religion and spirituality help foster those human strengths and virtues that lie at the heart of what makes a life well-lived. Conversely, are there religious elements that serve as impediments to the good life?

Dimensions of Positive Psychology

Seligman and Csikszentmihalyi (2000) have proposed that one way to think about positive psychology is to consider it at three levels: (1) the *subjective* level (subjective states, such as positive emotions and thoughts); (2) the *individual* level (individual traits, such as courage, or behavior patterns, such as helping those in need); and (3) the *societal or group* level (social institutions, such as positive civic and church communities, as well as positive work and home environments). The study of religion and spirituality, of course, cuts across all three levels, though we focus primarily on the second and (to a lesser extent) the first levels, since many religious teachings tend to focus on individual development. We should also note that although these three levels are a useful way of categorizing human experience, in reality the distinctions among the three levels become blurred. Many subjective states at the first level blend together into individual traits at the second level. Without a Level 2 trait, some Level 1 subjective experiences may occur less frequently. Also, throughout this book, we have maintained that individuals are not isolated from a Level 3 social context; they are surrounded, or surround themselves, with people and programs that help reinforce a value system (Hood et al., 2005; Watson, 1993). Hence the levels often interact with each other, and sometimes the unique interactions are what interest psychologists of religion the most.

---

[2]The popular use of the term "good life" may conjure a materialistic vision consisting of possessions and pleasure. Here the term is used in a more philosophical sense of what values constitute a life worth living, similar to Aristotle's concept of *eudaimonia* (flourishing).

Core Virtues

A useful framework for our discussion is Peterson and Seligman's (2004) characterological approach to positive psychology. They have identified six core virtues or character strengths, each of which is briefly discussed here. This is not to suggest that we promote some sense of global judgment that one person is virtuous while another is not. Rather, we should think in terms of virtues (plural) as "discrete, coordinated systems of thought, reason, emotion, motivation, and action" (McCullough & Snyder, 2000, p. 3). There are thus many virtues that fall within the six core broad categories discussed below.

There is a growing empirical literature surrounding each virtue, though the important connection with religion is still in its conceptual infancy. As a result, many ideas have yet to be empirically tested. What we can say, though, is that religion speaks considerably to what is right about people—specifically to the development of strengths of character, such as wisdom, courage, humanity, justice, temperance, and transcendence. As Exline (2002) has pointed out, if the psychological study of religion is to advance, we need to look "underneath the broad category of religious involvement to consider the effects of specific religious beliefs or doctrines. Even if psychological studies of religion cannot address 'ultimate matters,' they can address people's beliefs about such matters" (p. 246). Our discussion of positive psychology takes Exline's advice to heart.

Wisdom

Wisdom is defined as "cognitive strengths that entail the acquisition and use of knowledge" (Peterson & Seligman, 2004, p. 29); such strengths are "knowledge hard fought for, and then used for good" (p. 39). Wisdom is, in the words of Sternberg (2007), "in large part a decision to use one's intelligence, creativity, and knowledge for a common good" (p. 38). The presence of such "noble intelligence" makes no one resentful and everyone appreciative. Specific strengths of wisdom include creativity, curiosity, open-mindedness, love of learning, and seeing things in broad perspective (Peterson & Seligman, 2004).

Wisdom is a common theme in many religious traditions. Dahlsgaard, Peterson, and Seligman's (2005) study of the major writings of eight world philosophies (Confucianism and Taoism in China; Buddhism and Hinduism in south Asia; and Athenian philosophy, Judaism, Christianity, and Islam in the West) found that wisdom is explicitly named as a virtue in all but Buddhism (where it is thematically implied). For example, the authors point out that wisdom as a form of higher knowledge, including that gained through education and experience, was clearly taught as a specific virtue (*zhi*) by Confucius and is listed by Aquinas in his classic Christian enumeration of human strengths as the most important of the cardinal virtues. In contrast, Hindus and Buddhists view wisdom as an ideal attainment of transcendental knowledge of the self.

Wisdom is a broad construct, and therefore one that is difficult to test empirically (Bangen, Meeks, & Jeste, 2013). Research (e.g., Ardelt, 1997; Staudinger & Baltes, 1996; Wink & Helson, 1997) on wisdom has suggested that it is characterized by a highly developed form of thinking that involves dialectical reasoning, a recognition of limitations, and an openness both to difficult questions about the conduct and meaning of life (to which life goals and strategies may be mapped) and to different modes of experience (for reviews, see Baltes & Staudinger, 2000; Kramer, 2000). Though a minimal level of intelligence is a necessary condition for wisdom, it appears to be less of a predictor of wisdom-related performance than other components, such as life experience, chronological age, and certain personality characteristics (e.g., openness to experience, desire for personal growth) (Baltes & Staudinger, 2000; Staudinger & Leipold, 2003; see Bangen et al., 2013, for a literature review). Most of the research conducted to date has focused on the specific strengths of wisdom listed above, and a discussion of this research is beyond our scope here. What we should expect, however, is that religion, depending on its type, can both foster and inhibit wisdom. For example, to the extent that an I or E orientation keeps one from facing complex and difficult issues, then one's religiousness may be a barrier to wisdom. On the other hand, if an I orientation reflects an integrated crystallization of one's efforts to face the complexities of life, religiousness may be a hallmark of wisdom. At this point, the few studies that have directly investigated the relationship of religiousness and wisdom have not considered different religious orientations. In general, religiousness has been found to correlate positively with the cognitive and reflective dimensions of wisdom (Adamovová, 2013) and with a measure of "practical" wisdom (Krause & Hayward, 2014, 2015).

Courage

Defined by Peterson and Seligman (2004) as "emotional strengths that involve the exercise of the will to accomplish goals in the face of opposition, external or internal" (p. 36), courage includes such specific strengths as bravery, persistence, integrity, and vitality. Courage is likely to be a broader construct than what immediately comes to mind. Surely it includes courage in confronting physical danger, but it also includes moral courage, such as the expression of personal values in the face of rejection and even derision—the courage to stand up for one's beliefs. It also includes vital courage, such as the desire to live in the face of chronic illness.

Religious traditions too speak of courage, though it appears to be more representative theme in Western than in Eastern religious traditions. For example, Dahlsgaard et al.'s (2005) analysis found that courage is explicitly mentioned in all of the major Western traditions (Athenian philosophy, Christianity, Islam, and Judaism), but only in Hinduism among the major Eastern religions. The emphasis on courage in Hinduism may be due to the fact that the notions of caste in a stratified society are mingled with a sacred text, the Bhagavad Gita. The character strengths of courage are prescribed for the soldier caste, the second highest of four caste levels. In Greek philosophy, Aristotle saw virtue as a social practice lying between two extremes; in this case, courage is the mean between rashness and cowardliness.

Empirical research on courage, including its related character strengths, in relation to religiousness is just beginning to emerge. The research that has been conducted to date has largely centered around persistence, even in the face of difficult challenges. Toburen and Meier (2010) found that people persisted longer on stressful tasks when experimentally primed with God-related thoughts compared with non-God-related (neutral) thoughts. However, they also felt more anxiety—and, surprisingly, both of these tendencies were found regardless of whether the people identified themselves as Christians or as atheists/agnostic/others. Watterson and Geisler (2012) found that highly religious individuals were able to utilize their faith when other resources were depleted to persist on a strenuous task, suggesting that one's faith may enable greater self-regulatory ability. However, at least one study (Aruguete, Goodboy, Jenkins, Mansson, & McCutcheon, 2012) did not find religiousness to be associated with perseverance or better performance on an intellectual task.

Of course, there are historical examples of religious courage—martyrs who gave their lives because of religious conviction, or people like Mother Teresa who faced tremendous odds in carrying out their missional objectives. Perhaps the most indirect empirical indication of the religion–courage connection is the rather substantial literature investigating how religion serves as a source of courage in coping with difficult life circumstances. We explore that topic in Chapter 13.

Humanity

Defined by Peterson and Seligman (2004) as "interpersonal strengths that involve tending and befriending others" (p. 29), the virtue of humanity "relies on doing more than what is only fair—showing generosity when an equitable exchange would suffice, kindness even if it cannot (or will not) be returned, and understanding even when punishment is due" (p. 37). The character strengths of this virtue include love, kindness, and social intelligence.

Humanity was found by Dahlsgaard et al. (2005) to be among the most common in all of the eight religious traditions and philosophies they studied. Many Christians identify love as the hallmark virtue, primarily on the basis of the three theological virtues proposed by Saint Paul—faith, hope, and love, with love being held as the greatest. It is also stressed in the other Western religions; many Proverbs (Judaism) stress graciousness and kindness, and the importance of friendship and generosity is discussed in Aristotle's *Nicomachean Ethics*. Though humanity is not seemingly as heavily stressed in Eastern religious thought, Dahlsgaard et al. point out that this virtue is emphasized in all four of the major Western religions reviewed.

The well-established empirical tradition in the psychology of religion on helping behavior has already been discussed in this chapter. This is not to suggest that the virtue of humanity has been exhaustively covered by psychologists of religion, for helping behavior is but a small slice of the humanity "pie." Furthermore, as the reader may recall, there is little consensus from the empirical findings on the precise connection between religion and helping behavior. As a result, there should be no shortage of ideas for the psychologist of religion who wishes to investigate this virtue further.

Justice

Defined by Peterson and Seligman (2004) as "civic strengths that underlie healthy community life" (p. 30), justice implies the "shared notion that some standard should be in practice to protect intuitive notions of what is fair" (p. 37). The character strengths of justice include citizenship, fairness, and leadership. The principle of justice as a virtue is stressed by all of the eight traditions reviewed by Dahlsgaard et al. (2005), suggesting that it is perhaps a ubiquitous theme. However, Maltby and Hill (2008) maintain that justice as a virtue is especially applicable to Judaism:

> For the Jew, citizenship necessarily involves concerns for justice. Suggesting that a just God is indeed an imitable God, since humans were created in God's image (*imago dei*), Jewish law is structured to foster a sense of loyalty and social responsibility with a primary concern for justice. Indeed, following God's law prevents injustice gaps; it is the violation of such laws that leads to the need to respond to injustice, and to do so properly is yet another indication of citizenship as a developed character strength. (p. 128)

There is a considerable empirical research tradition centering around the theme of justice. For example, one of the more notable theories in social psychology, "equity" theory (Adams, 1965), proposes that although people desire to maximize self-interests in social relationships, they are happiest when there is an equitable distribution of benefits relative to the amount of effort put into the relationship. Research on organizational justice (Folger, 1977; Greenberg & Folger, 1983) has documented the importance in the procedural sense of justice of "voice" (Thibaut & Walker, 1975)—the opportunity to be heard, even if it has little desired influence on the outcome (Lind, Kanfer, & Earley, 1990). When these norms of justice are violated, an "injustice gap" (Worthington, 2006) occurs; the size and importance of this gap are determined by a number of factors, such as the intention behind the injustice and the injustice's severity (Hill, Exline, & Cohen, 2005).

The degree to which these notions of justice are applicable to one's religious identity is beginning to be empirically investigated. In a study of seminarians (supposedly a highly religious sample), a commitment to social justice was predicted by a trait of being forgiving via the personal characteristics of differentiation of self (the ability to balance one's autonomy with a relational harmony with others) and humility (Jankowski, Sandage, & Hill, 2013). Sandage and Morgan (2014) found that a sense of hope (which other research has shown may be influenced by one's religious commitment) and the ability to utilize positive religious coping predict social justice commitment. However, it has also been found that among white Christian students, social justice interest and commitment was negatively related to religious conservatism (Todd, McConnell, & Suffrin, 2014).

Transcendence

Defined by Peterson and Seligman (2004) as "strengths that forge connections to the larger universe and provide meaning" (p. 30), the virtue of transcendence includes appreciation of beauty and awe, gratitude, hope, humor, and spirituality. Perhaps surprisingly to some, transcendence—the notion that there is some greater meaning or purpose to life—is not as widespread among world traditions as might be expected. Dahlsgaard et al. (2005) claim that of the six core virtues discussed here, it may only exceed courage as a ubiquitous theme. Their review found transcendence to be explicitly named in five of the eight great traditions they reviewed, but with it at least thematically implied in the other three (Confucianism, Taoism, and Greek philosophy).

In Chapter 1, we have suggested that religion is uniquely capable of providing meaning and purpose. Indeed, it is around this theme that we have structured much of this book, so we do not review it further here. Maltby and Hill (2008), however, maintain that certain elements of transcendence are especially prominent in the theologies of Christianity and Islam. For example, they suggest that hope (along with optimism, future-mindedness, and future orientation), as one of the manifestations of transcendence, is a core personal characteristic strongly emphasized in Christianity. Such a sense of hope and significance may be one of the cohesive elements that helps make religion a unique meaning system (Silberman, 2005b). Emmons (2005) reminds us that for Christians, hope is one of the "Big Three" theological virtues, along with faith and love.

Snyder, Sigmon, and Feldman's (2002) review of the literature shows that hope has many positive effects on mental and even physical health. If hope is conceptualized—as it has been by Snyder and his colleagues (Snyder, 1994; Feldman & Snyder, 2005)—in terms of the ability to think of goals, to believe that one is capable of achieving those goals, and to perceive and apply pathways that lead to those goals, then religion is capable of fostering hope (Snyder et al., 2002). Indeed, Sethi and Seligman (1993) found that more conservative religious groups (whether Muslim, Jewish, or Christian) tended to be more hopeful and optimistic, perhaps because of specific religious teachings that, if taken literally, meet the conceptual criteria of hope stressed by Snyder and his colleagues. A more recent study (Marques, Lopez, & Mitchell, 2013) found that adolescents' life satisfaction was predicted by hope and spirituality, but not religious practice.

Temperance (and Self-Control)

Defined by Peterson and Seligman (2004) as "strengths that protect against excess" (p. 30), temperance includes such character strengths as forgiveness and mercy, humility and modesty, prudence and self-regulation. Temperance is explicitly identified in all of the eight great religious and philosophical traditions reviewed by Dahlsgaard et al. (2005) except for Confucianism, where it is thematically implied.

Consider, for example, Buddhism's Four Noble Truths. The first Noble Truth is that there is suffering (*dukkha*), which reflects the impermanence and imperfection of human existence. The second Noble Truth is that the cause of such suffering is the craving for pleasure or desire, which is inherent in the impermanence of our human condition. Thus what all humans should strive for is the cessation of desire, which results in the cessation of suffering, or *nirvana* (the third Noble Truth). The fourth Noble Truth is that a path leading to the cessation of desire can be achieved through the blueprint of the Eightfold Path: right views and right intent (which together constitute wisdom); right speech, right conduct, and right livelihood (which collectively make up morality); and right effort, right mindfulness, and right concentration (which together constitute mental discipline). This example shows not only that religion usually specifies a virtue (e.g., an end to the desire of impermanent things), but that it often prescribes a means by which that virtue can be obtained (e.g., the Eightfold Path).

One interesting approach to an understanding of positive psychology, much in line with the virtue of temperance, is that taken by Baumeister and Exline (1999). They argue that a core psychological function underlying many virtues is self-control as an internal restraining mechanism. A life of virtue, they maintain, frequently necessitates putting the collective interests of society and community above pure self-interest. In their estimation, the natural proclivity toward self-interest and personal gratification (the very definition in some religions of sin or personal evil), often at the expense of others, requires the necessity of self-regulation for the good of society; this makes self-control in some sense a master virtue—what they refer to as personality's "moral muscle." In fact, Baumeister and Exline claim that "virtues seem based on the positive exercise of self-control, whereas sin and vice often revolve around failures of self-control" (1999, p. 1175).

In Chapter 13, we discuss research indicating that religion is often associated with good physical and mental health. McCullough and Willoughby (2009) hypothesize that this is due in part to religion's influence on self-control and self-regulation. This hypothesis has generated a number of studies; these largely support the notion that religious thoughts and practices help (sometimes unconsciously) to foster self-regulation, which in turn leads to well-being (Briki et al., 2015; Koole, McCullough, Kuhl, & Roelofsma, 2010; Laurin, Kay, & Fitzsimmons, 2012; Rounding, Lee, Jacobson, & Ji, 2012).

Religion and Positive Psychology: Summary

The study of positive psychology is a relatively new development that has generated much enthusiasm among researchers. Though it has strong and obvious implications for the psychology of religion, there has not yet been much direct empirical research looking specifically at the association of religion and ordinary human strengths and virtues. What positive psychology does provide is a refreshingly new approach to understanding the role of religion in ordinary living—the extent to which it encourages and fosters the development of a virtuous character, as well as the possibility that it discourages or hinders such development. We have reviewed what positive researchers have identified as six core virtues, each of which includes more specific character strengths. These virtues and strengths have provided a useful categorical approach for researchers to investigate religious experience in light of research and thinking in positive psychology.

OVERVIEW

We have had something of a roller-coaster ride in this chapter. Religion does indeed seem to be related to some aspects of moral attitudes and behaviors, although there are almost always studies with contradictory findings. We have seen that in the areas of substance use/abuse, nonmarital sexual behavior, and (to a lesser extent) crime and delinquency, more religious persons generally report that they have stricter moral attitudes and are less likely to engage in behaviors that contravene societal (and especially religious) norms. The relationships are not always strong, but they do seem to be reasonably consistent, albeit qualified by various relevant factors as research progresses. However, faith is surprisingly unrelated to some other behaviors, such as cheating/dishonesty. There are indications that religious people *say* they are more honest, but the data do not always bear this out for actual behavior in a secular setting.

We have also found that the relationship of religiousness to helping behavior and prejudice is complex. Again, there are indications that religious people *say* they are more helpful, but the findings do not bear this out for actual behavior in a nonreligious setting. Within a religious context, the more faithful do indeed help more by giving money, time, and talent to religiously based causes. However, outside such a context, it becomes very difficult to distinguish helpers from nonhelpers on the basis of their religion. Batson and his colleagues have tried to build a case that I religiousness is only related to the *appearance* of helpfulness, not to actual behavior; however, some studies have failed to find any association between I scores and self-reported helping. The Q religious orientation is usually, but not always, positively associated with behavioral measures of giving assistance to others. The question of whether some religious orientations are more universally compassionate than others cannot be answered completely clearly. Though Batson's research suggests that questers are more likely to demonstrate universal compassion, there is evidence that they too may be more likely to demonstrate compassion to those with whom they agree than to others, especially if their compassionate acts are somehow likely to promote a view that violates their values.

The evidence is mixed, but it appears that religion is, in general, negatively associated with prejudice. However, those high in religiousness may hold negative attitudes toward proscribed behaviors, such as homosexuality. Whether individuals separate the behavior from the person performing the behavior (the "sin–sinner" issue) has yet to be fully resolved, and this question will undoubtedly generate new research in the years to come. At present, it seems that it is not religion per se that is linked to prejudice, but the ways in which one holds one's faith, the importance of one's religious *group* affiliation, and so on.

Finally, we have explored a promising new avenue for the psychology of religion—positive psychology. Though the implications are obvious, the research in this area to date is rather scarce.

In the end, we are left to puzzle over many things. Why do obtained relationships vary so much for different moral behaviors? Why doesn't religion have a stronger impact in *all* of these areas? How do we explain the "no relationship" findings? Can religion really be a source of criminal behavior, such as child sexual abuse or domestic violence? If so, can religion "right itself" and find within itself the cure for such problems? Does religion promote virtuous character development? These questions are difficult to answer, but they may serve as stimuli for future research efforts.

CHAPTER 13

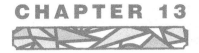

Religion, Health, Psychopathology, and Coping

Religion is comparable to a childhood neurosis.

There is a madness which is the special gift of heaven.

Religious anxiety is rarely, if ever, a cause of insanity. The
sublime faith of Christianity is rather a safeguard against it.

When misery is the greatest, God is the closest.

A mighty fortress is our God,
A bulwark never failing;
Our helper He amid the flood
Of mortal ills prevailing.

A little girl repeating the Twenty-Third Psalm said it this way:
"The Lord is my shepherd, that's all I want."[1]

R eligion and issues of mental health (particularly psychopathology) have had a long and
sometimes troubled relationship, often resulting in a tug-of-war over whose word was
final. In the West until the last four to five centuries, power was vested in the church, and
the medical profession took its orders from ecclesiastical authorities, which throughout history has combined kindness and compassion with cruelty and punishment (McNeill, 1951;
Zilboorg & Henry, 1941). Established religion reluctantly ceded power to medicine and psychiatry, and with similar reluctance, medicine has slowly yielded some control to psychology
and social work. Though the notion that sin and wrongdoing are the causes of mental problems remains—particularly in some conservative groups, but with occasional recurrences
even among the helping professions (Kirk & Kutchins, 1992)—religious groups increasingly
view psychology and related fields more positively.

Similarly, suspicion of and concern about religion within the psychological/psychiat-
ric community are abating. Historically, psychoanalysis and positivistic behaviorism either

---

[1] These quotations come, respectively, from the following sources: Freud (1927/1961b, p. 53); Jowett (1907,
p. 549); Caplan (1969, p. 132); Gross (1982, p. 242); Martin Luther, quoted in Bartlett (1955, p. 86); Mead
(1965, p. 166).

were openly antithetic toward religion or simply had no place for it in their views of mental life (Burnham, 1985; Farberow, 1963; Wulff, 1997). However, classic behaviorism has faded into psychological history, and psychoanalytic ideas (often in new garb) have become integral to the psychological study of religion and often the work of the clergy (Beit-Hallahmi, 1995; McDargh, 1983; Smith & Handelman, 1990). As part of this new awareness, religion and spirituality can be considered psychotherapeutic tools (Pargament, 2007). Antireligious statements, such as Albert Ellis's (1980) view that "the less religious [patients] are, the more emotionally healthy they will tend to be" (p. 637), are becoming passé. Ellis (2000) later came to feel that "religious beliefs which [he] once saw as irrational, are potentially helpful to some clients. Religious believers embrace some rational, self-helping beliefs as well" (p. 277).

Though we now realize that cooperation between religion and the behavioral sciences is essential to human betterment, challenges remain. Probably the most notable challenge is each field's lack of education and sophisticated knowledge about the other field. Many religious professionals, for example, may not be knowledgeable about psychology, particularly when it comes to distinguishing those psychological claims of a popular variety from those with scientific support. Similarly, many researchers, particularly those who are interested in the religion–health linkage, may be well trained in the field of health and health care, but may have a naïve understanding of religion and spirituality. For example, many studies (particularly those conducted prior to the 1980s) designated their respondents simply as "Catholic," "Protestant," "Jewish," and "other," or used such simplistic measures as church attendance to indicate the degree of religious commitment or salience. By now, we hope our readers can see that such measures are not likely to move our understanding of religious/ spiritual experience, including its relationship with mental and physical health, very far forward.

In Chapter 2, we have discussed the complexity of the religious domain, suggesting that categories such as the Intrinsic and Extrinsic or Committed and Consensual dimensions and measures (among other possibilities) may be useful. We have seen in other chapters how important it is to understand not just what a person believes or practices, but also *how* those beliefs are held and practiced. Simplistic indicators of religion often mask researchers' poor understanding of this highly complex realm. Still, consistency over multiple studies suggests reliable findings, and even where respondents have been poorly classified, clues may be present that will stimulate better research. Unfortunately, this is a costly and a time- and energy-consuming path to follow. A much more efficient approach entails the development of adequate theory to guide such studies; more exacting definitions on both sides of the religion–health linkage are essential prerequisites in such work.

THE RELIGION–HEALTH CONNECTION

Religion did not begin drawing sustained systematic attention from scientific researchers as a health-related factor until the 1980s (Oman & Thoresen, 2005). Since then, however, there has been an explosion of research—to the point that there have now been a number of reviews, the vast majority of which link religion and spirituality positively to physical health (e.g., Chida, Steptoe, & Powell, 2009; Ellison & Levin, 1998; Koenig, 2012; Koenig, King, & Carson, 2012; McCullough, Hoyt, Larson, Koenig, & Thoresen, 2000; W. R. Miller & Thoresen, 2003; Powell, Shahabi, & Thoresen, 2003; Steger, Fitch-Martin, Donnelly, & Richard,

2015) and even more so to mental health (e.g., Koenig, 1998, 2012; Koenig, King, & Carson, 2012; L. Miller & Kelley, 2005). For example, Koenig's (2012) systematic review of the literature on religion, spirituality, and health identified approximately 3,300 studies from 1872 to 2010, with 2,100 of those studies conducted since 2000. Approximately 80% of these studies involved mental health. In virtually all mental health domains—including depression, anxiety, suicide, psychotic disorders, substance abuse, and coping with adversity, as well as experiencing positive emotions (well-being and happiness, hope, optimism, etc.) and having positive character traits—the numbers of studies indicating that religion and spirituality are positively correlated with health exceed those of studies indicating a positive correlation with pathology. Also, some studies found no relationship between religion/spirituality and health, but even these were typically outnumbered by the studies that found a positive relationship.

There have also been those (e.g., Sloan & Bagiella, 2002; Sloan, Bagiella, & Powell, 1999) who question, primarily on the basis of procedural concerns, the strength of the alleged religion–health linkages. Criticizing the methodology of much of this research, these researchers believe that the claims of religion's beneficial effects are greatly exaggerated. However, as the field matures and more studies are being published, meta-analytic studies (in which analyses are conducted on combined data from many studies) are being increasingly conducted, and the evidence continues to point to an association between religion and spirituality on the one hand and positive health on the other. Occasional negative health effects, however, are found.

Before we delve into what the research says, four concerns should be noted. First, most of the studies investigating the religion–health connection rely on self-report measures, although more objective physiological measures are sometimes used for the health variable. We know that self-reports sometimes present problems in obtaining valid responses. Second, most of the studies reported are cross-sectional studies (meaning that they compare groups at one point in time), from which cause-and-effect relationships cannot be determined. Thus most of the research is correlational in nature. Third, as Chapters 1 and 2 have made clear, both religion and spirituality are multidimensional, and it may be that only certain aspects of being religious or spiritual are associated with health. Furthermore, the health variable (whether it is some aspect of mental or physical health) is also multidimensional, thus leading to an overwhelming array of possible relationships. So it should not be surprising that results vary tremendously; in fact, we should only expect that, at best, certain patterns may emerge. Perhaps we all have to be reminded from time to time that science is a slow and laborious process. Fourth, most of the research has focused on Christianity (and Judaism to a far lesser extent), with other major world religions and other groups largely neglected (Park & Slattery, 2013). It is not clear whether the findings to date would be that much different if we had many more studies with other religious (or nonreligious groups).

Religion and Physical Health

In a review that is somewhat dated but still highly regarded and considered definitive, Powell et al. (2003) concluded that the relationship between religion and physical health does exist, though it "may be more limited and more complex than has been suggested by others" (p. 50). These reviewers acknowledge the "file drawer effect"—the unknown impact of unpublished results that may weaken the relationship (since "no effect" findings are less likely to get published), but also the fact that the strength of the relationship may be *underestimated* due to imprecise measurement of religion or spirituality (see Hill & Pargament, 2003).

Koenig (2012) found the relationship of religion/spirituality with physical health to be slightly more mixed than the relationship with mental health, largely due to more studies' finding no relationship with physical health. As Koenig points out, the fact that there are more "no relationship" studies is not surprising, given that the existential and moral issues addressed by religion and spirituality are often less closely related to physical health than to mental health. Furthermore, many physical health effects build up over time and are only indirectly related to religion and spirituality through intermediary psychological, social, and behavioral pathways. That is, the positive relationship of religion and spirituality with mental health (e.g., less anxiety) may have long-term implications for physical health, but these are often difficult to determine. Still, however, Koenig found that the number of studies showing a positive relationship with physical health exceeded the "no relationship" findings (and the positive relationship findings with physical pathology) in such domains as coronary heart disease, hypertension, cerebrovascular disease (stroke), Alzheimer disease, cancer, immune/endocrine functioning, physical function, pain/somatic symptoms, and self-rated health. Even with the ultimate measure of health, mortality, those who were religious or spiritual were likely to live longer (as found in 75% of the studies).

Why might there be any connection at all between religiousness or spirituality and physical (as well as emotional) health? Oman and Thoresen (2005; see also Thoresen, 2007) suggest four broad mechanisms that may operate independently or in combination, all of which have received at least some empirical support (see Koenig et al., 2012, for a more extensive discussion of each mechanism and the empirical research).

- *Health behaviors.* Religion in general or specific religious groups may encourage healthy practices, such as exercise (Oman & Reed, 1998; Hill, Burdette, Ellison, & Musick, 2006; Gillum, King, Obisesan, & Koenig, 2008), use of seat belts (Oman & Thoresen, 2006), or dietary health (Hart, Bowen, Kuniyuki, Hannon, & Campbell, 2007; King, 1990; Obisesan, Livingston, Trulear, & Gillum, 2006). Religious involvement may also discourage unhealthy practices, such as smoking, drinking, drug use, or risky sexual behavior (Benjamins & Buck, 2008; Feinstein, Liu, Ning, Fitchett, & Lloyd-Jones, 2010; King, 1990; Levin & Schiller, 1987; Sarafino, 1990; Whooley, Boyd, Gardin, & Williams, 2002; see Chapter 12 for a more complete discussion). A comparison of highly religious mothers with their less committed counterparts revealed that the former were significantly more likely to engage in active illness prevention behaviors than the latter group (Ameika, Eck, Ivers, Clifford, & Malcarne, 1994). Still, the more religious mothers felt that they had less control over illness. Since a major prevention category was to "go to the doctor," this finding may suggest an inclination for religion to promote deference both to God and to medical authorities. This possibility merits further assessment, as it may also imply a more general obeisance to authority.

- *Psychological states.* Involvement in religion may foster more positive psychological states, such as joy or hope (Maltby & Hill, 2008), which are perhaps useful in buffering stress (Ai, Park, Huang, Rodgers, & Tice, 2007; Cole & Pargament, 1999). It may also protect against negative psychological states, such as fear, sadness, or anger. Reviewing over 300 studies that examined religiousness/spirituality and well-being, Koenig (2012) found a statistically significant positive correlation between the two constructs in almost 80% of the studies (e.g., Cohen, 2002; Ferriss, 2002; Francis & Kaldor, 2002; Fry, 2001; Krause, 2004b; Laurencelle, Abell, & Schwartz, 2002), though some studies have found no relationship (Hunsberger, Pratt, & Pancer, 2001b) or a weak relationship (Diener & Clifton, 2002; Tsuang, Williams, Simpson, & Lyons, 2002).

- *Coping.* Religious and spiritual involvement may provide additional ways of dealing with life's stressors by complementing nonreligious coping. Like other effective coping, religious coping can lead to stress-related personal growth (Park, 2005) and may be a unique source of meaning and purpose to life (Oman & Thoresen, 2003; Paloutzian & Park, 2013b). Religion seems to enhance one's self-regulation or sense of control (Fiori, Brown, Cortina, & Antonucci, 2006; Loewenthal & Cornwall, 1993; McCullough & Willoughby, 2009; Saroglou, 2010), which in turn appears to be associated with better health practices such as less substance abuse (McCullough & Carter, 2013; for a comprehensive review on self-regulation, see Vohs & Baumeister, 2011). However, some research suggests that the Extrinsic orientation to religion, in particular, may be negatively associated with self-control (Vitell et al., 2009). We go into greater detail on religious coping later in this chapter.

- *Social support.* Involvement in religious groups may provide a greater social support network (Oman & Reed, 1998). In fact, religious attendance, though not a good measure of religiousness or spirituality, is one of the best predictors of health outcomes (Masters & Hooker, 2013), and the social support that one receives from religious attendance is one of the leading explanatory candidates. In general, positive social support has been shown to help create greater meaning in life (Krause, 2003, 2007a, 2007b, 2009). Koenig et al. (2012) reported that 61 of 74 studies they examined found a positive relationship between religious involvement and social support. Religious support has been associated with more positive affect or life satisfaction and with lower levels of depression (Fiala, Bjorck, & Gorsuch, 2002; Krause, Ellison, & Wulff, 1998); it has also been predictive of less emotional distress among people coping with stress from the early 1990s Gulf War (Pargament, Koenig, & Perez, 2000). Furthermore, social support from religious sources is a significant predictor of psychological adjustment, even after the effects of general social support are controlled for (VandeCreek, Pargament, Belavich, Cowell, & Friedel, 1999). However, research also shows that those most likely to receive the benefit of social support are those who are more religiously involved in their church or religious group (Krause, Ironson, & Hill, 2018).

Of course, these are broad categories of just some of the mediating factors between religion and both physical and mental health. But one can see even from this short list just how complex and difficult it is to explain why religion or spirituality may be at all related to health.

Religion, Stress, and the Immune System

Health is intimately connected to the defenses mobilized by the body when illness and infection are encountered. These stressors activate the body's immune system. One response is the release of a steroid hormone, cortisol. Secreted by the adrenal glands, cortisol has been called the "stress hormone." Too much or too little cortisol can be harmful to a broad spectrum of physiological activities. The negative effects of most interest here are elevated blood pressure, increased heart rate, indirect release of glucose for energy into the bloodstream, and possible problems with emotional control (Purves, Orians, & Heller, 1995; Stoppler, n.d.; Weber, n.d.). Especially in relation to the psychological effects, high levels of cortisol are considered undesirable.

Koenig et al. (2012) have reviewed an immense medical literature in the second edition of their *Handbook of Religion and Health.* For example, one study indicated that persons engaging in Buddhist meditation showed significant reductions in cortisol levels. In other work, female patients who resorted to prayer and religion while awaiting breast biopsies for possible cancer revealed less cortisol production than those not employing these methods. A study of women with metastatic breast cancer who evidenced religious activity and who considered faith important also showed lowered evening cortisol levels, but not reduced overall levels. In a number of other studies, the contributors to the *Handbook* found religion to be beneficial to the immune system with regard to other physiological indicators, such as interleukin. Apparently, therefore, religious and spiritual coping can reduce bodily expressions of stress.

Seeman, Dubin, and Seeman (2003) have provided a critical review of the evidence for biological pathways that may help us better understand the relationship of religion and spirituality with health. Most of the research they reviewed (see Table 1 on p. 55 of their review for a list of the actual empirical studies reviewed) investigated either Judeo-Christian practices or Zen, yoga, and other meditation/relaxation practices. Among Judeo-Christian practices, they found "reasonable" evidence for the association of religion/spirituality with lower blood pressure, less hypertension, and better immune functioning. They found only limited evidence supporting a link between Judeo-Christian practices and better lipid profiles. For Zen, yoga, and other meditation/relaxation practices, they found extensive evidence that such practices were associated with lower blood pressure and with better health outcomes in clinical patient populations; "reasonable" evidence that these practices were associated with lower cholesterol, lower stress hormone levels, and differential patterns of brain activity; but only limited evidence that such practices were associated with less oxidative stress, less blood pressure activity under challenge, and less stress hormone reactivity under challenge. In a more recent review of the literature (Aldwin, Park, Jeong, & Nath, 2014), a distinction was made between religiousness (defined in terms of such characteristics as religious affiliation and church attendance) and spirituality (defined in such terms as meditation and self-transcendence). Proposing that religiousness encourages better behavioral self-regulation, whereas spirituality involves more emotional regulation, these reviewers found that religiousness did in fact better predict practicing good health behaviors (e.g., less smoking and alcohol consumption, higher likelihood of getting health screenings), whereas spirituality was a better predictor of emotionally regulated biomarkers (e.g., lower blood pressure, less cardiac reactivity, and slower disease progression).

Though it is clearly safe to say that religiousness/spirituality and physiology are connected, it is far more difficult to put the particular pieces together to make much sense of this connection. One possibility goes back to a central thesis of this book—namely, that religion and spirituality offer meaning to individuals. The ability to find meaning in life is clearly related to better health (Krause, 2007a 2007b, 2009, 2012). First, the link between stress and poorer health is well documented (Thoits, 2010), in part due to suppressed immune system functioning. Though stress reduces meaning (Park, 2010), it is also true that finding meaning serves as a buffer to stress. One study (Van Tongeren, Hill, Krause, Ironson, & Pargament, 2017) found that people's self-reported sense of meaning in life (whether from religion or some other source) helped explain the relationship between stress and physical symptoms; that is, those people with a greater sense of meaning experienced fewer health symptoms in response to stress than did those people with a lesser sense of meaning. Furthermore, people with fewer self-reported health symptoms actually showed better immune system functioning, as measured by a test for latent Epstein–Barr virus.

Of course, there are many other indicators of health, and the evidence regarding the important role that meaning plays in health is just beginning to emerge in such domains as cardiovascular health (Cohen, Bavishi, & Rozanski, 2016), reduced mortality (Krause, 2009), and cancer survivorship (Canada, Murphy, Fitchett, & Stein, 2016). In short, a sense of meaning is related to a healthier immune system, to better cardiovascular health, and to surviving such serious illnesses as cancer—and since many people find meaning through religion, it is perhaps not so surprising that religion is related to better health. For a society that places great emphasis on physical health and longevity, but is also highly stressful, the implications of this research are significant.

Religion and Mortality

Of course, everyone dies at some point. But is the mortality rate different for those who are religious than for their less religious counterparts? Overall, it appears that religious people tend to live slightly longer lives (McCullough et al., 2000). Chida et al.'s. (2009) review of 69 studies of healthy populations found that religion or spirituality was an overall health protective factor in 27 studies, was a negative factor in 3 studies, and was a nonfactor in 39 studies. Furthermore, they discovered that stronger associations were found for more specific dimensions of religion and spirituality (e.g., religious involvement, social support, intrinsic religiousness or spirituality, religious or spiritual coping) than for more overall self-ratings of religiousness or spirituality. However, the overall protective effect of religion and spirituality was stronger in healthy populations than in nonhealthy populations. After reviewing the literature, Masters and Hooker (2013) concluded: "The literature suggests that R/S [religious/ spiritual] factors, particularly attendance, have a consistent protective relationship with risk for mortality in healthy populations" (p. 534). However, this is not necessarily due to religious content as much as simply to social participation on some regular basis, as discovered in a meta-analysis by Shor and Roelfs (2013). In other words, nonreligious social participation with similar frequency and commitment levels appears to have the same effect as religious participation. Using data from a historical sample, McCullough, Friedman, Enders, and Martin (2009) found a longevity difference between those who were more versus less religious among women, but not men. Furthermore, Moulton and Sherkat (2012) found in a large nationally representative sample that the positive association of religion with longevity was found only in the portion of the U.S. population that did not finish college. Among college graduates, those who participated in religion actually had *higher* mortality rates. Researchers are now left with the task of trying to further clarify why religiousness predicts longevity, as well as for whom this relationship does or does not apply.

Specific Health-Related Populations

Research on religion and spirituality in relation to health has been conducted in the context of specific populations of people facing major health issues such as heart disease, cancer, Alzheimer disease, and hypertension. Here we look at one population: people with cancer in its various forms. To demonstrate how vast this literature has become, one recent meta-analysis (Jim et al., 2015), investigating the relationship of religion and spirituality with physical health in patients with cancer only, found 497 analyses from 101 unique samples involving some 32,000 patients. Their statistical conclusion from this vast array of research was that, in general, religion and spirituality in patients with cancer is indeed positively associated with overall physical health, and more particularly with physical well-being, functional well-being, and physical symptoms. Furthermore, they found that the affective dimension of religion and spirituality (subjective emotional experiences such as a sense of transcendence, a sense of meaning and purpose, etc.), and to a lesser extent the cognitive dimension (religious or spiritual beliefs such a causal attributions to God, intrinsic beliefs, etc.), were more powerful predictors of health than the behavioral dimension (religious or spiritual practices such as praying or meditating, attending religious services, etc.). Beyond just believing or practicing one's faith, finding meaning through one's faith seems especially important to cancer survivors' physical health and overall quality of life (Canada et al., 2016).

Religion and Physical Health: Summary

Today, most researchers seem convinced that there is *some* relationship, mostly positive but sometimes negative, between religion and physical health. Now the questions facing researchers center on more specific issues about that relationship (e.g., whether religion has the same relationship with cardiovascular health as with cancer; whether it has the same relationship with different types of cancer; whether it matters what religion one adheres to or what one's religious beliefs are; etc.) and about the mediating mechanisms that help explain the relationship. Although the research to this point has been substantial, we have a long way to go before we can draw definitive conclusions that will explain the religion–physical health connection.

Religion and Mental Health

About 80% of the health studies summarized by Koenig (2012) linking religion and spirituality involved mental health. And, as already noted, the relationship of religion/spirituality with mental health appears to be stronger than it is with physical health. This should be expected, since religion more directly addresses several issues that are characterized as mental or emotional health issues (e.g., anxiety, depression, self-control, general well-being). Many of the same mechanisms that underlie the connection between religion and physical health are at work in religion's association with mental health as well. Lifestyle issues, social networks, psychological states, religious coping, and religion's general promotion of well-being are all important mediators between religion and mental or emotional health. We focus here primarily on the relationship between religion and positive emotions. This is not to say that religion causes people, for example, to be happy; most of the work is correlational in nature, and many people who are not at all religious or spiritual are happy people. Nor does it mean that there is only a rosy side to religious experience; we discuss some emotions that are not positive in nature. Finally, it also does not mean that religion is somehow synonymous with mental health. Later in this chapter, we explore religion's connection with psychopathology as well.

Before we explore specific emotions, it should be noted that until recently, psychologists of religion have neglected the affective basis of religion. This is somewhat surprising, given that (1) so many people find religious and spiritual experiences to have a strong emotional component; (2) emotions have long been recognized by theologians (e.g., Jonathan Edwards, Rudolph Otto, Friedrich Schleiermacher) to be prominent in religious experience; and (3) early psychologists of religion, particularly William James (1902/1985), placed emotions at the center of conscious religious experience. Some of this neglect is probably due to the fact that research on emotions has, as a whole, lagged behind research in other psychological domains, no doubt in part due to the difficulty of the subject matter. But there have been recent theoretical and methodological advances in the study of emotions, and psychologists of religion have been challenged to begin to apply these new understandings to their subject matter (Emmons, 2005; Hill, 1995, 2002).

Silberman (2003) proposes three ways in which religion can have an impact on emotional experience. First, religion helps define what is appropriate and inappropriate emotional expression, including its appropriate intensity. Second, the *content* of religious belief (e.g., the belief that God is loving vs. vengeful) will help determine the type of emotion experienced (e.g., security, gratitude, reciprocal love vs. insecurity, unpredictability, fear). Third, religion allows one to experience powerful emotions, such as closeness to the sacred (see also Hill & Pargament, 2003). To say that religion and emotion are intimately connected is hardly an overstatement.

Meaning, Purpose, and Self-Esteem

In Chapter 1, we have said that religion is in a unique position to provide what Park (2005, 2010) refers to as "global meaning"—a general sense of meaning to life that involves beliefs, goals, and subjective feelings. This may be the case because religion alone, so it seems to many, (1) is comprehensive, and therefore is capable of subsuming other sources of meaning, such as family, work, personal relationships, and enduring values; (2) is accessible to human understanding, often through a system of taught values compatible with a religious system; (3) is transcendent, in that it points "beyond me" to some greater being or ultimate authority; and (4) makes direct claims as a meaning provider through its sacred character. To this end, religion is unusually existentially satisfactory to many (Emmons, 1999; Hood, Hill, & Williamson, 2005; Park, 2005).

Empirical research supports the notion that religion is associated with a sense of meaning in life, though the association itself appears to be stronger among elderly persons (Ardelt, 2003; Hughes & Peake, 2002; Krause, 2003) and among ethnic minorities (Mattis, 2002; Moadel et al., 1999). It may serve as a form of "meaning making" (Park, 2005, 2010) because religion can offer the elderly a sense of hope and optimism (Krause, 2003, 2012), even if they may otherwise cycle downward in a sense of Eriksonian "despair" (Erikson, 1963). Those senior citizens especially prone to despair because of poverty, crime, and other losses disproportionately experienced by ethnic minorities may find religion as the sole source of life's meaning and purpose. Mattis (2002) conducted in-depth interviews with 23 African American women and found that religion/spirituality was the primary means by which they constructed meaning, especially in the face of adversity. She found eight faith-based meaning-making themes: Religion/spirituality helped these women to accept reality, to gain courage and insight, to confront and overcome limitations, to identify and grapple with existential questions, to recognize purpose and destiny, to define character and meaningful moral principles, to achieve growth, and to trust in transcendent sources of knowledge and communication.

The ability of religion and spirituality to define meaning and purpose in life even extends to adolescents and emerging adults (Bailey et al., 2016; Kimball, Cook, Boyatzis, & Leonard, 2016). This makes sense, given that the search for personal identity (Erikson, 1963) often involves existential issues. MacDonald and Holland (2002) used a five-dimensional measure of spirituality (the Expressions of Spirituality Inventory) to investigate the relationship between spirituality and boredom proneness among 296 undergraduates (several other studies have shown boredom to be negatively related to meaning and purpose in life). They found that spirituality significantly predicted lower boredom proneness, but only as a function of the inventory's dimensions of Existential Well-Being (comfort with oneself, confidence in one's ability to handle basic existential issues) and, for women only, Cognitive Orientation (belief in the existence of spirituality, perception of spirituality as having relevance to identity and daily functioning). The scale's other dimensions (Religiousness, Spiritual

Experience, and Spirituality) did not predict boredom. Francis (2000) found that among a sample of almost 26,000 teenagers in England and Wales, Bible reading had a small but clearly detectable effect on adolescents' sense of purpose, even after gender, age, personality, church attendance, and belief in God were accounted for.

High scores on the measure of Intrinsic religion (but not on the Quest or Extrinsic religion measure) have been found to be linked solidly with high scores on a measure of global self-esteem (Laurencelle et al., 2002; Ryan, Rigby, & King, 1993). A study of almost 1,000 people in Australia found that belief in God, attending church, and praying were correlated positively with self-esteem and well-being (Francis & Kaldor, 2002).

A religious person's level of self-esteem, however, may be influenced by other related factors. For example, Benson and Spilka (1973) showed that a positive outlook toward oneself corresponded to a similar perception of God. It is, however, well established that God concepts are multidimensional (Gorsuch, 1968; Spilka, Armatas, & Nussbaum, 1964). One long-standing dichotomy that is basic to Western religion is the one between notions of a loving God and a controlling God (Benson & Spilka, 1973; Spilka, Addison, & Rosensohn, 1975), or between what have more recently been alluded to as benevolent God and authoritarian God representations (Johnson, Okun, & Cohen, 2015). Examining this dichotomy, Culbertson (1996) expected these images to relate to one's sense of personal shame. A controlling God concept was found to be positively affiliated with shame, but a loving God concept was independent of shame. Other research has shown that an authoritarian God is associated with depression (Rosmarin, Krumrei, & Andersson, 2009), aggression (Bushman, Ridge, Das, Key, & Busath, 2007) and decreased forgiveness (Johnson, Li, Cohen, & Okun, 2013). Pargament et al. (1990) have observed that viewing God in a positive and benevolent light can buttress meaning, self-esteem, and one's sense of control in life. Subsequent research by Johnson and colleagues (Johnson, Cohen, & Okun, 2016; Johnson et al., 2013) has shown that a benevolent concept of God is positively associated with a benevolent self-identity and a sense of moral obligation, such as forgiveness, intentions to volunteer, and willingness to aid others (including people from outside one's own religious group).

Foster and Keating (1990) conducted a rather ingenious investigation into the relationships between male and female God images for men and women. They observed greater self-esteem when women interacted with a female God, while males viewed themselves more favorably when their God was masculine.

Optimism and Hope

Maltby and Hill (2008) have suggested that the perceived provision of hope is a key positive psychological ingredient of the Christian religion. Indeed, Koenig et al. (2012) found that of 72 studies investigating the relationship of religion or spirituality to optimism or hope, only 17 found no relationship. All of the other studies found positive relationships between religion and greater hope or optimism. Markstrom's (1999) survey of 125 high school juniors in West Virginia (half of the sample was African American and half was European American) found that greater religious involvement was associated with such ego strengths as hope, will, purpose, love, care, and fidelity. Unlike most studies comparing European Americans with other racial groups, this study found the religious associations to be stronger among the European American students. Krause (2002) discovered from his sample of 1,500 senior citizens that perceived closeness to God was a significant predictor of optimism, especially among African Americans. Religious belief, but not religious behavior, was found to be the best predictor of hope in a study of 271 clinically depressed patients (Murphy et al., 2000).

Some research suggests that optimism is associated with religious conservatism (Sethi & Seligman, 1993, 1994). This suggestion runs contrary to the common hypothesis that religious conservatism or fundamentalism should be associated with a negative self-concept and low self-esteem, because of an emphasis on personal sin and guilt (Hood, 1992b). Sethi and Seligman (1993) compared members of three different religious groups (liberal, moderate, and "fundamentalist"—though their measure of fundamentalism would be better described as one of religious conservatism or orthodoxy) on a variety of measures from which they derived indices of optimism and pessimism. Optimism was greatest among the members of the fundamentalist group, followed by those from the moderate group. The members of the liberal group evidenced the least optimism. Religious leaders were interviewed with regard to distinguishing the prayers and hymns typically used by the different faiths. A content analysis of these materials showed that theory paralleled the level of group optimism. In other words, the fundamentalist group was exposed to the most optimistic religious content, and the liberal group to the least. In related work, it was concluded that fundamentalism stresses the most hopefulness, the least hopelessness, and the least self-blame for negative happenings (Sethi & Seligman, 1994). It should be noted, however, that questions have been raised about the validity of the optimism–pessimism measures used (Kroll, 1994).

Snyder, Sigmon, and Feldman (2002) suggest that religion is uniquely capable of providing hope because it provides adherents with explicit goals, promotes pathways (including pathway thoughts) to achieve those goals, and supplies incentives for motivation to reach those goals. Emmons (2005) states: "In its religious context, hope provides respite during trials, brings perseverance during challenges, and provides assurance of eternal joy" (p. 242).

"Sacred" Emotions and Attitudes

Emmons (2005) suggests that the characteristics of certain emotions allow us to consider them as "sacred" emotions or attitudes. Attitudes such as gratitude, hope, humility, awe, and reverence are more likely to occur in religious or spiritual *settings*, to be elicited by religious or spiritual *practices*, to be experienced by people who *self-identify* as religious or spiritual, to be cultivated in adherents by religious and spiritual *systems*, and to be experienced when apparent secular aspects of lives are imbued with spiritual *significance*. If, in fact, the search for the sacred is a defining feature of religion and spirituality, as suggested by many (Hill et al., 2000; Pargament, 1997, 1999; Zinnbauer et al., 1997), then we might expect such sacred attitudes to be generated when the sacred is encountered. Here we look at two such attitudes: gratitude and humility.

GRATITUDE

Understood as an emotional response to a gift (Emmons, 2005), gratitude has been shown to have a significant impact on emotional well-being (Emmons & McCullough, 2003; Watkins, Woodward, Stone, & Kolts, 2003). Emmons and McCullough (2003) found that an intervention of a daily and weekly practice of gratitude caused increases in a general sense of subjective well-being and hope. Based on their findings, Watkins et al. (2003) maintained that people who are grateful have a general sense of abundance, appreciate the simple everyday pleasures of life, and appreciate the contribution of others to their well-being. Watkins (2004) proposed that the relationship between gratitude and subjective well-being may very well reflect a "cycle of virtue," whereby gratitude enhances happiness, which in turn promotes further gratitude; this is an example of what Fredrickson (2001) has called the "upward spiral" of positive affect. There is now an abundance of evidence suggesting that gratitude is linked to many positive psychological states, including expanded and stronger social relationships (Algoe, 2012)—in part because people who exhibit gratitude are motivated to behave more prosocially (DeSteno, Bartlett, Baumann, Williams, & Dickens, 2010; McCullough, Kimeldorf, & Cohen, 2008), in that they may see more good in those around them (McCullough, Emmons, & Tsang, 2002). Emmons and Stern (2013, p. 847) suggest that gratitude is a "healing affect" that may decrease lifetime risks of depression, anxiety, and substance abuse. In general, gratitude is good for one's overall well-being (Watkins, 2014; Watkins & McCurrach, 2016; Wood, Froh, & Geraghty, 2010) and for one's physical health (Algoe & Way, 2014; Davis et al., 2016; Huffman et al., 2016; Krause & Ellison, 2009; Krause, Emmons, & Ironson, 2015; Krause, Hayward, Bruce, & Woolever, 2014).

It is clear that most religions extol the virtue of gratitude (Carlisle & Tsang, 2013; Emmons & Crumpler, 2000; Emmons & Kneezel, 2005). But are religious people any more grateful than others? Watkins et al. (2003) found religiousness to be positively correlated with gratitude, and those who scored high in religiousness also acknowledged the contribution of the divine to their sense of well-being. Similarly, McCullough et al. (2002) found that gratitude, as part of daily mood, was positively associated with various measures of religiousness, including scores on Intrinsic (but not Extrinsic or Quest) religious orientation, interest level in religion, and general religiousness. Gratitude is also associated with prayer frequency (Lambert, Fincham, Braithwaite, Graham, & Beach, 2009). People who are more involved in their church not only sense a greater cohesiveness and social support, but they also feel more grateful to God, and these findings last over time (3 years in one study; Krause & Ellison, 2009).

Are religious people just naturally grateful? Maybe so, but research suggests that there is something unique about religious gratefulness. Rosmarin, Pirutinsky, Cohen, Galler, and Krumrei (2011) found that religious gratitude predicted mental well-being over and above general gratitude, but only among those who were more religiously committed.

HUMILITY

Many people think of humility as a "religious-type" trait (Exline & Geyer, 2004). Indeed, there is good reason for this, since humility is a highly valued virtue found in many religious traditions (Bollinger & Hill, 2012). Given such dictionary definitions and popular conceptions as "lowliness," self-abasement," and "submission," it is also a trait not encouraged in Western society. As C. S. Lewis (1942/2000, p. 153) once said, "Thousands of humans have been brought to think that humility means pretty people trying to believe they are ugly and clever men trying to believe they are fools." However, the psychological literature provides a different picture. For example, Furey (1986) defined "humility" as

> the acceptance of our imperfection. It does not prohibit self-expression. Nor does it rule out pride in one's accomplishments. Humility in no way limits human potential. Rather humility allows us to accept the limitations of our potential. Psychologically, humility implies the acceptance of ourselves. (p. 7)

Understood as "a nondefensive willingness to see the self accurately" (Exline & Rose, 2005, p. 320) and a willingness to own one's limitations (Whitcomb, Battaly, Baehr, & Howard-Snyder, 2017), a feeling of humility is often promoted when one contemplates the mysteries of the universe. In so doing, some of the components of humility delineated by Tangney (2009) may be activated: a willingness to see oneself accurately, an accurate perspective of one's place in the world, an ability to acknowledge personal mistakes and limitations, an openness to new ideas and perspectives, a low self-focus, and an appreciation of the value of all things.

Most research on humility has been conducted in the past decade, and we are just now beginning to see a pattern of results suggesting that a number of positive tendencies are associated with being humble (see Hill & Laney, 2017, for a more complete review). Some of these findings include such prosocial characteristics as gratitude (Dwiwardani et al., 2014; Exline, 2012), forgiveness (Exline, Baumeister, Zell, Kraft, & Witvliet, 2008), helpfulness (LaBouff, Rowatt, Johnson, Tsang, & McCullough, 2012), honesty (Ashton & Lee, 2005), generosity (Exline & Hill, 2012), and commitment to social justice (Jankowski, Sandage, & Hill, 2013), as well as appreciating others' strengths and accomplishments (Tangney, 2009) and being cooperative (Hilbig & Zettler, 2009).

Exline and Geyer (2004) found that undergraduate students, regardless of how religious they were, consistently saw humility as a positive characteristic, associated humility with good psychological adjustment, reported that humble people were more likely to be religious or spiritual, and reported experiences of personal success associated with positive emotion when recalling situations where they felt humbled. However, religiousness was positively associated with each of these findings (i.e., each association was stronger among those who scored higher in religiousness). High religiousness was also positively associated with the desire to become more humble.

But are religious people actually more humble, as the common perceptions from Exline and Geyer's (2004) sample would suggest? We would predict this to be the case, given that humility is a virtue espoused by many religious traditions, including Christianity. Indeed, some evidence in the Exline and Geyer study suggests that more religious people *desire* to be humble. Furthermore, religious people report being more humble (Rowatt, Kang, Haggard, & LaBouff, 2014), and humility predicts less religious struggle (Grubbs & Exline, 2014a). Rowatt, Ottenbreit, Nesselroade, and Cunningham (2002), however, found evidence of a religious pride—a "holier-than-thou" attitude—in their student samples at a medium-sized church-affiliated university. This religious pride was greatest among those with high Intrinsic scores and least among those with high Quest scores. It is likely that many religious people understand humility in terms of a vertical relationship—as a proper attitude in relation to God (Bollinger & Hill, 2012)—whereas most research on humility has investigated it as a horizontal relationship among people.

Religion and Mental Health: Summary

Perhaps even more than they facilitate physical health, religion and spirituality seem to facilitate mental health. Park and Slattery's (2013) literature review identifies 11 possible mechanisms or pathways, each with empirical support, through which religion positively influences mental or emotional health: social support; social identity (a distinctive world view and sense of membership); guidelines for healthy living; the promotion of forgiveness (which has been shown to be positively related to health); a positive relationship with a transcendent being; religious coping resources and strategies; religious practices such as prayer that may influence a sense of well-being; positive affect; sense of meaning; emotional regulation; and afterlife beliefs. This is quite a list. Park and Slattery also pointed out that there are negative pathways (largely negative utilization of many of these same mechanisms such as negative social interactions that decrease a sense of social support), but it appears that the positive pathways tend to outweigh the negative for most people.

RELIGION AND PSYCHOPATHOLOGY

As indicated thus far in this chapter, religion is usually associated with good health, both psychologically and physically. But there also may be many ways in which faith and psychological problems may be related. Not all of the studies in Koenig's (2012) review of the literature on religion and spirituality in relation to both physical and mental health showed a positive relationship. Sometimes religion and spirituality showed no association with health, and sometimes they were inversely related to health. It is an overgeneralization to say that religion is necessarily good or bad for one's health.

How might faith be associated with psychological problems? We consider five possible relationships:

1. Religion may be an expression of mental disorder.
2. Institutionalized faith can be a socializing and suppressing force, aiding people to cope with their life stresses and mental aberrations.
3. Religion can serve as a haven—a protective agency for some mentally disturbed people.
4. Spiritual commitment and involvement may perform therapeutic roles in alleviating mental distress.
5. Religion can be a stressor, a source of problems; in a sense, it can be "a hazard to one's mental health."[2]

Religion as an Expression of Mental Disorder

Many years ago, when one of us (Bernard Spilka) was an undergraduate, he and his fellow students were regularly harassed and challenged by two street corner evangelists. Actually, only one was capable of presenting his Biblically based arguments; the other stood to the side, reading from a large open Bible in an unintelligible mumble. The students never saw him do anything else. It was evident that his contact with reality was extremely poor, and he illustrates what books on psychopathology frequently suggest—namely, that any aspect of religious belief, experience, or behavior can be meaningful to a seriously disturbed mind.

Disturbed Religious Beliefs, Thoughts, and Behavior

It is not uncommon that a person suffering from major mental illness who is delusional and possibly hallucinating feels chosen by God to do certain things. Proportions of severely disturbed inpatients with religious delusions vary from 6% in Pakistan to about 20% in Europe to 36% in North America (Mohr, 2013). Delusions may be manifested in the belief that one is an angel of God—or, on the other side of the coin, that one is cursed by God—and can lead to tragic behavior such as homicide (Kraya & Patrick, 1997) or cutting off body parts (Field & Waldfogel, 1995).

One form of mental pathology that is manifested in religious thinking and behavior has been termed "scrupulosity" (Mora, 1969). Askin, Paultre, White, and Van Ornum (1993, p. 3) call it "the religious manifestation of Obsessive–Compulsive Disorder." They specifically

---

[2]With the exception of the last role for religion, we are deeply indebted to James E. Dittes for this framework, which was first used in Spilka and Werme (1971).

define scrupulosity as "a condition involving continuous worry about religious issues or compulsions to perform religious rituals" (Askin et al., 1993, pp. 3–4). Primary among the expressions associated with scrupulosity are a fear of sin and compulsive doubt (Nolan, 1990), and scrupulosity is often found in those with perfectionistic tendencies (Allen, Wang, & Stokes, 2015). Although it is associated with personal uncertainty that may influence fear of sin and fear of God (Fergus & Rowatt, 2014a, 2014b), Witzig and Pollard (2013) found that, contrary to expectations, scrupulosity is not significantly related to religious fundamentalism.

In addition, scrupulous persons engage in rigid ritualistic observances and practices in order to gain some sense of purification. However, they can never feel clean and accepted by God, because they make attributions to themselves as bad and sinful, and to the deity as unforgiving and tolerating no deviation from extreme religious strictures. Such a concern can result in excessive religious shame over moral failings—a shame that can be exacerbated by afterlife beliefs such as an excessive fear of hell (Exline & Yali, 2006) or bad karma. Less extreme forms may be resolved by efforts to combat perfectionism, such as facilitating humility or self-forgiveness (Hall & Fincham, 2005). Though scrupulosity is not restricted to the teenage years, there is evidence that its peak period of occurrence in life is adolescence (Nolan, 1990; Wulff, 1997), thus providing support for Freudian theory suggesting that scrupulosity is related to sexual impulse control. Those suffering from this condition continually seek assurances from religious authorities and tend to reject psychotherapy. It is possible, however, for an involved cleric to work with a therapist to help alleviate the problem (Nolan, 1990).

Religious and Mystical Experiences

The often extremely unusual and graphic nature of religious or mystical experiences can easily lead one to conclude that they are signs of mental disturbance. The association of religious and mystical episodes with the use of drugs has been widely noted (Batson, Schoenrade, & Ventis, 1993; Bridges, 1970; see also the discussion of entheogens in Chapters 10 and 11). Insofar as drug use may reflect abnormality, psychedelic experiences with a religious flavor can be regarded as expressing deviance in personality. Hood (1995a), however, details a wide variety of avenues to religious experience, further suggesting that such experience is not a common result of psychopathology.

Before we too readily label religious and mystical experiences as indicating mental deviance, let us recall from Chapters 10 and 11 that considerable percentages of the U.S. and British populations report such encounters (Greeley, 1974; Hardy, 1979; Hay & Morisy, 1978; Thomas & Cooper, 1978), most (70–80%) of whom are identified as religious (Spilka, Ladd, McIntosh, Milmoe, & Bickel, 1996). In a highly significant theoretical and research paper, Rodney Stark (1965) offered a breakdown of religious and mystical experiences ranging from the normal to the possibly pathological. For example, his "salvational" type is said to be motivated by a sense of "sin and guilt" (p. 102). Of a more extreme nature, with much potential for illustrating mental disturbance, is Stark's "revelational" experience. It is the rarest and most deviant form he discusses, and is expressed in visual and auditory hallucinations that the individual regards as messages from the divine, angels, or Satan. It has also received some confirmation from work showing that personality and adjustment problems may be associated with religious experiences involving extreme physical–emotional reactions and/or hallucinations (Jackson & Spilka, 1980). Similar connections have been offered by other scholars (Boisen, 1936; Spilka, Brown, & Cassidy, 1993).

There is no doubt that religious and mystical encounters may reflect mental disturbance; however, the weight of the evidence suggests that most such experiences are not pathological, and that many even have beneficial effects (Clark, Malony, Daane, & Tippett, 1973; Heriot-Maitland, 2008; Francis, Ziebertz, Robbins, & Reindl, 2015; McCallister, 1995). Furthermore, Kohls and his colleagues have demonstrated that among persons who have mystical experiences, those who are adept at spiritual practices are more prone to experience these states as positive (Kohls & Walach, 2007; Kohls, Hack, & Walach, 2008; Kohls, Walach, & Wirtz, 2009).

Glossolalia

Glossolalia, or "speaking in tongues" (discussed in greater detail in Chapter 10), can be quite impressive in its effects and may be expressive of mental disorder. Glossolalia is a worldwide phenomenon (Bourguignon, 1992; Greenberg & Witztum, 1992). One estimate suggests that at least 2 million persons in the United States engage in glossolalia (Greenberg & Witztum, 1992). Psychiatry and psychology are slowly accepting the idea that it is not pathological behavior. There is currently little doubt that it is learned behavior, which is reinforced in certain group settings into which glossolalic individuals are socialized (Goodman, 1972; Lynn, 2013; Samarin, 1959). It continues to play a role in Pentecostalism. Schumaker (1995) speaks of the dissociation of learned associations, but then identifies dissociation with a broad range of mental problems. At worst, glossolalia might be termed a "mild psychopathological disorder" (Greenberg & Witztum, 1992, p. 306), but this may be more the exception than the rule. A representative example of research in this area is presented in Research Box 13.1.

RESEARCH BOX 13.1. The Psychology of Speaking in Tongues
(Kildahl, 1972)

In this study, two groups—one of 20 persons who spoke in tongues, the other of 20 people who did not—were interviewed in depth about their lives and tongue-speaking experiences. The groups were equated for religiosity, which was evidently high. Three projective tests (the Rorschach inkblot, the Thematic Apperception Test, and the Draw-a-Person) and one objective test (the Minnesota Multiphasic Personality Inventory) were administered to the participants.

It was observed that the nonglossolalic individuals tended to be more independent and autonomous, but also more depressed, than their glossolalic peers. Speaking in tongues was associated with strong trust in a religious group leader. Though no real differences existed between the two groups in well-being, the glossolalic participants were characterized as being more dependent on the guidance of a valued religious authority. They were inclined to relinquish personal independence and control to this leader, and usually ceased engaging in glossolalia when they lost faith in their spiritual guide.

Kildahl cited one researcher who asserted that "more than 85 percent of tongue-speakers had experienced a clearly defined anxiety crisis preceding their speaking in tongues" (p. 57). In this study, the glossolalia seemed to be constructive and anxiety-reducing.

Religion as a Socializing and Suppressing Agent

The Control Functions of the Religious Community

Marty (1975) details how "religious America has been and is conducive to the building of human community" (p. 35). Churches and congregations thus strive to create and strengthen a natural human desire to belong; this is sociality par excellence. To maintain and reinforce the group's bonds, a religious community actively functions to socialize, suppress, and inhibit what the community considers deviant and unacceptable behavior—whether these functions emanate from scriptural guidance, clerical pressure, or the social reinforcement of congregants (Koenig, McCullough, & Larson, 2001).

Churchgoers overwhelmingly represent the more conservative and conforming members of the North American social order (Glock & Stark, 1965; Herberg, 1960; McGuire, 1992; Stark & Glock, 1968). Stark and Glock (1968) refer to churches as "moral communities" (p. 163); as such, mental deviance is often redefined as a moral problem, since it threatens social cohesion. Whether a religious institution is liberal or conservative, it attempts to suppress conflict among its adherents, even if this increases dissension in the larger community (McGuire, 1992). This suppression can extend into all aspects of an individual's life—not the least of which are child-rearing practices that attempt to control displeasing and socially inappropriate behaviors, such as aggression (Bateman & Jensen, 1958).

These socializing forces will be effective to the degree that mentally disturbed persons attend religious services, have contact with others in this setting, and are exposed to their traditional outlooks. The research supports such an inference: Improvements in mental health among those with mental disorders go along with church or temple attendance (Strawbridge, Shema, Cohen, & Kaplan, 2001). Church attendance apparently strengthens impulse control and counters a variety of deviant tendencies (Rohrbaugh & Jessor, 1975). This is evidently true even for Hare Krishna members, whose overall adjustment improves with the length of time that they are affiliated with this group. The social controls exercised by this cult constitute a learning environment for its adherents (Ross, 1983).

Stark (1971) has shown that mentally disturbed persons who live outside a hospital setting assign less personal importance to religion and are less religiously active than nondisturbed citizens are. He has theorized that "psychopathology seems to *impede* the manifestation of conventional religious beliefs and activities" (p. 175; emphasis in original). This notable study is detailed in Research Box 13.2. It confirms other findings indicating that the faith of mentally disordered individuals is itself disturbed and deviant (Hardt, 1963; Lowe, 1955; Lowe & Braaten, 1966; Reifsnyder & Campbell, 1960). There are also indications that the more severe an individual's psychopathology is, the less the individual is involved in both personal and organized religious activity (MacDonald & Luckett, 1983).

The Control Functions of Religious Ideas and Institutions

In the preceding section, we have looked at the control functions of religion that emanate from church affiliation. The implication is that mental disturbance may be socially shaped and focused by religious ideas and the ways churches, synagogues, or mosques present them. Institutionalized faith lives by both formal and informal rules and referents—the Ten Commandments, the Golden Rule, the Bible, Papal statements, interpretations and decisions of denominational conclaves, and so forth. Scripture is replete with statements that associate religious devotion with bodily and mental health (Koenig et al., 2001). The ecclesiastical

---

RESEARCH BOX 13.2. Psychopathology and Religious Commitment
(Stark, 1971)

Theorizing that conventional religious involvement would be incompatible with deviant thinking and behavior, Rodney Stark hypothesized a negative relationship between these two variables. In his study, 100 mentally disturbed persons were carefully matched with 100 nondisturbed individuals and compared on a variety of religious items. The basic findings were as follows.

Percentage claiming:	Mentally disturbed	Nondisturbed
No religious affiliation	16	3
Religion not important at all	16	4
Not belonging to any church	54	40
Never attending church	21	5

Note. Adapted from Stark (1971). Copyright © 1971 the Religious Research Association. Adapted by permission.

The hypothesis was clearly confirmed, as the mentally disturbed persons demonstrated less conventional religious involvement than the nondisturbed sample. In another part of this study, Protestants and Catholics from a national sample who scored low on indices of psychic difficulties were more likely to be religiously orthodox and to attend church frequently than those revealing such problems. Again, the hypothesis was supported.

---

climate also sponsors notions of how a "good Jew" or a "good Christian" thinks and acts. These notions are supported by images of God's love, mercy, or vengeance—which are not taken lightly by faithful people, whether they be nondisturbed or disturbed individuals. When adopted as guides for personal action, these rules and referents may be very effective forces for the suppression and socialization of abnormal impulses. Even if psychopathology comes to the surface, the argument has often been made that the use of religion may prevent worse things from happening. One paper suggests that "occasionally religiosity in paranoid schizophrenia might itself be a mechanism to control underlying hostility and aggressive behavior" (MacDonald & Luckett, 1983, p. 33).

In summary, Mowrer (1958) quoted Feifel on the socializing function of religious doctrine: "Religion . . . tries to school us in those wise restraints—self-discipline, the capacity for sacrifice and service to others—that make the repressive control of impulses unnecessary" (p. 579). This is an ideal that many disturbed people attempt to realize.

Religious Role Models

Both children and adults often learn how to behave by modeling themselves after people whom they admire or who purvey ideas and ideals relevant to success in attaining desired goals (Bandura, 1977, 1986). In other words, they learn by observing others and emulating their thoughts and behavior. These others may be people with whom they interact or about whom they read, hear, or are informed. Social learning theory suggests that "the power of a moral model . . . can be an important component in the development of self-control" (Casey

& Burton, 1986, p. 82). Within limits, people can learn to be what is generally defined as "normal" or "abnormal" by emulating others.

Ministers, priests, rabbis, Biblical heroes, Jesus and his apostles, saints, significant others from churches (e.g., youth group leaders), and even family members may stand as spiritual exemplars to be imitated (see Oman & Thoresen, 2003). Explicitly and implicitly, these figures enact roles that may significantly influence the behavior and thinking of religious people along approved lines. In local settings, clergy may stand as greatly admired models. In one study of over 3,000 children and adolescents, clerics were rated as more supportive than parents, suggesting the potential of priests and ministers as positive role models (Nelsen, Potvin, & Shields, 1976). In all likelihood, these images can be meaningful referents for some mentally disturbed individuals. As Bandura (1977) has affirmed, "modeling influences can strengthen or weaken inhibitions over behavior" (p. 49).

Such a behavioral role model approach has been formalized by the Swedish scholar Hjalmar Sundén. As noted in earlier chapters, his role theory appears applicable to religious behavior in general, since it stresses experience, perception, motivation, and learning. Holm (1987a) notes that "when an individual in a certain religious tradition absorbs descriptions from sacred history, he learns models for his attitudes toward the supernatural" (p. 41); he adds that "this description will function as a structuring role pattern" (p. 41). Here is a theoretical framework that usefully connotes religious role models with the socialized control of thinking and behavior on the part of mentally distressed persons.

It is evident that religious systems and their supporters can suppress abnormal thinking and behavior, and can help mentally disordered people become part of the larger community. Such social and ideological sustenance may also contribute to ego strength and integration. Stated differently, adherence to a faith that is in line with cultural norms can constructively influence psychopathology.

Religion as a Haven

Religion can offer mentally distressed individuals refuge from the stresses of daily life—a safe harbor from the turmoil and turbulence of living. This can take place in three ways: (1) Everyday existence may be circumscribed and controlled by rules that leave little doubt about how to behave; (2) being part of a religious organization may alleviate fears of social isolation and rejection; and (3) strong identification with a religious body can provide the perceived security of divine protection. These processes can also take place within different types of religious organizations, including groups or movements that are out of the religious mainstream (so-called "sects" or "cults," which are frequently referred to as "new religious movements").

Though many reasons exist for the formation of new religious bodies, particularly sects and cults, such movements often attract a disproportionate number of mentally disturbed individuals. As noted earlier, if such persons are not socialized by mainline churches, they may become estranged from traditional religion. This is a two-way street: The average churchgoer is probably sympathetic to the plight of mentally disordered individuals, but may still prefer not to be associated with such people. The inability of mentally disturbed persons to fit in may cause them to respond in a reciprocal manner and to reject conventional beliefs and believers. They may, however, find a home in religious or spiritual subcultures in sects or cults, which are by definition out of the mainstream. Since members of these bodies often feel that they are ostracized by society (and in many instances they actually are), they may find common cause with others who are similarly rejecting or rejected for reasons of individual mental deviance (Coates, 2012a).

It is important to recognize that the majority of members of what are socially regarded as deviant religious groups are quite "normal" and mentally healthy (Richardson, 1995). Some disturbed individuals may, of course, find a haven that functions as a source of meaning and a framework of needed control in these religious groups, but they probably constitute the exception and not the rule (Ross, 1983). Nevertheless, new religious movements are often functioning in a positive manner for individuals who experience previous vulnerabilities (Coates, 2012b).

Alienated individuals may be attracted by a wide variety of religious and ecclesiastical elements. Unquestioning attachment to a spiritual leader may reflect emotional immaturity and strong dependency needs. The charismatic quality of some of the founders of these groups can also entice persons whose reality contacts are weak. One study of members of the Unification Church (pejoratively called "Moonies") revealed that over 40% admitted having had mental difficulties prior to joining the church; many of these had sought professional help, and a few had been hospitalized (Galanter, Rabkin, Rabkin, & Deutsch, 1979). The researchers concluded that the outcome of affiliation with the Unification Church was psychologically beneficial.

Another example of the way in which sects or cults may serve a temporary haven function is implied by work showing that some young people, but by no means all, who affiliate themselves with these bodies come from troubled homes and families (Schwartz & Kaslow, 1979). Such a religious group can act as a substitute family until a person is able to cope with a North American milieu that highly values personal autonomy; the group can offer needed social and psychological backing, with positive acceptance and support. We see this in Kildahl's (1972) description of the fellowship among glossolalic individuals. He described them as exhibiting "a tremendous openness, concern, and care for one another . . . they bore each other's burdens . . . were with each other in spirit and in physical presence" (p. 299).

Finding a spiritual haven is not easy. Particularly among the cults and sects, troubled people move rather easily from one such group to another. The unstable membership of these bodies is well documented (McLoughlin, 1978; Sasaki, 1979; Wood, 1965), possibly as seekers continue their search for meaning and control. Although we have focused upon the more negative mental health aspects of some of those attracted to cults, the more psychologically healthy aspects of those attracted to cults and sects must not be forgotten, as discussed in Chapter 9.

Religion as Therapy

For the last half century, the role of faith as therapeutic has been increasingly recognized on a number of levels. Not only do religious and spiritual practices exercise such a role, but clergy themselves are now explicitly undertaking psychological training as therapists. As part of what has become known as "clinical pastoral education," churches have been able to avail themselves of theologically sophisticated counselors and therapists who can utilize the doctrines of their faith when working with parishioners. We describe this and similar developments in greater detail later in the chapter (see "Religion and Psychotherapy," below).

We have seen that the suppression/socialization functions of religion may work to inhibit deviant mental expression, if not to improve disordered mental states. However, moving beyond the suppression/socialization functions of religion can be actively therapeutic. Some of the activities and phenomena that we have discussed as possible expressions of mental disorders, such as religious experiences and glossolalia, may also perform remedial roles. Sometimes these work directly; at other times, they work indirectly by involving friends and congregants as socializers and suppressors. We have already reviewed an extensive literature, for example, showing that some religious and spiritual experiences have been associated with such positive emotions as optimism and hope. Furthermore, one must consider the social context of the experience. Prince (1992) notes that religious experiences may be defined as pathological or therapeutic, depending on culture and group values. In situations where such experiences are valued, he claims that some "may be channeled into socially valuable roles" (p. 289). This is true among Pentecostal sects that encourage religious mysticism. Hine (1969) suggests that these experiences aid adjustment and integrate people into their groups, which also provide quite supportive environments.

Conversion

The beneficial and therapeutic effects of conversion have been celebrated for millennia. We hear about being "born again," being "twice born," "finding God," "coming home," and so forth. Well over a century ago, Starbuck (1899) claimed that for converts "the joy, the relief, and the acceptance are qualities of feeling, perhaps, which give the truest picture of what is going on in conversion—the free exercise of new powers, and escape from something, and the birth into Larger Life" (p. 122). Though clinicians might employ different language, these are unquestionably therapeutic goals. Hill (2002) points out how spiritual transformation can create changes in meaning systems that yield a positive affective state through a new or renewed sense of purpose, value, efficacy, and self-worth. Although there may be many reasons for conversion, clinicians are becoming increasingly sensitive to the potential benefits of conversion experiences (Bergman, 1953; Levin & Zegans, 1974).

Ritual

Perhaps nowhere are the therapeutic aspects of religion better realized than through ritual. The role of ritual in ceremony and prayer cannot be minimized, for it is considered a means of contacting the supernatural and concurrently oneself and others. It is often a call for vicarious control by a deity when a supplicant is unable to exercise mastery (Brown, 1994). Prayer is probably the most common ritual and is discussed later in this chapter as a form of religious coping. Even though the following comments present ritual in the broadest perspective, let us keep in mind that these remarks are fully appropriate to religion. Though some aspects of ritual may involve mental disturbance, the use of religious rituals per se is not necessarily abnormal or unhealthy.

Since the evidence overwhelmingly confirms that the roots of ritual run deep in both biology and the evolutionary process, it is easy to believe that it must perform some important function (Huxley, 1966, 1968). This inference is further supported by the apparent fact that there are no known cultures without ritual (Helman, 1994). Wulff (1997) cites Lorenz to the effect that ritualization is involved in "communicating, restricting aggression, and increasing pair and group cohesion" (p. 155). All of these may involve facets of mental disturbance. Rituals are also said to manage life's uncertainties (Horner & Dobb, 1997). They counter ambiguity, increase control over oneself and the environment, enhance meaning, reduce stress, decrease anxiety, and curb impulsivity (Erikson, 1966). Social bonding is also facilitated. Several noted clinical scholars add that rituals channel destructive and extreme emotions into controllable forms (Benson & Stark, 1996; Pargament, 1997; Pruyser, 1968). Kiev (1966) has pointed out that ritual explicitly promotes "therapeutic emotional reactions" via the opportunity to "express in socially approved ways ordinarily inhibited impulses and desires" (p. 170). Pruyser (1968) has suggested that ritual is adaptive when it creates a "structure for emotional expression" or performs "dynamically as a defense against the intensity of any emotion or the unpleasantness of some" (p. 143). Through its emotion-regulating and control functions, ritual (and specifically religious ritual) works to increase self-control and to counter disordered thinking and behavior.

The ubiquitous nature of religious ritual is well demonstrated by Moberg (1971), who covers the range from the individual level through family, churches, and synagogues to literally nationwide forms that utilize the mass media. Given such possibilities, the healing and therapeutic possibilities inherent in rites and ceremonies appear quite impressive.

There can be little doubt about the importance of ritual. The observations of astute anthropologists and clinicians concerning its effects are quite striking; however, objective empirical work in this realm is lacking. It is a topic worthy of rigorous research by psychologists.

Religion as a Hazard to Mental Health

As we have already commented, the dominant traditional view of faith in psychology has been to associate it with psychopathology. We have shown that the opposite is often true; however, religious institutions and doctrines can create stress and cause psychological problems. Indeed, there is some truth in the title of a book written well over four decades ago, *Religion May Be Hazardous to Your Health* (Chesen, 1972). Similarly, the noted psychologist Paul W. Pruyser (1977) referred in an article title to "The Seamy Side of Current Religious Beliefs." Albert Ellis (1988) indicated 11 ways in which religion seems to create and support mental disorder, although he later modified his position, as noted earlier in this chapter. The problem has been considered of such magnitude that Koenig et al. (2001), in the first edition of their definitive *Handbook of Religion and Health*, devoted a chapter to "Religion's Negative Effects." The message is simply this: Religion does contain elements that can adversely affect the mental well-being of its adherents.

Religion as a Source of Abnormal Mental Content

The doctrines and sources of institutional faith sometimes contain the seeds of psychopathology. Though most individuals who accept religious mandates live happy and fruitful lives, there are those who misinterpret and misapply the core elements of their faith. Others are, in a sense, victimized by parents, clergy, or influential others who misuse religion to gain power and personal gratification. This can happen when people treat religious precepts in a rigid and inflexible manner (Stifoss-Hanssen, 1994). One study dealing with some mental disorder correlates of "rigid religiosity" is detailed in Research Box 13.3. In essence, clinicians believe that a strict religious upbringing contributes to the development of emotional disorders, depression, suicidal potential, and a generally fearful response to life (Culver, 1988).

RESEARCH BOX 13.3. Rigid Religiosity and Mental Health: An Empirical Study
(Stifoss-Hanssen, 1994)

Religious bodies possess rules and regulations that people can often interpret in ways ranging from an easy flexibility to a rigid absolutism. The latter has been defined in one major
study as a "law-orientation" (Strommen, Brekke, Underwager, & Johnson, 1972). In the
present study, a scale assessing rigid–flexible religiosity was developed and administered
to 56 volunteer hospitalized patients with neuroses and a control group of 70 nonpatients.
The patients scored significantly higher than the controls on this scale, demonstrating that
rigid religiosity is a correlate of severely neurotic thinking and behavior. The author also
suggested a positive relationship between mental disturbance and an Extrinsic religious
orientation.

The inability to adapt church tenets and scripture to modern life is an accusation usually directed at fundamentalist groups and conservative religious bodies, often in an unbal-
anced manner. In fact, research, particularly on fundamentalism, suffers from a wide variety
of biases. At the same time, some individuals are attracted to these bodies because of what
Ostow (1990) has called an "illusory defense against reality" (p. 122). The great reliance of
orthodox groups on a literalist interpretation of scripture may be one of those defenses (Hood
et al., 2005). In addition, the authoritarian structure of many fundamentalist groups endows
its leaders (who are often seen as having a special relationship with the deity) with the power
to control and suppress dissent. The argument is made that the absolutist structure and dictates of these institutions produce a "fundamentalist mindset" that creates adjustment problems for their members (Kirkpatrick, Hood, & Hartz, 1991). This mindset has been further
described as involving extreme dogmatism and a need for simplistic "quick fixes for problems
involving marriage, children, sexuality, or society" (Hartz & Everett, 1989, p. 208). These
factors have been used to explain the anxiety, "guilt, low self-esteem, sexual inhibitions, and
vivid fears of divine punishment" noted among individuals who leave these groups (Hartz &
Everett, 1989, p. 209).

Despite all of these unpleasant inferences, research supporting such ideas is rather
sparse. In fact, as noted earlier, fundamentalism is positively associated with an optimistic
outlook on life (Sethi & Seligman, 1993). Other research has failed to find evidence for any
adverse effects on the ego development or the adaptive capacity of fundamentalists (Weaver,
Berry, & Pittel, 1994). When such contradictions exist, the only answer is to call for more
research; however, we must keep in mind that this is a troubling and controversial area, and
objectivity is imperative.

Religious and Spiritual Struggle

Religious and spiritual content that results in a personal struggle has the potential to become
a severe hazard (Exline, 2013). For example, a person's moral failings or spiritual doubts may
invoke an obsession with divine punishment. This is not to suggest that all people who experience struggle in their spiritual lives are doomed, but if such struggles are extreme, they
may become debilitating. At the least, spiritual struggle appears to be a modest but significant predictor of poor adjustment (Ano & Vasconcelles, 2005).

Religion and Psychotherapy

No treatment of the domain of religion and mental disorder would be complete without recognizing the increasing role of religion and spirituality in treating psychological problems. Many years ago, Bergin (1980) poignantly observed the need for clinical psychology to broaden its perspective, as the religious outlooks of clients and therapists are often markedly discrepant in regard to religion. In 2005, the American Psychological Association (APA) adopted an evidence-based approach to professional practice as its health care standard—which, in principle, has huge implications for how religion and spirituality are to be treated in clinical practice. This approach means that clinical psychologists must integrate the "best available research with clinical expertise in the context of patient characteristics, culture, and preferences" (APA Presidential Task Force on Evidence-Based Practice, 2006, p. 273). Thus therapists should be responsive to the religious and spiritual proclivities that may be part of their clients' identities, and should approach such inclinations on the basis of what the research says rather than their own personal faith commitments (Shafranske, 2013), including those that may be antagonistic to religion.

As a result, the educational curricula of many mental health professionals are increasingly including training to increase awareness of clients' and patients' religious and spiritual concerns. This is matched in the seminary training of clergy-to-be and in programs for those already working in religious institutions; both groups are now becoming extensively familiar with the psychological complexities they must confront when dealing with congregants' mental problems (Koenig et al., 2001; Richards & Bergin, 1997).

The result of these developments has been an alliance between psychiatry and psychology on the one hand, and religion on the other (Academy of Religion and Mental Health, 1959; Group for the Advancement of Psychiatry [GAP], 1960; Klausner, 1964). This alliance has resulted in serious efforts to integrate the basic principles underlying these disciplines. Those working in this interdisciplinary realm have proposed a variety of approaches to enhancing people's well-being and adaptive thinking/behavior. Some themes and approaches intended particularly for clerical counselors and therapists include "pastoral counseling" (Hiltner, 1949; Wicks, Parsons, & Capps, 1985), "clinical pastoral education" (Thornton, 1970), "spiritual psychotherapy" (Karasu, 1999), "reframing in pastoral care" (Capps, 1990), "Christotherapy" (Tyrrell, 1985), and "ethical therapy" (Andrews, 1987). Psychotherapists' appreciation of the need for spiritual perspectives and understanding in their work has also been greatly enhanced (W. R. Miller, 1999; Richards & Bergin, 2000). Mutuality and coordination to realize common goals are increasingly sought as the barriers separating religious from psychological and psychiatric professionals are reduced.

RELIGION AND COPING

Police shootings of innocent civilians. Civilian shootings of innocent police. Terrorist attacks around the world. Raging wildfires. Earthquakes and tsunamis. Hurricanes and tornadoes. Gang violence. We live in a world that is beyond our control. To cope effectively, we often must marshal all available personal resources. In this section, we examine religion as one of those resources.

In the week following the tragedy of September 11, 2001, there was a spike in religious emotions and sentiments (Savage & Torgler, 2011), and U.S. national polling organizations reported increases in church attendance of 6–24% (Walsh, 2002). This trend continued through October into November. Members of many religious bodies sensed a revival of faith. People were turning to their deity for support and comfort. Was this indeed a new revival of faith? Apparently not, as 3 months later, the influx of churchgoers had receded to pre-September 11 levels. Uecker's (2008b) analysis from a national study of adolescents concluded that there was no faith revival among that age group following 9/11. Still, however, religious resources were available and were immediately utilized to help people cope with a national tragedy of monumental proportions.

Following September 11, Presbyterian clergy reported that they intentionally increased their sense of reliance upon God for strength, support, and guidance to help cope (Meisenhelder & Marcum, 2004). A study by Ai, Tice, Peterson, and Huang (2005) of 453 students found 3 months after the September 11 attacks that many resorted to prayer as a primary coping mechanism—particularly those with an initially high negative emotional reaction. The researchers found that the use of prayer for coping was related to less subsequent distress, largely through the sense of spiritual support and positive attitudes that the praying seemed to provide. In a different line of research, prayer was also found to be a frequent means of coping with trauma among Muslim refugees from Kosovo and Bosnia (Ai, Tice, Huang, & Ishisaka, 2005; see also Ai, Peterson, & Huang, 2003). Eighty-six percent of this sample reported praying, with 77% of the total sample using prayer so that their enemies "would pay for what they have done" (Ai, Tice, Huang, & Ishisaka, 2005, p. 291). As suggested by this latter finding, religious coping can take many forms.

Most of the research on religious coping reported in this section is based on Christian samples in the United States. However, research on coping is beginning to expand to other cultures and religious traditions, including Islam (Abu-Raiya, Pargament, & Mahoney, 2011; Khan, Sultana, & Watson, 2009: Khan & Watson, 2006), Buddhism (Falb & Pargament, 2013; Phillips, Cheng, Oemig, Hietbrink, & Vonnegut, 2012; Phillips et al., 2009), Judaism (Pirutinsky, Rosmarin, Pargament, & Midlarsky, 2011: Rosmarin, Pargament, & Flannelly, 2009; Rosmarin, Pargament, Krumrei, & Flannelly, 2010), and Hinduism (Tarakeshwar, Pargament, & Mahoney, 2003). In their review of religious coping among diverse populations, Abu-Raiya and Pargament (2015) arrived at four general conclusions. First, religious coping is common in virtually all religious traditions thus far studied. Second, both positive and negative religious coping approaches are used in diverse religious traditions. Third, positive religious coping methods are used more frequently than negative religious coping methods in the other religious groups studied (i.e., those other than U.S. Christian samples). Fourth, despite these commonalities in the use of religious coping, there are some distinct variations based on the nature and tenets of each faith tradition. Thus there are many similarities across traditions with regard to religious coping, but we cannot claim that "one size fits all."

The Process of Coping

Coping is at the heart of life. From its biological and evolutionary roots to complex human social behavior, it is the essence of living. In individualistically oriented Western society in particular, people are usually judged on their ability to cope with what is demanded of them. In many cases, personal trials prompt people to turn to their faith for help. Religion may be an especially important resource when individuals must deal with those "times that try the soul"—when crisis strikes and options are limited.

In order to understand how people handle life's problems, some researchers have emphasized coping *styles* or *traits*—relatively long-lasting, if not permanent, characteristics of individuals. Others have looked to the *process* of coping, and to change in the way difficulties are handled (Lazarus & Folkman, 1984). Though it may be argued that personal religiosity is commonly treated as if it were an aspect of personality, those who have studied the role of religion in coping are mostly concerned with it as a process variable, asking what it does for the person and how it functions when problems arise.

How Religion Enters into the Coping Process

People do not face stressful situations without resources. They rely on a system of beliefs, practices, and relationships which affects how they deal with difficult situations. In the coping process, this orienting system is translated into concrete situation-specific appraisals, activities, and goals. Religion is part of this general orienting system. A person with a strong religious faith who suffers a disabling injury, must find a way to move from the generalities of belief to the specifics of dealing with the injury. (Silverman & Pargament, 1990, p. 2)

Pargament (1997) suggests that people engaged in coping are searching for a "sense of significance" (p. 92). This is especially cogent for a theory that emphasizes religious coping, since religion is an exclusively human venture. "Significance" is a complex composite of values, beliefs, feelings, and conceptual schemas that defines the phenomenological essence of a person. Significance is thus a unified, holistic pattern of orientations toward oneself, others, and the world—and the search for significance is part of a meaning-making process. Pargament (1997) also speaks of an "orienting system, a frame of reference, a blueprint of oneself and the world that is used to anticipate and come to terms with life's events" (p. 100). It therefore contributes to and is part of the search for significance. Needless to say, religion, for many if not most people, is an important part of this orienting system.

The Coping Functions of Religion

In our view, stress, whether it involves harm/loss, threat, or challenge, reflects a situation in which meaning and control are in jeopardy. We may have difficulty making sense out of a situation, or be unable to master it. Religion is one way these needs are met, and the worldwide prevalence of religion may testify in part to the success of faith in attaining these goals. In Chapter 1, we have offered a framework for conceptualizing the psychology of religion in terms of meaning and control. We now further enlarge the scope of this framework, in order to understand the functions of religion for coping with life.

The Need for Meaning

Simply put, being able to comprehend tragedy—to make it meaningful—probably constitutes the core of successful coping and adjustment. For most people, religion performs this role quite well, especially in times of personal crisis. Fichter (1981) asserts that "religious reality is the only way to make sense out of pain and suffering" (p. 20), though not everyone is likely to agree with this point. That this struggle to understand tragedy via religion may last for a long time is evidenced by one extensive study (Echterling, 1993). Interviews with flood disaster survivors over a 7-year period led the researcher to infer that "they became theologians by asking how God could have allowed such tragedies to occur to them and their loved ones. They became philosophers by asking the meaning of life when they knew how frail and ephemeral life could be" (Echterling, 1993, p. 5). In other words, they searched for meaning in their moment of trial. Many survivors of Hurricane Katrina in 2005 showed the same pattern (Aten, Bennett, Hill, Davis, & Hook, 2012).

Faith habitually conveys the meaning that life's difficulties can be overcome. Whether or not people control objective conditions may be less important than their belief that even insurmountable obstacles can be mastered. As noted in earlier chapters, in much of life the sense of control is really an illusion; yet it is one that can be a powerful force supporting constructive coping behavior (Lefcourt, 1973).

The Importance of Control

The idea of control is complex—so complex that Skinner (1996) was able to identify 88 control constructs. There is great overlap among these concepts, but one elemental scheme that is pertinent to our concern speaks of two basic forms: (1) "primary control," or "being in charge" (i.e., having the ability to change the situation); and (2) "secondary control," or being able to effect change in oneself. The famous writer Nikos Kazantzakis (1961) noted this latter potential when he quoted a mystic's prescription: "Since we cannot change reality, let us change the eyes which see reality" (p. 45). Faith may play an important role in stimulating both primary and secondary forms of control, and the two forms are probably not independent of each other. In psychological circles, however, religion is largely regarded as functioning as a form of secondary control.

Pargament (1997) has posited three approaches to the issue of control in religious coping. A "deferring" mode of relationship—for example, praying in order to put the problem totally in the hands of God—does not appear to be as helpful as when a "collaborative" mode of relationship is manifested, in which God and the supplicant work together. Here prayer may keep the individual working on the problem while seeking the support of the deity. In a "self-directive" approach, God is acknowledged, but the problem is regarded as requiring personal rather than divine solution. Gorsuch and his colleagues have proposed a fourth style, which they term "surrender" (Maynard, Gorsuch, & Bjorck, 2001; Wong-McDonald & Gorsuch, 1997). This is similar to the deferring approach, but the deferring mode is akin to assigning *all* control to the external power of God, whereas the surrender style occupies a middle ground (some or most personal control is "surrendered" to God). In both self-direction and collaboration, by contrast, internal control is present. Petitioning for aid from God (i.e., the collaborative approach) is best for the individual who feels that personal responsibility cannot be deferred or surrendered. The collaborative and self-directive modes involve more of an internal locus of control, which research has shown to be generally beneficial (Phares, 1976); these modes have been found to relate to more positive coping outcomes than does the deferring approach, which employs a more external locus of control (Harris, Spilka, & Emrick, 1990; McIntosh & Spilka, 1990; Pargament et al., 1988).

As noted in Chapter 6, Jacobson, Luckhaupt, Delaney, and Tsevat (2006) conducted a qualitative study of how patients with HIV/AIDS interpreted their religious and spiritual experiences to their sense of self and adaptation while facing an HIV diagnosis. That is, how did religion and spirituality serve as a meaning-making framework for their current predicament? In-depth interviews with 19 patients resulted in four distinct patterns of religious/spiritual coping, three of which neatly corresponded with Pargament et al.'s (1988) religious coping styles: (1) "deferring believers," who believed that God had a reason for their illness;

(2) "collaborative believers," who found a working relationship with God as a means for new global meaning; (3) "spiritual/religious seekers," who were spiritually oriented but adrift or unfulfilled, and thus in a stage of struggle; and (4) "self-directed believers," who stressed very subjective and individualized spiritual experiences not grounded in traditional religion.

The need for meaning and the importance of control are interrelated. As Baumeister (1991) noted, "meaning is used to predict and control the environment" (p. 183), and religious meaning can help people regulate their emotions. A wonderful anecdotal example of how religion can realize this role was provided by a patient with breast cancer, who stated, "I had no idea that God could answer so many of my questions" (Johnson & Spilka, 1988, p. 12). Here we consider how religious meaning making can help us by facilitating three forms of secondary control. Rothbaum, Weisz, and Snyder (1982) have termed these "interpretive," "predictive," and "vicarious" control; all three are especially significant for understanding how religion helps people deal with the problems they confront both in everyday living and in troubled times.

INTERPRETIVE CONTROL

When people are in great difficulty, it is natural for them to feel that there is no way out of their predicament. In seeking to understand such an event and to achieve some degree of control over what seems hopeless, people often reinterpret what is taking place. They exercise interpretive control and construe a distressing situation in less troubling or even positive terms. They may claim that "things could be worse" or that "I have it better than a lot of other people." For example, in one study a patient with cancer concluded, "I looked upon cancer as a detour in the road, but not a roadblock" (Johnson & Spilka, 1988, p. 13). Religion is often invoked under such conditions, and through such interpretations, people gain control over their emotions and may thus become better able to handle their difficulties in a constructive way.

PREDICTIVE CONTROL

The perpetual human dream is to foretell the future. The idea of precognition fascinates people. If they could predict what would happen on future rolls of dice, who would win horse races, what the stock market might do, or whether their efforts in general would result in success or failure, they would expect to become the beneficiaries of unlimited wealth and happiness. The Bible has said, "The Lord himself shall give you a sign" (Isaiah 7:14).

Predictive control assures a person that things will turn out all right in the end. For example, another patient with cancer stated, "Because of my relationship with God, I had faith that this cancer was not going to take my life" (Johnson & Spilka, 1988, p. 12). There is a poignant example of predictive control in Eliach's (1982) *Hasidic Tales of the Holocaust*. Eliach tells the story of a devout Jew who during World War II was brought by the Nazis into the death camp at Auschwitz. The number 145053 was tattooed on his arm. He looked at it and suddenly concluded that he would live. He reached this conclusion by adding the digits together and finding that they totaled 18; 18 is a number that within Judaism means life, and thus he felt assured of survival. It was as if God had offered an omen signifying a secure future. Such predictive control gives the person confidence that the morrow will be good. We must keep in mind, however, that the critical element here is *perception* of the future; what actually occurs is independent of this aspiration.

VICARIOUS CONTROL

When people feel that they may not be able to cope with their troubles—particularly in cases of serious illness, where death is a possibility—they often turn to their God, and vicariously, the deity becomes a support or substitute for their own efforts. The essence of such vicarious control was stated by one woman with cancer, who declared, "I could talk to my God and ask for his help in healing" (Johnson & Spilka, 1988, p. 12). Identifying with her God gave her the strength to face potential death through her perceived divine connection. She thus attained a measure of vicarious control over her circumstances.

What Factors Prompt People to Turn to Religion?

The "availability" hypothesis or heuristic raises the question of why, in specific circumstances, certain things have a higher likelihood than others of coming to people's minds (Fiske & Taylor, 1991). Pargament and Abu-Raiya (2007) identified six key characteristics of individuals as predictors of persons for whom religion as a coping method may be more available: greater religiousness, lower socioeconomic status, gender (females more than males), older age, minority status, and critical life events (e.g., terminal illness, major disasters).

People turn to religion because it often works for them. Levin and Schiller (1987) raise the interesting possibility that "perhaps the nervous system represents the locus of a mechanism by which religious faith or religious beliefs . . . promote well-being" (p. 24). The mechanism may well be the sense of control that is often promoted by religion (McIntosh, Kojetin, & Spilka, 1985). Specifically, the perceptions that one is personally in control of life situations and that God is in overall control (i.e., Pargament's "collaborative" mode) relate to good health (Loewenthal & Cornwall, 1993; McIntosh & Spilka, 1990). Another possibility has been advanced by Benson (1975)—namely, that certain religious rituals (prayer, meditation, etc.) may stimulate a "relaxation response" that is broadly healthful (Goleman, 1984). In other words, not only may religion promote an increased sense of control; its rituals themselves may reduce stress and tension.

Futhermore, Bjorck and Cohen (1993) claim that the greater the stress, the more religious coping takes place. For example, religious coping is common among war veterans (Aflakseir & Coleman, 2009). Further threats (defined as the anticipation of more damage) elicit greater use of religion than actual harm/losses, which require acceptance. Since events that challenge people call upon personal effort and resources, they are seen as most controllable. Resorting to faith as a coping aid is thus least often employed in these situations.

Religious and spiritual coping has generated far too much research to report here (for reviews, see Cummings & Pargament, 2010; Gall & Guirguis-Younger, 2013; Pargament, 2011; Pargament, Falb, Ano, & Wachholtz, 2013). In the sections below, we highlight some of the major findings from this research.

Varieties of Religious Coping

Religion provides many possible ways of coping with the stresses of life. Table 13.1 mainly includes the work of Pargament, Poloma, and Tarakeshwar (2001), yet permits a consideration of various religious devices and roles. Pargament et al.'s (2001) approach is one way in which the various coping functions may be described. Others may see many of these devices as aspects of prayer, such as confession, thanksgiving, pleading, meditation, or self-improvement

TABLE 13.1. Various Means of Using Religion for Coping with the Stresses of Life

Variety of coping	Typical statement
Self-directive coping	"It's my problem to solve, not God's."
Collaborative coping	"God helps those who help themselves."
Deferring coping	"It's in God's hands."
Pleading religious coping	"Please, God, help me through this terrible time."
Benevolent religious reappraisal	"God gives me these trials to test me."
Punishing God reappraisal	"I have sinned and deserve to suffer."
Demonic reappraisal	"It is the work of the Devil."
Reappraisal of God's powers	"Nothing is too small for God not to notice and help."
Seeking spiritual support	"I know I can rely on God's love."
Spiritual discontent	"How could God do this to me?"
Seeking congregational support	"I know I can depend on my minister and other church members for help."
Interpersonal religious discontent	"I feel as if the church has deserted me."
Religious forgiving	"Father, help me be a better person; let me not be angry and afraid."
Rites of passage	"Now I am a man."
Religious conversion	"I have seen the light; I have found the way; I am born again."

Note. From Snyder (2001). *Coping with stress: Effective people and processes.* Copyright © 2000 Oxford University Press, Inc. Reprinted with permission.

(David, Ladd, & Spilka, 1992; see also the discussion of prayer below). An excellent example of coping research in this tradition is presented in Research Box 13.4.

Prayer as a Coping Method

For many, prayer is at the core of faith (Brown, 1994; Buttrick, 1942; Heiler, 1932). It is easy to perform, is intensely personal, can be kept private, and is widely employed. Approximately 90% of U.S. residents indicate that they pray, and 76% regard it as very important in everyday life (McCullough & Larson, 1999; Poloma & Gallup, 1991). As Trier and Shupe (1991) have observed, "prayer [is] the most often practiced form of religiosity" (p. 354). One reason why it may be so popular is that it helps people cope with their problems.

Religious activities, especially prayer, are usually regarded as positive coping devices directed toward both solving problems and facilitating personal growth (Folkman, Lazarus, Dunkel-Schetter, De Longis, & Gruen, 1986). Some psychologists, however, see religious ritual, including prayer, as a means of controlling one's emotions (Koenig, George, & Siegler, 1988). Others see it as an effective problem-focused mechanism, in that praying may be the only practical way of dealing with many tragedies, such as the death of a loved one (Bjorck & Cohen, 1993; Harris et al., 2010). Apparently, it can perform both problem- and emotion-focused functions (Carver, Scheier, & Pozo, 1992).

RESEARCH BOX 13.4. God Help Me: I. Coping Efforts as Predictors of the Outcomes to Significant Negative Life Events (Pargament et al., 1990)

In this landmark research, a very basic question was addressed: "What kinds of religious coping are helpful, harmful, or irrelevant to people dealing with significant negative events?" (p. 798). The authors also attempted to find out whether measures of religious coping techniques would predict outcomes of coping better than measures of nonreligious coping techniques.

A sample of 586 Christian church members responded to questionnaires assessing religious and nonreligious coping activities and outcomes in regard to negative events that they had experienced during the preceding year. Six kinds of religious coping and four kinds of nonreligious coping were identified. Three outcome measures were assessed: mental health status, general outcome of the negative event, and its religious outcome. The religious variables, to varying degrees, predicted all three of the outcomes. This was most evident for spiritually based activities and for faith and trust in God. Religious discontent and concern with punishment from God hindered coping and adjustment. Positive effects were predictable from perceptions of a just, loving, and supportive deity; involvement in religious rituals, such as attendance at services; prayer; Bible reading; focusing on the afterlife, living a good life; and having support from clergy and church members. It was also observed that an extrinsic, utilitarian faith was helpful. The authors concluded that at least among church members, religious coping is an important and beneficial part of the overall process of coping with stress.

Forms of Prayer

This simple concept, "prayer," covers many possibilities. Foster (1992) conceptually identified 21 different forms of prayer. A survey of seven empirical efforts resulted in from four to nine kinds of prayer (Ladd & Spilka, 2002). The most stable types identified have been "petitionary," "ritualistic," "meditational," "confessional," "thanksgiving," "intercessory," "self-improvement," and "habitual." All have been confirmed and measured by separate, reliable scales (David et al., 1992). One U.S. national study discussed "contemplative," "conversational," "colloquial," "ritual," "petitionary," and "meditative" prayers (Poloma & Gallup, 1991). There is considerable overlap among the various proposed schemes—a condition that has not been helped by the lack of a coordinating theory. If any generalities may be inferred from the data on prayer, it would appear that the more people pray, the more forms of prayer they utilize (David et al., 1992). In addition, frequency of prayer goes with praying for more things—health, interpersonal concerns, and financial matters (Trier & Shupe, 1991).

In order to provide some theoretical footing for conceptualizing prayer, Ladd and Spilka (2002) surveyed the literature and attempted to create a categorizing structure for the forms of prayer that have been empirically identified. Their model conceptualizes prayer as consisting of three directions of cognitive connections: inward (self-connection), outward (human–human connection), and upward (human–divine connection). Subsequent work (Ladd & Spilka, 2006) has resulted in a measurement scale that meets scientific criteria and supports this model.

Usage and Efficacy of Different Forms of Prayer

Overall, more prayers are offered in the name of health than anything else (Wachholtz & Sambamoorthi, 2011). However, people are selective in their praying, and the different forms of prayer they use may be employed in different circumstances. For example, patients who have survived more than 5 years since an initial diagnosis of breast cancer are likely to stress prayers of thanksgiving (Ladd, Milmoe, & Spilka, 1994). Petitionary prayers, which are said to be the oldest and most common prayers, are employed to counter frustration and threat, whereas contemplative prayers (attempts to relate deeply to one's God) seem to aid internal integration of the self (Janssen, de Hart, & den Draak, 1990; Poloma & Gallup, 1991). Meditational prayers (which are concerned with one's relationship to God) seem to reduce anger, to lessen anxiety, and to aid relaxation (Carlson, Bacaseta, & Simanton, 1988). Contemplative prayers have also been shown to aid psychotherapy by lessening distress and specific kinds of complaints (Finney & Malony, 1985a, 1985b, 1985c). By contrast, there is some suggestion that mechanical, ritualized prayers may relate negatively to well-being (McCullough & Larson, 1999).

Little coping research has been done on most forms of prayer; however, a few, such as intercessory and petititionary prayer, are deserving of further exploration.

INTERCESSORY PRAYER

Intercessory prayer is a particularly controversial issue. The idea that prayers in behalf of another person can influence the health of that other person has a long history. Research has generally not supported this notion. No differences were found between "treatment" groups (those who were prayed for by others) and control groups in studies of deteriorating rheumatic and psychological illness (Joyce & Weldon, 1965) and of alcohol consumption by individuals with alcohol abuse or dependence (Walker, Tonigan, Miller, Comer, & Kahlich, 1997). Small differences were found in studies of children's leukemia (Colipp, 1969) and adult coronary disease (Byrd, 1988). More recently, a meta-analysis of 14 studies by Masters, Spielmans, and Goodson (2006) concluded that no scientifically discernible effect of distant intercessory prayer was found. We must conclude that at this stage of research on intercessory prayer, its power and significance have yet to be demonstrated. Frequently throughout this book, we have encouraged that further research on a topic be conducted. Here, however, we concur with the contention of Masters (2005) that scientific experimental methodology is not well suited to study divine intervention; as a result, such studies are probably draining resources from other important research on the religion–health connection.

That said, there is some evidence that intercessory prayer can have a profound positive influence on close relationships, including on the person who is offering the prayer on behalf of another. For example, research has shown that praying for a romantic partner predicts relationship satisfaction (Fincham, Beach, Lambert, Stillman, & Braithwaite, 2008) and trust (Lambert, Fincham, LaVallee, & Brantley, 2012); increases relationship commitment (Fincham & Beach, 2014); increases forgiveness by motivating changes in relationships (Lambert, Fincham, et al., 2010); and reduces infidelity (Fincham, Lambert, & Beach, 2010). Apparently, there is some truth to the old adage that "the family that prays together, stays together."

PETITIONARY PRAYER

As noted above, petitionary prayer is the most common kind of prayer offered, and though it is treated negatively by some religionists, others have repeatedly averred that "petition is the heart of prayer" (Capps, 1982, p. 130). Capps (1982) further terms it "the crux of the psychology of religion" (p. 131). Simply said, prayers of petition ask for something. One content analysis of 227 petitionary prayers (Brown, 1994) showed that most requested something for family members (37%); next came prayers for alleviation of illness (21%). (The latter, though petitionary, were also intercessory when the illness was that of someone else, not the person doing the praying.) In third place were petitionary prayers for persons who had died (Brown, 1994). Obviously, people can plead for anything—one reason for the popularity of petitionary prayers. Earlier work by Brown (1966) with children and adolescents led to the conclusion that on the average, the more serious a situation is, the more strongly young people feel that petitionary prayer is appropriate. An egocentric belief in the direct efficacy of petitionary prayer decreases with increasing age. There is reason to believe that as the belief in the material effectiveness of these prayers lessens, it is replaced by a belief in nonspecific effects, such as "granting courage, improving morale or producing other psychological changes" (Brown, 1968, p. 77).

Contextual Coping Concerns

The concept of coping seems to have no limits. The content of this field varies from dealing with one's own outlook on life, to handling relations with others at home, work, school, and play, to dealing with the most tragic crisis situations that may be encountered. One person's petty annoyances can be another's sources of deep distress and depression. Therefore, it is necessary to consider contextual issues (both external and internal) that affect coping.

Faith and Coping with Daily Hassles

Coping begins with the needs of daily living, and is not restricted to handling crises. Some researchers have thus asked whether faith might play a role in adapting to the "hassles" of everyday life (Belavich, 1995). Noting that a number of adaptive coping strategies might be utilized, Belavich administered a carefully selected battery of tests to over 200 college students, and controlled for a variety of demographic variables. Sophisticated data analyses revealed that "religion plays a significant role in a person's experience with minor stressors on a day-to-day basis" (p. 24). Specifically, faith aids coping by diverting individuals from stress, and by enabling them to call upon the social support provided by other religious people and figures. Some aspects of religious coping were, however, related to poorer adjustment. The latter indicators—pleading and spiritual coping—implied a negative function. Conceptual efforts to explain these adverse findings call for further research.

Spirituality and Coping

Some valuable insights may be derived from the work of Socha (1999) on spirituality and coping. Emphasizing the "human existential situation," Socha goes beyond religion to a broader spiritual scheme. (See the discussions of "religion" vs. "spirituality" in several previous chapters.) He offers a holistic, growth-oriented view, in which a person recognizes the transitory nature of situations and acknowledges his or her own coping limits. Such awareness implies knowing when to define circumstances in terms of "sacredness"—a religious or secular notion of placing things in broader perspective. Belavich's (1995) work indicates what is done on a day-to-day basis; Socha's outlook suggests why, and introduces a different theoretical frame—a phenomenological approach that emphasizes how the individual perceives and explains the situation. This takes us back to the question of the meanings that precede the actions people take (another direction for research on coping and religion).

In other work relating to spirituality, Kennedy, Rosati, Spann, Neelon, and Rosati (n.d.), like Socha (1999), broaden the notion of coping from a focused pattern of responses to a broader approach based on making lifestyle changes. Working within a medically based program, these workers felt that their therapeutic procedures would constructively affect well-being and spirituality. Though they did not distinguish between religion-based and non-religion-based spiritualities, half of the participants in their program evidenced an increase in spirituality, and close to 100% reported an increase in their subjective sense of well-being. Positive and significant correlations were obtained among spirituality, well-being, and meaning. Distinguishing between faith-oriented and non-faith-oriented spiritualities should provide a substantive direction for further research, and may enable participants to utilize such avenues more effectively to make the desired lifestyle changes.

Religion and Positive–Negative Life Orientation

Another factor that contributes to effective coping behavior is whether a person takes a generally positive or generally negative perspective on life and its problems. This dimension is often treated as a general characteristic that includes attitudes toward both oneself and the world (Myers, 1992). Primarily viewed as trait-dependent, it is largely conceptualized in terms of optimism–pessimism. Its significance is well illustrated by a longitudinal study in which a pessimistic explanatory style manifested in early life predicted poor health in middle and old age (Peterson, Seligman, & Vaillant, 1988). Faith has been shown to be a significant component of optimism.

The association of religion with personal happiness is apparently a major function of faith in general (Ellison, 1991). Extensive surveys of thousands of people in 14 countries have also shown a positive association between religiousness and feelings of well-being (Myers, 1992). Utilizing a variety of religious measures in national samples in the United States, Pollner (1989) concluded that "relations with a divine other are a significant correlate of well-being" (p. 100). In his system, religion's effectiveness results from the following: (1) It brings a sense of order and coherence to stressful situations; (2) it has been found to counter feelings of shame or anger that are aroused by stress; (3) it also creates positive feelings about oneself, simply as a result of having a perceived relationship with the deity; lastly, (4) religion fosters a general tendency to see the self and the world in positive terms. In addition, there is strong evidence that religion, in offering a sense of meaning, control, and esteem, does support an optimistic outlook. This in turn helps people deal constructively with life, and seems to have long-range beneficial effects.

Religious/Spiritual Struggles

Most people report that religion and spirituality are powerful resources for joy, purpose, and meaning—themes that we have used as an important framework throughout this book. We have also reviewed the literature on religious and spiritual coping largely from a positive coping perspective. However, as we have mentioned earlier, there are negative approaches to religious coping. Religious and spiritual experiences can be sources of difficulty, tension, and struggle. Exline (2013) discusses four types of religious and spiritual struggles: struggles with the divine, intrapersonal struggles, interpersonal struggles, and struggles related to perceptions of supernatural evil.

STRUGGLES WITH THE DIVINE

As Exline and Rose (2005) point out, when a person is faced with suffering, the natural response is to engage in an attributional search similar to what we have described in Chapter 1. To the degree that God is held responsible for the suffering, anger and mistrust may occur (Exline, Park, Smyth, & Carey, 2011; Exline, Yali, & Lobel, 1999). However, people who report a close, committed relationship with God and/or who have more positive God images are less likely to express such anger. Some people view anger at God as morally wrong and may be unwilling to admit, even to themselves, such anger. Research has also shown that a small percentage of those who do blame God for negative events often find that their basic beliefs about God's existence are shaken (Altemeyer & Hunsberger, 1997; Exline & Martin, 2005). However, some may see the suffering as a lesson from God that is ultimately good (Exline & Rose, 2005).

INTRAPERSONAL STRUGGLES

The conflictual nature of wanting to do right, but struggling with other natural inclinations that may be interpreted by a religious person as sin, is often a recipe for perceived failure (Exline, 2013). This appraisal of moral imperfection can lead to shame or low self-esteem and thereby decrease one's sense of spiritual self-efficacy (Hill, 2002); in more extreme cases, it can increase frightening afterlife beliefs such as a fear of hell (Exline & Yali, 2006). Such struggles may lead to doubts about one's salvation, for example, or (conversely) doubts about the validity of one's religious beliefs (Hunsberger, Pratt, & Pancer, 2002).

However, many people report that the challenges of such struggles can lead to growth. For some, the result is a greater self-discipline, the practice of which may lead to a strengthened "moral muscle" (Baumeister & Exline, 1999). For others, it may mean focusing and relying on God's power for transformation (something akin to the Christian theological doctrine of grace); this may result in humbly accepting God's love and forgiveness—a process that has been empirically demonstrated to be associated with self-forgiveness (Carfaro & Exline, cited in Exline & Rose, 2005). For yet others, it may mean the act of surrender or submission to the authority of some higher power—a potentially adaptive coping style under some circumstances (Wong-McDonald & Gorsuch, 2000, 2004). In any case, the fact remains that most religious and spiritual traditions, even if individually determined rather than imposed by some external system of beliefs, prescribe moral guidelines that are often difficult to live up to. Such guidelines can thus constitute a source of struggle.

INTERPERSONAL STRUGGLES

Given that religion provides an important sense of meaning, disagreements between people about religion are sometimes intense. This may be especially true with people we care the most about, such as family members (Curtis & Ellison, 2002). Such tensions may occur over social issues that are sometimes addressed by religious teachings such as, for example, gay marriage or the ordination of gay/lesbian clergy.

Psychologists of religion should be sensitive to the social context of faith. For example, the faith experience of minority groups, especially if they threaten the teachings of the dominant societal religion, may create tension. The minority group members themselves may experience stigma or even forms of social discrimination (Dubow, Pargament, Boxer, & Tarakeshwar, 2000). Rosenberg (1962) observed that people who practiced a minority religion usually felt isolated from their larger social context. The long-range effects of such isolation were likely to include lower self-esteem, depressive feelings, and psychosomatic symptoms.

STRUGGLES RELATED TO PERCEPTIONS OF SUPERNATURAL EVIL

Spiritual experience is by and large a positive experience (Hardy, 1979; Exline, Yali, & Sanderson, 2000), though many people of religious conviction perceive oppression and attack as part of the spiritual realm. Attributions to Satan are rare, but when they do occur, they are most often in response to negative life-altering events (Lupfer, Tolliver, & Jackson, 1996) and are often indices of spiritual distress (Exline et al., 2000). For example, Krumrei, Mahoney, and Pargament (2011) found that demonic appraisals following divorce are not unusual.

Religion and Coping with Major Stress

We have pictured living as a process of continual coping. Clearly, religion can play a constructive role in handling the problems of daily life, but the real test of faith comes when common hassles are supplemented by the major trials of human existence—aging, catastrophic illness, or disability; family, social, and economic difficulties; the loss of loved ones; and, of course, confronting our own death. We have looked at some of these issues in prior chapters. In this section, we look at some of the religious coping research surrounding three major sets of stressors: aging, serious illness, and the loss of a child.

Religion and Coping with Age-Related Stressors

The many types of stressors that elderly individuals must confront—social, economic, emotional, and health-related—have been described in Chapter 7. As that chapter notes, research has consistently revealed that religious coping mechanisms, especially prayer, are most frequently employed when senior citizens are dealing with health-related stress (Conway, 1985–1986; Manfredi & Pickett, 1987). Turning to a deity for support appears to be the most effective strategy available to elderly persons with health problems. This holds true across different ethnic groups, socioeconomic statuses, and levels of education (Koenig, George, & Siegler, 1988; Krause & Van Tranh, 1989).

Furthermore, whether the religious variables examined are attendance at services, beliefs, prayer, or church social support, all are correlated negatively with depression and loneliness among elderly persons (Johnson & Mullins, 1989; Koenig, Kvale, & Ferrel, 1988; Pressman, Lyons, Larson, & Strain, 1990). Faith not only fosters long-range hope, but also creates optimism for the short-term future (Myers, 1992). Among senior citizens, religious involvement is a solid correlate of happiness (Myers, 1992).

One study of religiosity and time perspective found that religious people are more willing to look into the distant future and confront their eventual death than their nonreligious peers are (Hooper & Spilka, 1970). One's own impending demise is obviously a threat, and thinking about personal death is positively correlated with participation in religious activities by elderly persons (Fry, 1990). In addition, the salience of an individual's religion to self-image increases with age (Moberg, 1965).

To sum up, the findings are clear: Religion is a powerful buffer against stress among elderly people. As Myers (1992) has stated, "the happiest of senior citizens are those who are actively religious" (p. 75).

Religion and Coping with Serious Illness

Hayden (1991) researched the utility of religion in helping patients with arthritis cope with pain—an important feature of this illness. He noted tendencies for a conservative religiousness and a sense of meaning in life to counter pain perceptions. These worked best with individuals who were not very depressed to begin with, and who believed that their faith could address their pain effectively. That there is a significant psychological component in the perception of pain goes without saying. Physical and psychological pain often go together, and a strong faith combined with being religiously active seems to counter pain-related distress, depression, and anxiety (Ross, 1990).

When serious, potentially fatal illness strikes, one can expect religion to be invoked rapidly and with telling effect. This is especially true when the problem is cancer. There is apparently a pervasive tendency to avoid blaming God for the bad things that happen to people, and to credit God for positive possibilities and outcomes (Johnson & Spilka, 1991; Spilka & Schmidt, 1983b). To the degree that patients with cancer view God as being in control of things, their sense of threat to life lessens, and their self-esteem improves (Jenkins & Pargament, 1988). An Intrinsic religious orientation also counteracts feelings of anger, hostility, and social isolation (Acklin, Brown, & Mauger, 1983). In addition, patients may receive much social support from their coreligionists.

The literature on the role of faith as a coping mechanism in serious illness covers a broad range of maladies. In order to gain some perspective, we confine ourselves to the literature on religious coping with cancer and HIV/AIDS.

RELIGIOUS COPING WITH CANCER

In their systematic review of the literature linking physical health with religion, Powell et al. (2003) concluded that there is insufficient evidence to suggest that religion either protects against contracting cancer or slows the progression of cancer, other than in certain groups (e.g., Mormons) that place restrictions on such behaviors as smoking, alcohol, and sexual practices. However, the issue of using one's faith to cope with cancer appears to be another story.

A number of interview-based studies (e.g., Feher & Maly, 1999; Gall, de Renart, & Boonstra, 2000; Strang & Strang, 2001) have shown the importance, often by spontaneous reporting, of religion and spirituality in coping with cancer. Other studies (e.g., Brady, Peterman, Fitchett, Mo, & Cella, 1999; Cotton, Levine, Fitzpatrick, Dold, & Targ, 1999; Tate & Forchheimer, 2002) have used a quantitative approach and have concluded that faith is an important predictor to the quality of life among patients with cancer.

Why might religion be such a successful coping mechanism? If a child contracts cancer, for instance, how do the child, siblings, parents, and other family members react? The child victim is likely to experience hospitalizations involving separations from others, as well as to experience much pain (both from the illness and from efforts to counter it). The effects of possible surgical procedures and chemotherapy can be particularly devastating. The predominant child responses are depression and anxiety (Spilka, Zwartjes, & Zwartjes, 1991). Though the age of the child is a factor, fear of death and a wide variety of other anxieties indicate extreme stress. The basic problems have been pictured as those of meaning and mastery (Hart & Schneider, 1997; Spinetta, 1977), and religion appears to meet these needs rather well (Spilka et al., 1991). Psychiatrist Robert Coles (1990) has written of the efficacy of prayer, religious ritual, and Biblical readings in helping children with cancer cope with their trials. Pargament (1997) points out how religion may also constructively deal with the mechanism of denial—a common factor in these circumstances.

Religion plays a role in helping parents and siblings cope as well. With regard to parents, the list of reactions to children's cancer is extensive, ranging from anxiety and fear to extreme marital distress and breakup (Enskar, Carlsson, Golsater, Hamrim, & Kreuger, 1997; Grootenhuis & Last, 1997; Leyn, 1976). Church social support and religion's potential for meaning and control can provide strong backing to parents in dealing with their children's illness and their own reactions (Zwartjes, Spilka, Zwartjes, Heideman, & Cilli, 1979).

RELIGIOUS COPING WITH HIV/AIDS

Several studies on religious coping have involved patients with HIV/AIDS. Earlier in this chapter, we have reviewed a qualitative study (Jacobson et al., 2006) that found three of the religious coping strategies outlined by Pargament et al. (1988) to be commonly used by people diagnosed with HIV. A number of other studies document the frequency with which religion is employed as a coping resource. Cotton et al. (2006) found that the use of religion and spirituality was common in their sample of 450 patients with HIV/AIDS: Almost one-fourth of their sample attended weekly religious services, and one-third prayed or meditated daily. Positive coping strategies (e.g., "sought God's love and care") were significantly more common than negative strategies (e.g., "wondered whether God has abandoned me"), and spirituality levels remained stable over a period of 12–18 months. Ironson, Stuetzle, and Fletcher (2006) found a self-reported increase in spirituality and religiousness over a 4-year time period in 45% of their sample after HIV diagnosis (vs. 13% who reported a decrease in spirituality/religiousness). This research team further discovered that those who reported an increase in religiousness or spirituality also showed slower disease progression, even after such other potential mediating factors as church attendance, initial disease status, age, gender, health behaviors (e.g., risky sex, use of cocaine), social support, and other factors were controlled for. These two studies are but a small representation of a suddenly vast research literature suggesting that when faced with such dire circumstances as an HIV diagnosis, many people turn to religion or spirituality.

Religion and Coping with the Death of a Child

We expect the old to die; we painfully acknowledge that younger people do die, mostly by accident; but the death of youngsters is something we want to deny. Still, it occurs, and the death of infants who have not yet had a chance to enjoy life is particularly upsetting. With all the publicity that sudden infant death syndrome (SIDS) has received in recent years, new parents often worry about such a possibility. (Fortunately, however, the death rate from SIDS declined from 1.5 per 1,000 in 1980 to 0.55 per 1,000 infants in 2004; U.S. Bureau of the Census, 2007.)

McIntosh, Silver, and Wortman (1993) have examined the role of faith following the death of an infant from SIDS (see Research Box 13.5). They found that religious participation elicited social support, and that religion helped bereaved parents for whom it was important to derive meaning from this calamity. In other words, parental faith supported the parents' efforts at cognitively processing the death of their child.

The McIntosh et al. (1993) study suggests that religion as a coping device may be especially important when a devastating, uncontrollable event such as the death of a child occurs. Naturalistic explanations of a child's death are unsatisfactory for most people, because they imply no future, no hope—simply complete and total termination. In contrast, religious interpretations offer not only the potential of future life and other-worldly gratification for the deceased, but this-worldly answers that offer a measure of contentment for survivors. McIntosh et al.'s (1993) study indicates this for parents who suddenly lose an infant to SIDS, and it has also been demonstrated for those who anticipate the death of a child from illness (Friedman, Chodoff, Mason, & Hamburg, 1963). Similar findings hold when parents have to deal with the deaths of premature and newborn infants (Palmer & Noble, 1986).

Three different "theodicies" (attempts to defend God's goodness in the face of tragedy) have been observed among bereaved parents: "1) reunion with the deceased in an afterlife; 2) death as a purposive event; and 3) death as punishment for wrong-doing on the part of survivors" (Cook & Wimberly, 1983, p. 237). These are regarded as attempts to make the death meaningful, and even to experience guilt feelings. Attributions to a purposeful God are also invoked when a friend dies, but people with an Intrinsic religious orientation may undergo

---

RESEARCH BOX 13.5. Religion's Role in Adjustment to a Negative Life Event: Coping with the Death of a Child (McIntosh, Silver, & Wortman, 1993)

This significant study examined how religion helped parents who lost an infant to SIDS adjust to this tragedy. A sample of 124 parents was studied; each set of parents was interviewed within 15–30 days after their child's death, and reinterviewed 18 months later. Adjustment and coping were related to four factors: religion, social support, cognitive processing, and meaning. The researchers hypothesized that religious participation would promote perceptions of social support and adjustment. They also expected that when religion per se was important to the parents, it would help them find meaning in the loss and aid cognitive processing of the event, and would enhance adjustment through these avenues. These hypotheses were supported. In addition, religious participation helped the parents derive meaning from their loss.

This study revealed that religion may not affect adjustment and distress directly; rather, it may work indirectly by bolstering perceptions of social support, aiding cognitive processing, and increasing the meaningfulness of an infant's death, probably by putting it in the context of a positive religious framework. Research such as this indicates the complexity of the role of religion in the coping process, and clarifies some of the mechanisms that are operative when a person's faith is tested by crisis and tragedy.

much cognitive restructuring in order to understand what has occurred, possibly because of their positive image of the deity. There is also the possibility that it is cognitively easier to deal with one's own death than that of another valued person (Park & Cohen, 1993; Schoenrade, Ludwig, Atkinson, & Shane, 1990).

OVERVIEW

As we have seen, the issue of religion and health is an extremely complex topic on many levels, from cause to expression. The amount of research on religion and health has grown significantly over the past two decades, and only a small representation could be covered in this chapter. We have, however, attempted to provide what we believe to be a fair representation.

Serious defects that often stemmed from antireligious perspectives exist in many early studies of relationships between religion and psychopathology. The more modern view is that religion functions largely as a means of countering rather than contributing to psychopathology, though severe forms of unhealthy religion will probably have serious psychological and perhaps even physical consequences. In most instances, faith buttresses people's sense of control and self-esteem, offers meanings that oppose anxiety, provides hope, sanctions socially facilitating behavior, enhances personal well-being, and promotes social integration. Probably the most hopeful sign is the increasing recognition by both clinicians and religionists of the potential benefits each group has to contribute. Awareness of the need for a spiritual perspective has opened new and more constructive possibilities for working with mentally disturbed individuals and resolving adaptive issues.

A central theme throughout this book is that religion "works" because it offers people meaning and control, and brings them together with like-thinking others who provide social support. This theme is probably nowhere better represented than in the section of this chapter on how people use religious and spiritual resources to cope. Religious beliefs, experiences, and practices appear to constitute a system of meanings that can be applied to virtually every situation a person may encounter. People are loath to rely on chance. Fate and luck are poor referents for understanding, but religion in all its possible manifestations can fill the void of meaninglessness admirably. There is always a place for one's God—simply watching, guiding, supporting, or actively solving a problem. In other words, when people need to gain a greater measure of control over life events, the deity is there to provide the help they require.

CHAPTER 14

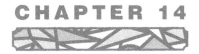

Epilogue

One of the most devastating examples of the danger of religion, is of course, September 11, 2001.

Dear God, save us from the people who believe in you.

For those who regard a transcendental explanation as inadequate, or feel that an appeal to supernatural explanations involves a sacrifice of intellectual integrity, the phenomena of religious observance must be aligned with what is known of other aspects of human psychological functioning.

Some significant portion of traditional supernatural belief is associated with accurate observations interpreted rationally.

We have yet to fully understand the profound and mysterious religious experiences of human everywhere, experiences that shape attitudes toward life and arouse hopes for transcendence and personal immortality.[1]

A t the end of our review of the ever-increasing literature on the psychology of religion, it is fitting to take stock of the field—both as it is now and as it is likely to develop in the immediate future. There is a heavy dose of evaluation in the former effort, and a bit of prophecy in the latter. Yet, as in our epilogue to the fourth edition, we wish at least to go on record so that our prophecies can be judged empirically.

The problems and possibilities of the psychology of religion continue to be functions of the notable personalities involved in the field. To these we now add the considerable influence in shaping the field by funding linked to the interests of the late Sir John Templeton, who, with his considerable wealth, established the John Templeton Foundation. The rise of positive psychology, as well as studies reflecting his interests in unlimited love, forgiveness, and spiritual transformation—all these efforts are guided by the monies his foundation provided. As has often been true in the history of this field, single individuals can be immensely important in determining not simply whether religion will be studied, but, if so, what aspects will be examined (Hood, 2000a). Even more than the fourth edition of this work, this fifth edition reveals that differences in emphasis and orientation among us authors reflect the diversity that characterizes contemporary psychology in general and the current psychology

---

[1] These quotations come, respectively, from the following sources: Albacete (2002, p. 166); Dowd (2002); Hinde (1999, p. 233); Hufford (1982, p. xviii); and Wiebe (1997, p. 222).

of religion in particular. This diversity may well be restrained as major funding from individuals or foundations influences the field. The future psychology of religion may largely be one of funded research projects (Coon, 1992; Hood, 2000a). That many of these will surely be Templeton-funded projects concerns some commentators (Wulff, 2003). However, researchers are free to explore any aspects of religion, not simply those that are funded by Templeton interests. We address this issue below.

RESEARCH IN THE PSYCHOLOGY OF RELIGION

Our immediate focus has been upon the empirical psychology of religion, because it most adequately characterizes the academic study of religion in North American psychology departments. As we have seen, the empirical psychology of religion is as old as scientific psychology itself. Yet, from its inception, scientific psychology has often been more of an ideal than a fact. The term "empirical" has undergone a curious change over time, so that entire orientations historically identified as empirical are not granted that description today by mainstream psychologists (Belzen & Hood, 2006). For many psychologists, classical psychoanalytic, object relations, Jungian, and phenomenological psychologies are not empirical. "Empirical" has come to mean relying upon the triad of observation, experimentation, and measurement. This is the paradigm that, according to Gorsuch (1988), identified the resurgence of interest in the psychology of religion beginning about 1960. Hill and Pargament (2003) claim the same for the psychology of religion and spirituality. These investigators place the study of both religion and spirituality within a natural-scientific framework. In the past, this has not always been the case (Hamlyn, 1967; Hearnshaw, 1987). Porpora (2006) has noted how the explicit stance of "methodological atheism," or what we have identified in Chapter 1 as the "methodological exclusion of the transcendent," actually empirically limits the study of religion. Thus we welcome the call for a new interdisciplinary paradigm that is both multilevel and nonreductive (Emmons & Paloutzian, 2003). This new paradigm is evident in many places in this fifth edition, and is likely to guide the future of research on the psychology of religion.

A Historical Reminder

The Two Stances of Wilhelm Wundt

Authorities such as Robinson (1981) remind us that psychology as a natural science emerged in the 19th century, and that its success was largely a North American phenomenon associated with professionalization of the field (Coon, 1992; Hood, 2000a; Taves, 1999). Its roots, however, had been laid down by philosophical developments utilizing natural-scientific assumptions to describe phenomena in the light of principles based upon observation, measurement, and experimentation. Textbooks commonly cite Wilhelm Wundt's establishment of his psychological laboratory at Leipzig in 1879 as the beginning of scientific psychology. This event indicated that psychology was moving from speculative philosophy to natural science. The bridge was experimentation, which involved measurement, manipulation, and observation. Yet Wundt (1901) actually fostered two psychologies—limiting the applicability of natural-scientific assumptions to some phenomena, but applying different assumptions and methods to other, more social "folk" expressions (Wundt, 1916). The same can be said of William James, who, as Robinson (2002, p. 37) reminds us, had a psychological laboratory that preceded Wundt's by at least 4 years. Indeed, James was unique among the early psychologists for his genuine openness to questions concerning religion and the supernatural.

From the beginning, psychology struggled with natural-scientific assumptions. Even less could psychology maintain its grasp on the entire range and scope of religion with natural-scientific hands—aspects of religion, maybe, but not religion itself. The reduction of religion to categories of science, a persistent goal of early Enlightenment philosophers, can be judged to have failed (Bowker, 1973; Porpora, 2006; Preus, 1987). The identity of psychology as a natural science has always been and remains problematic (Robinson, 2002). Psychology as a natural science is restricted to accepting the principle of the methodological exclusion of the transcendent, and hence is only minimally concerned with two of the four options noted by Dittes (1969; see Chapter 1). Thus the need is for even more interdisciplinary research, as well as acceptance of the widest variety of methodological options for increasing our scientific understanding of religion (Hood & Belzen, 2005; Belzen & Hood, 2006).

Sir John Templeton sought not to have a natural science replace religion, but rather to rescue religion from the narrow perspectives of the "new atheists" or "anti-theists" discussed in Chapter 9. Like James, Sir John Templeton was genuine in his concern for *both* religion and science:

> My own hope for rescuing various religions from obsolescence would be for the visions and teaching of the great prophets and teachers of the past not to be disputed. Rather they should be studied again and considered together with recent concepts of reality as springboards toward creating new and even expanded understanding of divinity in worship and ritual. (Templeton, 2000, p. 9)

Almost every major topic reviewed in this text now has a handbook devoted to it, resulting in too many volumes to list here. However, one need only compare handbooks that avoid the methodological inclusion of the transcendent (e.g., Paloutzian & Park, 2013a) with those that do not (e.g., Miller, 2012a) to note what a difference this makes. The same can be seen in introductory textbooks in the psychology of religion that avoid this approach (e.g., Beit-Hallahmi, 2015) and those that do not (e.g., Sisemore, 2016).

The Two Stances of William James

William James, a contemporary of Wundt and a founder of North American psychology, also failed to apply laboratory measurement-based methodologies to the study of religion. Twice president of the American Psychological Association (APA), James also helped establish the American Society of Psychical Research. The two organizations made strange bedfellows. Coon (1992) reminds us that psychology gained its professional roots in North America within a population that equated psychology ("psychical") with things spiritual. The study of things psychical was a bridging concept that allowed psychologists to gain popular support for their science, while aiming to use natural-scientific methods to debunk the claims of spiritualists. James's refusal to accept this debunking is why Charles Taylor, in his own Gifford Lecture, claimed of him that "this long-dead author is in striking ways a contemporary" (2002, p. vii) James's most consistently psychological work, *The Principles of Psychology* (1890/1950), took a rigorous stance that psychology was to be a natural science. However, as Hood (2000a) has emphasized, James took this stance provisionally, seeking to expose its limits. These limits were both revealed and transcended in James's confrontation with religion. Religious experience was the subject matter of his Gifford Lectures and the basis for James's other undisputed classic text in the psychology of religion.

James's *The Varieties of Religious Experience* (1902/1985) explored the range and depth of religious experience, using personal documents placed within the context of their development so that their fruits could be assessed. The stress upon measurement and the use of questionnaires, already established by such notables as Hall (1900) and Starbuck (1899), were ignored by James in favor of the existential thrust of experience, defined and interpreted within a more historical, narrative context. In modern terms, James's research was qualitative, not quantitative. His psychological treatment of religion specifically expanded the boundaries of the natural-science-based psychology articulated in *The Principles* (Hood, 1995c). *The Varieties* still remains the single most frequently assigned text in the psychology of religion (Vande Kemp, 1976). This should not convey the idea that the contemporary empirical psychology of religion has been heavily influenced by James; however, he remains the most significant figure in identifying the tensions between a psychology of religion and the tendency to move toward a religious psychology.

Despite the fact that many empirical psychologists of religion tend to be social psychologists, they come from the *psychological* tradition of social psychology, not the *sociological* tradition. Ironically, as Schellenberg (1990) has noted, the latter has been influenced more strongly by James than the former has been. The natural-scientific assumptions of psychology remain firm for most of the psychologically oriented social psychologists who do empirical research. Those who confine themselves to natural-scientific assumptions tend to produce what Beit-Hallahmi (1991) identifies as a "psychology of religion" rather than a "religious psychology" per se. A psychology of religion places psychological categories at the forefront, and would have psychology explain religion only insofar as its phenomena can be captured within natural-scientific constructs from mainstream psychology. On the other hand, religious psychology gives supremacy to religious constructs, and expects psychology to follow from and to be constrained within the conceptual limits of a natural science whose explanatory power is superseded by religion. There is an uneasy tension between psychologists of religion and religious psychologists, which promises to persist in the foreseeable future. It is further complicated as the psychology of religion becomes entangled in efforts to tease out differences and similarities between religion at both conceptual and measurement levels, as we have noted throughout this fifth edition. Furthermore, new interdisciplinary frameworks such as the cognitive science of religion (CSR; see Chapters 4 and 9) tend to be fiercely split on the ontological status of the objects of their studies.

As we have noted in this text, the ontological status assigned to what is measured is crucial in developing theory within the psychology of religion (Porpora, 2006). Psychologists of religion must begin with a rich and accurate description of religion from the believer's perspective (Vergote, 1997). To do this, psychologists of religion will need to participate more in the actual religious and spiritual practices of their subjects. Examples of this more culturally sensitive means of gathering relevant data can be found in Belzen's (1999; Belzen & Hood, 2006, pp. 23–24) study of conversion among the *"bevindelijken"* in the Netherlands, and Poloma's (2003) study of a Pentecostal revival group known as the Toronto Blessing and Reviving. Furthermore, such culturally sensitive participatory studies do not negate the ability to gather measurement data as well, as illustrated by Hood and Williamson's (2008a, 2008b) study of the Christian serpent handlers of Appalachia; Poloma and Hood's (2008) study of a Pentecostal emerging church in Atlanta, Georgia; and Luhrmann's (2012) study of American evangelicals who communicate with God. While scientific explanations of aspects of religion have been explored in this text, we are not so brash as to think we have exhaustively "explained" religion. These approaches remain as their own valid ways of knowing, similar in many ways to scientific knowing (Miles, 2007).

The Measurement Paradigm in the Psychology of Religion

Hood (1994) has argued for a compromise position—neither a psychology of religion and spirituality nor a religious and spiritual psychology, but rather psychology *and* religion in interactive dialogues, where all of the four options articulated by Dittes (1969; again, see Chapter 1) stay genuinely in play. This is also what we take to be the spirit of the new paradigm for the psychology of religion, which we have referred to throughout this text. This stance admits the possible validity of both vertical and horizontal transcendent concepts (Streib & Hood, 2016). At odds is the extent to which a genuine interaction can occur, given the limited empirical characteristics of many religious and spiritual constructs. Still, one can identify the empirical consequences of many such constructs. The psychology of religion is both broadened and challenged by newer orientations such as transpersonal psychology and the human sciences, both of which accept a broader definition of "empirical," including much that is compatible with religious and spiritual traditions.

The hostility of some of those who identify themselves as "spiritual but not religious" is directed not only toward a narrowly conceived religion, but a narrowly conceived natural science as well. Perhaps this is best illustrated by reactions to well-established claims of parapsychology, which are simply ignored by psychologists as fraud, attribution errors, or superstition (Sheldrake, 2012). The irony is that if one accepts as the gold standard for psychological research double-blind experimentation among three disciplines (psychology, medicine, and parapsychology), psychology has by far the lowest frequency of double-blind studies and parapsychology the highest (Watt & Nagtegaal, 2004). Our point here is to note that is unlikely that any method, however rigorous, will persuade those whose metaphysical beliefs are fixed regarding the reality of something intuitively unacceptable. It is perhaps ironic that using double-blind studies becomes a curious pandering to an inappropriate method when it is dogmatically applied to an area such as petitionary prayer for healing, where the notion of double-blinding God is at best paradoxical. The issue is simply that methodological diversity implies both ontological and epistemological considerations appropriate to the nature of the object studied (Hood, 2012a).

The numbers of journals, both in print and online, are now so extensive that few can read even a fraction of what is relevant to the psychology of religion. Furthermore, boundaries among these journals promise to become more permeable as social scientists sympathetic to both religious and spiritual phenomena begin to develop scientific theories compatible with concepts central to religion. Likewise, as proponents of more traditionally measurement-based experimental psychology broaden their theoretical horizons, new measurement and experimental techniques are likely to be developed to permit more adequate assessment of variables that are religiously and spiritually relevant.

Moreover, some of the newer journals—such as *The International Journal for the Psychology of Religion* and *Mental Health, Religion and Culture*—emphasize by their titles alone that the psychology of religion can no longer be simply North American. As we have seen in Chapters 4 and 9, the new CSR is less restricted in its range of sampling than mainstream psychology of religion is. The originators of a widely popular acronym, Henrich, Heine, and Norenzayan (2010), have noted that much of social science in the West is based upon sampling from Western, educated, industrialized, rich, democratic (WEIRD) societies. The acronym has been deliberately chosen and can be interpreted to apply not only to those studied, but to those who study them. And even when research in either the mainstream psychology of religion or CSR is not sampling from WEIRD societies (i.e., when such research is genuinely cross-cultural in focus), researchers from both perspectives are still collecting data mainly from university students. As Shweder et al. (2006) remind us, "The Western institution of the university carries with it many features of an elite cosmopolitan culture wherever it has diffused around the world" (p. 722). Hence university students and those researching them are more homogeneous than are their respective societies.

Thus the psychology of religion will become more humble as it takes methodological pluralism seriously. It will be forced to accept what Pickren (2009) observes that many psychologists have failed to recognize: Namely, there are psychologies that are "functionally incommensurate in epistemology, methods, and practices" (p. 88). This is not only humbling, but also exciting, and it bodes well for the future exploration of religion and its vicissitudes.

When one considers the explosion of literature in the psychology of religion, it is obvious that no psychologist can master even a small portion of it. Part of what we have done in this fifth edition is to assure that securely established data and findings need not be replicated. It has been over 30 years since Hearnshaw (1987) noted that writing in psychology since 1950 exceeded the total output of works on the subject produced since the time of the Greeks. Although the literature since 1987 has continued to increase exponentially, it has produced no agreed-upon theoretical integration. Despite the vast amount of research produced in the North American resurgence of interest in the psychology of religion since 1950, much of it is, in Dittes's (1971a) view, a "promiscuous empiricism" (p. 393). The rigors of measurement and the cleverness of experimental designs fail if at the end the results are trivial or uninformative. The psychology of religion is likely to become more like a quilt, in which measurement will at best sew together patches derived from diverse theoretical perspectives. This is in the best spirit of the call for a new paradigm: interdisciplinary, nonreductive, and multilevel.

THE NEED FOR THEORY IN THE PSYCHOLOGY OF RELIGION

There is no all-encompassing theory in general psychology, much less in the psychology of religion. Calls for evolutionary psychology as a grand narrative to integrate all of psychology echo a trend that has occurred in almost every generation of researchers. CSR is not new in this regard. Throughout this text, we have noted how evolutionary psychology has been used in support of religious and spiritual views, and by some as a not-so-humble claim to have reductively explained religion. Yet even the most vocal defenders of evolutionary psychology note that it is not a monolithic enterprise or a single enterprise (Kirkpatrick, 2006a, p. 78). Critics have argued that it is not even clear that evolutionary theory is a genuine empirical theory, failing as it does to permit falsification and, in the words of Watts (2006, p. 63), "not being really testable." No doubt much empirical work will be done under the umbrella of some form of evolutionary theory, but it is likely to be done in the tradition of hypothesis testing, assuring that hypotheses derived from evolutionary theory will be "verified." However, verification has long been abandoned as a defensible philosophy of science (Belzen & Hood, 2006). Evolutionary theories thus have their place in the psychology of religion, but must be cautiously evaluated as a grand narrative. Evolution does not demand a denial either of God or of some *teleos* or directionality inherent in the process (Watts, 2002, pp. 17–31). Evolutionary psychology's success in providing a fuller understanding of religion and spirituality as part of the new paradigm will depend upon its openness to a truly interdisciplinary effort, including a willingness to give theology its due.

Consistent with theory development in the psychology of religion is similar growth in general psychology as it is forced to confront religious issues. Religion is no longer a marginal concern of psychology; whether in the challenges of therapy or in the collective confrontation with cults (and, more recently, with groups advocating terrorism as a tactic), it occupies much of the center stage of general culture. Mainstream psychology will begin to confront religion in terms of its theories, if for no other reason than to show the meaningful relevance of psychology to the interests of a culture that supports and in the process seeks guidance from this science, natural or otherwise. In many cases, the vacuum left by some religions will be filled by psychology. Vitz (1977) has made the case that for some people, psychology has become a religion. Some areas, such as transpersonal psychology, blur the boundaries between psychology as science and as a spiritual discipline. In the future, religionists will probably need to be more psychologically skilled, and psychologists will need to be more religiously and spiritually sophisticated, if there are to remain identifiable but permeable boundaries between psychology on the one hand and spirituality/religion on the other.

In a similar vein, journals devoted to a faith commitment—either by constraining their psychology within the more narrow confines of a particular faith tradition (e.g., the *Journal of Psychology and Christianity*, the *Journal of Psychology and Judaism*), or by interrelating or integrating psychology and religion (e.g., the *Journal of Psychology and Theology*)—will assure that psychology itself appropriately reflects on its own limits. Religion and psychology may confront similar questions, but how they are asked defines what constitutes an appropriate answer. Precisely what it is within religion or spirituality that admits of an empirical answer must be more clearly theoretically determined. So, too, the limits of empiricism must be acknowledged theoretically as new empirical methods are created.

The discussion of mysticism in Chapter 11 indicates the interface between phenomenological and measurement psychology, in which the results of phenomenological analysis can be operationalized and fulfill the requirements of a measurement paradigm that can in turn lead to quasi-experimental designs. This is the possibility of "the empirical validation of phenomenologically derived classifications" argued by Seigfried (1990, p. 12) in her study of William James. Once again, the issue is not only that multiple methods can be of value in the psychology of religion, but that measurement can be based upon a variety of theoretical and even alternative methodological perspectives. It is long past the time when the psychological illumination of religious issues can be assumed to deny the validity of the religious nature that is illuminated psychologically (Vergote, 1997, p. 208). Boundaries must be identified theoretically, even if they are to be crossed.

If there is a forthcoming change in the psychology of religion, it is likely to be most evident in the North American dominance of the field. The success of psychology in the United States and Canada has always been associated with its development as a profession. Contemporary psychology has witnessed a split in allegiances between the APA, long the dominant organization for psychologists (whether teachers, researchers, or practitioners), and the more recently formed Association for Psychological Science (originally the American Psychological Society), which focuses more upon research and teaching than upon practice. This apparent dichotomy suggests that even within North American psychology, tensions between research and practice, and between knowledge and application, are considerable. The tension is reflected in religion as a specialty in the Association for Psychological Science and religion as a division within the APA. Practitioners are more likely to foster a religious psychology than researchers are. It is unlikely that this emphasis will gain as strong an academic foothold in North American universities as a research-based empirical psychology of religion.

Compared to North American psychologists of religion, Europeans are less measurement-oriented and more receptive to phenomenological, psychodynamic, hermeneutical, and cultural studies. These cultures are also less overtly committed to institutional religion. Thus the European psychology of religion promises to challenge the supremacy of the North American psychology of religion, both because of European psychology's greater breadth and scope, and because of North American psychology's tendency to take apologetic religious-psychological stances. While much of European psychology of religion follows a more restricted empirical model common to American psychology, globalization promises to become a two-way street, with American psychology of religion in the spirit of the new paradigm seeking insights from the more qualitative European psychologies noted above. In addition, Asian studies in the psychology of religion are emerging—with much less distinct lines among psychology, religion/spirituality, and science. To date, mainly transpersonal psychologists have examined these traditions, but their influence will undoubtedly affect measurement-based psychology. Again, the challenge to a psychology of religion premised upon measurement and experimentation is for theoretical meaningfulness as well as greater breadth and scope. We prophesied in the second edition of this book that another *Annual Review of Psychology* would be unlikely to "include a review of psychology of religion in which the data base consists exclusively of convenience samples of Protestant Christians selected primarily from North American universities" (Hood, Spilka, Hunsberger, & Gorsuch, 1996, p. 448). Unfortunately, this optimistic prophecy has not been borne out, as we have noted above and throughout the text. The only other *Annual Review of Psychology* (Emmons & Paloutzian, 2003) article moves beyond a focus on measurement, but its database is very much like that of Gorsuch's (1988) earlier review. Advancements in statistical methods have not paralleled advances in theory, despite the call for a new paradigm. For many reasons, this situation is even less acceptable now than we found it to be in our fourth edition.

However, this fifth edition does suggest movement toward a more reflective and humble psychology of religion—one that accepts spirituality as an integral aspect of our discipline, insofar as individuals define themselves as spiritual beings (Miller, 2012b; Streib & Hood, 2016). The future looks promising as psychologists of religion seek greater conceptual depth, more comprehensive models, and more inclusive approaches (Reich & Hill, 2008).

EXTREMISM, CONFLICT, AND THE PSYCHOLOGY OF RELIGION

The urgency of the need to consider the global dimensions of psychology and religion has been highlighted by recent world events. After September 11, 2001, few would disagree that we live in seriously troubled times. Perhaps for some there is a renewed call to faith, but for others it appears that religion itself may be the problem. The great faith traditions of Christianity, Islam, and Judaism find themselves in both direct and indirect conflict. Whether it be the imagery of "Onward Christian Soldiers" or the cries of "*Jihad!*", a sense of being wronged is succeeded by hate, usually legitimated by carefully selected scriptural prescriptions.

The problem extends well beyond armed violence. There is a psychology of religious extremism that has not yet been empirically understood. It appears to be associated with a sense of righteousness and the need to demonize other points of view. However, as we have discussed in Chapter 9, the psychology of religion has a firm database (beginning well before the events of September 11, 2001) that can and should serve as a basis for examining conversion to and exit from extreme religious groups. Virtually all of the current "anti-" trends in religion—those targeting abortion, evolution, women, homosexuality, science, medicine, and progress in general—are clothed in anti-Satan beliefs and rhetoric. In North American Christianity, this tradition began with the Salem witch trials in 17th-century colonial Massachusetts, which reflected medieval religious views of women. The title of Karlsen's (1989) history, *The Devil in the Shape of a Woman*, places the trials in a religious framework. Others have focused upon extreme aspects of Islam (Kressel, 2007). However, we must be careful not to link religious extremism with any one faith tradition, much less to use it as a necessary defining criterion of religious fundamentalism (Hood, Hill, & Williamson, 2005).

Extremists may take refuge in ethnocentrism, creating ingroup–outgroup distinctions and reinforcing these with alienating rhetoric. Abortion is likely to be countered with sexism; prayer in the schools may take on an anti-Semitic tint; and brotherhood can be restricted to one's fellow believers. "True believing" knows few bounds, especially when religion is an organizing force. Believers in "conspiracy" ask who is behind pornography, evolutionary theory, secular humanism, women's rights, or opposition to prayer in the schools—and the approved answers too often excite bigotry.

This is not to say that there may not be extremists on both sides of all these issues. Those who consider themselves "warriors in God's name" find their counterparts in atheistic networks. The advocates of science in the *Skeptical Inquirer* journal commonly take on conservative religionists. The editors, publisher, and writers of the now-defunct *Science and Spirit* made a commendable effort to struggle for a middle ground by subtitling the magazine as "connecting science, religion, and life." Of course, this stance may itself be regarded as extreme by those who polarize these issues.

One does not have to look far to find religious roots for the events of September 11, 2001. These illustrate the extremes to which religious traditions are able to motivate true believers (Nielsen, 2001). Unhappily, the actions of extremist Muslims on that tragic September day have created much distress among moderate Muslims in the United States. Equally extremist Christians have directed indiscriminate hate speech against Islam and its representatives (Sachs, 2002b). The Palestinian–Israeli conflict, when seized upon by extremists on either side, has often been reduced to a conflict between Islam and Judaism, but this tendency has intensified since the September 11 events (Karsh, 2002; Sachs, 2002a). Extremism blunts perception and cognition, so that unreasonable and false generalizations simplify and polarize thinking.

Perceptions of science as the enemy, particularly where evolution is concerned, seem as strong today as they were with the Scopes trial in Tennessee over 90 years ago. State school boards in Ohio, Kansas, and Georgia, among others, have generally given up on replacing Darwinian theory with creationism, and now argue for equal time in the classroom. Whereas creationism was relatively easily rejected as religion rather than science, arguments from "intelligent design" have since been introduced into this classic fray (Clines, 2002; Holt, 2002). The backers of this more sophisticated position are often highly trained scientists themselves (Nelson, 2002).

It is not difficult to give many more examples of extreme behaviors connected to religion. However, the extremism–religion association is not well understood and merits both the development of theory and the undertaking of research. It will require a global approach— one not restricted to sampling North American university undergraduates. We need to know a great deal more than is currently understood about the cognitive and motivational aspects of the kind of religious commitment that supports extreme behavior, so that we can empirically engage Dionne's (2001) question: "Is religion the cause or the solution?" (p. B11).

FINAL THOUGHTS: NEEDS FOR TODAY AND THE FUTURE

Once again, what appears the clearest need in social-scientific work that will assure the vigor, relevance, and compatibility of the psychology of religion with mainstream psychology is theory. Our prophecy in the third and fourth editions that the psychology of religion will no longer be atheoretical, piecemeal, and lacking in sustained development has not yet been proven false. Mainstream psychology has proposed a variety of theories that integrate and guide meaningful empirical research, and many of them are beginning to influence the study of religion. Likewise, more restricted theories are being developed within our field that can sustain significant research (Hill & Gibson, 2008). In any case, whether broad or narrow, the demand for theory will guide the future psychology of religion. We suspect that theory will be revitalized precisely to the extent that it is genuinely interdisciplinary and nonreductive. To cite an example discussed in Chapter 9, attachment theory and psychoanalysis (especially object relations theory) can no longer stand in isolation from one another. They are best viewed as complementary theories that are not incompatible (Fonagy, 2001).

Closely related to the issue of theory is the need for more sophisticated theological literacy among researchers in the psychology of religion (Hunter, 1989). For instance, Gorsuch (1994) has emphasized that if the Intrinsic religious orientation is treated as a motivational construct, then assessing it independently of belief content is essential. Low correlations between measures of general Intrinsic religiousness (such as the Allport–Ross Intrinsic scale) and other variables may be due to the fact that only when specific beliefs are taken into account can more powerful predictions be made. That is, whether one is intrinsically motivated may be a less powerful predictor than one's intrinsic motivation within a particular belief context. In a similar vein, Hood (1992b) has argued that empirically identified psychological processes are of little use in making predictions unless the content of specific faith traditions is taken into account. The psychology of religion, even when it is not a "religious psychology" in Beit-Hallahmi's (1991) sense, needs to be religiously and spiritually informed in order to make meaningful empirical predictions (Gorsuch, 2008; Porpora, 2006).

Finally, concern for theory is not unrelated to training in the professional practice of psychology. The need for clinicians and counselors to be sensitive to cultural, gender, and religious differences makes the understanding of religion necessary. Jones (1994) has made a case for the inclusion of religious values and perspectives within modern clinical psychology. At a minimum, sensitivity to clients' values, including religious ones, is an ethical imperative for clinicians and other care providers working within the social sciences.

In many cases, psychotherapy takes place within a religious framework. Clinical and counseling psychologists have begun to explore the integration of religion in psychotherapy. Titles such as *A Spiritual Strategy for Counseling and Psychotherapy* (Richards & Bergin,

1997), *Incorporating Spirituality in Counseling and Psychotherapy* (Miller, 2003), and *Spiritually Integrated Psychotherapy* (Pargament, 2007) attest to the fact that the new paradigm seeks genuine integration and that theology and religion must be in dialogue (Watts, 2002). The two-volume handbook published by the APA (Pargament, Exline, & Jones, 2013; Pargament, Mahoney, & Shafranske, 2013) discusses extensive examples of diverse theologies and their clinical integration in actual practice. If much of the funding for research in the psychology of religion is funded by what some see as the conservative vision of Sir John Templeton (Wulff, 2003), it remains true that this vision can generate empirically testable hypotheses. Those with other visions can do the same. The standards by which research is evaluated need not be hampered by the source of funding. That conservative religion seeks to defend itself in the face of more liberal opposition is part of the dynamic that social psychologists of religion have long studied, as we have noted in Chapter 9. The tension between transformation and tradition is likely to characterize the study of religion for the foreseeable future.

It has long been established that things believed and acted upon as true have real consequences, whether they are true or not in some ultimate sense. Understanding religious perspectives, however different from our own, is another tool for effectively interacting with those whose religiously based views provide them with meaning, security, and mastery. Theory, empirically supported, ought properly to dominate the future of the psychology of religion. Psychology is itself a product of culture, and as we remember the events of September 11, 2001, we are keenly aware that we are North American psychologists who wish greater illumination of religious and spiritual phenomena—phenomena that, with our current knowledge, can be seen only "through a glass darkly." We also are aware that, as Pickren (2009) notes, "the 21st century is unlikely to be another American century in psychology" (p. 87). And this state alone reminds us of Sir John Templeton's insight that both religion and science progress best under the penumbra of humility.

References

Aarson, B., & Osmond, H. (1970). *Psychedelics: The use and implications of psychedelic drugs.* Garden City, NY: Doubleday.

Abu-Raiya, H. (2013). The psychology of Islam: Current empirically based knowledge, potential challenges, and directions for future research. In K. I. Pargament, J. Exline, & J. Jones (Eds.), *APA handbook of psychology, religion, and spirituality* (Vol. 1, pp. 681–695). Washington, DC: American Psychological Association.

Abu-Raiya, H., & Pargament, K. I. (2015). Religious coping among diverse religions: Commonalities and divergences. *Psychology of Religion and Spirituality, 7,* 24–33.

Abu-Raiya, H., Pargament, K. I., & Mahoney, A. (2011). Examining coping methods with stressful interpersonal events experienced by Muslims living in the United States following the 9/11 attacks. *Psychology of Religion and Spirituality, 3,* 1–14.

Academy of Religion and Mental Health. (1959). *Religion, science, and mental health.* New York, NY: New York University Press.

Acevedo, G. A. (2014). Review: *The Oxford handbook of religious conversion. Journal for the Scientific Study of Religion, 53,* 853–854.

Ackerman, D. (1994). *A natural history of love.* New York, NY: Random House.

Acklin, M. W., Brown, E. C., & Mauger, P. A. (1983). The role of religious values in coping with cancer. *Journal of Religion and Health, 22,* 322–333.

Acock, A. C., & Bengtson, V. L. (1978). On the relative influence of mothers and fathers: A covariance analysis of political and religious socialization. *Journal of Marriage and the Family, 40,* 519–530.

Acock, A. C., & Bengtson, V. L. (1980). Socialization and attribution processes: Actual versus perceived similarity among parents and youth. *Journal of Marriage and the Family, 42,* 501–515.

Acredolo, C., & O'Connor, J. (1991). On the difficulty of detecting cognitive uncertainty. *Human Development, 34,* 204–223.

Adamczyk, A., & Hayes, B. E. (2012). Religion and sexual behaviors: Understanding the influence of Islamic cultures and religious affiliation for explaining sex outside of marriage. *American Sociological Review, 77,* 723–746.

Adamovová, L. (2013). Wise religiosity: The relationship between religiosity and wisdom moderated by personality traits. *Studia Psychologica, 55,* 181–194.

Adams, F., & Kelly, E. C. (1939). *The genuine works of Hippocrates.* Baltimore: Williams & Wilkins.

Adams, G. R., Bennion, L., & Huh, K. (1989). *Objective measure of ego identity status: A reference manual* (2nd ed.). Logan: Utah State University Press.

Adams, J. S. (1965). Inequity in social exchange. In L. Berkowitz (Ed.), *Advances in experimental social psychology* (Vol. 2, pp. 267–299). New York,s NY: Academic Press.

Aday, R. H. (1984–1985). Belief in afterlife and death anxiety: Correlates and comparisons. *Omega, 15,* 67–75.

Adelekan, M. L., Abiodun, O. A., Imouokhome-Obayan, A. O., Oni, G. A., & Ogunremi, O. O. (1993). Psychosocial correlates of alcohol, tobacco and cannabis use: Findings from a Nigerian university. *Drug and Alcohol Dependence, 33,* 247–256.

Adler, A. (1935). Introduction. *Journal of Invividual Psychology, 1*, 5–8.

Adorno, T. W., Frenkel-Brunswik, E., Levinson, D. J., & Sanford, R. N. (1950). *The authoritarian personality*. New York, NY: Harper & Row.

Aflakseir, A., & Coleman, P. G. (2009). The influence of religious coping on the mental health of disabled Iranian war veterans. *Mental Health, Religion and Culture, 12*, 175–190.

Aguilar-Vafaie, M. E., & Moghanloo, M. (2008). Dimension and facet personality correlates of religiosity among Iranian college students. *Mental Health, Religion and Culture, 11*, 461–483.

Ahern, G. (1990). *Spiritual/religious experience in modern society*. Oxford, UK: Alister Hardy Research Centre, Westminster College.

Ahmed, A. M. (2009). Are religious people more prosocial?: A quasi-evxperimental study with Madrasah pupils in a rural community in India. *Journal for the Scientific Study of Religion, 48*, 368–374.

Ahmed, A. M., & Salas, O. (2011). Implicit influences of Christian religious representations on dictator and prisoner's dilemma game decisions. *Journal of Socio-Economics, 40*, 242–246.

Ai, A. L., Dunkle, R. E., Peterson, C., & Bolling, S. F. (1998). The role of private prayer in psychological recovery among midlife and aged patients following cardiac surgery. *The Gerontologist, 38*, 591–601.

Ai, A. L., Dunkle, R. E., Peterson, C., & Bolling, S. F. (2000). Spiritual well-being, private prayer, and adjustment of older cardiac patients. In J. A. Thorson (Ed.), *Perspectives on spiritual well-being and aging* (pp. 98–119). Springfield, IL: Charles C Thomas.

Ai, A. L., Park, C. L., Huang, B., Rodgers, W., & Tice, T. N. (2007). Psychosocial mediation of religious coping styles: A study of short-term psychological distress following cardiac surgery. *Personality and Social Psychology Bulletin, 33*, 867–882.

Ai, A. L., Peterson, C., Bolling, S. F., & Koenig, H. (2002). Private prayer and optimism in middle-aged and older patients awaiting cardiac surgery. *The Gerontologist, 42*, 70–81.

Ai, A. L., Peterson, C., & Huang, B. (2003). The effect of religious-spiritual coping on positive attitudes of adult Muslim refugees from Kosovo and Bosnia. *International Journal for the Psychology of Religion, 13*, 29–47.

Ai, A. L., Tice, T. N., Huang, B., & Ishisaka, A. (2005). Wartime faith-based reactions among traumatized Kosovar and Bosnian refugees in the United States. *Mental Health, Religion and Culture, 8*, 291–308.

Ai, A. L., Tice, T. N., Peterson, C., & Huang, B. (2005). Prayers, spiritual support, and positive attitudes in coping with the September 11 national crisis. *Journal of Personality, 73*, 763–791.

Alaggia, R. (2001). Cultural and religious influences in maternal response to intrafamilial child sexual abuse: Charting new territory for research and treatment. *Journal of Child Sexual Abuse, 10*, 41–60.

Albacete, L. (2002). *God at the Ritz*. New York, NY: Crossroad.

Alberts, C. (2000). Identity formation among African late-adolescents in a contemporary South African context. *International Journal for the Advancement of Counselling, 22*, 23–42.

Albrecht, S. L., & Bahr, H. M. (1983). Patterns of religious disaffiliation: A study of lifelong Mormons, Mormon converts, and former Mormons. *Journal for the Scientific Study of Religion, 22*, 366–379.

Albrecht, S. L., & Cornwall, M. (1989). Life events and religious change. *Review of Religious Research, 31*, 23–38.

Albrecht, S. L., Cornwall, M., & Cunningham, P. H. (1988). Religious leave-taking: Disengagement and disaffiliation among Mormons. In D. G. Bromley (Ed.), *Falling from the faith: Causes and consequences of religious apostasy* (pp. 62–80). Newbury Park, CA: SAGE.

Aldridge, D. (2000). *Spirituality, healing and medicine*. London, UK: Jessica Kingsley.

Aldwin, C. M., Park, C. L., Jeong, Y., & Nath, R. (2014). Differing pathways between religiousness, spirituality, and health: A self-regulation perspective. *Psychology of Religion and Spirituality, 6*, 9–21.

Alem, A., Kebede, D., & Kullgren, G. (1999). The epidemiology of problem drinking in Butajira, Ethiopia. *Acta Psychiatrica Scandinavica, 100*(Suppl. 397), 77–83.

Alexander, M. W., & Judd, B. B. (1986). Differences in attitudes toward nudity in advertising. *Psychology: A Quarterly Journal of Behavior, 23*, 26–29.

Algoe, S. B. (2012). Find, remind, and bind: The functions of gratitude in everyday relationships. *Social and Personality Psychology Compass, 6*, 455–469.

Algoe, S. B., & Way, B. (2014). Evidence for a role of the oxytocin system, indexed by genetic variation in CD38, in the social bonding effects of expressed gratitude. *Social Cognitive and Affective Neuroscience, 9*, 1855–1861.

Ali, H. K., & Naidoo, A. (1999). Sex education sources and attitudes about premarital sex of Seventh Day Adventist youth. *Psychological Reports, 84*, 312.

Al-Issa, I. (1977). Social and cultural aspects of hallucinations. *Psychological Reports, 84*, 570–587.

Allegro, J. M. (1971). *The sacred mushroom and the cross*. New York, NY: Bantam.

Allen, G. E. K., Wang, K. T., & Stokes, H. (2015).

Examining legalism, scrupulosity, family perfectionism, and psychological adjustment among LDS individuals. *Mental Health, Religion and Culture, 18,* 246–258.

Allen, R. O., & Spilka, B. (1967). Committed and consensual religion: A specification of religion–prejudice relationships. *Journal for the Scientific Study of Religion, 6,* 191–206.

Allison, J. (1961). Recent empirical studies of conversion experiences. *Pastoral Psychology, 17,* 21–33.

Allport, G. W. (1950). *The individual and his religion.* New York, NY: Macmillan.

Allport, G. W. (1954). *The nature of prejudice.* Cambridge, MA: Addison-Wesley.

Allport, G. W. (1959). Religion and prejudice. *The Crane Review, 2,* 1–10.

Allport, G. W. (1966). The religious context of prejudice. *Journal for the Scientific Study of Religion, 5,* 447–457.

Allport, G. W., Gillespie, J. M., & Young, J. (1948). The religion of the post-war college student. *Journal of Psychology, 25,* 3–33.

Allport, G. W., & Ross, J. M. (1967). Personal religious orientation and prejudice. *Journal of Personality and Social Psychology, 5,* 432–443.

Almond, G. A., Appleby, S. R., & Sivan, E. (2002). *Strong religion: The rise of fundamentalisms around the world.* Chicago, IL: University of Chicago Press.

Alsdurf, P., & Alsdurf, J. M. (1988). Wife abuse and scripture. In A. L. Horton & J. A. Williamson (Eds.), *Abuse and religion: When praying isn't enough* (pp. 221–227). Lexington, MA: Lexington Books.

Altemeyer, B. (1981). *Right-wing authoritarianism.* Winnipeg, Canada: University of Manitoba Press.

Altemeyer, B. (1988). *Enemies of freedom: Understanding right-wing authoritarianism.* San Francisco, CA: Jossey-Bass.

Altemeyer, B. (1996). *The authoritarian specter.* Cambridge, MA: Harvard University Press.

Altemeyer, B. (2003). Why do religious fundamentalists tend to be prejudiced? *International Journal for the Psychology of Religion, 13,* 17–28.

Altemeyer, B., & Hunsberger, B. (1992). Authoritarianism, religious fundamentalism, quest, and prejudice. *International Journal for the Psychology of Religion, 2,* 113–133.

Altemeyer, B., & Hunsberger, B. (1993). Response to Gorsuch. *International Journal for the Psychology of Religion, 3,* 33–37.

Altemeyer, B., & Hunsberger, B. (1997). *Amazing conversions: Why some turn to faith and others abandon religion.* Amherst, NY: Prometheus Books.

Altemeyer, B., & Hunsberger, B. (2004). A revised Religious Fundamentalism Scale: The short and

sweet of it. *International Journal for the Psychology of Religion, 14,* 47–54.

Altemeyer, B., & Hunsberger, B. (2005). Fundamentalism and authoritarianism. In R. F. Paloutzian & C. L. Park (Eds.), *Handbook of the psychology of religion and spirituality* (pp. 378–393). New York, NY: Guilford Press.

Altemeyer, S., Klein, C., Keller, B., Silver, C. F., Hood, R. W., Jr., & Streib, H. (2015). Subjective definitions of spirituality and religion: An explorative study in Germany and the USA. *International Journal of Corpus Linguistics, 20,* 526–552.

Alvarado, K. A., Templer, D. I., Bresler, C., & Thomas-Dobson, S. (1995). The relationship of religious variables to death depression and death anxiety. *Journal of Clinical Psychology, 51,* 202–204.

Ameika, C., Eck, N. H., Ivers, B. J., Clifford, J. M., & Malcarne, V. (1994, April 22). *Religiosity and illness prevention.* Paper presented at the annual convention of the Rocky Mountain Psychological Association, Las Vegas, NV.

American Psychiatric Association. (1987). *Diagnostic and statistical manual of mental disorders* (3rd ed., rev.). Washington, DC: Author.

American Psychiatric Association. (1994). *Diagnostic and statistical manual of mental disorders* (4th ed.). Washington, DC: Author.

American Psychiatric Association. (2000). *Diagnostic and statistical manual of mental disorders* (4th ed., text rev.). Washington, DC: Author.

American Psychiatric Association. (2013). *Diagnostic and statistical manual of mental disorders* (5th ed.). Arlington, VA: Author.

American Psychological Association (APA) Presidential Task Force on Evidence-Based Practice. (2006). Evidence-based practice in psychology. *American Psychologist, 61,* 271–285.

Ames, E. S. (1910). *The psychology of religious experience.* Boston, MA: Houghton Mifflin.

Amey, C. H., Albrecht, S. L., & Miller, M. K. (1996). Racial differences in adolescent drug use: The impact of religion. *Substance Use and Misuse, 31,* 1311–1332.

Anderson, K. (2008). *Baby boomerangs.* Richardson, TX: Probe Ministries.

Anderson, L. R., & Mellor, J. M. (2009). Religion and cooperation in a public goods experiment. *Economics Letters, 105,* 58–60.

Andresen, J. (2001). Introduction: Towards a cognitive science of religion. In J. Andresen (Ed.), *Religion in mind: Cognitive perspectives on religious belief, ritual, and experience* (pp. 1–44). New York, NY: Cambridge University Press.

Andrews, L. M. (1987). *To thine own self be true.* Garden City, NY: Doubleday/Anchor.

Ano, G. G., & Vasconcelles, E. B. (2005). Religious

coping and psychological adjustment to stress: A meta-analysis. *Journal of Clinical Psychology, 61,* 461–480.

Anthony, D., Ecker, B., & Wilbur, K. (Eds.). (1987). *Spiritual choices.* New York, NY: Paragon House.

Anthony, D., & Robbins, T. (1974). The Meher Baba movement: Its effect on post-adolescent social alienation. In I. I. Zaretsky & M. P. Leone (Eds.), *Religious movements in contemporary America* (pp. 228–243). Princeton, NJ: Princeton University Press.

Anthony, D., & Robbins, T. (1992). Law, social science and the "brainwashing" exception to the First Amendment. *Behavioral Sciences and the Law, 10,* 5–29.

Anthony, D., & Robbins, T. (1994). Brainwashing and totalitarian influence. In U. S. Ramachdran (Ed.), *Encyclopaedia of human behavior* (Vol. 1, pp. 457–471). New York, NY: Academic Press.

Anthony, F. V., Hermans, C. A., & Sterkens, C. (2010). A comparative study of mystical experience among Christian, Muslim, and Hindu students in Tamil Nadu, India. *Journal for the Scientific Study of Religion, 49,* 264–277.

Antonovsky, A. (1987). *Unraveling the mystery of health: How people measure stress and stay well.* San Francisco, CA: Jossey-Bass.

Apolito, P. (1998). *Apparitions of the Madonna at Oliveto Citra: Local visions and cosmic drama* (A. William, Jr., Trans.). University Park: Pennsylvania State University Press.

Appelle, S. (1996). The abduction experience: A critical evaluation of theory and evidence. *Journal of UFO Studies, 6,* 29–79.

Appelle, S., Lynn, S. J., & Newman, L. (2000). Alien abduction experiences. In E. Cardeña, S. J. Lynn, & S. Krippner (Eds.), *Varieties of anomalous experience* (pp. 253–282). Washington, DC: American Psychological Association.

Archer, S. L. (1989). Gender differences in identity development: Issues of process, domain and timing. *Journal of Adolescence, 12,* 117–138.

Ardelt, M. (1997). Wisdom and life satisfaction in old age. *Journal of Gerontology, 52B,* 15–27.

Ardelt, M. (2003). Effects of religion and purpose in life on elders' subjective well-being and attitudes toward death. *Journal of Religious Gerontology, 14,* 55–77.

Arendt, H. (1979). *The origins of totalitarianism.* San Diego, CA: Harcourt Brace Jovanovich.

Argue, A., Johnson, D. R., & White, L. K. (1999). Age and religiosity: Evidence from a three-wave panel analysis. *Journal for the Scientific Study of Religion, 38,* 423–435.

Argyle, M. (1959). *Religious behavior.* Glencoe, IL: Free Press.

Argyle, M., & Hills, P. (2000). Religious experiences and their relation with happiness and personality. *International Journal for the Psychology of Religion, 10,* 157–172.

Aries, P. (1974). *Western attitudes toward death from the Middle Ages to the present.* Baltimore: Johns Hopkins University Press.

Arnold, M. (1897). A wish. In *The poetical works of Matthew Arnold* (pp. 288–289). New York, NY: Thomas Y. Crowell. (Original work published 1853)

Arnold, R., Avants, S. K., Margolin, A., & Marcotte, D. (2002). Patient attitudes concerning the inclusion of spirituality into addiction treatment. *Journal of Substance Abuse Treatment, 23,* 319–326.

Aruguete, M. S., Goodboy, A. K., Jenkins, W. J., Mansson, D. H., & McCutcheon, L. E. (2012). Does religious faith improve test performance? *North American Journal of Psychology, 14,* 185–196.

Ashtari, S. (2014, July 21). Children exposed to religion have difficulty distinguishing fact from fiction, study finds. *The Huffington Post.* Retrieved from *www.huffingtonpost.com/2014/07/21/children-religion-fact-fiction_n_5607009.html.*

Ashton, M. C., & Lee, K. (2005). Honesty–humility, the Big Five, and the five-factor model. *Journal of Personality, 73,* 1321–1353.

Askin, H., Paultre, Y., White, R., & Van Ornum, W. (1993, August). *The quantitative and qualitative aspects of scrupulosity.* Paper presented at the annual convention of the American Psychological Association, Toronto, Ontario, Canada.

Assanangkornchai, S., Conigrave, K. M., & Saunders, J. B. (2002). Religious beliefs and practice, and alcohol use in Thai men. *Alcohol and Alcoholism, 37,* 193–197.

Association of Statisticians of American Religious Bodies (ASARB). (2014). *U.S. religion census 1952 to 2010.* Retrieved from *www.usreligioncensus.org/compare.php.*

Astin, A. W., Astin, H. S., & Lindholm, J. A. (2011). *Cultivating the spirit: How college can enhance students' inner lives.* San Francisco, CA: Jossey-Bass.

Aten, J. D., Bennett, P. R., Hill, P. C., Davis, D. E., & Hook, J. N. (2012). Predictors of God concept and God control after Hurricane Katrina. *Psychology of Religion and Spirituality, 4,* 182–192.

Aten, J. D., & Hernandez, B. C. (2005). A 25-year review of qualitative research published in spirituality and psychologically oriented journals. *Journal of Psychology and Christianity, 24,* 266–277.

Atkins, D. C., Baucom, D. H., & Jacobson, N. S. (2001). Understanding infidelity: Correlates in a national random sample. *Journal of Family Psychology, 15,* 735–749.

Atkins, D. C., & Kessel, D. E. (2008). Religiousness

and infidelity: Attendance, but not faith and prayer, predict marital fidelity. *Journal of Marriage and Family, 70*, 407–418.

Atran, S. (2002). *In gods we trust.* New York, NY: Oxford University Press.

Austin, W. H. (1980). Are religious beliefs "enabling mechanisms for survival"? *Zygon, 15*(2), 193–201.

Avants, S. K., Warburton, L. A., & Margolin, A. (2001). Spiritual and religious support in recovery from addiction among HIV-positive injection drug users. *Journal of Psychoactive Drugs, 33*, 39–45.

Awn, P. J. (1994). Indian Islam: The Shah Bano affair. In J. S. Hawley (Ed.), *Fundamentalism and gender* (pp. 63–78). New York, NY: Oxford University Press.

Azari, N. P. (2006). Neuroimaging studies of religious experience: A critical review. In P. McNamara (Ed.), *Where God and science meet* (Vol. 2, pp. 34–54). Westport, CT: Praeger.

Azari, N. P., Missimer, J., & Seitz, R. J. (2005). Religious experience and emotion: Evidence for distinctive cognitive neural patterns. *International Journal for the Psychology of Religion, 15*, 263–281.

Azari, N. P., Nickel, J., Wunderlich, G., Niedeggen, M., Hefter, H., Tellman, L., et al. (2001). Neural correlates of religious experience. *European Journal of Neuroscience, 13*, 649–652.

Bach, G. R., & Wyden, P. (1969). *The intimate enemy.* New York, NY: Morrow.

Back, K. W., & Bourque, L. (1970). Can feelings be enumerated? *Behavioral Science, 15*, 487–496.

Badcock, C. R. (1980). *Psychoanalysis of culture.* Oxford, UK: Blackwell.

Bader, C. (1999). New perspectives on failed prophecy. *Journal for the Scientific Study of Religion, 38*, 119–131.

Badham, P. (1976). *Christian beliefs about life after death.* London, UK: Macmillan.

Baetz, M., Larson, D. B., Marcoux, G., Bowen, R., & Griffin, R. (2002). Canadian psychiatric inpatient religious commitment: An association with mental health. *Canadian Journal of Psychiatry, 47*, 159–166.

Bahr, H. M., & Albrecht, S. L. (1989). Strangers once more: Patterns of disaffiliation from Mormonism. *Journal for the Scientific Study of Religion, 28*, 180–200.

Bahr, H. M., & Harvey, C. D. (1980). Correlates of morale among the newly widowed. *Journal of Social Psychology, 110*, 219–233.

Bahr, S. J., Maughan, S. L., Marcos, A. C., & Li, B. (1998). Family, religiosity, and the risk of adolescent drug use. *Journal of Marriage and the Family, 60*, 979–992.

Baier, C. J., & Wright, B. R. E. (2001). "If you love me, keep my commandments": A meta-analysis of the effect of religion on crime. *Journal of Research in Crime and Delinquency, 38*, 3–21.

Bailey, K. L., Jones, B. D., Hall, T. W., Wang, D. C., McMartin, J., & Fujikawa, A. M. (2016). Spirituality at a crossroads: A grounded theory of Christian emerging adults. *Psychology of Religion and Spirituality, 8*, 99–109.

Bailey, L. W., & Yates, J. (1996). *The near-death experience: A reader.* New York, NY: Routledge.

Bainbridge, W. S. (1997). *The sociology of religious movements.* New York, NY: Routledge.

Bainbridge, W. S., & Stark, R. (1980a). Client and audience cults in America. *Sociological Analysis, 41*, 199–214.

Bainbridge, W. S., & Stark, R. (1980b). Sectarian tension. *Review of Religious Research, 22*, 105–124.

Bakalar, J., & Grinspoon, L. (1989). Testing psychotherapies and drug therapies: The case of psychedelic drugs. In S. Peroutka (Ed.), *Ecstasy: The clinical, pharmacological, and neurotoxicological effects of the drug MDMAS.* Norwell, MA: Kluwer Academic.

Bakalar, N. (2016, June 14). Churchgoers may live longer. *The New York Times*, p. D4.

Baker-Brown, G., Ballard, E. J., Bluck, S., de Vries, B., Suedfeld, P., & Tetlock, P. E. (1992). The conceptual integrative complexity scoring manual. In C. P. Smith (Ed.), *Motivation and personality: Handbook of thematic content analysis* (pp. 401–418). Cambridge, UK: Cambridge University Press.

Baker-Sperry, L. (2001). Passing on the faith: The father's role in religious transmission. *Sociological Focus, 34*, 185–198.

Balch, R. W. (1980). Looking behind the scenes in a religious cult: Implications for the study of conversion. *Sociological Analysis, 45*, 301–314.

Balch, R. W., Farnsworth, G., & Wilkins, S. (1983). When the bombs dropped: Reactions to disconfirmed prophecy in a millennial sect. *Sociological Perspectives, 26*, 137–158.

Balk, D. E. (1995). *Adolescent development: Early through late adolescence.* Pacific Grove, CA: Brooks/Cole.

Ballard, S. N., & Fleck, J. R. (1975). The teaching of religious concepts: A three stage model. *Journal of Psychology and Theology, 3*, 164–171.

Baltes, P. B., & Staudinger, U. M. (2000). Wisdom: A metaheuristic (pragmatic) to orchestrate mind and virtue toward excellence. *American Psychologist, 55*, 122–135.

Bandura, A. (1977). *Social learning theory.* Englewood Cliffs, NJ: Prentice-Hall.

Bandura, A. (1986). *Social foundations of thought and action.* Englewood Cliffs, NJ: Prentice-Hall.

Bandura, A. (2003). On the psychosocial impact and

mechanism of spiritual modeling: Comment. *International Journal for the Psychology of Religion, 13,* 167–173.

Banergee, K., & Bloom, P. (2013). Would Tarzan believe in God?: Conditions for the emergence of religious belief. *Trends in Cognitive Science, 17,* 7–8.

Bangen, K. J., Meeks, T. W., & Jeste, D. V. (2013). Defining and assessing wisdom: A review of the literature. *American Journal of Geriatric Psychiatry, 21,* 1254–1266.

Banister, P., Burman, E., Parker, I., Taylor, M., & Tindall, C. (1994). *Qualitative methods in psychology: A research guide.* Buckingham, UK: Open University Press.

Bänziger, S., Janssen, J., & Scheeps, P. (2008). Praying in a secularized society: An empirical study of praying practices and varieties. *International Journal for the Psychology of Religion, 18,* 256–265.

Bao, W. N., Whitbeck, L. B., Hoyt, D. R., & Conger, R. D. (1999). Perceived parental acceptance as a moderator of religious transmission among adolescent boys and girls. *Journal of Marriage and the Family, 61,* 362–374.

Barber, N. (2012, August 9). The God Spot revisited: Spirituality arises as an evolved function of the brain. *Psychology Today: The Human Beast.* Retrieved from *www.psychologytoday.com/blog/the-human-beast/2012/08/the-god-spot-revisited.*

Barber, T. X. (1970). *LSD, marijuana, yoga, and hypnosis.* Chicago, IL: Aldine.

Barkan, S. E. (2006). Religiosity and premarital sex in adulthood. *Journal for the Scientific Study of Religion, 45,* 407–417.

Barkan, S. E., & Greenwood, S. F. (2003). Religious attendance and subjective well-being among older Americans: Evidence from the General Social Survey. *Review of Religious Research, 45,* 116–129.

Barker, E. (1983). Supping with the devil: How long a spoon does the sociologist need? *Sociological Analysis, 44,* 197–206.

Barker, E. (1984). *The making of a Moonie.* Oxford, UK: Blackwell.

Barker, E. (1986). Religious movements: Cult and anticult since Jonestown. *Annual Review of Sociology, 12,* 329–346.

Barker, I. R., & Currie, R. F. (1985). Do converts always make the most committed Christians? *Journal for the Scientific Study of Religion, 24,* 305–313.

Barkow, J. H. (1982). Culture and sociobiology. In T. C. Weigele (Ed.), *Biology and the social sciences* (pp. 59–73). Boulder, CO: Westview Press.

The Barna Group. (2007, September 24). A new generation expresses its skepticism and frustration with Christianity. Retrieved November 21, 2008, from *www.barna.org/FlexPage.aspx?Page=BarnaUpdate&BarnaUpdateII.*

The Barna Group. (2014, February 4). Barna FRAMES: Three major faith and culture trends for 2014. Retrieved from *www.barna.com/research/three-major-faith-and-culture-trends-for-2014.*

Barna, G., & Kinnaman, D. (2015). Do you really know why they're avoiding church? Retrieved from *www.barna.com/churchless.*

Barnard, G. W. (1997). *Exploring unseen worlds: William James and the philosophy of mysticism.* Albany, NY: State University of New York Press.

Barnes, H., & Becker, H. (1938). *Social thought from lore to science.* New York, NY: Heath.

Barnes, K., & Gibson, N. J. S. (2013). Supernatural agency: Individual difference predictors and situational correlates. *International Journal for the Psychology of Religion, 23,* 42–62.

Barr, H. L., Langs, R. J., Holt, R. R., Goldberger, L., & Klein, C. S. (1972). *LSD, personality and experience.* New York, NY: Wiley.

Barrett, H. C. (2015). *The shape of thought: How mental adaptations evolve.* Oxford, UK: Oxford University Press.

Barrett, J. B., DaVanzo, J., Ellison, D. G., & Grammich, G. (2014). Religion and attitudes toward family planning issues among US Adults. *Review of Religious Research, 56,* 161–188.

Barrett, J. L. (2000). Exploring the natural foundations of religion, *Trends in Cognitive Sciences, 4,* 29–34.

Barrett, J. L. (2004). *Why would anyone believe in God?* Lanham, MD: Altamira.

Barrett, J. L. (2007). Is the spell really broken?: Biopsychological explanations of religion and theistic belief. *Theology and Science, 5,* 58–72.

Barrett, J. L. (2010). The relative unnaturalness of atheism: On why Geertz and Markusson are both right and wrong. *Religion, 40,* 169–172.

Barrett, J. L. (2011). Cognitive science of religion: Looking back, looking forward. *Journal for the Scientific Study of Religion, 50,* 229–239.

Barrett, J. L. (2012). *Born believers: The science of children's religious belief.* New York, NY: Free Press.

Barrett, J. L. (2013). Exploring religion's basement: The cognitive science of religion. In R. F. Paloutzian & C. L. Park (Eds.), *Handbook of the psychology of religion and spirituality* (2nd ed., pp. 234–255). New York, NY: Guilford Press.

Barrett, J. L., & Keil, F. C. (1996). Conceptualizing a non-natural entity: Anthropomorphism in God concepts. *Cognitive Psychology, 31,* 219–247.

Barrett, J. L., & Richard, R. A. (2003). Anthropomorphism or preparedness?: Exploring children's God concepts. *Review of Religious Research, 44,* 300–312.

Barrett, J. L., Richert, R. A., & Driesenga, A. (2001). God's beliefs versus mother's: The development of non-human agent concepts. *Child Development, 72,* 50–65.

Barron, F. (1953). An ego-strength scale which predicts response to psychotherapy. *Journal of Consulting Psychology, 17,* 327–333.

Barry, C. M., Willoughby, B. J., & Clayton, K. (2015). Living your faith: Associations between family and personal religious practices and emerging adults' sexual behavior. *Journal of Adult Development, 22,* 159–172.

Bartlett, J. (Ed.). (1955). *Familiar quotations by John Bartlett* (13th ed.). Boston, MA: Little, Brown.

Bassett, R. L., Baldwin, D., Tammaro, J., Mackmer, D., Mundig, C., Wareing, A., & Tschorke, D. (2002). Reconsidering intrinsic religion as a source of universal compassion. *Journal of Psychology and Theology, 30,* 131–143.

Bassett, R. L., Hodak, E., Allen, J., Bartos, D., Grastorf, J., Sittig, L., & Strong, J. (2000). Homonegative Christians: Loving the sinner but hating the sin. *Journal of Psychology and Theology, 19,* 258–269.

Bassett, R. L., Miller, S., Anstey, K., Crafts, K., Harmon, J., Lee, Y., et al. (1990). Picturing God: A nonverbal measure of God concept for conservative Protestants. *Journal of Psychology and Christianity, 9,* 73–81.

Bassett, R. L., Smith, A., Thrower, J., Tindall, M., Barclay, J., Tiuch, K., et al. (2005). One effort to measure implicit attitudes toward spirituality and religion. *Journal of Psychology and Christianity, 24,* 210–218.

Bassett, R. L., van Nikkelen-Kuyper, M., Johnson, D., Miller, A., Carter, A., & Grimm, J. P. (2005). Being a good neighbor: Can students come to value homosexual persons? *Journal of Psychology and Theology, 33,* 17–26.

Bateman, M. M., & Jensen, J. S. (1958). The effect of religious background on modes of handling anger. *Journal of Social Psychology, 47,* 133–141.

Batson, C. D. (1976). Religion as prosocial: Agent or double agent? *Journal for the Scientific Study of Religion, 15,* 29–45.

Batson, C. D. (1977). Experimentation in psychology of religion: An impossible dream? *Journal for the Scientific Study of Religion, 16,* 413–418.

Batson, C. D. (1979). Experimentation in the psychology of religion: Living with or in a dream? *Journal for the Scientific Study of Religion, 18,* 90–93.

Batson, C. D. (1990). Good Samaritans—or priests and Levites?: Using William James as a guide in the study of religious prosocial motivation. *Personality and Social Psychology Bulletin, 16,* 758–768.

Batson, C. D., & Burris, C. T. (1994). Personal religion: Depressant or stimulant of prejudice and discrimination? In M. P. Zanna & J. M. Olson (Eds.), *The Ontario Symposium: Vol. 7. The psychology of prejudice* (pp. 149–169). Hillsdale, NJ: Erlbaum.

Batson, C. D., Denton, D. M., & Vollmecke, J. T. (2008). Quest religion, anti-fundamentalism, and limited versus universal compassion. *Journal for the Scientific Study of Religion, 47,* 135–145.

Batson, C. D., Eidelman, S. H., Higley, S. L., & Russell, S. A. (2001). "And who is my neighbor?": II. Quest religion as a source of universal compassion. *Journal for the Scientific Study of Religion, 40,* 39–50.

Batson, C. D., Flink, C. H., Schoenrade, P. A., Fultz, J., & Pych, V. (1986). Religious orientation and overt versus covert racial prejudice. *Journal of Personality and Social Psychology, 50,* 175–181.

Batson, C. D., & Flory, J. D. (1990). Goal-relevant cognitions associated with helping by individuals high on intrinsic, end religion. *Journal for the Scientific Study of Religion, 29,* 346–360.

Batson, C. D., Floyd, R. B., Meyer, J. M., & Winner, A. L. (1999). "And who is my neighbor?": Intrinsic religion as a source of universal compassion. *Journal for the Scientific Study of Religion, 38,* 445–457.

Batson, C. D., & Gray, R. A. (1981). Religious orientation and helping behavior: Responding to one's own or to the victim's needs? *Journal of Personality and Social Psychology, 40,* 511–520.

Batson, C. D., Naifeh, S. J., & Pate, S. (1978). Social desirability, religious orientation, and racial prejudice. *Journal for the Scientific Study of Religion, 17,* 31–41.

Batson, C. D., Oleson, K. C., Weeks, J. L., Healy, S. P., Reeves, P. J., Jennings, P., & Brown, T. (1989). Religious prosocial motivation: Is it altruistic or egoistic? *Journal of Personality and Social Psychology, 57,* 873–884.

Batson, C. D., & Raynor-Prince, L. (1983). Religious orientation and complexity of thought about existential concerns. *Journal for the Scientific Study of Religion, 22,* 38–50.

Batson, C. D., & Schoenrade, P. A. (1991a). Measuring religion as quest: 1. Validity concerns. *Journal for the Scientific Study of Religion, 30,* 416–429.

Batson, C. D., & Schoenrade, P. A. (1991b). Measuring religion as quest: 2. Reliability concerns. *Journal for the Scientific Study of Religion, 30,* 430–447.

Batson, C. D., Schoenrade, P., & Pych, V. (1985). Brotherly love or self-concern?: Behavioural consequences of religion. In L. B. Brown (Ed.), *Advances in the psychology of religion* (pp. 185–208). New York, NY: Oxford University Press.

Batson, C. D., Schoenrade, P., & Ventis, W. L. (1993). *Religion and the individual: A social-psychological perspective.* New York, NY: Oxford University Press.

Batson, C. D., & Ventis, W. L. (1982). *The religious experience: A social-psychological perspective.* New York, NY: Oxford University Press.

Baumard, N., & Boyer, P. (2013). Religious beliefs as reflective elaborations on intuitions: A modified dual process model. *Current Directions in Psychological Science, 22*, 295–300.

Baumeister, R. F. (1991). *Meanings of life.* New York, NY: Guilford Press.

Baumeister, R. F., & Exline, J. J. (1999). Virtue, personality, and social relations: Self-control as the moral muscle. *Journal of Personality, 67*, 1165–1194.

Baumeister, R. F., & Leary, M. R. (1995). The need to belong: Desire for interpersonal attachments as a fundamental human motivation. *Psychological Bulletin, 117*, 497–529.

Baumeister, R. F., Vohs, K. D., & Tice, D. M. (2007). The strength model of self-control. *Current Directions in Psychological Science, 16*, 351–355.

Baumrind, D. (1967). Child care practices anteceding three patterns of preschool behavior. *Genetic Psychology Monographs, 75*, 43–88.

Baumrind, D. (1991). Parenting styles and adolescent development. In R. M. Lerner, A. C. Petersen, & J. Brooks-Gunn (Eds.), *The encyclopedia of adolescence* (Vol. 2, pp. 746–758). New York, NY: Garland Press.

Bazargan, S., Sherkat, D. E., & Bazargan, M. (2004). Religion and alcohol use among African-American and Hispanic inner-city emergency care patients. *Journal for the Scientific Study of Religion, 43*, 419–428.

Bear, D. M., & Fedio, P. (1977). Quantitative analysis of interictal behavior in temporal lobe epilepsy. *Archives of Neurology, 34*(8), 454–467.

Bear, M. F., Connors, B. W., & Paradiso, M. A. (1996). *Neuroscience: Exploring the brain.* Baltimore: Williams & Wilkins.

Beaudoin, T. (1998). *Virtual faith: The irreverent spiritual quest of Generation X.* San Francisco, CA: Jossey-Bass.

Beck, R., & Haugen, A. D. (2013). The Christian religion: A theological and psychological review. In K. I. Pargament, J. J. Exline, & J. W. Jones (Eds.), *APA handbook of psychology, religion, and spirituality* (Vol. 1, pp. 697–711). Washington, DC: American Psychological Association.

Beck, R., & McDonald, A. (2004). Attachment to God: The Attachment to God Inventory, tests of working model correspondence, and an exploration of faith group differences. *Journal of Psychology and Theology, 32*, 92–103.

Beck, S. H., Cole, B. S., & Hammond, J. A. (1991). Religious heritage and premarital sex: Evidence from a national sample of young adults. *Journal for the Scientific Study of Religion, 30*, 173–180.

Becker, H. S. (1963). *Outsiders.* New York, NY: Free Press.

Beckford, J. A. (1978). Accounting for conversion. *British Journal of Sociology, 29*, 249–262.

Beckford, J. A. (1979). Politics and the anti-cult movement. *Annual Review of the Social Sciences of Religion, 3*, 169–190.

Beckford, J. A., & Richardson, J. T. (1983). A bibliography of social scientific studies of new religious movements. *Social Compass, 30*, 111–135.

Beckstead, R. T. (2007, August). Restoration and the sacred mushroom: Did Joseph Smith use psychedelic substances to facilitate visionary experiences? Retrieved September 2, 2008, from *www.mormonselixirs.org.*

Begley, S. (2001a, January 28). Searching for the God within. *Newsweek.* Retrieved from *www.newsweek.com/searching-god-within-150935.*

Begley, S. (2001b, May 7). Religion and the brain: In the new field of neurotheology, scientists seek the biological basis of spirituality: Is God all in our heads? *Newsweek,* pp. 50–57.

Begley, S. (2009, August 12). (Un)wired for God. *Newsweek.* Retrieved from *www.newsweek.com/why-religion-may-not-be-hard-wired-78555.*

Begue, L. (2000). Social practices, religion and moral judgment: New results. *Cahiers Internationaux de Psychologie Sociale, 445*, 67–76.

Beit-Hallahmi, B. (1977). Curiosity, doubt, and devotion: The beliefs of psychologists and the psychology of religion. In H. N. Malony (Ed.), *Current perspectives in the psychology of religion* (pp. 381–391). Grand Rapids, MI: Eerdmans.

Beit-Hallahmi, B. (1989). *Prolegomena to the psychological study of religion.* Lewisburg, PA: Bucknell University Press.

Beit-Hallahmi, B. (1991). Goring the sacred ox: Towards a psychology of religion. In H. N. Malony (Ed.), *Psychology of religion: Personalities, problems, possibilities* (pp. 189–194). Grand Rapids, MI: Baker.

Beit-Hallahmi, B. (1995). Object relations theory and religious experience. In R. W. Hood, Jr. (Ed.), *Handbook of religious experience* (pp. 254–268). Birmingham, AL: Religious Education Press.

Beit-Hallahmi, B. (2007). Atheists: A psychological profile. In M. Martin (Ed.), *The Cambridge companion to atheism* (pp. 300–317). New York, NY: Cambridge University Press.

Beit-Hallahmi, B. (2015). *Psychological perspectives on religion and religiosity.* New York, NY: Routledge.

Beit-Hallahmi, B., & Argyle, M. (1997). *The psychology of religious behaviour, belief, and experience.* London, UK: Routledge.

Belavich, T. G. (1995, August). *The role of religion in coping with daily hassles.* Paper presented at the annual convention of the American Psychological Association, New York, NY.

Bellah, R. N., Marsden, R., Sullivan, W. M., Swidler, A., & Tipton, S. M. (1996). *Habits of the heart* (rev. ed.). Berkeley: University of California Press.

Belzen, J. A. (1997). *Hermeneutical approaches in the psychology of religion*. Amsterdam: Rodopi.

Belzen, J. A. (1999). Religion as embodiment: Cultural-psychological concepts and methods in the study of conversion among "bevindelijken." *Journal for the Scientific Study of Religion, 36*, 358–371.

Belzen, J. A., & Hood, R. W. (2006). Methodological issues in the psychology of religion: Toward another paradigm? *Journal of Psychology, 140*, 5–28.

Benda, B. B. (1997). An examination of a reciprocal relationship between religiosity and different forms of delinquency within a theoretical model. *Journal of Research in Crime and Delinquency, 34*, 163–186.

Benda, B. B., & Corwyn, R. F. (1997). Religion and delinquency: The relationship after considering family and peer influences. *Journal for the Scientific Study of Religion, 36*, 81–92.

Benda, B. B., & Corwyn, R. F. (1999). Abstinence and birth control among rural adolescents in impoverished families: A test of theoretical discriminators. *Child and Adolescent Social Work Journal, 16*, 191–214.

Benda, B. B., & Corwyn, R. F. (2000). A theoretical model of religiosity and drug use with reciprocal relationships: A test using structural equation modeling. *Journal of Social Service Research, 26*, 43–67.

Benefiel, M., Fry, L. W., & Geigle, D. (2014). Spirituality and religion in the workplace: History, theory, and research. *Psychology of Religion and Spirituality, 6*, 175–187.

Bengtson, V. L., & Troll, L. (1978). Youth and their parents: Feedback and intergenerational influence in socialization. In R. M. Lerner & G. B. Spanier (Eds.), *Child influences on marital and family interaction: A life-span perspective* (pp. 215–240). New York, NY: Academic Press.

Benjamins, M. R., & Buck, A. C. (2008). Religion: A sociocultural predictor of health behaviors in Mexico. *Journal of Aging and Health, 20*, 290–305.

Benson, H. (1975). *The relaxation response*. New York, NY: Morrow.

Benson, H., & Stark, M. (1996). *Timeless healing: The power and biology of belief*. New York, NY: Scribner.

Benson, P. L. (1988a, October). *The religious development of American Protestants: Overview of the National Research Project*. Paper presented at the annual convention of the Religious Research Association, Chicago, IL.

Benson, P. L. (1988b, October). *The religious development of adults*. Paper presented at the annual convention of the Religious Research Association, Chicago, IL.

Benson, P. L. (1992a). Patterns of religious development in adolescence and adulthood. *Psychologists Interested in Religious Issues Newsletter, 17*, 2–9.

Benson, P. L. (1992b). Religion and substance use. In J. F. Schumaker (Ed.), *Religion and mental health* (pp. 211–220). New York, NY: Oxford University Press.

Benson, P. L., Dehority, J., Garman, L., Hanson, E., Hochschwender, M., Lebold, C., et al. (1980). Intrapersonal correlates of nonspontaneous helping behavior. *Journal of Social Psychology, 110*, 87–95.

Benson, P. L., Donahue, M. J., & Erickson, J. A. (1989). Adolescence and religion: A review of the literature from 1970 to 1986. *Research in the Social Scientific Study of Religion, 1*, 153–181.

Benson, P. L., Donahue, M. J., & Erickson, J. A. (1993). The Faith Maturity Scale: Conceptualization, measurement, and empirical validation. In M. L. Lynn & D. O. Moberg (Eds.), *Research in the social scientific study of religion* (Vol. 5, pp. 1–26). Greenwich, CT: JAI Press.

Benson, P. L., Masters, K. S., & Larson, D. B. (1997). Religious influences on child and adolescent development. In N. E. Alessi (Ed.), *Handbook of child and adolescent psychiatry: Vol. 4. Varieties of development* (pp. 206–219). New York, NY: Wiley.

Benson, P. L., & Spilka, B. (1973). God image as a function of self-esteem and locus of control. *Journal for the Scientific Study of Religion, 13*, 297–310.

Benson, P. L., Williams, D. L., & Johnson, A. L. (1987). *The quicksilver years: The hopes and fears of young adolescents*. San Francisco, CA: Harper & Row.

Benson, P. L., Yeager, P. K., Wood, M. J., Guerra, M. J., & Manno, B. V. (1986). *Catholic high schools: Their impact on low-income students*. Washington, DC: National Catholic Educational Association.

Bentall, R. P. (1990). The illusion of reality: A review and integration of psychological research on hallucinations. *Psychological Bulletin, 107*, 82–95.

Bentall, R. P. (2000). Hallucinatory experiences. In E. Cardeña, S. J. Lynn, & S. Krippner (Eds.), *Varieties of anomalous experience* (pp. 85–120). Washington, DC: American Psychological Association.

Berenbaum, H., Kerns, J., & Raghavan, C. (2000). Anomalous experiences, peculiarity, and psychopathology. In E. Cardeña, S. J. Lynn, & S. Krippner (Eds.), *Varieties of anomalous experience* (pp. 25–46). Washington, DC: American Psychological Association.

Berger, P. (1979). *The heretical imperative: Contemporary possibilities of religious affirmation*. Garden City, NY: Doubleday/Anchor.

Berger, P., & Luckmann, T. (1967). *The social construction of reality: A treatise in the sociology of knowledge*. Garden City, NY: Doubleday.

Bergin, A. E. (1964). Psychology as a science of inner experience. *Journal of Humanistic Psychology, 4,* 95–103.

Bergin, A. E. (1980). Psychotherapy and religious values. *Journal of Consulting and Clinical Psychology, 48,* 95–105.

Bergling, K. (1981). *Moral development: The validity of Kohlberg's theory*. Stockholm, Sweden: Almqvist & Wiksell.

Bergman, B. (2001, April 9). The kids are all right. *Maclean's, 114*(15), 42–48.

Bergman, P. (1953). A religious conversion in the course of psychotherapy. *American Journal of Psychotherapy, 7,* 41–58.

Bergman, R. L. (1971). Navajo peyote use: Its apparent safety. *American Journal of Psychiatry, 128,* 695–699.

Bergson, H. L. (1911). *Creative evolution*. New York, NY: Henry Holt.

Bering, J. M. (2006). The cognitive psychology of belief in the supernatural. *Scientific American, 94,* 142–149.

Bering, J. M. (2009, January 19). Is religion adaptive?: It's complicated. *Scientific American.* Retrieved from *https://blogs.scientificamerican.com/bering-in-mind/is-religion-adaptive-it-8217-s-complicated.*

Bering, J. M. (2011a, March 13). Signs, signs, everywhere signs: Seeing God in tsunamis and everyday events. *Scientific American.* Retrieved from *https://blogs.scientificamerican.com/bering-in-mind/signs-signs-everywhere-signs-seeing-god-in-tsunamis-and-everyday-events.*

Bering, J. (2011b). *The belief instinct*. New York, NY: Norton.

Bering, J. M., & Bjorkland, D. F. (2004). The natural emergence of reasoning about the afterlife as a developmental regularity. *Developmental Psychology, 40,* 217–233.

Berkhofer, R. F., Jr. (1963). Protestants, pagans, and sequences among the North American Indians, 1760–1860. *Ethnohistory, 10,* 201–232.

Berlyne, D. E. (1960). *Conflict, arousal, and curiosity*. New York, NY: McGraw-Hill.

Bernard, L. L. (1924). *Instinct*. New York, NY: Henry Holt.

Bernhardt, W. H. (1958). *A functional philosophy of religion*. Denver, CO: Criterion Press.

Bernstein, B. (1964). Aspects of language and learning in the genesis of the social process. In D. Hymes (Ed.), *Language in culture and society* (pp. 251–263). New York, NY: Harper & Row.

Bernt, F. M. (1989). Being religious and being altruistic: A study of college service volunteers. *Personality and Individual Differences, 10,* 663–669.

Berzonsky, M. D., & Kuk, L. S. (2000). Identity status, identity processing style, and the transition to university. *Journal of Adolescent Research, 15,* 81–98.

Bettelheim, B. (1976). *The uses of enchantment*. New York, NY: Knopf.

Bibby, R. W. (1987). *Fragmented gods: The poverty and potential of religion in Canada*. Toronto, Ontario, Canada: Irwin.

Bibby, R. W. (1993). *Unknown gods: The ongoing story of religion in Canada*. Toronto, Ontario, Canada: Stoddart.

Bibby, R. W. (2001). *Canada's teens: Today, yesterday, and tomorrow*. Toronto, Ontario, Canada: Stoddart.

Bibby, R. W., & Weaver, H. R. (1985). Cult consumption in Canada: A further criticism of Stark and Bainbridge. *Sociological Analysis, 46,* 445–460.

Biello, D. (2007). Searching for God in the brain. *Scientific American Mind, 18,* 38–45.

Bieser, V. (1995, February 23). Dying of shame. *The Jerusalem Report,* pp. 30–32.

Billiet, J. B. (1995). Church involvement, individuals, and ethnic prejudice among Flemish Roman Catholics: New evidence of a moderating effect. *Journal for the Scientific Study of Religion, 34,* 224–233.

Bird, F., & Remier, B. (1982). Participation rates in new religious movements and para-religious movements. *Journal for the Scientific Study of Religion, 21,* 1–14.

Birnbaum, J. H. (1995, May 15). The gospel according to Ralph. *Time,* pp. 18–27.

Bivens, A. J., Neimeyer, R. A., Kirchberg, T. M., & Moore, M. K. (1994–1995). Death concern and religious beliefs among gays and bisexuals of variable proximity to AIDS. *Omega, 30,* 105–120.

Bjorck, J. P., & Cohen, L. H. (1993). Coping with threats, losses, and challenges. *Journal of Social and Clinical Psychology, 12,* 56–72.

Black, H. K. (1999). Poverty and prayer: Spiritual narratives of elderly African-American women. *Review of Religious Research, 40,* 359–374.

Blackford, R., & Schüklenk, U. (2009). *50 voices of disbelief: Why we are atheists*. Chichester, UK: Wiley-Blackwell.

Blackmore, S. (1991). Near death experiences: In or out of the body. *Skeptical Inquirer, 16,* 34–45.

Blaine, B. E., Trivedi, P., & Eshleman, A. (1998). Religious belief and the self-concept: Evaluating the implications for psychological adjustment. *Personality and Social Psychology Bulletin, 24,* 1040–1052.

Blake, W. (1967). The garden of love. In *Songs of*

innocence and experience (Plate 44). New York, NY: Orion Press. (Original work published 1789)

Blanton, H., & Jaccard, J. (2006). Arbitrary metrics in psychology. *American Psychologist, 61,* 27–41.

Bloch, J. P. (1988). *New spirituality, self, and belonging: How new agers, and neo-pagans talk about themselves.* Westport, CT: Praeger.

Blogowska, J., & Saroglou, V. (2013). For better or worse: Fundamentalists' attitudes toward outgroups as a function of exposure to authoritative religious texts. *International Journal for the Psychology of Religion, 23,* 103–125.

Blomquist, J. M. (1985). The effect of divorce experience on spiritual growth. *Pastoral Psychology, 34,* 82–91.

Bloom, P. (2004). *Descartes' baby: How the science of child development explains what makes us human.* New York, NY: Basic Books.

Bloom, P. (2007). Religion is natural. *Developmental Science, 10,* 147–151.

Blumberg, A. (2015, May 14). Son of gay dads will be baptized at Florida Episcopal Church after initial denial (UPDATE). *The Huffington Post.* Retrieved from *www.huffingtonpost.com/2015/05/06/gay-dads-baptism_n_7223744.html.*

Bock, D. C., & Warren, N. C. (1972). Religious belief as a factor in obedience to destructive demands. *Review of Religious Research, 13,* 185–191.

Bock, E. W., & Radelet, M. L. (1988). The marital integration of religious independents: A reevaluation of its significance. *Review of Religious Research, 29,* 228–241.

Bohannon, J. R. (1991). Religiosity related to grief levels of bereaved mothers and fathers. *Omega, 23,* 153–159.

Boisen, A. T. (1936). *Exploration of the inner world.* Chicago, IL: Willet, Clark.

Boisen, A. T. (1960). *Out of the depths: An autobiographical study of mental disorder and religious experience.* New York, NY: Harper.

Bollinger, R. A., & Hill, P. C. (2012). Humility. In T. G. Plante (Ed.), *Religion, spirituality, and positive psychology: Understanding the psychological fruits of faith* (pp. 31–47). Westport, CT: Praeger.

Bondurant, J. V. (1965). *Conquest of violence: The Gandhian philosophy of conflict.* Berkeley: University of California Press.

Booth, L. (1991). *When God becomes a drug: Breaking the chains of religious addiction and abuse.* New York, NY: Perigee.

Borders, T. F., Curran, G. M., Mattox, R., & Booth, B. M. (2010). Religiousness among at-risk drinkers: Is it prospectively associated with the development or maintenance of an alcohol-use disorder? *Journal of Studies on Alcohol and Drugs, 71,* 136–142.

Boswell, J. (n.d.). *The life of Samuel Johnson, LL.D.*

New York, NY: Modern Library. (Original work published 1791)

Botero, C. A., Gardner, B., Kirby, K. R., Bulbulia, J., Gavin, M. C., & Gray, R. D. (2014). The ecology of religious beliefs. *Proceedings of the National Academy of Sciences of the USA, 11,* 16784–16789.

Bottomley, F. (1979). *Attitudes toward the body in Western Christendom.* London, UK: Lupus.

Bottoms, B. L., Nielsen, M., Murray, R., & Filipas, H. (2003). Religion-related child physical abuse: Characteristics and psychological outcomes. *Journal of Aggression, Maltreatment and Trauma, 8,* 87–114.

Bottoms, B. L., Shaver, P. R., Goodman, G. S., & Qin, J. (1995). In the name of God: A profile of religion-related child abuse. *Journal of Social Issues, 51,* 85–111.

Bouchard, T. J., Jr. (1996a). IQ similarity in twins reared apart: Findings and responses to critics. In R. Sternberg & C. Grigorenko (Eds.), *Intelligence: Heredity and environment* (pp. 126–160). New York, NY: Cambridge University Press.

Bouchard, T. J., Jr. (1996b). Behavior genetic studies of intelligence, yesterday and today: The long journey from plausibility to proof. *Journal of Biosocial Science, 28,* 527–555.

Bouchard, T. J., Jr. (2004). Genetic influence on human psychological traits. *Current Directions in Psychological Science, 13,* 148–151.

Bouchard, T. J., Jr., & McGue, M. (2003). Genetic and environmental influences on human psychological differences. *Journal of Neurobiology, 54,* 4–45.

Bouma, G. D. (1979). The real reason one conservative church grew. *Review of Religious Research, 20,* 127–137.

Bourguignon, E. (1970). Hallucinations and trance: An anthropologist's perspective. In W. Keup (Ed.), *Origins and mechanisms of hallucination* (pp. 83–90). New York, NY: Plenum Press.

Bourguignon, E. (1992). Religion as a mediating factor in culture change. In J. F. Schumaker (Ed.), *Religion and mental health* (pp. 259–269). New York, NY: Oxford University Press.

Bourque, L. B. (1969). Social correlates of transcendental experience. *Sociological Analysis, 30,* 151–163.

Bourque, L. B., & Back, K. W. (1971). Language, society, and subjective experience. *Sociometry, 34,* 1–21.

Bouyer, L. (1980). Mysticism: An essay in the history of the word. In R. Woods (Ed.), *Understanding mysticism* (pp. 42–55). Garden City, NY: Image.

Bowker, J. (1973). *The sense of God: Sociological, anthropological, and psychological approaches to the origin of the sense of God.* Oxford, UK: Clarendon Press.

Bowland, S. E., Foster, K., & Vosler, A. N. (2013).

Culturally competent and spiritually sensitive therapy with Lesbian and Gay Christians. *Social Work, 58,* 321–332.

Bowlby, J. (1969). *Attachment and loss: Vol. 1. Attachment.* New York, NY: Basic Books.

Bowlby, J. (1973). *Attachment and loss: Vol. 2. Separation: Anxiety and anger.* New York, NY: Basic Books.

Bowlby, J. (1980). *Attachment and loss: Vol. 3. Loss.* New York, NY: Basic Books.

Boyatzis, C. J. (2005). Religious and spiritual development in childhood. In R. F. Paloutzian & C. L. Park (Eds.), *Handbook of the psychology of religion and spirituality* (pp. 123–243). New York, NY: Guilford Press.

Boyatzis, C. J. (2006). Advancing our understanding of the dynamics of religion in the family and parent–child relationship. *International Journal for the Psychology of Religion, 16,* 245–251.

Boyatzis, C. J. (2012). Spiritual development during childhood and adolescence. In L. Miller (Ed.), *The Oxford handbook of psychology and spirituality* (pp. 151–164). New York, NY: Oxford University Press.

Boyatzis, C. J., & Janicki, D. (2003). Parent–child communication about religion: Survey and diary data on unilateral transmission and bi-directional reciprocity styles. *Review of Religious Research, 44,* 252–270.

Boyer, P. (1994). *The naturalness of religious ideas.* Berkeley: University of California Press.

Boyer, P. (2001). *Religion explained: The evolutionary origins of religious thought.* New York, NY: Basic Books.

Boyer, P. (2003). Religious thought and behaviour as by-products of brain function. *Trends in Cognitive Sciences, 7,* 119–124.

Boyer, P., & Walker, S. (2000). Intuitive ontology and cultural input in the acquisition of religious concepts. In K. S. Rosengren, C. N. Johnson, & P. L. Harris (Eds.), *Imagining the impossible: Magical, scientific, and religious thinking in children* (pp. 130–156). Cambridge, UK: Cambridge University Press.

Brabant, S., Forsyth, C., & McFarlain, G. (1995). Life after the death of a child: Initial and long term support from others. *Omega, 31,* 67–85.

Bradshaw, M., & Ellison, C. O. (2008). Do genetic factors influence religious life?: Findings from a behavior genetic analysis of twin siblings. *Journal for the Scientific Study of Religion, 47,* 529–544.

Bradshaw, M., Ellison, C. G, & Marcum, J. P. (2010). Attachment to God, images of God, and psychological distress in a nationwide sample of Presbyterians. *International Journal for the Psychology of Religion, 20,* 130–147.

Brady, M. J., Peterman, A. H., Fitchett, G., Mo, M., & Cella, D. (1999). A case for including spirituality in quality of life measurement in oncology. *Psychooncology, 8,* 417–428.

Braun, K. L., & Zir, A. (2001). Roles for the church in improving end-of-life care: Perceptions of Christian clergy and laity. *Death Studies, 25,* 685–705.

Brehm, S. S. (1992). *Intimate relationships.* New York, NY: McGraw-Hill.

Brewer, M. B. (1997). On the social origins of human nature. In C. McGarty & S. A. Haslam (Eds.), *The message of social psychology* (pp. 54–62). Cambridge, MA: Blackwell.

Brickhead, J. (1997). Reading "snake handling": Critical reflections. In S. G. Glazer (Ed.), *Anthropology of religion* (pp. 1–84). Westport, CT: Greenwood Press.

Bridges, H. (1970). *American mysticism from William James to Zen.* New York, NY: Harper & Row.

Briki, W., Aloui, A., Bragazzi, N. L., Chaouachi, A., Patrick, T., & Chamari, K. (2015). Trait self-control, identified-introjected religiosity and health-related-feelings in healthy Muslims: A structural equation model analysis. *PLOS One, 10*(5), e0126193.

Brinkerhoff, M. B., & Burke, K. L. (1980). Disaffiliation: Some notes on "falling from the faith." *Sociological Analysis, 41,* 41–54.

Brinkerhoff, M. B., Grandin, E., & Lupri, E. (1992). Religious involvement and spousal violence: The Canadian case. *Journal for the Scientific Study of Religion, 31,* 15–31.

Brinkerhoff, M. B., & Mackie, M. M. (1993). Casting off the bonds of organized religion: A religious-careers approach to the study of apostasy. *Review of Religious Research, 34,* 235–257.

Brinthaupt, T. M., & Lipka, R. P. (Eds.). (1994). *Changing the self.* Albany, NY: State University of New York Press.

Bristol, F. M. (1904). *The religious instinct of man.* Cincinnati, OH: Jennings & Pye.

Britton, W. B., & Bootzin, R. R. (2004). Near-death experiences and the temporal lobe. *Psychological Science, 15,* 254–258.

Broadway, B. (2004, September 4). Do we have a genetic propensity for religious belief? Retrieved December 4, 2004, from *archives.seattletimes.nwsource.com/cgi-bin/texis.cgi/web/vortex/display.*

Brody, G. H., Stoneman, Z., & Flor, D. (1996). Parental religiosity, family processes, and youth competence in rural, two-parent African American families. *Developmental Psychology, 32,* 696–706.

Bromley, D. G. (1988). Religious disaffiliation: A neglected social process. In D. G. Bromley (Ed.), *Falling from the faith: Causes and consequences of religious apostasy* (pp. 9–25). Newbury Park, CA: SAGE.

Bromley, D. G. (1998). Linking social structure and the exit process in religious organizations: Defectors, whistle-blowers and apostates. *Journal for the Scientific Study of Religion, 37*, 145–160.

Bromley, D. G., & Breschel, E. F. (1992). General population and institutional support for social control of new religious movements: Evidence from national survey data. *Behavioral Sciences and the Law, 10*, 39–52.

Bromley, D. G., & Richardson, J. T. (Eds.). (1983). *The brainwashing/deprogramming controversy: Sociological, psychological, legal and historical perspectives.* Lewiston, NY: Edwin Mellen Press.

Bronson, L., & Meadow, A. (1968). The need for achievement orientation of Catholic and Protestant Mexican-Americans. *Revista Interamericana de Psicologia, 2*, 159–168.

Brown, D. E. (1991). *Human universals.* New York, NY: McGraw-Hill.

Brown, F. C. (1972). *Hallucinogenic drugs.* Springfield, IL: Charles C Thomas.

Brown, F., & McDonald, J. (2000). *The serpent handlers: Three families and their faith.* Winston-Salem, NC: Blair.

Brown, J., Cohen, P., Johnson, J. G., & Salzinger, S. (1998). A longitudinal analysis of risk factors for child maltreatment: Findings of a 17-year prospective study of officially recorded and self-reported child abuse and neglect. *Child Abuse and Neglect, 22*, 1065–1078.

Brown, L. B. (1966). Egocentric thought in petitionary prayer: A cross-cultural study. *Journal of Social Psychology, 68*, 197–210.

Brown, L. B. (1968). Some attitudes underlying petitionary prayer. In A. Godin (Ed.), *From cry to word: Contributions toward a psychology of prayer* (pp. 65–84). Brussels, Belgium: Lumen Vitae Press.

Brown, L. B. (1987). *The psychology of religious belief.* London, UK: Academic Press.

Brown, L. B. (1994). *The human side of prayer: The psychology of praying.* Birmingham, AL: Religious Education Press.

Brown, T. L., Parks, G. S., Zimmerman, R. S., & Phillips, C. M. (2001). The role of religion in predicting adolescent alcohol use and problem drinking. *Journal of Studies on Alcohol, 62*, 696–705.

Bruce, S. (1999). *Choice and religion: A critique of rational choice theory.* Oxford, UK: Oxford University Press.

Bruggeman, E. L., & Hart, K. J. (1996). Cheating, lying, and moral reasoning by religious and secular high school students. *Journal of Educational Research, 89*, 340–344.

Bruni, F. (2015a, May 6). Catholicism undervalues women. *The New York Times*, p. A23.

Bruni, F. (2015b, May 27). On same-sex marriage, Catholics are leading the way. *The New York Times*, p. A19.

Brunner, B. (Ed.). (2003). *Time almanac 2004.* Needham, MA: Pearson Education.

Bryan, J. W., & Freed, F. W. (1993). Abortion research: Attitudes, sexual behavior, and problems in a community college population. *Journal of Youth and Adolescence, 22*, 1–22.

Bryant, A. N., Choi, J. Y., & Yasuno, M. (2003). Understanding the religious and spiritual dimensions of students' lives in the first year of college. *Journal of College Student Development, 44*, 723–745.

Buber, M. (1965). *Between man and man.* New York, NY: Macmillan.

Bucher, A. A. (1991). Understanding parables: A developmental analysis. In F. K. Oser & W. G. Scarlett (Eds.), *Religious development in childhood and adolescence* (New Directions for Child Development, No. 52, pp. 101–105). San Francisco, CA: Jossey-Bass.

Bucke, R. M. (1961). *Cosmic consciousness: A study of the evolution of the human mind.* Hyde Park, NY: University Books. (Original work published 1901)

Budd, S. (1973). *Sociologists and religion.* London, UK: Macmillan.

Bufe, C. (1991). *Alcoholics Anonymous: Cult or cure?* San Francisco, CA: Sharp Press.

Buglios, V., & Gentry, C. (1974). *Helter Skelter: The true story of the Manson murders.* New York, NY: Norton.

Bulbulia, J. (2004). The cognitive and evolutionary psychology of religion. *Biology and Philosophy, 19*, 655–686.

Bulbulia, J. (2005). Are there any religions?: An evolutionary exploration. *Method and Theory in Religion, 17*, 71–100.

Bullard, T. E. (1987). *UFO abductions: The measure of a mystery.* Mount Rainier, MD: Fund for UFO Research.

Bulliet, R. W. (1979). *Conversion to Islam in the medieval period: An essay in quantitative history.* Cambridge, MA: Harvard University Press.

Bullivant, S. (2013). Defining "atheism." In S. Bullivant & M. Ruse (Eds.), *The Oxford handbook of atheism* (pp. 11–21). Oxford, UK: Oxford University Press.

Bullivant, S., & Ruse, M. (Eds.). (2013). *The Oxford handbook of atheism.* Oxford, UK: Oxford University Press.

Bulman, R. J., & Wortman, C. B. (1977). Attributions of blame and coping in the real world: Severe accident victims react to their lot. *Journal of Personality and Social Psychology, 35*, 351–363.

Burdette, A. M., Ellison, C. G., Sherkat, D. E., & Gore, K. A. (2007). Are there religious variations in marital infidelity? *Journal of Family Issues, 28,* 1553–1581.

Buri, J. R., Louiselle, P. A., Misukanis, T. M., & Mueller, R. A. (1988). Effects of parental authoritarianism and authoritativeness on self-esteem. *Personality and Social Psychology Bulletin, 14,* 271–282.

Burkert, W. (1996). *Creation of the sacred: Tracks of biology in early religions.* Cambridge, MA: Harvard University Press.

Burkimsher, M. (2014). Is religious attendance bottoming out?: Examination of current trends across Europe. *Journal for the Scientific Study of Religion, 53,* 432–445.

Burnham, J. C. (1985). The encounter of Christian theology with deterministic psychology and psychoanalysis. *Bulletin of the Menninger Clinic, 49,* 321–352.

Burris, C. T., Harmon-Jones, E., & Tarpley, W. R. (1997). "By faith alone": Religious agitation and cognitive dissonance. *Basic and Applied Social Psychology, 19,* 17–31.

Burris, C. T., & Jackson, L. M. (1999). Hate the sin/ love the sinner, or love the hater?: Intrinsic religion and responses to partner abuse. *Journal for the Scientific Study of Religion, 38,* 160–174.

Burris, C. T., & Jackson, L. M. (2000). Social identity and the true believer: Responses to marginalization among the intrinsically religious. *British Journal of Social Psychology, 39,* 257–278.

Burris, C. T., Jackson, L. M., Tarpley, W. R., & Smith, G. J. (1996). Religion as quest: The self-directed pursuit of meaning. *Personality and Social Psychology Bulletin, 22,* 1068–1076.

Burris, J. L., Sauer, S. E., & Carlson, C. R. (2011). A test of religious commitment and spiritual transcendence as independent predictors of underage alcohol use and alcohol-related problems. *Psychology of Religion and Spirituality, 3,* 231–240.

Burton, T. (1993). *Serpent-handling believers.* Knoxville: University of Tennessee Press.

Bushman, B. J., Ridge, R. D., Das, E., Key, C. W., & Busath, G. L. (2007). When God sanctions killing: Effects of scriptural violence. *Psychological Science, 18,* 204–207.

Button, T. M. M., Hewitt, J. K., Rhee, S. H., Corley, R. P., & Stallings, M. C. (2010). The moderating effect of religiosity on the genetic variance of problem alcohol use. *Alcoholism: Clinical and Experimental Research, 34,* 1619–1624.

Buttrick, G. A. (1942). *Prayer.* New York, NY: Abingdon-Cokesbury.

Buxant, C., & Saroglou, V. (2008). Joining and leaving a new religious movement: A study of ex-members'

mental health. *Mental Health, Religion and Culture, 11,* 251–271.

Byman, D. (2015). *Al Qaeda, the Islamic state, and the global jihadist movement: What everyone needs to know.* New York, NY: Oxford University Press.

Byrd, R. C. (1988). Positive therapeutic effects of intercessory prayer in a coronary care unit population. *Southern Medical Journal, 81,* 826–829.

Byrom, G. (2009). Differential relationships between experiential and interpretive dimensions of mysticism and magical ideation in a university sample. *Archive for the Psychology of Religion, 31,* 127–150.

Caird, D. (1988). The structure of Hood's Mysticism Scale: A factor analytic study. *Journal for the Scientific Study of Religion, 27,* 122–127.

Caird, E. (1969). *The evolution of religion.* New York, NY: Kraus. (Original work published 1893)

Caldwell-Harris, C. L., Wilson, A., LoTempio, E., & Beit-Hallahmi, B. (2011). Exploring the atheist personality: Well-being, awe, and magical thinking in atheists, Buddhists, and Christians. *Mental Health, Religion and Culture, 14,* 659–672.

Camargo, R. J., & Loftus, J. A. (1993, August 20). *Clergy sexual involvement with young people: Distinctive characteristics.* Paper presented at the annual convention of the American Psychological Association, Toronto, Ontario, Canada.

Campbell, R. A., & Curtis, J. E. (1994). Religious involvement across societies: Analyses for alternative measures in national surveys. *Journal for the Scientific Study of Religion, 33,* 217–229.

Canada, A. L., Murphy, P. E., Fitchett, G., & Stein, K. (2016). Re-examining the contributions of faith, meaning, and peace to quality of life: A report from the American Cancer Society's Study of Cancer Survivors-II (SCS-II). *Annals of Behavioral Medicine, 50,* 79–86.

Caplan, A. L. (Ed.). (1978). *The sociobiology debate.* New York, NY: Harper & Row.

Caplan, R. B. (1969). *Psychiatry and the community in nineteenth century America.* New York, NY: Basic Books.

Caplovitz, D., & Sherrow, F. (1977). *The religious drop-outs: Apostasy among college graduates.* Beverly Hills, CA: SAGE.

Capps, D. (1982). The psychology of petitionary prayer. *Theology Today, 39,* 130–141.

Capps, D. (1990). *Reframing: A new method in pastoral care.* Minneapolis, MN: Fortress.

Capps, D. (1992). Religion and child abuse: Perfect together. *Journal for the Scientific Study of Religion, 31,* 1–14.

Capps, D. (1994). An Allportian analysis of Augustine. *International Journal for the Psychology of Religion, 4,* 205–228.

Capps, D. (1995). *The child's song: The religious abuse of children.* Louisville, KY: Westminster John Knox Press.

Capps, D., & Dittes, J. E. (Eds.). (1990). *The hunger of the heart: The confessions of Augustine.* West Lafayette, IN: Society for the Scientific Study of Religion.

Cardeña, E., Lynn, S. J., & Krippner, S. (2000a). Introduction: Varieties of anomalous experience. In E. Cardeña, S. J. Lynn, & S. Krippner (Eds.), *Varieties of anomalous experience* (pp. 3–21). Washington, DC: American Psychological Association.

Cardeña, E., Lynn, S. J., & Krippner, S. (Eds.). (2000b). *Varieties of anomalous experience.* Washington, DC: American Psychological Association.

Cardeña, E., Lynn, S. J., & Krippner, S. (Eds.). (2014). *Varieties of anomalous experience: Examining the scientific evidence* (2nd ed.). Washington, DC: American Psychological Association.

Cares, A. C., & Cusick, G. R. (2012). Risks and opportunities of faith and culture: The case of abused Jewish women. *Journal of Family Violence, 27,* 427–435.

Carey, R. G. (1971). Influence of peers in shaping religious behavior. *Journal for the Scientific Study of Religion, 10,* 157–159.

Carey, R. G. (1979–1980). Weathering widowhood: Problems and adjustment of the widowed during the first year. *Omega, 10,* 163–174.

Carey, R. G., & Posavec, E. J. (1978–1979). Attitudes of physicians on disclosing information to and maintaining life for terminal patients. *Omega, 10,* 163–174.

Carlisle, R. D., & Tsang, J. (2013). The virtues: Gratitude and forgiveness. In K. I. Pargament, J. J. Exline, & J. W. Jones (Eds.), *APA handbook of psychology, religion, and spirituality* (Vol. 1, pp. 423–437). Washington, DC: American Psychological Association.

Carlson, C. R., Bacaseta, P. E., & Simanton, D. A. (1988). A controlled evaluation of devotional meditation and progressive relaxation. *Journal of Psychology and Theology, 16,* 362–368.

Carlson, S. M., Taylor, M., & Levin, G. R. (1998). The influence of culture on pretend play: The case of Mennonite children. *Merrill–Palmer Quarterly, 44,* 538–565.

Carlsson, B. G. (1997). Religion and cultural attitudes toward homosexuality: An emancipatory study. *Nordisk Sexologi, 15,* 143–147. [Abstract used]

Carmody, D., & Carmody, J. (1996). *Mysticism: Holiness East and West.* New York, NY: Oxford University Press.

Carroll, J. B. (Ed.). (1956). *Language, thought, and reality: Selected writings of Benjamin Lee Whorf.* New York, NY: Wiley.

Carroll, M. P. (1983). Vision of the Virgin Mary: The effects of family structures on Marian apparitions. *Journal for the Scientific Study of Religion, 22,* 205–221.

Carroll, M. P. (1986). *The cult of the Virgin Mary: Psychological origins.* Princeton, NJ: Princeton University Press.

Carroll, R. P. (1979). *When prophecy failed: Cognitive dissonance in the prophetic traditions of the Old Testament.* New York, NY: Seabury Press.

Carroll, S. T. (2013). Addressing religion and spirituality in the workplace. In K. I. Pargament, A. Mahoney, & E. P. Shafranske (Eds.), *APA handbook of psychology, religion, and spirituality* (Vol. 2, pp. 595–612). Washington, DC: American Psychological Association.

Cartwright, R. H., & Kent, S. A. (1992). Social control in alternative religions: A familial perspective. *Sociological Analysis, 53,* 345–361.

Carver, C. S., Scheier, M. F., & Pozo, C. (1992). Conceptualizing the process of coping with health problems. In H. S. Friedman (Ed.), *Hostility, coping, and health* (pp. 167–199). Washington, DC: American Psychological Association.

Casey, W. M., & Burton, R. V. (1986). The social-learning theory approach. In G. L. Sapp (Ed.), *Handbook of moral development* (pp. 74–91). Birmingham, AL: Religious Education Press.

Cassiba, R., Granqvist, P., & Constantini, A. (2013). Mothers' attachment security predicts their children's sense of God's closeness. *Attachment and Human Development, 15,* 51–64.

Cather, W. (1990). *My mortal enemy.* New York, NY: Vintage. (Original work published 1926)

Catton, W. R., Jr. (1966). *From animistic to naturalistic sociology.* New York, NY: McGraw-Hill.

Cecil, Lord D. (1966). *Melbourne.* Indianapolis, IN: Bobbs-Merrill.

Chadwick, B. A., & Top, B. L. (1993). Religiosity and delinquency among LDS adolescents. *Journal for the Scientific Study of Religion, 32,* 51–67.

Chancellor, J. D. (2000). *Life in the family: An oral history of the children of God.* Syracuse, NY: Syracuse University Press.

Chandy, J. M., Blum, R. W., & Resnick, M. D. (1996). Female adolescents with a history of sexual abuse: Risk outcome and protective factors. *Journal of Interpersonal Violence, 11,* 503–518.

Chatters, L. M., Taylor, R. J., & Lincoln, K. D. (2002). Advances in the measurement of religiosity among older African Americans: Implications for health and mental health researchers. In J. H. Skinner & J. A. Teresi (Eds.), *Multicultural measurement in older populations* (pp. 199–220). New York, NY: Springer.

Chau, L. L., Johnson, R. C., Bowers, J. K., Darvill,

T. J., & Danko, G. P. (1990). Intrinsic and extrinsic religiosity as related to conscience, adjustment, and altruism. *Personality and Individual Differences, 11,* 397–400.

Chaves, M. (1989). Secularization and religious revival: Evidence for U.S. church attendance rates, 1972–1986. *Journal for the Scientific Study of Religion, 28,* 464–477.

Chaves, M. (1991). Family structure and Protestant church attendance: The sociological basis of cohort and age-effects. *Journal for the Scientific Study of Religion, 30,* 501–514.

Chaves, M. (1997). *Ordaining women: Culture and conflict in religious organizations.* Cambridge, MA: Harvard University Press.

Chaves, M., & Cavendish, J. C. (1994). More evidence on U.S. Catholic church attendance. *Journal for the Scientific Study of Religion, 33,* 376–381.

Chaves, M., & Garland, D. (2009). The prevalence of clergy sexual advances toward adults in their congregations. *Journal for the Scientific Study of Religion, 48,* 817–824.

Chawla, N., Neighbors, C., Lewis, M. A., Lee, C. M., & Larimer, M. E. (2007). Attitudes and perceived approval of drinking as mediators of the relationship between the importance of religion and alcohol use. *Journal of Studies on Alcohol and Drugs, 68,* 410–418.

Chen, Z., Hood, R. W., Jr., Yang, L., & Watson, P. J. (2011). Mystical experience among Tibetan Buddhists: The common core thesis revisited. *Journal for the Scientific Study of Religion, 50,* 328–338.

Chen, Z., Qi, W., Hood, R. W., Jr., & Watson, P. J. (2011). Common core thesis and qualitative and quantitative analysis of mysticism in Chinese Buddhist monks and nuns. *Journal for the Scientific Study of Religion, 50,* 654–670.

Chen, Z., Zhang, Y., Hood, R. W., Jr., & Watson, P. (2012). Mysticism in Christians and non-Christians: Measurement invariance of the Mysticism Scale and implications for the mean differences. *International Journal for the Psychology of Religion, 22,* 155–168.

Chesen, E. S. (1972). *Religion may be hazardous to your health.* New York, NY: Wyden.

Chida, Y., Steptoe, A., & Powell, L. H. (2009). Religiosity/spirituality and mortality. *Psychotherapy and Psychosomatics, 78,* 81–90.

Childs, E. (2010). Religious attendance and happiness: Examining gaps in the current literature—A research note. *Journal for the Scientific Study of Religion, 49,* 550–560.

Christ, C. P., & Plaskow, J. (1979). *Womanspirit rising.* New York, NY: Harper & Row.

Clark, E. T. (1929). *The psychology of religious awakening.* New York, NY: Macmillan.

Clark, J. (1978). Problems in the referral of cult members. *Journal of the National Association of Private Psychiatric Hospitals, 9,* 19–21.

Clark, J. (1979). Cults. *Journal of the American Medical Association, 242,* 279–281.

Clark, J. H. (1983). *A map of mental states.* London, UK: Routledge & Kegan Paul.

Clark, J. M., Brown, J. C., & Hochstein, L. M. (1989). Institutional religion and gay/lesbian oppression. *Marriage and Family Review, 14,* 265–284.

Clark, J., Langone, M. D., Schacter, R., & Daly, R. C. G. (1981). *Destructive cult conversion: Theory, research and practice.* Weston, MA: American Family Foundation.

Clark, R. W. (1984). The evidential value of religious experiences. *International Journal for Philosophy of Religion, 16,* 189–201.

Clark, W. H. (1958). *The psychology of religion.* New York, NY: Macmillan.

Clark, W. H. (1969). *Chemical ecstasy: Psychedelic drugs and religion.* New York, NY: Sheed & Ward.

Clark, W. H., Malony, H. N., Daane, J., & Tippett, A. R. (1973). *Religious experience: Its nature and function in the human psyche.* Springfield, IL: Charles C Thomas.

Clark, W. R., & Grunstein, M. (2000). *Are we hardwired?* New York, NY: Oxford University Press.

Clarke, R.-L. (1986). *Pastoral care of battered women.* Philadelphia, PA: Westminster Press.

Clines, F. X. (2002, March 12). Ohio board hears debate on an alternative to Darwinism. *The New York Times,* p. A16.

Cloninger, C. R., & Yokoyama, S. (1981). The channeling of social behavior. *Science, 213,* 749–751.

Clouse, B. (1986). Church conflict and moral stages: A Kohlbergian interpretation. *Journal of Psychology and Christianity, 5,* 14–19.

Clouse, B. (1991). Religious experience, religious belief and moral development of students at a state university. *Journal of Psychology and Christianity, 10,* 337–349.

Coates, D. D. (2012a). "Cult commitment" from the perspective of former members: Direct rewards of membership versus dependency inducing practices. *Deviant Behavior, 33,* 168–184.

Coates, D. D. (2012b). "I'm now far healthier and better able to manage the challenges of life": The mediating role of New Religious Movement membership and exit. *Journal of Spirituality in Mental Health, 14,* 181–208.

Cobb, N. J. (2001). *Adolescence: Continuity, change, and diversity* (4th ed.). Mountain View, CA: Mayfield.

Cobb, N. J., Ong, A. D., & Tate, J. (2001). Reason-based evaluations of wrongdoing in religious and moral narratives. *International Journal for the Psychology of Religion, 11*, 259–276.

Cochran, G., Hardy, J., & Harpending, H. (2005). Natural history of Ashkenazi intelligence. *Journal of Biosocial Science, 38*, 659–693.

Cochran, J. K. (1993). The variable effects of religiosity and denomination on adolescent self-reported alcohol use by beverage type. *Journal of Drug Issues, 23*, 479–491.

Cochran, J. K., & Beeghley, L. (1991). The influence of religion on attitudes toward nonmarital sexuality: A preliminary assessment of reference group theory. *Journal for the Scientific Study of Religion, 30*, 45–62.

Cochran, J. K., Chamlin, M. B., Beeghley, L., & Fenwick, M. (2004). Religion, religiosity, and nonmarital sexual conduct: An application of reference group theory. *Sociological Inquiry, 74*, 102–127.

Cochran, J. K., Chamlin, M. B., Wood, P. B., & Sellers, C. S. (1999). Shame, embarrassment, and formal sanction threats: Extending the deterrence/rational choice model to academic dishonesty. *Sociological Inquiry, 69*, 91–105.

Coe, G. A. (1900). *The spiritual life: Studies in the science of religion.* New York, NY: Eaton & Mains.

Coe, G. A. (1916). *The psychology of religion.* Chicago, IL: University of Chicago Press.

Cohen, A. B. (2002). The importance of spirituality in well-being for Jews and Christians. *Journal of Happiness Studies, 3*, 287–310.

Cohen, A. B. (2009). Many forms of culture. *American Psychologist, 64*, 194–204.

Cohen, A. B., Gorvine, B. J., & Gorvine, H. (2013). The religion, spirituality, and psychology of Jews. In K. I. Pargament, J. J. Exline, & J. W. Jones (Eds.), *APA handbook of psychology, religion, and spirituality* (Vol. 1, pp. 665–679). Washington, DC: American Psychological Association.

Cohen, A. B., & Hill, P. C. (2007). Religion as culture: Religious individualism and collectivism among American Catholics, Jews, and Protestants. *Journal of Personality, 75*, 709–742.

Cohen, A. B., & Rozin, P. (2001). Religion and the morality of mentality. *Journal of Personality and Social Psychology, 81*, 697–710.

Cohen, A. B., Shariff, A. F., & Hill, P. C. (2008). The accessibility of religious beliefs. *Journal of Research in Personality, 42*, 1408–1417.

Cohen, R., Bavishi, C., & Rozanski, A. (2016). Purpose in life and its relationship to all-cause mortality and cardiovascular events: A meta-analysis. *Psychosomatic Medicine, 78*, 122–133.

Coker, A. L., Smith, P. H., Thompson, M. P., McKeown, R. E., Bethea, L., & Davis, K. E. (2002). Social support protects against the negative effects of partner violence on mental health. *Journal of Women's Health and Gender-Based Medicine, 11*, 465–476.

Colantonio, A., Kasl, S. V., & Ostfeld, A. M. (1992). Depressive symptoms and other psychosocial factors as predictors of stroke in the elderly. *American Journal of Epidemiology, 136*, 884–894.

Cole, B. S., Hopkins, C. M., Tisak, J., Steel, J. L., & Carr, B. I. (2008). Assessing spiritual growth and spiritual decline following a diagnosis nof cancer: Reliability and validity of the spiritual transformation scale. *Psych-Oncology, 17*, 112–121.

Cole, B. S., & Pargament, K. I. (1999). Spiritual surrender: A paradoxical path to control. In W. R. Miller (Ed.), *Integrating spirituality into treatment* (pp. 179–198). Washington, DC: American Psychological Association.

Cole, S. W., Hawkley, L. C., Arevalo, J. M., Sung, C. Y., Rose, R. M., & Cacioppo, J. T. (2007). Social regulation of gene expression in human leukocytes. *Genome Biology, 8*, R189.

Coleman, P. (2001). Elderly find it harder to cope with bereavement as they lose faith in religion. Retrieved October 20, 2007, from *www.soton.ac.uk/~pubaffrs01111.htm*.

Coleman, T. J., & Arrowood, R. B. (2015). Only we can save ourselves: An atheist's "salvation." In H. Bacon, W. Dossett, & S. Knowles (Eds.), *Alternative salvations: Engaging the sacred and the secular* (pp. 11–20). London, UK: Bloomsbury.

Coleman, T. J., & Hood, R. W., Jr. (2015). Reconsidering everything from folk categories to existential theory of mind. *Religion and Society: Advances in Research, 6*, 18–22.

Coleman, T. J., Hood, R. W., Jr., & Shook, J. R. (2015). An introduction to atheism, secularity, and science. *Science, Religion, and Culture, 2*(3), 1–14.

Coles, R. (1990). *The spiritual life of children.* Boston, MA: Houghton Mifflin.

Colipp, P. J. (1969). The efficacy of prayer: A triple-blind study. *Medical Times, 97*, 201–204.

Collins, M. A. (2007). Religiousness and spirituality as possible recovery variables in treated and natural recoveries: A qualitative study. *Alcoholism Treatment Quarterly, 24*, 119–135.

Comte-Sponville, A. (2007). *The little book of atheistic spirituality* (N. Houston, Trans.). New York, NY: Viking.

Condran, J. G., & Tamney, J. B. (1985). Religious "nones": 1957–1982. *Sociological Analysis, 46*, 415–423.

Conn, J. W. (Ed.). (1986). *Women's spirituality: Resources for Christian development.* New York, NY: Paulist Press.

Connors, G. J., Tonigan, J. S., & Miller, W. R. (1996). A measure of religious background and behavior for use in behavior change research. *Psychology of Addictive Behaviors, 10,* 90–96.

Conrad, P., & Schnelder, J. W. (1980). *Deviance and medicalization: From badness to sickness.* St. Louis, MO: Mosby.

Conway, F., & Siegelman, J. (1978). *Snapping: America's epidemic of sudden personality change.* Philadelphia, PA: Lippincott.

Conway, K. (1985–1986). Coping with the stress of medical problems among black and white elderly. *International Journal of Aging and Human Development, 21,* 39–48.

Cook, A. S., & Oltjenbruns, K. A. (1989). *Dying and grieving.* New York, NY: Holt, Rinehart & Winston.

Cook, T., & Wimberly, D. (1983). If I should die before I wake: Religious commitment and adjustment to the death of a child. *Journal for the Scientific Study of Religion, 22,* 222–238.

Coon, D. J. (1992). Testing the limits of sense and science: American experimental psychologists combat spiritualism, 1880–1920. *American Psychologist, 47,* 143–151.

Coopersmith, S., Regan, M., & Dick, L. (1975). *The myth of the generation gap.* San Francisco, CA: Albion.

Corcoran, K. E., Pettinicchio, D., & Robbins, B. (2012). Religion and the acceptability of white-collar crime: A cross-national analysis. *Journal for the Scientific Study of Religion, 51,* 542–567.

Cornwall, M. (1987). The social bases of religion: A study of factors influencing religious belief and commitment. *Review of Religious Research, 29,* 44–56.

Cornwall, M. (1988). The influence of three agents of religious socialization: Family, church, and peers. In D. L. Thomas (Ed.), *The religion and family connection* (pp. 207–231). Provo, UT: Religious Studies Center, Brigham Young University.

Cornwall, M. (1989). The determinants of religious behavior: A theoretical model and empirical test. *Social Forces, 68,* 572–592.

Cornwall, M., & Thomas, D. L. (1990). Family, religion, and personal communities: Examples from Mormonism. *Marriage and Family Review, 15,* 229–252.

Corssan, J. D. (1975). *The dark interval.* Niles, IL: Argus Communication.

Cortes, A. de J. (1999). Antecedents to the conflict between religion and psychology in America. *Journal of Psychology and Theology, 27,* 20–32.

Corveleyn, J., & Luyten, P. (2005). Psychodynamic psychologies and religion: Past, present, and future. In R. F. Paloutzian & C. L. Parks (Eds.), *Handbook of the psychology of religion and spirituality* (pp. 80–100). New York, NY: Guilford Press.

Corwyn, R. F., & Benda, B. B. (2000). Religiosity and church attendance: The effects on use of "hard drugs" controlling for sociodemographic and theoretical factors. *International Journal for the Psychology of Religion, 10,* 241–258.

Corwyn, R. F., Benda, B. B., & Ballard, K. (1997). Do the same theoretical factors explain alcohol and other drug use among adolescents? *Alcoholism Treatment Quarterly, 15,* 47–62.

Cota-McKinley, A. L., Woody, W. D., & Bell, P. A. (2001). Vengeance: Effects of gender, age, and religious background. *Aggressive Behavior, 27,* 343–350.

Cotton, S. P., Levine, E. G., Fitzpatrick, C. M., Dold, K. H., & Targ, E. (1999). Exploring the relationships among spiritual well-being, quality of life, and psychological adjustment in women with breast cancer. *Psycho-Oncology, 8,* 429–438.

Cotton, S. P., Puchalski, C. M., Sherman, S. N., Mrus, J. M., Peterman, A. H., Feinberg, J., et al. (2006). Spirituality and religion in patients with HIV/AIDS. *Journal of General Internal Medicine, 21*(Suppl. 5), S5–S13.

Coward, H. (1986). Intolerance in the world's religions. *Studies in Religion, 15,* 419–431.

Coyle, B. R. (2001). Twelve myths of religion and psychiatry: Lessons for training psychiatrists in spiritually sensitive treatments. *Mental Health, Religion and Culture, 4,* 147–174.

Cragun, R. T., Kosmin, B., Keysar, A., Hammer, J. H., & Nielsen, M. E. (2012). On the receiving end: Discrimination toward the non-religious in the U.S. *Journal of Contemporary Religion, 27,* 105–127.

Crisler, C. R. (1994). An evolutionist looks at the origin of religion. Retrieved May 20, 2007, from *www.banned-books.com/truth seeker/1994/archive/121_1/ts211q.html.*

Crooks, E. B. (1913). Professor James and the psychology of religion. *Monist, 23,* 122–130.

Crosby, R. A., & Yarber, W. L. (2001). Perceived versus actual knowledge about correct condom use among U.S. adolescents: Results from a national study. *Journal of Adolescent Health, 28,* 415–420.

Crowne, D. P., & Marlowe, D. (1964). *The approval motive: Studies in evaluative dependence.* New York, NY: Wiley.

Crumbaugh, J. C. (1977). The Seeking of Noetic Goals test (SONG): A complementary scale to the Purpose in Life Test (PIL). *Journal of Clinical Psychology, 33,* 900–907.

Crumbaugh, J. C., & Maholick, L. T. (1964). An experimental study in existentialism: The psychometric approach to Frankl's concept of noogenic neurosis. *Journal of Clinical Psychology, 20,* 200–207.

Culbertson, B. (1996, June). *The correlation between shame and the concept of God among intrinsically religious Nazarenes.* Unpublished master's thesis, Southern Nazarene University, Bethany, OK.

Culver, V. (1988, April 17). Emotional upset linked to strictness in religion. *The Denver Post,* pp. 1B–2B.

Culver, V. (1994, May 11). Clergy sex misconduct prevalent. *The Denver Post,* pp. 1B, 8B.

Culver, V. (2001, November 6). Methodist court bars openly gay ministers. *The Denver Post,* p. 11A.

Cummings, J. P., & Pargament, K. I. (2010). Medicine for the spirit: Religious coping in individuals with medical conditions. *Religions, 1,* 28–53.

Cunningham, J. P., & Yu, B. M. (2014). Dimensionality reduction for large-scale neural recordings. *Nature Neuroscience, 17,* 1500–1509.

Curtis, K. T., & Ellison, C. G. (2002). Religious heterogamy and marital conflict: Findings from the national survey of families and households. *Journal of Family Issues, 23,* 551–576.

Cutten, G. B. (1908). *The psychological phenomena of Christianity.* New York, NY: Scribner.

Dahl, K. E. (1999). Religion and coping with bereavement. *Dissertation Abstracts International, 59*(7), 3686B.

Dahlsgaard, K., Peterson, C., & Seligman, M. E. P. (2005). Shared virtue: The convergence of valued human strengths across culture and history. *Review of General Psychology, 9,* 203–213.

Dannaway, F. R., Piper, A., & Webster, P. (2006). Bread of heaven or wines of light: Entheogenic legacies and esoteric cosmologies. *Journal of Psychoactive Drugs, 38,* 493–503.

Danso, H., Hunsberger, B., & Pratt, M. (1997). The role of parental religious fundamentalism and right-wing authoritarianism in child-rearing goals and practices. *Journal for the Scientific Study of Religion, 36,* 496–511.

d'Aquili, E. G. (1978). The neurobiological bases of myth and concepts of deity. *Zygon, 13,* 257–275.

d'Aquili, E. G., Laughlin, C. D., Jr., & McManus, J. (Eds.). (1979). *The spectrum of ritual: A biogenetic analysis.* New York, NY: Columbia University Press.

d'Aquili, E. G., & Newberg, A. B. (1993). Religious and mystical states: A neuropsychological model. *Zygon, 28,* 177–200.

d'Aquili, E. G., & Newberg, A. B. (1999). *The mystical mind: Probing the biology of mystical experience.* Minneapolis, MN: Fortress Press.

Darley, J. M., & Batson, C. D. (1973). "From Jerusalem to Jericho": A study of situational and dispositional variables in helping behavior. *Journal of Personality and Social Psychology, 27,* 100–108.

Darley, J. M., & Shultz, T. R. (1990). Moral rules: Their content and acquisition. *Annual Review of Psychology, 41,* 525–556.

Darling, N., & Steinberg, L. (1993). Parenting style as

context: An integrative model. *Psychological Bulletin, 113,* 487–496.

Darwin, C. (1972). *The origin of species.* New York, NY: Dutton. (Original work published 1859)

David, J., Ladd, K., & Spilka, B. (1992). *The multidimensionality of prayer and its role as a source of secondary control.* Paper presented at the annual convention of the American Psychological Association, Washington, DC.

Davidson, J. D., & Caddell, D. P. (1994). Religion and the meaning of work. *Journal for the Scientfic Study of Religion, 33,* 135–147.

Davidson, L., & Griel, A. L. (2007). Characters in search of a script: The exit narratives of formerly ultra-Orthodox Jews. *Journal for the Scientific Study of Religion, 46,* 201–216.

Davis, C. F. (1989). *The evidential force of religious experience.* Oxford, UK: Clarendon Press.

Davis, D. E., Choe, E., Meyers, J., Wade, N. Varjas, K., Gifford, A., et al. (2016). Thankful for the little things: A meta-analysis of gratitude interventions. *Journal of Counseling Psychology, 63,* 20–31.

Davis, D. E., Worthington, E. L., Jr., Hook, J. N., & Hill, P. C. (2013). Research on religion/spirituality and forgiveness: A meta-analytic review. *Psychology of Religion and Spirituality, 5,* 233–241.

Davis, J. A., & Smith, T. W. (1994). *General social surveys, 1972–1994* [Machine-readable data file]. Chicago, IL: National Opinion Research Center [Producer]; Storrs, CT: Roper Center for Public Opinion Research, University of Connecticut [Distributor].

Davis, P. (Ed.). (1976). *The American heritage dictionary.* New York, NY: Dell.

Dawkins, R. (1976). *The selfish gene.* New York, NY: Oxford University Press.

Dawkins, R. (1986). *The blind watchmaker.* New York, NY: Norton.

Dawkins, R. (2006). *The God delusion.* Boston, MA: Houghton Mifflin.

Dawson, L. (1999). When prophecy fails and faith persists: A theoretical overview. *Nova Religio, 3,* 60–82.

Day, J. M. (1991). Narrative, psychology and moral education. *American Psychologist, 46,* 167–178.

Day, J. M. (1994). Moral development, belief, and unbelief: Young adult accounts of religion in the process of moral growth. In J. Corveleyn & D. Hutsebaut (Eds.), *Belief and unbelief: Psychological perspectives* (pp. 155–173). Atlanta, GA: Rodopi.

Day, J. M. (2001). From structuralism to eternity?: Re-imagining the psychology of religious development after the cognitive-developmental paradigm. *International Journal for the Psychology of Religion, 11,* 173–183.

de Chardin, P. T. (1959). *The phenomenon of man* (B. Wall, Trans.). New York, NY: Harper & Row.

De Frain, J. D., Jakub, D. K., & Mendoza, B. L. (1991–1992). The psychological effects of sudden infant death on grandmothers and grandfathers. *Omega, 24,* 165–182.

De Haan, L. G., & Schulenberg, J. (1997). The covariation of religion and politics during the transition to adulthood: Challenging global identity assumptions. *Journal of Adolescence, 20,* 537–552.

de Jonge, J. (1995). On breaking wills: The theological roots of violence in families. *Journal of Psychology and Christianity, 14,* 26–36.

de Mello, A. (1984). *Sadhana: A way to God.* New York, NY: Image Books.

De Roos, S. A., Miedema, S., & Iedema, J. (2001). Attachment, working models of self and others, and God concept in kindergarten. *Journal for the Scientific Study of Religion, 40,* 607–618.

de Vaus, D. A. (1983). The relative importance of parents and peers for adolescent religious orientation: An Australian study. *Adolescence, 18,* 147–158.

De Vellis, B. M., De Vellis, R. F., & Spilsbury, J. C. (1988). Parental actions when children are sick: The role of belief in divine influence. *Basic and Applied Social Psychology, 9,* 185–196.

de Visser, R. O., Smith, A. M. A., Richters, J., & Rissel, C. E. (2007). Associations between religiosity and sexuality in a representative sample of Australian adults. *Archives of Sexual Behavior, 36,* 33–46.

Deconchy, J.-P. (1965). The idea of God: Its emergence between 7 and 16 years. In A. Godin (Ed.), *From religious experience to a religious attitude* (pp. 97–108). Chicago, IL: Loyola University Press.

Degelman, D., Mullen, P., & Mullen, N. (1984). Development of abstract religious thinking: A comparison of Roman Catholic and Nazarene youth. *Journal of Psychology and Christianity, 3,* 44–49.

Deikman, A. (1966). Implications of experimentally produced contemplative meditation. *Journal of Nervous and Mental Disease, 142,* 101–116.

Dein, S. (1997). Lubavitch: A contemporary messianic movement. *Journal of Contemporary Religion, 12,* 191–204.

Dein, S. (2001). What really happens when prophecy fails: The case of Lubavitch. *Sociology of Religion, 62,* 383–401.

Dein, S., & Littlewood, R. (2000). Apocalyptic suicide. *Mental Health, Religion and Culture, 3,* 109–114.

Dekmejian, R. H. (1985). *Islam in revolution: Fundamentalism in the Arab world.* Syracuse, NY: Syracuse University Press.

Delgado, R. (1977). Religious totalism. *University of Southern California Law Review, 15,* 1–99.

Delgado, R. (1982). Cult and conversions: The case for informed consent. *Georgia Law Review, 16,* 533–574.

Demerath, N. J. (1965). *Social class and American Protestantism.* Chicago, IL: Rand McNally.

DeNicola, K. (1997). Response to Reich's "Do we need a theory for the religious development of women?" *International Journal for the Psychology of Religion, 7,* 93–97.

Dennett, D. (2006). *Breaking the spell: Religion as a natural phenomenon.* New York, NY: Viking.

Dennett, D. C., & LaScola, L. (2010). Preachers who are not believers. *Evolutionary Psychology, 8,* 122–150.

The Denver Post. (2001, November 19). Church's gay pastor a first for Lutherans. p. 9A.

The Denver Post. (2015, April 30). Pope calls gender pay gap "pure scandal." p. 14A.

Desmond, S., Ulmer, J. T., & Bader, C. D. (2013). Religion, self-control, and substance use. *Deviant Behavior, 34,* 384–406.

DeSteno, D., Bartlett, M. Y., Baumann, J., Williams, L. A., & Dickens, L. (2010). Gratitude as moral sentiment: Emotion-guided cooperation in economic exchange. *Emotion, 10,* 289–293.

DeWall, C. N., Pond, R. S., Jr., Carter, E. C., McCullough, M. E., Lambert, N. M., Fincham, F. D., & Nezlek, J. B. (2014). Explaining the relationship between religiousness and substance use: Self-control matters. *Journal of Personality and Social Psychology, 107,* 339–351.

Dewhurst, K., & Beard, A. W. (1970). Sudden religious conversions in temporal lobe epilepsy. *British Journal of Psychiatry, 117,* 497–507.

DeYoung, C. G. (2006). Higher-order factors of the Big Five in a multi-informant sample. *Journal of Personality and Social Psychology, 91,* 1138–1151.

DeYoung, C. G., Peterson, J. B., & Higgins, D. M. (2002). Higher-order factors of the Big Five predict conformity: Are there neuroses of health? *Personality and Individual Differences, 33,* 533–553.

Dickie, J. R., Eshleman, A. K., Merasco, D. M., Shepard, A., Vander Wilt, M., & Johnson, M. (1997). Parent–child relationships and children's images of God. *Journal for the Scientific Study of Religion, 36,* 25–43.

Diener, E., & Clifton, D. (2002). Life satisfaction and religiosity in broad probability samples. *Psychological Inquiry, 13,* 206–209.

Dienstbier, R. A. (1979). Emotion-attribution theory: Establishing roots and exploring future perspectives. In R. A. Dienstbier (Ed.), *Nebraska Symposium on Motivation* (Vol. 26, pp. 237–306). Lincoln: University of Nebraska Press.

Dillon, M. (2014). Asynchrony in attitudes toward abortion and gay rights: The challenge to values alignment. *Journal for the Scientific Study of Religion, 53,* 1–16.

Dillon, M., & Wink, P. (2007). *In the course of a lifetime: Tracing religious belief, practice, and change.* Berkeley: University of California Press.

Dionne, E. J. (2001, September 19). Is religion the cause or the solution? *The Denver Post*, p. B11.

Ditman, K. S., Moss, T., Forgy, E. W., Zunin, L. M., Lynch, R. D., & Funk, W. A. (1969). Dimensions of the LSD, methylphenidate and chlordiazepoxide experiences. *Psychopharmacologia, 14*, 1–11.

Dittes, J. E. (1969). The psychology of religion. In G. Lindzey & E. Aronson (Eds.), *The handbook of social psychology* (Vol. 5, pp. 602–659). Reading, MA: Addison-Wesley.

Dittes, J. E. (1971a). Conceptual derivation and statistical rigor. *Journal for the Scientific Study of Religion, 10*, 393–395.

Dittes, J. E. (1971b). Typing the typologies: Some parallels in the career of church–sect and extrinsic—intrinsic religion. *Journal for the Scientific Study of Religion, 10*, 375–383.

DizzyBoy.com. (n.d.). Aging quotes. Retrieved December 11, 2008, from *www.dizzyboy.com/quotes/aging_quotes.html*.

Dobkin de Rios, M. (1984). *Hallucinogens: Cross-cultural perspectives.* Albuquerque: University of New Mexico Press.

Doblin, R. (1991). Pahnke's "Good Friday" experiment: A long-term follow-up and methodological critique. *Journal of Transpersonal Psychology, 23*, 1–28.

Dollahite, D. C. (2003). Fathering for eternity: Generative spirituality in Latter-Day Saint fathers of children with special needs. *Review of Religious Research, 44*, 237–251.

Dollahite, D. C., & Lambert, N. M. (2007). Forsaking all others: How religious involvement promotes marital fidelity in Christian, Jewish, and Muslim couples. *Review of Religious Research, 48*, 290–307.

Dollahite, D. C., & Marks, L. D. (2005). How highly religious families strive to fulfill sacred purposes. In V. L. Bengtson, D. Klein, A. Acock, K. Allen, & P. Dilworth-Anderson (Eds.), *Sourcebook of family theory and research* (pp. 533–537). Thousand Oaks, CA: SAGE.

Domino, G., & Miller, K. (1992). Religiosity and attitudes toward suicide. *Omega, 25*, 271–282.

Donahue, M. J. (1985). Intrinsic and extrinsic religiousness: Review and meta-analysis. *Journal of Personality and Social Psychology, 48*, 400–419.

Donahue, M. J. (1998, August). *There is no true spirituality apart from religion.* Paper presented at the annual convention of the American Psychological Association, Chicago, IL.

Donahue, M. J., & Benson, P. L. (1995). Religion and the well-being of adolescents. *Journal of Social Issues, 51*, 145–160.

Donelson, E. (1999). Psychology of religion and adolescents in the United States: Past to present. *Journal of Adolescence, 22*, 187–204.

D'Onofrio, B., Eaves, L. J., Murrelle, L., Maes, H. H., & Spilka, B. (1999). Understanding biological and social influences on religious affiliation, attitudes, and behaviors: A behavior-genetic perspective. *Journal of Personality, 67*, 953–984.

Dover, H., Miner, M., & Dowson, M. (2007). The nature and structure of Muslim religious reflection. *Journal of Muslim Mental Health, 2*, 189–210.

Dovidio, J. F., & Fazio, R. H. (1992). New technologies for the direct and indirect assessment of attitudes. In J. M. Tanur (Ed.), *Questions about questions: Inquiries into the cognitive bases of surveys* (pp. 204–237). New York, NY: Russell Sage Foundation.

Dowd, M. (2002, April 7). Sacred cruelties. *The New York Times.* Retrieved April 8, 2002, from *www.nytimes.com/2002/04/07/opinion07DOWD.html?todaysheadlines.*

Downton, J. V., Jr. (1980). An evolutionary theory of spiritual conversion and commitment: The case of the Divine Light Mission. *Journal for the Scientific Study of Religion, 19*, 381–396.

Doxey, C., Jensen, L., & Jensen, J. (1997). The influence of religion on victims of childhood sexual abuse. *International Journal for the Psychology of Religion, 7*, 179–183.

Dresser, H. W. (1929). *Outlines of the psychology of religion.* New York, NY: Crowell.

Dublin, L. I. (1963). *Suicide.* New York, NY: Ronald Press.

Dubose, E. R. (2000, November). Spiritual care at the end of life. *Bulletin of the Park Ridge Center for the Study of Health, Faith, and Ethics*, p. 18.

Dubow, E. F., Pargament, K. I., Boxer, P., & Tarakeshwar, N. (2000). Initial investigation of Jewish early adolescents' ethnic identity, stress, and coping. *Journal of Early Adolescence, 20*, 418–441.

Duck, R. J., & Hunsberger, B. (1999). Religious orientation and prejudice: The role of religious proscription, right-wing authoritarianism and social desirability. *International Journal for the Psychology of Religion, 9*, 157–179.

Dudley, M. G., & Kosinski, F. A., Jr. (1990). Religiosity and marital satisfaction: A research note. *Review of Religious Research, 32*, 78–86.

Dudley, R. L. (1978). Alienation from religion in adolescents from fundamentalist religious homes. *Journal for the Scientific Study of Religion, 17*, 389–398.

Dudley, R. L., & Dudley, M. G. (1986). Transmission of religious values from parents to adolescents. *Review of Religious Research, 28*, 3–15.

Dufour, L. R. (2000). Sifting through tradition: The creation of Jewish feminist identities. *Journal for the Scientific Study of Religion, 39*, 90–106.

Dulin, P. L., Hill, R. D., & Ellingson, K. (2006). Relationships among religious factors, social support and alcohol abuse in a Western U.S. college student sample. *Journal of Alcohol and Drug Education, 50,* 5–14.

Dunn, K. S., & Horgas, A. L. (2000). The prevalence of prayer as a spiritual self-care modality in elders. *Journal of Holistic Nursing, 18,* 337–351.

Dunn, M. S. (2005). The relationship between religiosity, employment, and political beliefs on substance use among high school seniors. *Journal of Alcohol and Drug Education, 49,* 73–88.

Duriez, B., & Hutsebaut, D. (2000). The relation between religion and racism: The role of postcritical beliefs. *Mental Health, Religion and Culture, 3,* 85–102.

Durkheim, E. (1915). *The elementary forms of the religious life: A study in religious sociology* (J. W. Swain, Trans.). London, UK: Allen & Unwin.

Durr, R. A. (1970). *Poetic vision and the psychedelic experience.* New York, NY: Dell.

Dwiwardani, C., Hill, P. C., Bollinger, R. A., Marks, L. E., Steele, J. R., Doolin, H. N., et al. (2014). Virtues develop from a secure base: Attachment and resilience as predictors of humility, gratitude, and forgiveness. *Journal of Psychology and Theology, 42,* 83–90.

Dynes, R. R. (1955). Church–sect typology and socioeconomic status. *American Sociological Review, 20,* 555–660.

Eaton, J. W., & Weil, R. J. (1955). *Culture and mental disorders.* Glencoe, IL: Free Press.

Echterling, L. G. (1993, August). *Making do and making sense: Long-term coping of disaster survivors.* Paper presented at the annual convention of the American Psychological Association, Toronto, Ontario, Canada.

Ecklund, E. H., & Lee, K. S. (2011). Atheists and agnostics negotiate religion and family. *Journal for the Scientific Study of Religion, 50,* 728–743.

Ecklund, E. H., & Park, J. Z. (2009). Conflict between religion and science among academic scientists? *Journal for the Scientific Study of Religion, 48,* 276–292.

Edgell, P., Gerteis, J., & Hartmann, D. (2006). Atheists as "others": Moral boundaries and cultural membership in American society. *American Sociological Review, 71,* 211–234.

Edwards, A. C., & Lewis, M. J. (2008a). Attitudes to mysticism: Relationship with personality in Western and Eastern traditions. *Spirituality and Health International, 9,* 145–160.

Edwards, A. C., & Lewis, M. J. (2008b). Construction and validation of a scale to assess attitudes to mysticism: The need for a new scale for research in the psychology of religion. *Spirituality and Health International, 9,* 16–31.

Egan, K. M., Trichopoulos, D., Stampfer, M. J.,

Willett, W. C., Newcomb, P. A., Trentham-Dietz, A., et al. (1996). Jewish religion and the risk of breast cancer. *Lancet, 347,* 1645–1646.

Einstein, A. (1931). Religion and science. In A. M. Drummond & R. H. Wagner (Eds.), *Problems and opinions* (pp. 355–358). New York, NY: Century.

Eisinga, R., Billiet, J., & Felling, A. (1999). Christian religion and ethnic prejudice in cross-national perspective: A comparative analysis of the Netherlands and Flanders (Belgium). *International Journal of Comparative Sociology, 40,* 375–393.

Eisinga, R., Konig, R., & Scheepers, P. (1995). Orthodox religious beliefs and anti-Semitism: A replication of Glock and Stark in the Netherlands. *Journal for the Scientific Study of Religion, 34,* 214–223.

Eister, A. W. (1973). H. Richard Niebuhr and the paradox of religious organizations: A radical critique. In C. Y. Glock & P. E. Hammond (Eds.), *Beyond the classics?: Essays in the scientific study of religion* (pp. 355–408). New York, NY: Harper & Row.

Eliach, Y. (1982). *Hasidic tales of the Holocaust.* New York, NY: Avon.

Elkind, D. (1961). The child's concept of his religious denomination: I. The Jewish child. *Journal of Genetic Psychology, 99,* 209–225.

Elkind, D. (1962). The child's concept of his religious denomination: II. The Catholic child. *Journal of Genetic Psychology, 101,* 185–193.

Elkind, D. (1963). The child's conception of his religious denomination: III. The Protestant child. *Journal of Genetic Psychology, 103,* 291–304.

Elkind, D. (1964). Piaget's semi-clinical interview and the study of spontaneous religion. *Journal for the Scientific Study of Religion, 4,* 40–46.

Elkind, D. (1970). The origins of religion in the child. *Review of Religious Research, 12,* 35–42.

Elkind, D. (1971). The development of religious understanding in children and adolescents. In M. P. Strommen (Ed.), *Research on religious development* (pp. 655–685). New York, NY: Hawthorn Books.

Elkins, D. N. (2001). Beyond religion: Toward a humanist spirituality. In K. J. Schneider, J. T. Bugenthal, & J. F. Pierson (Eds.), *The handbook of humanistic psychology* (pp. 201–212). Thousand Oaks, CA: SAGE.

Elkind, D., & Elkind, S. (1970). Varieties of religious experience in young adolescents. *Journal for the Scientific Study of Religion, 2,* 102–112.

Elkins, D. N., Hedstrom, L. J., Hughes, L. L., Leaf, J. A., & Saunders, C. (1988). Toward a humanistic–phenomenological spirituality. *Journal of Humanistic Psychology, 28,* 5–18.

Ellenberger, H. F. (1970). *The discovery of the unconscious: The history and evolution of dynamic psychiatry.* New York, NY: Basic Books.

Ellens, J. H. (Ed.). (2014). *Seeking the sacred with psychoactive substances: Chemical paths to spirituality and God* (2 vols.). Santa Barbara, CA: Praeger/ABC-CLIO.

Elliott, D. M. (1994). The impact of Christian faith on the prevalence and sequelae of sexual abuse. *Journal of Interpersonal Violence, 9*, 95–108.

Ellis, A. (1980). Psychotherapy and atheistic values: A response to A. E. Bergin's "Psychotherapy and religious issues." *Journal of Consulting and Clinical Psychology, 48*, 635–639.

Ellis, A. (1986). Do some religious beliefs help create emotional disturbance? *Psychotherapy in Private Practice, 4*, 101–106.

Ellis, A. (1988). Is religiosity pathological? *Free Inquiry, 18*, 27–32.

Ellis, A. (2000). Spiritual goals and spirited values in psychotherapy. *Journal of Individual Psychology, 56*, 277–284.

Ellis, L., & Wahab, E. A. (2013). Religiosity and fear of death: A theory-oriented review of the empirical literature. *Review of Religious Research, 55*, 149–189.

Ellison, C. G. (1991). Religious involvement and subjective well-being. *Journal of Health and Social Behavior, 32*, 80–89.

Ellison, C. G., & Anderson, K. L. (2001). Religious involvement and domestic violence among U.S. couples. *Journal for the Scientific Study of Religion, 40*, 269–286.

Ellison, C. G., Bartkowski, J. P., & Anderson, K. L. (1999). Are there religious variations in domestic violence? *Journal of Family Issues, 20*, 87–113.

Ellison, C. G., Bartkowski, J. P., & Segal, M. L. (1996). Do conservative Protestant parents spank more often?: Further evidence from the National Survey of Families and Households. *Social Science Quarterly, 77*, 663–673.

Ellison, C. G., & Levin, J. S. (1998). The religion–health connection: Evidence, theory, and future directions. *Health Education and Behavior, 24*, 700–720.

Ellison, C. G., & McFarland, M. J. (2011). Religion and gambling among U.S. adults: Exploring the role of traditions, beliefs, practices, and networks. *Journal for the Scientific Study of Religion, 50*, 82–102.

Ellison, C. G., & McFarland, M. J. (2013). The social context of religion and spirituality in the United States. In K. I. Pargament, J. J. Exline, & J. W. Jones (Eds.), *APA handbook of psychology, religion, and spirituality* (Vol. 1, pp. 21–50). Washington, DC: American Psychological Association.

Ellison, C. G., & Sherkat, D. E. (1993). Obedience and autonomy: Religion and parental values reconsidered. *Journal for the Scientific Study of Religion, 32*, 313–329.

Ellison, C. G., & Taylor, R. J. (1996). Turning to prayer: Social and situational antecedents of religious coping among African-Americans. *Review of Religious Research, 38*, 111–131.

Ellwood, R. (1986). The several meanings of cult. *Thought, 61*, 212–224.

Elms, A. C. (1976). *Personality in politics.* New York, NY: Harcourt Brace Jovanovich.

Elson, B. D., Hauri, P., & Cunis, D. (1977). Physiological changes in yoga meditation. *Psychophysiology, 14*, 52–57.

Emanuel, E. J. (2002). Euthanasia and physician-assisted suicide. *Archives of Internal Medicine, 162*, 142–152.

Emavardhana, T., & Tori, C. D. (1997). Changes in self-concept, ego defense mechanisms, and religiosity following seven-day Vipassana meditation retreats. *Journal for the Scientific Study of Religion, 36*, 194–206.

Emmons, N. A., & Kelemen, D. (2014). The development of children's prelife reasoning: Evidence from two cultures. *Child Development, 85*, 1617–1633.

Emmons, R. A. (1995). Levels and domains in personality: An introduction. *Journal of Personality, 63*, 341–364.

Emmons, R. A. (1999). *The psychology of ultimate concerns.* New York, NY: Guilford Press.

Emmons, R. A. (2005). Emotion and religion. In R. F. Paloutzian & C. L. Park (Eds.), *Handbook of the psychology of religion and spirituality* (pp. 235–252). New York, NY: Guilford Press.

Emmons, R. A., & Crumpler, A. (1999). Religion and spirituality?: The roles of sanctification and the concept of God. *International Journal for the Psychology of Religion, 9*, 17–24.

Emmons, R. A., & Kneezel, T. T. (2005). Giving thanks, spiritual and religious correlates of gratitude. *Journal of Psychology and Christianity, 24*, 140–148.

Emmons, R. A., & McCullough, M. E. (2003). Counting blessings versus burdens: An experimental investigation of gratitude and subjective well-being in daily life. *Journal of Personality and Social Psychology, 84*, 377–389.

Emmons, R. A., & Paloutzian, R. (2003). Psychology of religion. *Annual Review of Psychology, 54*, 377–402.

Emmons, R. A., & Schnitker, S. A. (2013). Gods and goals: Religion and purposeful action. In R. F. Paloutzian & C. L. Park (Eds.), *Handbook of the psychology of religion and spirituality* (2nd ed., pp. 256–273). New York, NY: Guilford Press.

Emmons, R. A., & Stern, R. (2013). Gratitude as a psychotherapeutic intervention. *Journal of Clinical Psychology: In Session, 69*, 846–855.

Engs, R. C., & Mullen, K. (1999). The effect of religion

and religiosity on drug use among a selected sample of post secondary students in Scotland. *Addiction Research, 7,* 149–170.

Enskar, K., Carlsson, M., Golsater, M., Hamrin, E., & Kreuger, A. (1997). Parental reports of changes and challenges that result from parenting a child with cancer. *Journal of Pediatric Oncology Nursing, 14*(3), 156–163.

Epstein, S., & O'Brien, E. J. (1985). The person-situation debate in historical and current perspective. *Psychological Bulletin, 98,* 513–537.

Erickson, D. A. (1964). Religious consequences of public and sectarian schooling. *School Review, 72,* 21–33.

Erickson, J. A. (1992). Adolescent development and commitment: A structural equation model of the role of family, peer group, and educational influences. *Journal for the Scientific Study of Religion, 31,* 131–152.

Erikson, E. H. (1963). *Childhood and society* (2nd ed.). New York, NY: Norton.

Erikson, E. H. (1964). *Insight and responsibility.* New York, NY: Norton.

Erikson, E. H. (1965). Youth: Fidelity and diversity. In E. H. Erikson (Ed.), *The challenge of youth* (pp. 1–28). Garden City, NY: Doubleday/Anchor.

Erikson, E. H. (1966). Ontogeny of ritualization in man. *Philosophical Transactions of the Royal Society of London, Series B, Biological Sciences, 251,* 337–349.

Erikson, E. H. (1968). *Identity: Youth and crisis.* New York, NY: Norton.

Erikson, E. H. (1969). Identity and the life cycle [Special issue]. *Psychological Issues, 1.*

Ernsberger, D. J., & Manaster, G. J. (1981). Moral development, intrinsic/extrinsic religious orientation and denominational teachings. *Genetic Psychology Monographs, 104,* 23–41.

Eshleman, A. K., Dickie, J. R., Merasco, D. M., Shepard, A., & Johnson, M. (1999). Mother God, Father God: Children's perceptions of God's distance. *International Journal for the Psychology of Religion, 9,* 139–146.

Esposito, J. L. (1998). *Islam: The straight path.* New York, NY: Oxford University Press.

Etxebarria, I. (1992). Sentimientos de culpa y abandono de los valores paternos [Guilt feelings and abandoning parental values]. *Infancia y Aprendizaje, 57,* 67–88.

Evans, E. M. (2000). Beyond Scopes: Why creationism is here to stay. In K. S. Rosengren, C. N. Johnson, & P. L. Harris (Eds.), *Imagining the impossible: Magical, scientific, and religious thinking in children* (pp. 305–333). Cambridge, UK: Cambridge University Press.

Evans, J. H. (2013). The growing social and moral conflict between conservative Protestantism and science. *Journal for the Scientific Study of Religion, 52,* 368–385.

Evans, R., McIntosh, D. N., & Spilka, B. (1986). *Marital adjustment and form of personal faith.* Paper presented at the convention of the Rocky Mountain Psychological Association, Denver, CO.

Exline, J. J. (2002). The picture is getting clearer, but is the scope too limited?: Three overlooked questions in the psychology of religion. *Psychological Inquiry, 13,* 245–247.

Exline, J. J. (2012). Humility and the ability to receive from others. *Journal of Psychology and Christianity, 31,* 40–50.

Exline, J. J. (2013). Religious and spiritual struggles. In K. I. Pargament, J. J. Exline, & J. W. Jones (Eds.), *Handbook of the psychology of religion and spirituality* (Vol. 1, pp. 459–475). Washington, DC: American Psychological Association.

Exline, J. J., Baumeister, R. F., Zell, A. L., Kraft, A. J., & Witvliet, C. V. O. (2008). Not so innocent: Does seeing one's own capability for wrongdoing predict forgiveness? *Journal of Personality and Social Psychology, 94,* 495–515.

Exline, J. J., & Geyer, A. L. (2004). Perceptions of humility: A preliminary study. *Self and Identity, 3,* 95–114.

Exline, J. J., & Hill, P. C. (2012). Humility: A consistent and robust predictor of generosity. *Journal of Positive Psychology, 7,* 208–218.

Exline, J. J., & Martin, A. (2005). Anger toward God: A new frontier in forgiveness research. In E. I. Worthington, Jr. (Ed.), *Handbook of forgiveness* (pp. 73–88). New York, NY: Routledge.

Exline, J. J., Pargament, K. I., Grubbs, J. B., & Yali, A. M. (2014). The Religious and Spiritual Struggles Scale: Development and initial validation. *Psychology of Religion and Spirituality, 6,* 208–222.

Exline, J. J., Park, C. L., Smyth, J. M., & Carey, M. P. (2011). Anger toward God: Social-cognitive predictors, prevalence, and links with adjustment to bereavement and cancer. *Journal of Personality and Social Psychology, 100,* 129–148.

Exline, J. J., & Rose, E. (2005). Religious and spiritual struggles. In R. F. Paloutzian & C. L. Parks (Eds.), *Handbook of the psychology of religion and spirituality* (pp. 315–330). New York, NY: Guilford Press.

Exline, J., & Rose, J. (2013). Religious and spiritual struggles. In R. F. Paloutzian & C. L. Park (Eds.), *Handbook of the psychology of religion and spirituality* (2nd ed., pp. 380–398). New York, NY: Guilford Press.

Exline, J. J., & Yali, A. M. (2006). Heaven's gates and hell's flames: Afterlife beliefs of Catholic and

Protestant undergraduates. *Research in the Social Scientific Study of Religion, 17,* 235–260.

Exline, J. J., Yali, A. M., & Lobel, M. (1999). When God disappoints: Difficulty forgiving God and its role in negative emotion. *Journal of Health Psychology, 4,* 365–379.

Exline, J. J., Yali, A. M., & Sanderson, W. C. (2000). Guilt, discord, and alienation: The role of religious strain in depression and suicidality. *Journal of Clinical Psychology, 56,* 1481–1496.

Eysenck, H. J. (1981). *A model for personality.* New York, NY: Springer.

Faber, H. (1972). *Psychology of religion.* Philadelphia, PA: Westminster.

Faber, M. B. (2002). *The magic of prayer: An introduction to the psychology of faith.* Westport, CT: Praeger.

Fahs, S. L. (1950). The beginnings of mysticism in children's growth. *Religious Education, 45,* 139–147.

Falb, M. D., & Pargament, K. I. (2013). Buddhist coping predicts psychological outcomes among end-of-life caregivers. *Psychology of Religion and Spirituality, 5,* 252–262.

Falconer, D. S. (1981). *Introduction to quantitative genetics* (2nd ed.). New York, NY: Longmans.

Falkenheim, M. A., Duckro, P. N., Hughes, H. M., Rossetti, S. J., & Gfeller, J. D. (1999). Cluster analysis of child sexual offenders: A validation with Roman Catholic priests and brothers. *Sexual Addiction and Compulsivity, 6,* 317–336.

Farah, C. E. (1987). *Islam.* New York, NY: Barrons.

Farb, P. (1978). *Humankind.* New York, NY: Bantam Books.

Farberow, N. L. (1963). *Taboo topics.* New York, NY: Atherton.

Farias, M. (2013). The psychology of atheism. In S. Bullivant & M. Ruse (Eds.), *The Oxford handbook of atheism* (pp. 468–482). Oxford, UK: Oxford University Press.

Farias, M., Newheiser, A. K., Kahane, G., & de Toledo, Z. (2013). Scientific faith: Belief in science increases in the face of stress and existential anxiety. *Journal of Experimental Social Psychology, 49*(6), 1210–1213.

Faulkner, J. E., & DeJong, G. F. (1966). Religiosity in 5-D: An empirical analysis. *Social Forces, 45,* 246–254.

Fay, J. W. (1939). *American psychology before William James.* New Brunswick, NJ: Rutgers University Press.

Fazzino, L. L. (2014). Leaving the church behind: Applying a deconversion perspective to evangelical exit narratives. *Journal of Contemporary Religion, 29,* 249–266.

Feher, S., & Maly, R. C. (1999). Coping with breast cancer in later life: The role of religious faith. *Psycho-Oncology, 8,* 408–416.

Feierman, J. R. (Ed.). (2009). *The biology of religious behavior.* Santa Barbara, CA: ABC-CLIO.

Feierman, J. R. (2016). Religion's possible role in facilitating eusocial human societies. A behavioral biology (ethological) perspective. *Studia Humana, 5,* 5–33.

Feifel, H. (Ed.). (1959). *The meaning of death.* New York, NY: McGraw-Hill.

Feinstein, M., Liu, K., Ning, H., Fitchett, G., & Lloyd-Jones, D. M. (2010). Burden of cardiovascular risk factors, subclinical atherosclerosis, and incident cardiovascular events across dimensions of religiosity: The multi-ethnic study of atherosclerosis. *Circulation, 121,* 659–666.

Feldman, D. B., & Snyder, C. R. (2005). Hope and the meaningful life: Theoretical and empirical associations between goal-directed thinking and life meaning. *Journal of Social and Clinical Psychology, 24,* 401–421.

Feldman, D. H. (2004). Piaget's stages: The unfinished symphony of cognitive development. *New Ideas in Psychology, 22,* 175–231.

Feldman, K. A. (1969). Change and stability of religious orientations during college: Part I. Freshman–senior comparisons. *Review of Religious Research, 11,* 40–60.

Feldman, K. A., & Newcomb, T. M. (1969). *The impact of college on students.* San Francisco, CA: Jossey-Bass.

Fergus, T. A., & Rowatt, W. C. (2014a). Personal uncertainty strengthens associations between scrupulosity and both the moral appraisals of intrusive thoughts and beliefs that God is upset with sins. *Journal of Social and Clinical Psychology, 33,* 51–74.

Fergus, T. A., & Rowatt, W. C. (2014b). Examining a purported association between attachment to God and scrupulosity. *Psychology of Religion and Spirituality, 6,* 230–236.

Fernhout, H., & Boyd, D. (1985). Faith in autonomy: Development in Kohlberg's perspectives in religion and morality. *Religious Education, 80,* 287–307.

Ferrer, J. N. (2003). Integral transformative practices: A participatory perspective. *Journal of Transpersonal Psychology, 35,* 21–42.

Ferriss, A. L. (2002). Religion and the quality of life. *Journal of Happiness Studies, 3,* 199–215.

Festinger, L. (1957). *A theory of cognitive dissonance.* Stanford, CA: Stanford University Press.

Festinger, L., Riecken, H. W., & Schachter, S. (1956). *When prophecy fails.* Minneapolis, MN: University of Minnesota Press.

Fetchenhauer, D. (2009). Evolutionary perspectives on religion: What they can and what they cannot explain (yet). In E. Voland & W. Schiefenhovel (Eds.), *The biological evolution of religious mind and behavior* (pp. 275–291). New York, NY: Springer.

Feuerstein, G. (1992). *Holy madness.* New York, NY: Arcana.

Fiala, W. E., Bjorck, J. P., & Gorsuch, R. L. (2002). The Religious Support Scale: Construction, validation, and cross-validation. *American Journal of Community Psychology, 30,* 761–786.

Fichter, J. H. (1981). *Religion and pain.* New York, NY: Crossroads.

Field, H. L., & Waldfogel, S. (1995). Severe ocular self-injury. *General Hospital Psychiatry, 17,* 224–227.

Filsinger, E. E., & Wilson, M. R. (1984). Religiosity, socioeconomic rewards, and family development: Predictors of marital adjustment. *Journal of Marriage and the Family, 46,* 663–670.

Fincham, F. D., & Beach, S. R. H. (2013). Can religion and spirituality enhance prevention programs for couples? In K. I. Pargament, A. Mahoney, & E. P. Shafranske (Eds.), *APA handbook of psychology, religion, and spirituality* (Vol. 2, pp. 461–479). Washington, DC: American Psychological Association.

Fincham, F. D., & Beach, S. R. H. (2014). I say a little prayer for you: Praying for partner increases commitment in romantic relationships. *Journal of Family Psychology, 28,* 587–593.

Fincham, F. D., Beach, S. R. H., Lambert, N., Stillman, T., & Braithwaite, S. R. (2008). Spiritual behaviors and relationship satisfaction: A critical analysis of the role of prayer. *Journal of Social and Clinical Psychology, 27,* 362–388.

Fincham, F. D., Lambert, N., & Beach, S. R. H. (2010). Faith and unfaithfulness: Can praying for your partner reduce infidelity? *Journal of Personality and Social Psychology, 99,* 649–659.

Finke, R., & Stark, R. (2001). The new holy clubs: Testing church-to-sect propositions. *Sociology of Religion, 62,* 175–189.

Finlay, B., & Walther, C. S. (2003). The relation of religious affiliation, service attendance, and other factors to homophobic attitudes among university students. *Review of Religious Research, 44,* 370–393.

Finney, J. R., & Malony, H. N. (1985a). Empirical studies of Christian prayer: A review of the literature. *Journal of Psychology and Theology, 13,* 104–115.

Finney, J. R., & Malony, H. N. (1985b). An empirical study of contemplative prayer as an adjunct to psychotherapy. *Journal of Psychology and Theology, 13,* 284–290.

Finney, J. R., & Malony, H. N. (1985c). Contemplative prayer and its use in psychotherapy: A theoretical

model. *Journal of Psychology and Theology, 13,* 172–181.

Fiori, K. I., Brown, E. E., Cortina, K. S., & Antonucci, T. C. (2006). Locus of control as a mediator of the relationship between religiosity and life satisfaction: Age, race, and gender differences. *Mental Health, Religion and Culture, 9,* 239–263.

Firebaugh, G., & Harley, B. (1991). Trends in U.S. church attendance: Secularization and revival, or merely life cycle effects? *Journal for the Scientific Study of Religion, 30,* 487–500.

Fischer, R. (1969). The perception–hallucination continuum (a re-examination). *Diseases of the Nervous System, 30,* 161–171.

Fischer, R. (1971). A cartography of ecstatic and meditative states. *Science, 174,* 897–904.

Fischer, R. (1978). Cartography of conscious states: Integration of East and West. In A. A. Sugerman & R. E. Tarter (Eds.), *Expanding dimensions of consciousness* (pp. 24–57). New York, NY: Springer.

Fisher, H. E. (1983). *The sex contract.* New York, NY: Morrow.

Fisher, R. D., Cook, I. J., & Shirkey, E. C. (1994). Correlates of support for censorship of sexual, sexually violent, and violent media. *Journal of Sex Research, 31,* 229–240.

Fisher, R. D., Derison, D., Polley, C. F., Cadman, J., & Johnston, D. (1994). Religiousness, religious orientation, and attitudes towards gays and lesbians. *Journal of Applied Social Psychology, 24,* 614–630.

Fishman, S. B. (2000). *Jewish life and American culture.* Albany, NY: State University of New York Press.

Fiske, J. (1885). *The idea of God as affected by modern knowledge.* Boston, MA: Houghton Mifflin.

Fiske, S. T., & Taylor, S. E. (1991). *Social cognition* (2nd ed.). New York, NY: McGraw-Hill.

Flanagan, E. (2015, March 2). Changing faith: Why it's not a bad thing. *The Huffington Post,* pp. 1–2.

Flatt, B. (1987). Some stages of grief. *Journal of Religion and Health, 26,* 143–148.

Florian, V., & Kravetz, S. (1985). Children's concepts of death: A cross-cultural comparison among Muslims, Cruze, Christians, and Jews in Israel. *Journal of Cross Cultural-Psychology, 16,* 174–189.

Flory, R. W. (2000). Conclusion: Toward a theory of Generation X religion. In R. W. Flory & D. E. Miller (Eds.), *Gen X religion* (pp. 231–249). New York, NY: Routledge.

Flournoy, T. (1903). Les principles de la psychologie religieuse. *Archives de Psychologie, 2,* 33–57.

Fogarty, J. A. (2000). *The magical thoughts of grieving children.* Amityville, NY: Baywood.

Folger, R. (1977). Distributive and procedural justice: Combined impact of "voice" and improvement on experienced inequity. *Journal of Personality and Social Psychology, 35,* 108–119.

Folkman, S., Lazarus, R. S., Dunkel-Schetter, C., De Longis, A., & Gruen, R. J. (1986). Dynamics of a stressful encounter: Cognitive appraisal, coping, and encounter outcomes. *Journal of Personality and Social Psychology, 50,* 992–1003.

Fonagy, P. (2001). *Attachment theory and psychoanalysis.* New York, NY: Random House.

Fones, C. S. L., Levine, S. B., Althof, S. E., & Risen, C. B. (1999). The sexual struggles of 23 clergymen: A follow-up study. *Journal of Sex and Marital Therapy, 25,* 183–195.

Fontaine, J. R. J., Duriez, B., Luyten, P., Corveleyn, J., & Hutsebaut, D. (2005). Consequences of a multidimensional approach to religion for the relationship between religiosity and value priorities. *International Journal for the Psychology of Religion, 15,* 123–143.

Ford, H. H., Zimmerman, R. S., Anderman, E. M., & Brown-Wright, L. (2001). Beliefs about the appropriateness of AIDS-related education for sixth and ninth grade students. *Journal of HIV/AIDS Prevention and Education for Adolescents and Children, 4,* 5–18.

Ford, J. A., & Hill, T. D. (2012). Religiosity and adolescent substance use: Evidence from the National Survey on Drug Use and Health. *Substance Use and Misuse, 47,* 787–798.

Ford, J., & Kadushin, C. (2002). Between sacral belief and moral community: A multidimensional approach to the relationship between religion and alcohol among whites and blacks. *Sociological Forum, 17,* 255–279.

Forliti, J. E., & Benson, P. L. (1986). Young adolescents: A national study. *Religious Education, 81,* 199–224.

Forman, R. K. C. (1990a). Mysticism, constructivism, and forgetting. In R. K. C. Forman (Ed.), *The problem of pure consciousness: Mysticism and philosophy* (pp. 3–49). New York, NY: Oxford University Press.

Forman, R. K. C. (Ed.). (1990b). *The problem of pure consciousness: Mysticism and philosophy.* New York, NY: Oxford University Press.

Forman, R. K. C. (Ed.). (1998). *The innate capacity: Mysticism, psychology and philosophy.* New York, NY: Oxford University Press.

Forte, R. (Ed.). (1997). *Entheogens and the future of religion.* San Francisco, CA: Council on Spiritual Practices.

Fortune, M. M., & Poling, J. N. (1994). *Sexual abuse by clergy: A crisis for the church* (JPCP Monograph No. 6). Eugene, OR: Wipf & Stock.

Foshee, V. A., & Hollinger, B. R. (1996). Maternal religiosity, adolescent social bonding, and adolescent alcohol use. *Journal of Early Adolescence, 16,* 451–468.

Foster, K. A., Bowland, S., & Vosler, A. N. (2015). All the pain along with all the joy: Spiritual resilience in lesbian and gay Christians. *American Journal of Community Psychology, 55*(1–2), 191–201.

Foster, L. (1984). *Religion and sexuality: The Shakers, the Mormons, and the Oneida community.* Urbana: University of Illinois Press.

Foster, R. A., & Babcock, R. L. (2001). God as a man versus God as a woman: Perceiving God as a function of the gender of God and the gender of the participant. *International Journal for the Psychology of Religion, 11,* 93–104.

Foster, R. A., & Keating, J. P. (1990, November). *The male God-concept and self-esteem: A theoretical framework.* Paper presented at the annual convention of the Society for the Scientific Study of Religion, Virginia Beach, VA.

Foster, R. A., & Keating, J. P. (1992). Measuring androcentrism in the Western God-concept. *Journal for the Scientific Study of Religion, 31,* 366–375.

Foster, R. J. (1992). *Prayer: Finding the heart's true home.* San Francisco, CA: Harper.

Fowler, J. W. (1981). *Stages of faith: The psychology of human development and the quest for meaning.* San Francisco, CA: Harper & Row.

Fowler, J. W. (1991a). Stages in faith consciousness. In F. K. Oser & W. G. Scarlett (Eds.), *Religious development in childhood and adolescence* (New Directions for Child Development, No. 52, pp. 27–45). San Francisco, CA: Jossey-Bass.

Fowler, J. W. (1991b). *Weaving the new creation: Stages of faith and the public church.* San Francisco, CA: Harper.

Fowler, J. W. (1993). Response to Helmut Reich: Overview or apologetic? *International Journal for the Psychology of Religion, 3,* 173–179.

Fowler, J. W. (1994). Moral stages and the development of faith. In B. Puka (Ed.), *Moral development: A compendium: Vol. 2. Fundamental research in moral development* (pp. 344–374). New York, NY: Garland Press.

Fowler, J. W. (1996). *Faithful change: The personal and public challenges of postmodern life.* Nashville, TN: Abingdon Press.

Fowler, J. W. (2001). Faith development theory and the postmodern challenges. *International Journal for the Psychology of Religion, 11,* 157–172.

Fowler, J. W., & Dell, M. L. (2006). Stages of faith from infancy through adolescence: Reflections on three decades of faith development theory. In E. C. Roehlkepartain, P. E. King, L. Wenger, & P. L. Benson (Eds.), *The handbook of spiritual development in childhood and adolescence* (pp. 34–45). Thousand Oaks, CA: SAGE.

Fox, J. W. (1992). The structure, stability, and social antecedents of reported paranormal experiences. *Sociological Analysis, 53*, 417–431.

Francis, J. (1997). The psychology of gender differences in religion: A review of empirical research. *Religion, 27*, 81–96.

Francis, L. J. (1979). The priest as test administrator in attitude research. *Journal for the Scientific Study of Religion, 18*, 78–81.

Francis, L. J. (1980). Paths of holiness?: Attitudes towards religion among 9–11-year-old children in England. *Character Potential: A Record of Research, 9*, 129–138.

Francis, L. J. (1982). *Youth in transit: A profile of 16–25 year olds.* Aldershot, UK: Gower.

Francis, L. J. (1989). Monitoring changing attitudes towards Christianity among secondary school pupils between 1974 and 1986. *British Journal of Educational Psychology, 59*, 86–91.

Francis, L. J. (1993). Parental influence and adolescent religiosity: A study of church attendance and attitude toward Christianity among adolescents 11 to 12 and 15 to 16 years old. *International Journal for the Psychology of Religion, 3*, 241–253.

Francis, L. J. (1997a). The impact of personality and religion on attitude towards substance use among 13–15-year-olds. *Drug and Alcohol Dependence, 44*, 95–103.

Francis, L. J. (1997b). Personality, prayer, and church attendance among undergraduate students. *International Journal for the Psychology of Religion, 7*, 127–132.

Francis, L. J. (2000). The relationship between bible reading and purpose in life among 13–15-year-olds. *Mental Health, Religion and Culture, 3*, 27–36.

Francis, L. J. (2002). Psychological type and mystical orientation: Anticipating individual differences within congregational life. *Pastoral Sciences, 21*, 77–99.

Francis, L. J., & Astley, J. (Eds.). (2001). *Psychological perspectives on prayer: A reader.* Leominster, UK: Gracewing.

Francis, L. J., & Brown, L. B. (1990). The predisposition to pray: A study of the social influence on the predisposition to pray among eleven-year-old children in England. *Journal of Empirical Theology, 3*, 23–34.

Francis, L. J., & Brown, L. B. (1991). The influence of home, church and school on prayer among sixteen-year-old adolescents in England. *Review of Religious Research, 33*, 112–122.

Francis, L. J., & Gibbs, D. (1996). Prayer and self-esteem among 8- to 11-year-olds in the United Kingdom. *Journal of Social Psychology, 136*, 791–793.

Francis, L. J., & Gibson, H. M. (1993). Parental influence and adolescent religiosity: A study of church attendance and attitude toward Christianity among adolescents 11 to 12 and 15 to 16 years old. *International Journal for the Psychology of Religion, 3*, 241–253.

Francis, L. J., & Johnson, P. (1999). Mental health, prayer and church attendance among primary schoolteachers. *Mental Health, Religion and Culture, 2*, 153–158.

Francis, L. J., & Kaldor, P. (2002). The relationship between psychological well-being and Christian faith and practice in an Australian population sample. *Journal for the Scientific Study of Religion, 41*, 179–184.

Francis, L. J., & Katz, Y. I. (1992). The relationship between personality and religiosity in an Israeli sample. *Journal for the Scientific Study of Religion, 31*, 153–162.

Francis, L. J., & Lankshear, D. W. (2001). The relationship between church schools and local church life: Distinguishing between aided and controlled status. *Educational Studies, 27*, 425–438.

Francis, L. J., & Louden, S. H. (2000a). The Francis–Louden Mystical Orientation Scale (MOS): A study among Roman Catholic priests. *Research in the Social Scientific Study of Religion, 11*, 99–116.

Francis, L. J., & Louden, S. H. (2000b). Mystical orientation and psychological type: A study among students and adult churchgoers. *Transpersonal Psychology Review, 4*, 36–42.

Francis, L. J., & Louden, S. H. (2004). A Short Index of Mystical Orientation (SIMO): A study among Roman Catholic priests. *Pastoral Psychology, 53*, 49–51.

Francis, L. J., Pearson, P. R., & Kay, W. K. (1983). Are children bigger liars? *Psychological Reports, 52*, 551–554.

Francis, L. J., Pearson, P. R., & Kay, W. K. (1988). Religiosity and lie scores: A question of interpretation. *Social Behavior and Personality, 16*, 91–95.

Francis, L. J., & Thomas, T. H. (1996). Mystical orientation and personality among Anglican clergy. *Journal of Pastoral Psychology, 45*, 99–105.

Francis, L. J., Village, A., Robbins, M., & Ineson, K. (2007). Mystical orientation and psychological type: An empirical study of guests staying at a Benedictine abbey. *Studies in Spirituality, 17*, 207–223.

Francis, L. J., & Wilcox, C. (1996). Prayer, church attendance, and personality revisited: A study among 16- to 19-year-old girls. *Psychological Reports, 79*, 1266.

Francis, L. J., & Wilcox, C. (1998). Religiosity and feminity: Do women really hold a more positive attitude towards Christianity? *Journal for the Scientific Study of Religion, 37*, 462–469.

Francis, L. J., Ziebertz, H., Robbins, M., & Reindl, M. (2015). Mystical experience and psychopathology: A study among secular, Christian, and Muslim youth in Germany. *Pastoral Psychology, 64,* 369–379.

Frank, J. (1974). *Persuasion and healing: A comparative study of psychotherapy* (rev. ed.). New York, NY: Schocken Books.

Frankl, V. (1962). *Man's search for meaning* (rev. ed., I. Lasch, Trans.). Boston, MA: Beacon Press.

Frankl, V. E. (2000). *Man's search for ultimate meaning.* Cambridge, MA: Perseus.

Franks, K., Templer, D. I., Cappelletty, G. G., & Kauffman, I. (1990–1991). Exploration of death anxiety as a function of religious variables in gay men with and without AIDS. *Omega, 22,* 43–50.

Fredrickson, B. L. (2001). The role of positive emotions in positive psychology. *American Psychologist, 56,* 218–226.

Freud, S. (1919). *Totem and taboo* (A. A. Brill, Trans.). London, UK: Routledge. (Original work published 1913)

Freud, S. (1961a). *Civilization and its discontents* (J. Strachey, Trans.). New York, NY: Norton. (Original work published 1930)

Freud, S. (1961b). *The future of an illusion* (J. Strachey, Trans.). New York, NY: Norton. (Original work published 1927)

Friedenberg, E. (1969). Current patterns of a generation conflict. *Journal of Social Issues, 25,* 21–38.

Friedman, H. L. (2015). Judging another's spirituality: Comment on Sundararajan and Kim's (2014) claim that Müntzer was a false mystic. *The Humanistic Psychologist, 43,* 100–102.

Friedman, S. B., Chodoff, P., Mason, J. W., & Hamburg, D. A. (1963). Behavioral observations on parents anticipating the death of a child. *Pediatrics, 32,* 610–625.

Friedrich, C., & Brzezinski, Z. (1956). *Totalitarian dictatorship and autocracy.* New York, NY: Praeger.

Friedrichs, R. W. (1973). Social research and theology: End of the detente? *Review of Religious Research, 15,* 113–137.

Fromm, E. (1950). *Psychoanalysis and religion.* New Haven, CT: Yale University Press.

Frosk, P., Greenberg, C. R., Tennese, A. A. P., Lamont, R., Nylen, E., Hirst, E., et al. (2005). The most common mutation in FKRP causing limb girdle muscular dystrophy type 21 (LGMD21) may have occurred only once and is present in Hutterites and other populations. *Human Mutation, 25,* 38–44.

Fry, P. S. (1990). A factor analytic investigation of home-bound elderly individuals' concerns about death and dying, and their coping responses. *Journal of Clinical Psychology, 46,* 737–748.

Fry, P. S. (2001). The unique contribution of key existential factors to the prediction of psychological well-being of older adults following spousal loss. *Gerontologist, 41,* 69–81.

Fugate, J. R. (1980). *What the Bible says about . . . child training.* Tempe, AZ: Alpha Omega.

Fuller, R. C. (2000). *Stairways to heaven: Drugs in American religious history.* Boulder, CO: Westview Press.

Fuller, R. C. (2001). *Spiritual but not religious: Understanding unchurched America.* New York, NY: Oxford University Press.

Fullerton, J. T., & Hunsberger, B. (1982). A unidimensional measure of Christian orthodoxy. *Journal for the Scientific Study of Religion, 21,* 317–326.

Fulton, A. S. (1997). Identity status, religious orientation, and prejudice. *Journal of Youth and Adolescence, 26,* 1–11.

Fulton, A. S., Gorsuch, R. L., & Maynard, E. A. (1999). Religious orientation, antihomosexual sentiment, and fundamentalism among Christians. *Journal for the Scientific Study of Religion, 38,* 14–22.

Furey, R. J. (1986). *So I'm not perfect: A psychology of humility.* Staten Island, NY: Alba House.

Furnham, A. (1982). Locus of control and theological beliefs. *Journal of Psychology and Theology, 10,* 130–136.

Futterman, A., Dillon, J. J., Garand, F., III, & Haugh, J. (1999). Religion as a quest and the search for meaning in later life. In L. E. Thomas & S. A. Eisenhandler (Eds.), *Religion, belief and spirituality in late life* (pp. 153–176). New York, NY: Springer.

Gabbard, C. E., Howard, G. S., & Tageson, C. W. (1986). Assessing locus of control with religious populations. *Journal of Research in Personality, 20,* 292–308.

Gadamer, H.-G. (1986). *Truth and method* (G. Barden & J. Cumming, Trans.). New York, NY: Crossroad.

Galaif, E. R., & Newcomb, M. D. (1999). Predictors of polydrug use among four ethnic groups: A 12 year longitudinal study. *Addictive Behaviors, 24,* 607–631.

Galanter, M. (1980). Psychological induction into the large group: Findings from a large modern religious sect. *American Journal of Psychiatry, 137,* 1574–1579.

Galanter, M. (1983). Group induction techniques in a charismatic sect. In D. G. Bromley & J. T. Richardson (Eds.), *The brainwashing/deprogramming controversy: Sociological, psychological, legal and historical perspectives* (pp. 182–193). Lewiston, NY: Edwin Mellen Press.

Galanter, M. (1989a). *Cults: Faith, healing, and coercion.* New York, NY: Oxford University Press.

Galanter, M. (Ed.). (1989b). *Cults and new religious*

movements. Washington, DC: American Psychological Association.

Galanter, M. (2013). Charismatic groups and cults: A psychological and social analysis. In K. I. Pargament, J. J. Exline, & J. W. Jones (Eds.), *Handbook of the psychology of religion and spirituality* (Vol. 1, pp. 729–740). Washington, DC: American Psychological Association.

Galanter, M., & Buckley, P. (1978). Evangelical religion and meditation: Psychotherapeutic effects. *Journal of Nervous and Mental Disease, 166*, 685–691.

Galanter, M., Rabkin, R., Rabkin, J., & Deutsch, A. (1979). The Moonies: A psychological study of conversion and membership in a contemporary religious sect. *American Journal of Psychiatry, 136*, 165–169.

Galen, L. W. (2012). Does religious belief promote prosociality?: A critical examination. *Psychological Bulletin, 138*, 876–906.

Gall, T. L., de Renart, R. M. M., & Boonstra, B. (2000). Religious resources in long-term adjustment to breast cancer. *Journal of Psychosocial Oncology, 18*, 21–37.

Gall, T. L., & Guirguis-Younger, M. (2013). Religious and spiritual coping: Current theory and research. In K. I. Pargament, J. J. Exline, & J. W. Jones (Eds.), *APA handbook of psychology, religion, and spirituality* (Vol. 1, pp. 349–364). Washington, DC: American Psychological Association.

Gallup, G., Jr. (1978). *The Gallup Poll: Public opinion 1972–1977*. Washington, DC: Scholarly Resources.

Gallup, G., Jr. (1992). *The Gallup Poll: Public opinion 1991*. Wilmington, DE: Scholarly Resources.

Gallup, G., Jr., & Lindsay, D. M. (1999). *Surveying the religious landscape: Trends in U.S. beliefs*. Harrisburg, PA: Morehouse.

Gallup, G., Jr., & Proctor, W. (1982). *Adventures in immortality*. New York, NY: McGraw-Hill.

Gallup News. (2018). How important would you say religion is in your own life—very important, fairly important or not very important? Retrieved March 30, 2018, from *http://news.gallup.com/poll/1690/religion.aspx*.

The Gallup Poll. (2007, May 10–13). Religion. Retrieved July 17, 2007, from *www.pollingreport.com/religion.htm*.

The Gallup Poll. (2010a). Near-record high see religion losing influence in America. Retrieved from *www.gallup.com/poll/145409/Near-record-high-religion-losing-influence-america.aspx*.

The Gallup Poll. (2011). More than 9 in 10 Americans continue to believe in God. Retrieved from *www.gallup.com/poll/147887/Americans-Continue-Believe-God.aspx*.

The Gallup Poll. (2014, December 28). Religion and social trends. Retrieved from *www.gallup.com/topic/religion_and_social_trends.aspx*.

The Gallup Poll Monthly. (1992, December). No. 327, pp. 32–39.

Galton, F. (1869). *Hereditary genius: An inquiry into its laws and consequences* (2nd ed.). London, UK: Macmillan.

Gange-Fling, M., Veach, P. M., Kuang, H., & Houg, B. (2000). Effects of childhood sexual abuse on client spiritual well-being. *Counseling and Values, 44*, 84–91.

Gardella, P. (1985). *Innocent ecstasy*. New York, NY: Oxford University Press.

Garey, E., Siregar, J. R., Hood, R. W., Jr., Agustiani, H., & Setiono, K. (2017). Development and validation of Religious Attribution Scale: In association with religiosity and meaning in life among economically disadvantaged adolescents in Indonesia. *Mental Health, Religion and Culture, 19*(8), 818–832.

Garrett, W. R. (1974). Troublesome transcendence: The supernatural in the scientific study of religion. *Sociological Analysis, 35*, 167–180.

Garrett, W. R. (1975). Maligned mysticism: The maledicted career of Troeltsch's third type. *Sociological Analysis, 36*, 205–223.

Gartner, J., Larson, D. B., & Allen, G. D. (1991). Religious commitment and mental health: A review of the empirical literature. *Journal of Psychology and Theology, 19*, 6–25.

Gartrell, C. D., & Shannon, Z. K. (1985). Contacts, cognitions, and conversions: A rational choice approach. *Review of Religious Research, 27*, 32–48.

Garvey, M. (1998). *Searching for Mary: An exploration of Marian apparitions across the U.S.* New York, NY: Plume.

Gaustad, E. S. (1966). *A religious history of America* (rev. ed.). San Francisco, CA: Harper & Row.

Gazzaniga, M. S. (1985). *The social brain*. New York, NY: Basic Books.

Geffen, R. M. (2001, March–April). Intermarriage and the premise of American Jewish life. *Congress Monthly*, pp. 6–8.

Gelman, S. A., Manheim, B., Escalante, C., & Tapia, I. S. (2015). Teleological talk in parent–child conversations in Quechua. *First Language, 35*, 359–376.

General Social Survey (GSS). (2007). GSS cumulative datafile 1972–2006. Retrieved from *http://sda.berkeley.edu/D3/GSS06/Doc/gs060024.htm*.

General Social Survey (GSS). (2015). GSS cumulative datafile 1972–2014. Retrieved from *http://sda.berkeley.edu/sdaweb/analysis/;jsessionid=B34614FCCECACAB3F28AB964EC2B137F?dataset=gss14*.

Genia, V. (1997). The Spiritual Experience Index:

Revision and reformulation. *Review of Religious Research, 38,* 344–361.

Gentry, C. S. (1987). Social distance regarding male and female homosexuals. *Journal of Social Psychology, 127,* 199–208.

Gerlach, L. P., & Hine, V. H. (1970). *People, power, change: Movements of social transformation.* Indianapolis, IN: Bobbs-Merrill.

Gershoff, E. T., Miller, P. C., & Holden, G. W. (1999). Parenting influences from the pulpit: Religious affiliation as a determinant of parental corporal punishment. *Journal of Family Psychology, 13,* 307–320.

Gerson, G. S. (1977). The psychology of grief and mourning in Judaism. *Journal of Religion and Health, 16,* 260–274.

Gervais, W. M. (2013a). In godlessness we distrust: Using social psychology to solve the puzzle of anti-atheist prejudice. *Social and Personality Psychology Compass, 7,* 366–377.

Gervais, W. M. (2013b). Perceiving minds and gods: How mind perception enables, constrains, and is triggered by belief in gods. *Perspectives on Psychological Science, 8,* 380–394.

Gervais, W. M., Shariff, A. F., & Norenzayan, A. (2011). Do you believe in atheists?: Distrust is central to anti-atheist prejudice. *Journal of Personality and Social Psychology, 101,* 1189–1206.

Ghorbani, N., Watson, P. J., Amirbeigi, M., & Chen, Z. J. (2016). Religious schema within a Muslim ideological surround: Religious and psychological adjustment in Iran. *Archive for the Psychology of Religion, 38,* 253–277.

Ghorbani, N., Watson, P. J., Chen, Z., & Dover, H. (2013). Varieties of openness in Tehran and Qom: Psychological and religious parallels of faith and intellect oriented Islamic religious reflection. *Mental Health, Religion and Culture, 16,* 123–137.

Ghorbani, N., Watson, P. J., Ghramaleki, A. F., Morris, R. J., & Hood, R. W. (2002). Muslim–Christian religious orientation scales: Distinctions, correlations, and cross-cultural analysis in Iran and the United States. *International Journal for the Psychology of Religion, 12,* 69–91.

Ghorbani, N., Watson, P. J., Shamohammadi, K., & Cunningham, C. J. L. (2009). Post-critical beliefs in Iran: Predicting religious and psychological functioning. *Research in the Social Scientific Study of Religion, 20,* 217–237.

Ghorbani, N., Watson, P. J., Tavakoli, F., & Chen, Z. J. (2016). Self-control within a Muslim ideological surround: Empirical translation schemes and the adjustment of Muslim seminarians in Iran. *Research in the Social Scientific Study of Religion, 27,* 68–93.

Gibbons, D. E., & Jarnette, J. (1972). Hypnotic susceptibility and religious experience. *Journal for the Scientific Study of Religion, 11,* 152–156.

Gibbs, J. C. (1988). Three perspectives on tragedy and suffering: The relevance of near-death experience research. *Journal of Psychology and Theology, 16,* 21–33.

Gibbs, J. C. (2005a). What do near-death experiencers and Jesus have in common?: The near-death experience and Spong's new Christianity. *Journal of Near-Death Studies, 24,* 61–95.

Gibbs, J. C. (2005b). Reply to Michael Sabon's commentary. *Journal of Near-Death Studies, 24,* 105–107.

Gibbs, J. P. (1994). *A theory about control.* Boulder, CO: Westview Press.

Gibson, N. J. S. (2006). *The experimental investigation of religious cognition.* Unpublished doctoral dissertation, University of Cambridge, UK.

Gibson, T. (2008). Religion and civic engagement among America's youth. *Social Science Journal, 45,* 504–514.

Giesbrecht, N. (1995). Parenting style and adolescent religious commitment. *Journal of Psychology and Christianity, 14,* 228–238.

Giesbrecht, N., & Sevcik, I. (2000). The process of recovery and rebuilding among abused women in the conservative evangelical subculture. *Journal of Family Violence, 15,* 229–248.

Gilbert, K. (1992). Religion as a resource for bereaved parents. *Journal of Religion and Health, 31,* 19–30.

Gill, R., Hadaway, C. K., & Marler, P. L. (1998). Is religious belief declining in Britain? *Journal for the Scientific Study of Religion, 37,* 507–516.

Gilligan, C. (1977). In a different voice: Women's conceptions of self and morality. *Harvard Educational Review, 47,* 481–517.

Gillings, V., & Joseph, S. (1996). Religiosity and social desirability: Impression management and self-deceptive positivity. *Personality and Individual Differences, 21,* 1047–1050.

Gillum, R. F., King, D. E., Obisesan, T. O., & Koenig, H. G. (2008). Frequency of attendance at religious services and mortality in a U.S. national cohort. *Annals of Epidemiology, 18,* 124–129.

Gilmore, N., & Sommerville, M. A. (1994). Stigmatization, scapegoating and discrimination in sexually transmitted diseases: Overcoming "them" and "us." *Social Science and Medicine, 39,* 1339–1358.

Giovannoli, J. (2000). The biology of belief: How our biology biases our beliefs and perceptions. Retrieved from *www.2think.org/biology_belief.shtml.*

Girard, M., & Mullet, E. (1997). Forgiveness in adolescents, young, middle-age, and older adults. *Journal of Adult Development, 4,* 209–220.

Girard, R. (1977). *Violence and the sacred*. Baltimore: Johns Hopkins University Press.

Glass, J., Bengtson, V. L., & Dunham, C. C. (1986). Attitude similarity in three-generation families: Socialization, status inheritance or reciprocal influence? *American Sociological Review, 51*, 685–698.

Glick, I. O., Weiss, R. A., & Parkes, C. M. (1974). *The first year of bereavement*. New York, NY: Wiley.

Glock, C. Y. (1962). On the study of religious commitment. *Religious Education, 57*(Research Suppl.), S98–S110.

Glock, C. Y., & Stark, R. (1965). *Religion and society in tension*. Chicago, IL: Rand McNally.

Glock, C. Y., & Stark, R. (1966). *Christian beliefs and anti-Semitism*. New York, NY: Harper & Row.

Glover, R. J. (1997). Reltaionships in moral reasoning and religion among members of conservative, moderate, and liberal religious groups. *Journal of Social Psychology, 137*, 247–255.

Gochman, E. R. G., & Fantasia, S. C. (1979). *The concept of immortality as related to planning one's life*. Paper presented at the annual convention of the American Psychological Association, New York.

Godin, A. (1968). Genetic development of the symbolic function: Meaning and limits of the work of R. Goldman. *Religious Education, 63*, 439–445.

Godin, A. (1985). *The psychodynamics of religious experience*. Birmingham, AL: Religious Education Press.

Godin, A., & Hallez, M. (1964). Parental images and divine paternity. *Lumen Vitae, 19*, 253–284.

Goff, K. G. (2008, April). Why do Jews marry Catholics? Retrieved from *https://interfaithfamily.com/news_and_opinion/synagogues_and_the_jewish_community/Why_Do_Jews_Marry_Catholics*.

Goggin, K., Murray, T. S., Malcarne, V. L., Brown, S. A., & Wallston, K. A. (2007). Do religious and control cognitions predict risky behavior?: I. Development and validation of the Alcohol-related GodLocus of Control Scale for Adolescents (AGLOC-A). *Cognitive Therapy and Research, 31*, 111–122.

Goldfried, J., & Miner, M. (2002). Quest religion and the problem of limited compassion. *Journal for the Scientific Study of Religion, 41*, 685–695.

Goldman, M. S. (2006). Review essay: Cults, new religions, and the spiritual landscape: A review of four collections. *Journal for the Scientific Study of Religion, 45*, 87–96.

Goldman, R. (1964). *Religious thinking from childhood to adolescence*. New York, NY: Seabury Press.

Goldstein, S., & Goldscheider, G. (1968). *Jewish-Americans*. Englewood Cliffs, NJ: Prentice-Hall.

Goleman, D. (1977). *The varieties of meditative experience*. New York, NY: Dutton.

Goleman, D. (1984, May). The faith factor. *American Health*, pp. 48–53.

Goleman, D. (1988). *The meditative mind: The varieties of meditative experience*. Los Angeles, CA: Jeremy Tarcher/Perigee Books.

Goll, J., & Goll, M. A. (2006). *Dream language: The prophetic power of dreams, revelations, and the spirit of wisdom*. Shippensburg, PA: Destiny Image.

Golsworthy, R., & Coyle, A. (1999). Spiritual beliefs and the search for meaning among older adults following partner loss. *Mortality, 4*, 21–40.

Gong, F., Takeuchi, D. T., Agbayani-Siewert, P., & Tacata, L. (2003). Acculturation, psychological distress, and alcohol use: Investigating the effects of ethnic identity and religiosity. In K. M. Chun, P. B. Organista, & G. Marin (Eds.), *Acculturation: Advances in theory, measurement, and applied research*. Washington, DC: American Psychological Association.

Goodall, J. (1971). *In the shadow of man*. Boston, MA: Houghton Mifflin.

Goode, E. (2000, January–February). Two paranormalisms or two and a half?: An empirical formulation. *Skeptical Inquirer, 24*(1), 29–35.

Goodman, F. D. (1969). Phonetic analysis of glossolalia in four cultural settings. *Journal for the Scientific Study of Religion, 8*, 227–239.

Goodman, F. D. (1972). *Speaking in tongues: A cross-cultural study of glossolalia*. Chicago, IL: University of Chicago Press.

Goodman, F. D. (1988). *Ecstasy, religious ritual, and alternate reality*. Bloomington, IN: University of Indiana Press.

Goodman, F. D. (1990). *Where the spirits ride the wind: Trance journeys and other ecstatic experiences*. Bloomington, IN: University of Indiana Press.

Goodman, M. A., & Dollahite, D. C. (2006). How religious couples perceive the influence of God in their marriage. *Review of Religious Research, 48*, 141–155.

Goodman, R. M. (1979). *Genetic disorders among the Jewish people*. Baltimore: Johns Hopkins University Press.

Goodstein, L. (2015, March 15). Largest Presbyterian denomination gives final approval for same-sex marriage. *The New York Times*, p. A13.

Goodwill, K. A. (2000). Religion and the spiritual needs of gay Mormon men. *Journal of Gay and Lesbian Social Services, 11*, 23–27.

Gooren, H. (2007). Reassessing conventional approaches to conversion: Toward a new synthesis. *Journal for the Scientific Study of Religion, 46*, 337–353.

Gooren, H. (2010). *Religious conversion and disaffiliation: Tracing patterns of change in faith practices*. New York, NY: Palgrave Macmillan.

Gooren, H. (2011). Deconversion: Qualitative and

quantitative results from the cross-cultural research in Germany and the United States: A review essay. *Pastoral Psychology, 60,* 609–617.

Gordon, A. I. (1967). *The nature of conversion.* Boston, MA: Beacon Press.

Gordon, D. F. (1984). Dying to self: Self-control through self-abandonment. *Sociological Analysis, 5,* 41–56.

Gordon, M. S. (2002). *Islam: Origins, practices, holy texts, sacred persons, and sacred places.* New York, NY: Oxford University Press.

Gorelick, S. (1981). *City College and the Jewish poor.* New Brunswick, NJ: Rutgers University Press.

Gorsuch, R. L. (1968). The conceptualization of God as seen in adjective ratings. *Journal for the Scientific Study of Religion, 7,* 56–64.

Gorsuch, R. L. (1976). Religion as a significant predictor of important human behavior. In W. J. Donaldson, Jr. (Ed.), *Research in mental health and religious behavior* (pp. 206–221). Atlanta, GA: Psychological Studies Institute.

Gorsuch, R. L. (1984). Measurement: The boon and bane of investigating religion. *American Psychologist, 39,* 228–236.

Gorsuch, R. L. (1988). Psychology of religion. *Annual Review of Psychology, 39,* 201–221.

Gorsuch, R. L. (1993). Religion and prejudice: Lessons not learned from the past. *International Journal for the Psychology of Religion, 3,* 29–31.

Gorsuch, R. L. (1994). Toward motivational theories of intrinsic religious commitment. *Journal for the Scientific Study of Religion, 28,* 315–325.

Gorsuch, R. L. (1995). Religious aspects of substance abuse and recovery. *Journal of Social Issues, 51,* 65–83.

Gorsuch, R. L. (2002). *Integrating psychology and spirituality.* Westport, CT: Praeger.

Gorsuch, R. L. (2008). On the limits of scientific investigation: Miracles and intercessory prayer. In J. H. Ellens (Ed.), *Miracles: God, science, and psychology in the paranormal: Vol. 1. Religious and spiritual events* (pp. 280–299). Westport, CT: Greenwood Press.

Gorsuch, R. L., & Aleshire, D. (1974). Christian faith and ethnic prejudice: A review and interpretation of research. *Journal for the Scientific Study of Religion, 13,* 281–307.

Gorsuch, R. L., & Butler, M. C. (1976). Initial drug abuse: A review of predisposing social psychological factors. *Psychological Bulletin, 83,* 120–137.

Gorsuch, R. L., & McFarland, S. (1972). Single vs. multiple-item scales for measuring religious values. *Journal for the Scientific Study of Religion, 11,* 53–64.

Gorsuch, R. L., & McPherson, S. E. (1989). Intrinsic/extrinsic measurement: I/E-revised and single-item scales. *Journal for the Scientific Study of Religion, 28,* 348–354.

Gorsuch, R. L., & Miller, W. R. (1999). Assessing spirituality. In W. R. Miller (Ed.), *Integrating spirituality into treatment* (pp. 47–64). Washington, DC: American Psychological Association.

Gorsuch, R. L., & Smith, C. S. (1983). Attributions of responsibility to God: An interaction of religious beliefs and outcomes. *Journal for the Scientific Study of Religion, 22,* 340–352.

Gottschalk, S. (1973). *The emergence of Christian Science in American religious life.* Berkeley: University of California Press.

Gould, S. J. (1978). Biological potential vs. biological determinism. In A. L. Caplan (Ed.), *The sociobiology debate* (pp. 343–351). New York, NY: Harper & Row.

Gould, S. J. (1999). *Rocks of ages.* New York, NY: Ballantine.

Gould, S. J. (2002). *The structure of evolutionary theory.* Cambridge, MA: Harvard University Press.

Graebner, O. E. (1964). Child concepts of God. *Religious Education, 59,* 234–241.

Graham, R. (2015, April 30). Is it too late for evangelical Christians to honestly discuss same-sex marriage? Retrieved from *www.slate.com/articles/life/faithbased/2015/04/q_ideas_conference_2015_how_does_the_christian_ted_talks_deal_with_same.html.*

Grana Gomes, J. L., & Munoz-Rivas, M. (2000). Factores psicologicos de riesgo y de proteccion para el consumo de drogas en adolescents [Psychological risk and protection factors for drug use by adolescents]. *Psicologia Conductual, 8,* 249–269.

Granqvist, P. (1998). Religiousness and perceived childhood attachment: On the question of compensation or correspondence. *Journal for the Scientific Study of Religion, 37,* 350–367.

Granqvist, P. (2002a). *Attachment and religion: An integrative framework* (Comprehensive Summaries of Uppsala Dissertations from the Faculty of Social Sciences, No. 116). Uppsala, Sweden: Uppsala University.

Granqvist, P. (2002b). Attachment and religiosity in adolescence: Cross-sectional and longitudinal evaluations. *Personality and Social Psychology Bulletin, 28,* 260–270.

Granqvist, P. (2003). Attachment theory and religious conversions: A review and a resolution of the classic and contemporary paradigm chasm. *Review of Religious Research, 45,* 172–187.

Granqvist, P. (2006a). In the interests of intellectual humility: A rejoinder to Rizzuto and Wulff. *International Journal for the Psychology of Religion, 16,* 37–49.

Granqvist, P. (2006b). On the relation between secular and divine relationships: An emerging attachment perspective and a critique of the "depth" approaches. *International Journal for the Psychology of Religion, 16,* 1–18.

Granqvist, P., Fredrikson, M., Unge, P., Hagenfeldt, A., Valind, S., Larhammar, D., & Larsson, M. (2005). Sensed presence and mystical experiences are predicted by suggestibility, not by the application of transcranial weak complex magnetic fields. *Neuroscience Letters, 379,* 1–6.

Granqvist, P., & Hagekull, B. (1999). Religiousness and perceived childhood attachment: Profiling socialized correspondence and emotional compensation. *Journal for the Scientific Study of Religion, 38,* 254–273.

Granqvist, P., & Hagekull, B. (2001). Seeking security in the new age: On attachment and emotional compensation. *Journal for the Scientific Study of Religion, 40,* 527–545.

Granqvist, P., Ivarsson, T., Broberg, A. G., & Hagekull, B. (2007). Examining relations between attachment, religiosity, and New Age spirituality using the Adult Attachment interview. *Developmental Psychology, 43,* 590–601.

Granqvist, P., & Kirkpatrick, L. A. (2004). Religious conversion and perceived childhood attachment: A meta-analysis. *International Journal for the Psychology of Religion, 14,* 223–250.

Granqvist, P., & Kirkpatrick, L. A. (2008). Attachment and religious representations and behavior. In J. Cassidy & P. R. Shaver (Eds.), *Handbook of attachment: Theory, research, and clinical applications* (2nd ed., pp. 906–933). New York, NY: Guilford Press.

Granqvist, P., & Larsson, M. (2006). Contribution of religiousness in the prediction and interpretation of mystical experiences in a sensory deprivation context. *Journal of Psychology, 140,* 319–327.

Granqvist, P., Ljungdahl, C., & Dickie, J. R. (2007). God is nowhere, God is now here: Attachment activation, security attachment, and perceived closeness to God among 5–7 year old children from religious and non-religious homes. *Atttachment and Human Development, 9,* 55–71.

Grant, D., & Epp, L. (1998). The gay orientation: Does God mind? *Counseling and Values, 43,* 28–33.

Grasmick, H. G., Bursik, R. J., & Cochran, J. K. (1991). "Render unto Caesar what is Caesar's": Religiosity and taxpayers' inclinations to cheat. *Sociological Quarterly, 32,* 251–266.

Grasmick, H. G., Kinsey, K., & Cochran, J. K. (1991). Denomination, religiosity and compliance with the law: A study of adults. *Journal for the Scientific Study of Religion, 30,* 99–107.

Grasmick, H. G., Morgan, C. S., & Kennedy, M. B. (1992). Support for corporal punishment in the schools: A comparison of the effects of socioeconomic status and religion. *Social Science Quarterly, 73,* 177–187.

Graves, P. L., Wang, N.-Y., Mead, L. A., Johnson, J. V., & Klag, M. J. (1998). Youthful precursors of midlife social support. *Journal of Personality and Social Psychology, 74,* 1329–1336.

Gray, K., & Wegner, D. (2010). Blaming God for our pain: Human suffering and the divine mind. *Personality and Social Psychology Review, 14,* 7–16.

Grayling, A. C. (2007). *Against all gods.* London, UK: Oberon Books.

Greeley, A. M. (1963). *Religion and career: A study of college graduates.* New York, NY: Sheed & Ward.

Greeley, A. M. (1967). *The changing Catholic college.* Chicago, IL: Aldine.

Greeley, A. M. (1972). *The denominational society.* Glenview, IL: Scott, Foresman.

Greeley, A. M. (1974). *Ecstasy: A way of knowing.* Englewood Cliffs, NJ: Prentice-Hall.

Greeley, A. M. (1975). *Sociology of the paranormal: A reconnaissance* (Sage Research Papers in the Social Sciences, Vol. 3, No. 90-023). Beverly Hills, CA: SAGE.

Greeley, A. M. (2002). *Religion in Europe at the end of the second millennium.* New Brunswick, NJ: Transaction Books.

Greeley, A. M., & Gockel, G. L. (1971). The religious effects of parochial education. In M. P. Strommen (Ed.), *Research on religious development: A comprehensive handbook* (pp. 264–301). New York, NY: Hawthorne Books.

Greeley, A. M., & Hout, M. (1999). American's increasing belief in life after death: Religious competition and acculturation. *American Sociological Review, 64,* 813–835.

Greeley, A. M., & Rossi, P. H. (1966). *The education of Catholic Americans.* Chicago, IL: Aldine.

Green, E. (2014, November). Keeping the faith: How childhood influences churchgoing. *The Atlantic,* p. 32.

Greenberg, D., & Witztum, E. (1992). Content and prevalence of psychopathology in world religions. In J. F. Schumaker (Ed.), *Religion and mental health* (pp. 300–314). New York, NY: Oxford University Press.

Greenberg, J., & Folger, R. (1983). Procedural justice, participation, and the fair process effect in groups and organizations. In P. B. Paulus (Ed.), *Basic group processes* (pp. 235–256). New York, NY: Springer-Verlag.

Greenwald, A. G., & Banaji, M. (1995). Implicit social cognition: Attitudes, self-esteem, and stereotypes. *Psychological Review, 102,* 4–27.

Greenwald, A. G., & Harder, D. (2003). The dimensions of spirituality. *Psychological Reports, 92,* 975–980.

Greenwald, A. G., McGhee, D. E., & Schwartz, D. L. K. (1998). Measuring individual differences in implicit cognition: The Implicit Association Test. *Journal of Personality and Social Psychology, 74,* 1464–1480.

Greenwood, S. F. (1995). Transpersonal theory and religious experience. In R. W. Hood, Jr. (Ed.), *Handbook of religious experience* (pp. 495–519). Birmingham, AL: Religious Education Press.

Greer, J. E. (1983). A critical study of "Thinking about the Bible." *British Journal of Religious Education, 5,* 113–125.

Greil, A. L. (1993). Explorations along the sacred frontier: Notes on para-religions, quasi-religions, and other boundary phenomena. In D. G. Bromley & J. K. Hadden (Eds.), *Handbook of cults and sects in America: Assessing two decades of research and theory development* (pp. 153–172). Greenwich, CT: JAI Press.

Greil, A. L., & Robbins, T. (1994). Introduction: Exploring the boundaries of the sacred. In A. L. Greil & T. Robbins (Eds.), *Between sacred and secular: Research and theory on quasi-religion* (pp. 1–23). Greenwich, CT: JAI Press.

Greil, A. L., & Rudy, D. R. (1990). On the margins of the sacred. In T. Robbins & D. Anthony (Eds.), *In gods we trust: New patterns of religious pluralism in America* (pp. 219–232). New Brunswick, NJ: Transaction Books.

Greven, P. (1991). *Spare the child: The religious roots of punishment and the psychological impact of physical abuse.* New York, NY: Knopf.

Griffin, G. A. E., Gorsuch, R., & Davis, A.-L. (1987). A cross-cultural investigation of religious orientation, social norms, and prejudice. *Journal for the Scientific Study of Religion, 26,* 358–365.

Griffiths, A. J. F., Miller, J. H., Suzuki, D. T., Lewontin, R. C., & Gelbart, W. M. (2000). *An introduction to genetic analysis.* New York, NY: Freeman.

Griffiths, R. R., Richards, W. A., Johnson, M. W., McCann, U. D., & Jesse, R. (2008). Mystical-type experiences occasioned by psilocybin mediate the attribution of personal meaning and spiritual significance 14 months later. *Journal of Psychopharmacology, 22,* 621–632.

Griffiths, R. R., Richards, W. A., McCann, U. D., & Jesse, R. (2006). Psilocybin can occasion mystical experiences having substantial and sustained personal meaning and spiritual significance. *Psychopharmacology, 187,* 268–283.

Groebel, J. (1989). The problems and challenges of research on terrorism. In J. Goebel & J. H. Goldstein (Eds.), *Terrorism: Psychological perspectives* (pp. 15–38). Seville, Spain: University of Seville.

Grof, S. (1980). *LSD psychotherapy.* Pomona, CA: Hunter House.

Grootenhuis, M. A., & Last, B. F. (1997). Parents' emotional reactions related to different prospects for the survival of their children with cancer. *Journal of Psychosocial Oncology, 15*(1), 43–62.

Gross, L. (1982). *The last Jews in Berlin.* New York, NY: Simon & Schuster.

Gross, M. L. (1978). *The psychological society.* New York, NY: Random House.

Grossman, J. D. (1975). *The dark interval.* Nile, IL: Argus Communications.

Groth-Marnat, G. (1992). Buddhism and mental health: A comparative analysis. In J. F. Schumaker (Ed.), *Religion and mental health* (pp. 270–280). New York, NY: Oxford University Press.

Group for the Advancement of Psychiatry (GAP). (1960). *Psychiatry and religion* (Report No. 48, formulated by the Committee on Psychiatry and Religion). New York, NY: Author.

Group for the Advancement of Psychiatry (GAP). (1976, November). *Mysticism: Spiritual quest or psychic disorder?* (Report No. 97, formulated by the Committee on Psychiatry and Religion). New York, NY: Author.

Grubbs, J. B., & Exline, J. J. (2014a). Humbling yourself before God: Humility as a reliable predictor of lower divine struggle. *Journal of Psychology and Theology, 42,* 41–49.

Grubbs, J. B., & Exline, J. J. (2014b). Why did God make me this way?: Anger at God in context of personal transgression. *Journal of Psychology and Theology, 42,* 315–325.

Gruner, L. (1985). The correlation of private, religious devotional practices and marital adjustment. *Journal of Comparative Family Studies, 16,* 47–59.

Guralnik, D. B. (Ed.). (1986). *Webster's new world dictionary of the American language* (2nd college ed.). New York, NY: Prentice Hall Press.

Gurin, G., Veroff, J., & Feld, S. (1960). *Americans view their mental health: A nationwide interview study.* New York, NY: Basic Books.

Guthrie, S. E. (1993). *Faces in the clouds: A new theory of religion.* New York, NY: Oxford University Press.

Guthrie, S. E. (1996a). Religion: What is it? *Journal for the Scientific Study of Religion, 35,* 412–419.

Guthrie, S. E. (1996b). [Book reviews of P. Boyer, *The naturalness of religious ideas,* and S. N. Balagangadhara, *"The heathen in his blindness"—Asia, the West, and the dynamic of religion*]. *American Anthropologist, 98,* 162–163.

Guthrie, S. E. (2007). Opportunity, challenges and a definition of religion. *Journal for the Study of Religion, Nature, and Culture, 1,* 58–67.

Guttman, J. (1984). Cognitive morality and cheating behavior in religious and secular school children. *Journal of Educational Research, 77,* 249–254.

Haber, J. R., Grant, J. D., Sartor, C. E., Koenig, L. B., Heath, A., & Jacob, T. (2013). Religion/spirituality, risk, and the development of alcohol dependence in female twins. *Psychology of Addictive Behaviors, 27,* 562–572.

Hadaway, C. K. (1980). Denominational switching and religiosity. *Review of Religious Research, 21,* 451–461.

Hadaway, C. K. (1989). Identifying American apostates: A cluster analysis. *Journal for the Scientific Study of Religion, 28,* 201–215.

Hadaway, C. K., & Marler, P. L. (1993). All in the family: Religious mobility in America. *Review of Religious Research, 35,* 97–116.

Hadaway, C. K., Marler, P. L., & Chaves, M. (1993). What the polls don't show: A closer look at U.S. church attendance. *American Sociological Review, 58,* 741–752.

Hadaway, C. K., & Roof, W. C. (1988). Apostasy in American churches: Evidence from national survey data. In D. G. Bromley (Ed.), *Falling from the faith: Causes and consequences of religious apostasy* (pp. 29–46). Newbury Park, CA: SAGE.

Haddock, G. M., Zanna, M. P., & Esses, V. M. (1993). Assessing the structure of prejudicial attitudes: The case of attitudes toward homosexuals. *Journal of Personality and Social Psychology, 65,* 1105–1118.

Haerich, P. (1992). Premarital sexual permissiveness and religious orientation: A preliminary investigation. *Journal for the Scientific Study of Religion, 31,* 361–365.

Haidt, J. (2003). Elevation and the positive psychology of morality. In C. L. M. Keyes & J. Haidt (Eds.), *Flourishing: Positive psychology and the life well-lived* (pp. 275–289). Washington, DC: American Psychological Association.

Haj-Yahia, M. M. (2002). Attitudes of Arab women toward different patterns of coping with wife abuse. *Journal of Interpersonal Violence, 17,* 721–745.

Haldane, D. (2006, December 17). Hard-wired to see sacred. *The Denver Post,* p. 8A.

Haldane, J. B. S. (1931). In *Science and religion: A symposium* (pp. 37–53). New York, NY: Scribner.

Haldeman, D. C. (1991). Sexual orientation conversion therapy for gay men and lesbians: A scientific examination. In J. Gonsiorek & J. D. Weinrich (Eds.), *Homosexuality: Research implications for public policy* (pp. 149–160). Thousand Oaks, CA: SAGE.

Haldeman, D. C. (1994). The practice and ethics of sexual orientation conversion therapy. *Journal of Consulting and Clinical Psychology, 62,* 221–227.

Haldeman, D. C. (1996). Spirituality and religion in the lives of lesbians and gay men. In R. P. Cabaj & T. S. Stein (Eds.), *Textbook of homosexuality and mental health* (pp. 881–896). Washington, DC: American Psychiatric Press.

Hale, J. R. (1977). *Who are the unchurched?* Washington, DC: Glenmary Research Center.

Hale-Smith, A., Park, C. L., & Edmondson, D. (2012). Measuring beliefs about suffering: Development of the Views of Suffering Scale. *Psychological Assessment, 24,* 855–866.

Halford, L. J., Anderson, C. L., & Clark, E. (1981). Prophecy fails again and again: The Morrisites. *Free Inquiry in Creative Sociology, 9,* 5–10.

Hall, B. A. (1994). Ways of maintaining hope in HIV disease. *Research in Nursing and Health, 17,* 283–293.

Hall, D. L., Matz, D. C., & Wood, W. (2010). Why don't we practice what we preach?: A meta-analytic review of religious racism. *Personality and Social Psychology Review, 14,* 126–139.

Hall, G. S. (1900). The religious content of the child-mind. In N. M. Butler et al., *Principles of religious education* (pp. 161–189). New York, NY: Longmans, Green.

Hall, G. S. (1904). *Adolescence: Its psychology and relations to physiology, anthropology, sociology, sex, crime, religion and education* (2 vols.). New York, NY: Appleton.

Hall, G. S. (1917). *Jesus, the Christ, in the light of psychology* (2 vols.). Garden City, NY: Doubleday.

Hall, J. H., & Fincham, F. D. (2005). Self-forgiveness: The stepchild of forgiveness research. *Journal of Social and Clinical Psychology, 24,* 621–637.

Hall, J. R. (1989). *Gone from the promised land: Jonestown in American cultural history.* New Brunswick, NJ: Transaction Books.

Hall, K. S., Moreau, C., & Trussell, J. (2012). Lower use of sexual and reproductive health services among women with frequent religious participation, regardless of sexual experience. *Journal of Women's Health, 21,* 739–747.

Hall, T. A. (1995). Spiritual effects of childhood sexual abuse in adult Christian women. *Journal of Psychology and Theology, 23,* 129–134.

Hall, T. W., & Edwards, K. J. (1996). The initial development and factor analysis of the Spiritual Assessment Inventory. *Journal of Psychology and Theology, 24,* 233–246.

Halligan, F. R. (1995). Jungian theory and religious experience. In R. W. Hood, Jr. (Ed.), *Handbook of religious experience* (pp. 231–253). Birmingham, AL: Religious Education Press.

Hamberg, E. M. (1991). Stability and change in religious beliefs, practice, and attitudes: A Swedish panel study. *Journal for the Scientific Study of Religion, 30,* 63–80.

Hamer, D. (2004). *The God gene.* New York, NY: Doubleday.

Hamlyn, D. W. (1967). Empiricism. In P. Edwards (Ed.), *The encylopaedia of philosophy* (Vol. 2, pp. 499–504). New York, NY: Crowell, Collier & Macmillan.

Hands, D. (1992, Fall). Clergy sexual abuse. *Saint Barnabas Community Chronicle,* pp. 1–3.

Hanson, R. A. (1991). The development of moral reasoning: Some observations about Christian fundamentalism. *Journal of Psychology and Theology, 19,* 249–256.

Happold, F. C. (1991). *Mysticism: A study and an anthology* (3rd ed.). New York, NY: Penguin.

Hardt, H. D. (1963). *Mental health status and religious attitudes of hospitalized veterans.* Unpublished doctoral dissertation, University of Texas.

Hardy, A. (1965). *The living stream.* London, UK: Collins.

Hardy, A. (1966). *The divine flame.* London, UK: Collins.

Hardy, A. (1975). *The biology of God.* New York, NY: Taplinger.

Hardy, A. (1979). *The spiritual nature of man: A study of contemporary religious experience.* Oxford, UK: Clarendon Press.

Hardyck, J. A., & Braden, M. (1962). When prophecy fails again: A report of failure to replicate. *Journal of Abnormal and Social Psychology, 65,* 136–141.

Harley, B., & Firebaugh, G. (1993). Americans' belief in an afterlife: Trends over the past two decades. *Journal for the Scientific Study of Religion, 32,* 269–278.

Harms, E. (1944). The development of religious experience in children. *American Journal of Sociology, 50,* 112–122.

Harris, J. I., Erbes, C. R., Engdahl, B. E., Tedeschi, D. G., Olson, R. H., Winkowski, A. M. M., & McMahill, J. (2010). Coping functions of prayer and posttraumatic growth. *International Journal for the Psychology of Religion, 20,* 26–38.

Harris, N. A., Spilka, B., & Emrick, C. (1990, August 12). *Religion and alcoholism: A multidimensional approach.* Paper presented at the annual convention of the American Psychological Association, Boston, MA.

Harris, P. L. (2000). On not falling down to earth: Children's metaphysical questions. In K. S. Rosengren, C. N. Johnson, & P. L. Harris (Eds.), *Imagining the impossible: Magical, scientific, and religious thinking in children* (pp. 157–178). Cambridge, UK: Cambridge University Press.

Harris, S. (2004). *The end of faith: Religion, terror, and the future of reason.* New York, NY: Norton.

Harris, S. (2007). *Letter to a Christian nation.* London, UK: Bantam.

Hart, A., Jr., Bowen, D. J., Kuniyuki, A., Hannon, P., & Campbell, M. K. (2007). The relationship between the social environment within religious organizations and intake of fat versus fruits and vegetables. *Health Education and Behavior, 34,* 503–516.

Hart, D., & Schneider, D. (1997). Spiritual care for children with cancer. *Seminar in Oncological Nursing, 13*(4), 263–270.

Hartnett, K. (2013, February 15). Religion and premarital sex. *The Boston Globe.* Retrieved from *archive.boston.com/bostonglobe/ideas/brainiac/2013/02/religion_and_pr.html.*

Hartshorne, H., & May, M. A. (1928). *Studies in the nature of character: Vol. 1. Studies in deceit.* New York, NY: Macmillan.

Hartshorne, H., & May, M. A. (1929). *Studies in the nature of character: Vol. 2. Studies in service and self-control.* New York, NY: Macmillan.

Hartshorne, H., May, M. A., & Shuttleworth, F. K. (1930). *Studies in the nature of character: Vol. 3. Studies in the organization of character.* New York, NY: Macmillan.

Hartz, G. W., & Everett, H. C. (1989). Fundamentalist religion and its effect on mental health. *Journal of Religion and Health, 28,* 207–217.

Harvard Institute of Politics (IOP). (2008). The 14th Biannual Youth Survey of Politics and Public Service. Retrieved from *www.iop.harvard.edu/var/czp_site/storage/fekeditor/file/spring%20poll%2008%20-%20topline.pdf.*

Hassan, M. K., & Khalique, A. (1987). A study of prejudice in Hindu and Muslim college students. *Psychologia: An International Journal of Psychology in the Orient, 30,* 80–84.

Hastings, P. K., & Hoge, D. R. (1976). Changes in religion among college students, 1948 to 1974. *Journal for the Scientific Study of Religion, 15,* 237–249.

Haught, J. F. (2005). Science and scientism: The importance of a distinction. *Zygon, 40,* 363–368.

Haun, D. L. (1977). Perceptions of the bereaved, clergy, and funeral directors concerning bereavement. *Dissertation Abstracts International, 37,* 6791A.

Hawley, J. S. (1994a). Hinduism: *Sati* and its defenders. In J. S. Hawley (Ed.), *Fundamentalism and gender* (pp. 79–110). New York, NY: Oxford University Press.

Hawley, J. S. (Ed.). (1994b). *Sati, the blessing and the curse.* New York, NY: Oxford University Press.

Hay, D. (1979). Religious experience amongst a group of postgraduate students: A qualitative study. *Journal for the Scientific Study of Religion, 18,* 164–182.

Hay, D. (1987). *Exploring inner space: Scientists and religious experience* (2nd ed.). London, UK: Mowbray.

Hay, D. (1994). "The biology of God": What is the current status of Hardy's hypothesis? *International Journal for the Psychology of Religion, 4*, 1–23.

Hay, D., & Heald, G. (1987). Religion is good for you. *New Society, 80*, 20–22.

Hay, D., & Morisy, A. (1978). Reports of ecstatic, paranormal, or religious experience in Great Britain and the United States: A comparison of trends. *Journal for the Scientific Study of Religion, 17*, 255–268.

Hay, D., & Morisy, A. (1985). Secular society, religious meanings: A contemporary paradox. *Review of Religious Research, 26*, 213–227.

Hay, D., & Nye, R. (1998). *The spirit and the child.* London, UK: Fount/HarperCollins.

Hay, D., & Socha, P. M. (2005). Spirituality as a natural phenomenon: Bringing biological and psychological perspectives together. *Zygon, 40*, 589–612.

Hayden, J. J. (1991, August 18). *Rheumatic disease and chronic pain: Religious and affective variables.* Paper presented at the annual convention of the American Psychological Association, San Francisco, CA.

Hayes, B. C., & Hornsby-Smith, M. P. (1994). Religious identification and family attitudes: An international comparison. *Research in the Social Scientific Study of Religion, 6*, 167–186.

Hays, J. C., Meador, K. G., Branch, P. S., & George, L. K. (2001). The Spirituality History Scale in Four Dimensions (SHS-4): Validity and reliability. *Gerontologist, 41*, 239–249.

Hayward, R. D., & Krause, N. (2013). Patterns of change in prayer activity, expectancies, and contents during older adulthood. *Journal for the Scientific Study of Religion, 52*, 17–34.

Hearn, W. R. (1968). Biological science. In R. H. Bube (Ed.), *The encounter between Christianity and science* (pp. 199–223). Grand Rapids, MI: Eerdmans.

Hearnshaw, C. S. (1987). *The shaping of modern psychology.* New York, NY: Routledge.

Heelas, P., Woodhead, L., Steel, B., Szerszynski, B., & Trusting, K. (2005). *The spiritual revolutions: Why religion is giving way to spirituality.* Oxford, UK: Blackwell.

Hefner, P., & Koss-Chioino, J. D. (Eds.). (2006). *Spiritual transformation and healing: Anthropological, theological, neuroscientific, and clinical perspectives.* Lanham, MD: AltaMira Press.

Heiler, F. (1932). *Prayer: A study in the history and psychology of religion.* New York, NY: Oxford University Press.

Heintzelman, S. J., & King, L. A. (2013). On knowing more than we can tell: Intuition and the human experience of meaning. *Journal of Positive Psychology, 8*, 471–482.

Heintzelman, S. J., & King, L. A. (2014). Life is pretty meaningful. *American Psychologist, 69*, 561–574.

Heiphetz, L., Lane, J. D., Waytz, A., &Young, L. L. (2016). How children and adults represent God's mind. *Cognitive Science, 40*, 121–144.

Heirich, M. (1977). Change of heart: A test of some widely held theories of religious conversion. *American Sociological Review, 83*, 653–680.

Helfaer, P. (1972). *The psychology of religious doubt.* Boston, MA: Beacon Press.

Heller, D. (1986). *The children's God.* Chicago, IL: University of Chicago Press.

Helman, C. G. (1994). *Culture, health, and illness* (3rd ed.). Oxford, UK: Butterworth-Heinemann.

Helminiak, D. A. (1987). *Spiritual development: An interdisciplinary study.* Chicago, IL: Loyola University Press.

Helminiak, D. A. (1995). Non-religious lesbians and gays facing AIDS: A fully psychological approach to spirituality. *Pastoral Psychology, 43*, 301–318.

Helminiak, D. A. (1996a). A scientific spirituality: The interface of psychology and theology. *International Journal for the Psychology of Religion, 6*, 1–19.

Helminiak, D. A. (1996b). *The human core of spirituality.* Albany, NY: State University of New York Press.

Helminiak, D. A. (1998). *Religion and the human sciences.* Albany, NY: State University of New York Press.

Helminiak, D. (2000). *What the Bible really says about homosexuality.* Tajique, NM: Alamo Square Press.

Helminiak, D. A. (2015). *Brain, conscious, and God: A Lonerganian integration.* Albany, NY: State University of New York Press.

Henrich, J., Heine, S. J., & Norenzayan, A. (2010). The weirdest people in the world? *Behavioral and Brain Sciences, 33*, 61–83.

Herberg, W. (1960). *Protestant, Catholic, Jew.* Garden City, NY: Doubleday.

Herek, G. M. (1987). Religious orientation and prejudice: A comparison of racial and sexual attitudes. *Personality and Social Psychology Bulletin, 13*, 34–44.

Herek, G. M. (1988). Heterosexuals' attitudes toward lesbians and gay men: Correlates and gender differences. *Journal of Sex Research, 25*, 451–477.

Herek, G. M. (1994). Assessing heterosexuals' attitudes toward lesbians and gay men. In B. Greene & G. M. Herek (Eds.), *Lesbian and gay psychology: Theory, research and clinical applications* (pp. 206–228). Thousand Oaks, CA: SAGE.

Herek, G. M. (1998). Attitudes toward Lesbians and Gay Men Scale. In C. M. Davis (Ed.), *Handbook of sexuality-related measures* (pp. 392–394). Thousand Oaks, CA: SAGE.

Heriot-Maitland, C. P. (2008). Mysticism and madness: Different aspects of the same human experience? *Mental Health, Religion and Culture, 11*, 301–325.

Hernandez, G., Salerno, J. M., & Bottoms, B. L. (2010). Attachment to God, spiritual coping, and alcohol usage. *International Journal for the Psychology of Religion, 20*, 97–108.

Hernandez, K. M., Mahoney, A., & Pargament, K. I. (2011). Sanctification of sexuality: Implication for newlyweds' marital and sexual quality. *Journal of Family Psychology, 25*, 775–780.

Herold, E., Corbesi, B., & Collins, J. (1994). Psychosocial aspects of female topless behavior on Australian beaches. *Journal of Sex Research, 31*, 133–142.

Hertel, B. R. (1980). Inconsistency of beliefs in the existence of heaven and afterlife. *Review of Religious Research, 21*, 171–183.

Hertel, B. R., & Donahue, M. J. (1995). Parental influences on God images among children: Testing Durkheim's metaphoric parallelism. *Journal for the Scientific Study of Religion, 34*, 186–199.

Herzbrun, M. B. (1993). Father–adolescent religious consensus in the Jewish community: A preliminary report. *Journal for the Scientific Study of Religion, 32*, 163–168.

Hewstone, M. (Ed.). (1983a). *Attribution theory: Social and functional extensions.* Oxford, UK: Blackwell.

Hewstone, M. (1983b). Attribution theory and common-sense explanations: An introductory overview. In M. Hewstone (Ed.), *Attribution theory: Social and functional extensions* (pp. 1–27). Oxford, UK: Blackwell.

Hewstone, M., Islam, M. R., & Judd, C. M. (1993). Models of crossed categorization and intergroup relations. *Journal of Personality and Social Psychology, 64*, 779–793.

Heyman, D. K., & Gianturco, D. T. (1973). Long-term adaptation by the elderly to bereavement. *Journal of Gerontology, 28*, 359–362.

Hick, J. (1989). *An interpretation of religion.* New Haven, CT: Yale University Press.

Hick, J. (2010). *The new frontier of religion and science: Religious experience, neuroscience, and the transcendent.* New York, NY: Palgrave Macmillan. (Original work published 2006)

Higher Education Research Institute (HERI). (2005). *The spiritual life of college students: A national study of college students' search for meaning and purpose.* Los Angeles, CA: Graduate School of Education and Information Studies, University of California, Los Angeles.

Higher Education Research Institute (HERI). (2007, December 18). Spiritual changes in students during the undergraduate year: New longitudinal study shows growth in spiritual qualities from freshman to junior years. Retrieved February 16, 2009, from *www.spirituality.ucla.edu/news/report_back_dec07release_12.18.07.pdf.*

Hightower, P. R. (1930). Biblical information in relation to character and conduct. *University of Iowa Studies in Character, 3*(2), 72.

Hilbig, B. E., & Zettler, I. (2009). Pillars of cooperation: Honesty-humility, social value orientations, and economic behavior. *Journal of Research in Personality, 43*, 516–519.

Hill, D. R., & Persinger, M. A. (2003). Application of weak magnetic fields and mystical experiences. *Perceptual and Motor Skills, 97*, 1049–1050.

Hill, J. P. (2009). Higher education as moral community: Institutional influences on religious participation during college. *Journal for the Scientific Study of Religion, 48*, 515–534.

Hill, J. P. (2011). Faith and understanding: Specifying the impact of higher education on religious belief. *Journal for the Scientific Study of Religion, 50*, 533–551.

Hill, P. C. (1994). Toward an attitude process model of religious experience. *Journal for the Scientific Study of Religion, 33*, 303–314.

Hill, P. C. (1995). Affective theory and religious experience. In R. W. Hood, Jr. (Ed.), *Handbook of religious experience* (pp. 353–377). Birmingham, AL: Religious Education Press.

Hill, P. C. (1999). Giving religion away: What the study of religion offers psychology. *International Journal for the Psychology of Religion, 9*, 229–249.

Hill, P. C. (2002). Spiritual transformation: Forming the habitual center of personal energy. *Research in the Social Scientific Study of Religion, 13*, 87–108.

Hill, P. C. (2005). Measurement in the psychology of religion and spirituality. In R. F. Paloutzian & C. L. Park (Eds.), *Handbook of the psychology of religion and spirituality* (pp. 43–61). New York, NY: Guilford Press.

Hill, P. C. (2013). Measurement in the psychology of religion and spirituality. In R. F. Paloutzian & C. L. Park (Eds.), *Handbook of the psychology of religion and spirituality* (2nd ed., pp. 48–74). New York, NY: Guilford Press.

Hill, P. C., & Dwiwardani, C. (2010). Measurement at the interface of psychiatry and religion: Issues and existing measures. In P. J. Verhagen, H. M. van Praag, J. J. Lopez-Ibor, J. L. Cox, & D. Moussaoui (Eds.), *Religion and psychiatry: Beyond boundaries* (pp. 319–339). Chichester, UK: Wiley-Blackwell.

Hill, P. C., & Edwards, E. (2013). Measurement in the psychology of religiousness and spirituality: Existing measures and new frontiers. In K. I. Pargament, J. J. Exline, & J. W. Jones (Eds.), *APA handbook of psychology, religion, and spirituality* (Vol. 1, pp. 51–78). Washington, DC: American Psychological Association.

Hill, P. C., Exline, J. J., & Cohen, A. B. (2005). The social psychology of justice and forgiveness in civil and organizational settings. In E. L. Worthington, Jr. (Ed.), *Handbook of forgiveness* (pp. 477–490). New York, NY: Routledge.

Hill, P. C., & Gibson, N. J. S. (2008). Whither the roots?: Achieving conceptual depth in the psychology of religion. *Archiv für Religionspsychologie, 30,* 19–35.

Hill, P. C., & Hall, M. E. L. (2018). Uncovering the good in positive psychology: Toward a worldview conception that can help positive psychology flourish. In N. J. L. Brown, T. Lomas, & F. J. Eiroá-Orosa (Eds.), *The Routledge international handbook of critical positive psychology* (pp. 245–262). Abingdon, UK: Routledge.

Hill, P. C., & Hood, R. W., Jr. (1999a). *Measures of religiosity.* Birmingham, AL: Religious Education Press.

Hill, P. C., & Hood, R. W., Jr. (1999b). Religion, affect and the unconscious. *Journal of Personality, 67,* 1015–1046.

Hill, P. C., Jurkiewicz, C., Giacolone, R. A., & Fry, L. W. (2013). From concept to science: Continuing steps in workplace spirituality research. In R. F. Paloutzian & C. L. Park (Eds.), *Handbook of the psychology of religion and spirituality* (2nd ed., pp. 617–631). New York, NY: Guilford Press.

Hill, P. C., Kopp, K. J., & Bollinger, R. A. (2007). A few good measures: Assessing religion and spirituality in relation to health. In T. G. Plante & C. E. Thoresen (Eds.), *Spirit, science, and health: How the spiritual mind fuels physical wellness* (pp. 25–38). Westport, CT: Praeger.

Hill, P. C., & Laney, E. K. (2017). Beyond self-interest: Humility and the quieted self. In K. W. Brown & M. R. Leary (Eds.), *The Oxford handbook of hypoegoic phenomena: Theory and research on the quiet ego* (pp. 243–255). New York, NY: Oxford University Press.

Hill, P. C., & Pargament, K. I. (2003). Advances in the conceptualization and measurement of religion and spirituality: Implications for physical and mental health research. *American Psychologist, 58,* 64–74.

Hill, P. C., & Pargament, K. I. (2017). Measurement tools and issues in the psychology of religion and spirituality. In R. Finke & C. D. Bader (Eds.), *Faithful measures: New methods in the measurement of religion* (pp. 48–77). New York, NY: New York University Press.

Hill, P. C., Pargament, K. I., Hood, R. W., Jr., McCullough, M. E., Swyers, J. P., Larson, D. B.,

& Zinnbauer, B. J. (2000). Conceptualizing religion and spirituality: Points of commonality, points of departure. *Journal for the Theory of Social Behaviour, 30,* 51–77.

Hill, T. D., Burdette, A. M., Ellison, C. G., & Musick, M. A. (2006). Religious attendance and the health behaviors of Texan adults. *Preventative Medicine, 42,* 309–312.

Hill, T. D., & McCullough, M. E. (2008). Religious involvement and the intoxication trajectories of low-income urban women. *Journal of Drug Issues, 38,* 847–862.

Hiltner, S. (1949). *Pastoral counseling.* New York, NY: Abingdon-Cokesbury.

Hilty, D. M., & Morgan, R. L. (1985). Construct validation for the Religious Involvement Inventory: Replication. *Journal for the Scientific Study of Religion, 24,* 75–86.

Himmelfarb, H. S. (1979). Agents of religious socialization among American Jews. *Sociological Quarterly, 20,* 477–494.

Hinde, R. A. (1999). *Why gods persist: A scientific approach to religion.* London, UK: Routledge.

Hine, V. H. (1969). Pentecostal glossolalia: Toward a functional interpretation. *Journal for the Scientific Study of Religion, 8,* 211–226.

Hinkle, L. E., Jr., & Wolff, H. E. (1956). Communist interrogation and the indoctrination of "enemies of the states." *Archives of Neurology and Psychiatry, 76,* 117.

Hitchens, C. (2007). *God is not great: The case against religion.* London, UK: Atlantic Books.

Hochstein, L. M. (1986). Pastoral counselors: Their attitudes toward gay and lesbian clients. *Journal of Pastoral Care, 40,* 158–165.

Hodges, D. L. (1974). Breaking a scientific taboo: Putting assumptions about the supernatural into scientific theories of religion. *Journal for the Scientific Study of Religion, 13,* 393–408.

Hoebel, E. A. (1966). *Anthropology: The study of man.* New York, NY: McGraw-Hill.

Hoffman, B. (2006). *Inside terrorism* (2nd ed.). New York, NY: Columbia University Press.

Hoffman, D. H., Carter, D. J., Lopez, C. R. V., Benziller, H. L., Guo, A. X., Latifi, S. Y., & Craig, D. C. (2015, July 2). *Report to the Special Committee of the Board of Directors of the American Psychological Association: Independent review relating to APA ethics guidelines, national security interrogations, and torture.* Chicago, IL: Sidley Austin LLP.

Hoffman, S. J. (1992). *Prayers, piety, and pigskins: Religion in modern sports.* Paper presented at the annual convention of the Society for the Scientific Study of Religion, Washington, DC.

Hoffman, V. J. (1995). Muslim fundamentalists: Psychosocial profiles. In M. E. Marty & R. S. Appleby

(Eds.), *Fundamentalism comprehended* (pp. 199–230). Chicago, IL: University of Chicago Press.

Hoge, D. R. (1981). *Converts, dropouts, returnees: A study of religious change among Catholics.* New York, NY: Pilgrim Press.

Hoge, D. R. (1988). Why Catholics drop out. In D. G. Bromley (Ed.), *Falling from the faith: Causes and consequences of religious apostasy* (pp. 81–99). Newbury Park, CA: SAGE.

Hoge, D. R., Heffernan, E., Hemrick, E. F., Nelsen, H. M., O'Connor, J. P., Philibert, P. J., & Thompson, A. D. (1982). Desired outcomes of religious education and youth ministry in six denominations. *Review of Religious Research, 23,* 230–254.

Hoge, D. R., Johnson, B., & Luidens, D. A. (1993). Determinants of church involvement of young adults who grew up in Presbyterian churches. *Journal for the Scientific Study of Religion, 32,* 242–255.

Hoge, D. R., & Keeter, L. G. (1976). Determinants of college teachers' religious beliefs and participation. *Journal for the Scientific Study of Religion, 15,* 221–235.

Hoge, D. R., with McGuire, K., & Stratman, B. F. (1981). *Converts, dropouts, returnees: A study of religious change among Catholics.* New York, NY: Pilgrim Press.

Hoge, D. R., & Petrillo, G. H. (1978a). Determinants of church participation among high school youth. *Journal for the Scientific Study of Religion, 17,* 359–379.

Hoge, D. R., & Petrillo, G. H. (1978b). Development of religious thinking in adolescence: A test of Goldman's theories. *Journal for the Scientific Study of Religion, 17,* 139–154.

Hoge, D. R., Petrillo, G. H., & Smith, E. I. (1982). Transmission of religious and social values from parents to teenage children. *Journal of Marriage and the Family, 44,* 569–580.

Hoge, D. R., & Thompson, A. D. (1982). Different conceptualizations of goals of religious education and youth ministry in six denominations. *Review of Religious Research, 23,* 297–304.

Hoggatt, L., & Spilka, B. (1978). The nurse and the terminally ill patient. *Omega, 9,* 255–256.

Holden, G. W., & Edwards, L. A. (1989). Parental attitudes toward child rearing: Instruments, issues, and implications. *Psychological Bulletin, 106,* 29–58.

Holder, D. W., Durant, R. H., Harris, T. L., Daniel, J. H., Obeidallah, D., & Goodman, E. (2000). The association between adolescent spirituality and voluntary sexual activity. *Journal of Adolescent Health, 26,* 295–302.

Holland, J. C., Kash, K. M., Passik, S., Gronert, M. K., Sison, A., Lederberg, M., et al. (1998). A brief spiritual beliefs inventory for use in quality of life research in life-threatening illness. *Psycho-Oncology, 7,* 460–469.

Holley, P. (2015, May 11). Principal blames devil for her racist remarks. *The Denver Post,* p. 14A.

Holley, R. T. (1991). Assessing potential bias: The effects of adding religious content to the Defining Issues Test. *Journal of Psychology and Christianity, 10,* 323–336.

Holm, N. G. (1982). Mysticism and intense experiences. *Journal for the Scientific Study of Religion, 21,* 268–276.

Holm, N. G. (1987a). *Scandinavian psychology of religion.* Åbo, Finland: Åbo Akademi.

Holm, N. G. (1987b). Sundén's role theory and glossolalia. *Journal for the Scientific Study of Religion, 26,* 383–389.

Holm, N. G. (1991). Pentecostalism: Conversion and charismata. *International Journal for the Psychology of Religion, 1,* 135–151.

Holm, N. G. (1995). Role theory and religious experience. In R. W. Hood, Jr. (Ed.), *Handbook of religious experience* (pp. 397–420). Birmingham, AL: Religious Education Press.

Holm, N. G. (2008, June). *Mysticism and spirituality.* Keynote address presented at the 19th conference of the Donner Institute, Turku/Åbo, Finland.

Holm, N. G., & Belzen, J. A. (Eds.). (1995). *Sundén's role theory: An impetus to contemporary psychology of religion.* Åbo, Finland: Åbo Akademi.

Holmes, U. T. (1980). *A history of Christian spirituality.* New York, NY: Seabury Press.

Holt, J. (2002, April 14). "Intelligent design creationism and its critics": Supernatural selection. *The New York Times.* Retrieved April 14, 2002, from *www.nytimes.com/2002/04/14/books/review/14Holtlt.html?rd=hcmcp?p=042q.*

Holt, K., & Massey, C. (2012). Sexual preference or opportunity: An examination of situational factors by gender of victims of clergy abuse. *Sexual Abuse: A Journal of Research and Treatment, 25,* 606–621.

Holt, R. (1964). The return of the ostracized. *American Psychologist, 19,* 254–264.

Homan, K. J., & Boyatzis, C. J. (2010). Religiosity, sense of meaning, and health behavior in older adults. *International Journal for the Psychology of Religion, 20,* 173–186.

Hong, G.-Y. (1995). Buddhism and religious experience. In R. W. Hood, Jr. (Ed.), *Handbook of religious experience* (pp. 87–121). Birmingham, AL: Religious Education Press.

Honigmann, J. J. (1959). *The world of man.* New York, NY: Harper & Row.

Hood, R. W., Jr. (1970). Religious orientation and the report of religious experience. *Journal for the Scientific Study of Religion, 9,* 285–291.

Hood, R. W., Jr. (1973a). Hypnotic susceptibility and reported religious experience. *Psychological Reports, 33,* 549–550.

Hood, R. W., Jr. (1973b). Religious orientation and the experience of transcendence. *Journal for the Scientific Study of Religion, 12,* 441–448.

Hood, R. W., Jr. (1974). Psychological strength and the report of intense religious experience. *Journal for the Scientific Study of Religion, 13,* 65–71.

Hood, R. W., Jr. (1975). The construction and preliminary validation of a measure of reported mystical experience. *Journal for the Scientific Study of Religion, 14,* 29–41.

Hood, R. W., Jr. (1977). Eliciting mystical states of consciousness with semistructured nature experiences. *Journal for the Scientific Study of Religion, 16,* 155–163.

Hood, R. W., Jr. (1978a). Anticipatory set and setting: Stress incongruity as elicitors of mystical experience in solitary nature situations. *Journal for the Scientific Study of Religion, 17,* 278–287.

Hood, R. W., Jr. (1978b). The usefulness of the indiscriminately pro and anti categories of religious orientation. *Journal for the Scientific Study of Religion, 17,* 419–431.

Hood, R. W., Jr. (1980). Social legitimacy, dogmatism, and the evaluation of intense experiences. *Review of Religious Research, 21,* 184–194.

Hood, R. W., Jr. (1983). Social psychology and religious fundamentalism. In A. W. Childs & G. B. Melton (Eds.), *Rural psychology* (pp. 169–198). New York, NY: Plenum Press.

Hood, R. W., Jr. (1985). Mysticism. In P. Hammond (Ed.), *The sacred in a secular age* (pp. 285–297). Berkeley: University of California Press.

Hood, R. W., Jr. (1987). [Review of the book *The obedience experiments: A case study of controversy in social science*]. *Educational and Psychological Measurement, 47,* 840–845.

Hood, R. W., Jr. (1989). Mysticism, the unity thesis, and the paranormal. In G. K. Zollschan, J. F. Schumaker, & G. F. Walsh (Eds.), *Exploring the paranormal: Perspectives on belief and experience* (pp. 117–130). New York, NY: Avery.

Hood, R. W., Jr. (1991). Holm's use of role theory: Empirical and hermeneutical considerations of sacred text as a source of role adoption. *International Journal for the Psychology of Religion, 1,* 153–159.

Hood, R. W., Jr. (1992a). A Jamesian look at self and self loss in mysticism. *Journal of the Psychology of Religion, 1,* 1–14.

Hood, R. W., Jr. (1992b). Sin and guilt in faith traditions: Issues for self-esteem. In J. F. Schumaker (Ed.), *Religion and mental health* (pp. 110–121). New York, NY: Oxford University Press.

Hood, R. W., Jr. (1994). Psychology and religion. In U. S. Ramachdran (Ed.), *Encyclopaedia of human behavior* (Vol. 3, pp. 619–629). New York, NY: Academic Press.

Hood, R. W., Jr. (1995a). The facilitation of religious experience. In R. W. Hood, Jr. (Ed.), *Handbook of religious experience* (pp. 569–597). Birmingham, AL: Religious Education Press.

Hood, R. W., Jr. (Ed.). (1995b). *Handbook of religious experience.* Birmingham, AL: Religious Education Press.

Hood, R. W., Jr. (1995c). The soulful self of William James. In D. W. Capps & J. L. Jacobs (Eds.), The struggle for life: A companion to William James's *The varieties of religious experience* (Society for the Scientific Study of Religion Monograph Series, Whole No. 9, pp. 209–219). West Lafayette, IN: Society for the Scientific Study of Religion.

Hood, R. W., Jr. (1998). When the spirit maims and kills: Social psychological considerations of the history of serpent handling sects and the narrative of handlers. *International Journal for the Psychology of Religion, 8,* 71–86.

Hood, R. W., Jr. (2000a). American psychology of religion and the *Journal for the Scientific Study of Religion. Journal for the Scientific Study of Religion, 39,* 531–543.

Hood, R. W., Jr. (2000b, October). *The relationship between religion and spirituality.* Paper presented at the annual convention of the Society for the Scientific Study of Religion, Houston, TX.

Hood, R. W., Jr. (2002a). The mystical self: Lost and found. *International Journal for the Psychology of Religion, 12,* 1–14.

Hood, R. W., Jr. (2002b). *Dimensions of mystical experiences: Empirical studies and psychological links.* Amsterdam, The Netherlands: Rhodopi.

Hood, R. W., Jr. (2003). The relationship between religion and spirituality. In D. Bromley (Series Ed.) & A. L. Greil & D. Bromley (Vol. Eds.), *Defining religion: Investigating the boundaries between the sacred and the secular: Vol. 10. Religion and the social order* (pp. 241–265). Amsterdam, The Netherlands: Elsevier Science.

Hood, R. W., Jr. (2005a). *Handling serpents: Pastor Jimmy Morrow's narrative history of his Appalachian Jesus' Name tradition.* Mercer, GA: Mercer University Press.

Hood, R. W., Jr. (2005b). Mystical, spiritual, and religious experiences. In R. F. Paloutzian & C. L. Park (Eds.), *Handbook of the psychology of religion and spirituality* (pp. 348–364). New York, NY: Guilford Press.

Hood, R. W., Jr. (2006). The common core thesis in the study of mysticism. In P. McNamara (Ed.), *Where God and science meet* (Vol. 3, pp. 119–138). Westport, CT: Praeger.

Hood, R. W., Jr. (2007). Theories of ecstasy. In M.

McClymond (Ed.), *Encyclopedia of religious revivals in America* (Vol. 1, pp. 148–150). Westport, CT: Greenwood.

Hood, R. W., Jr. (2008a). Mysticism and the paranormal. In J. H. Ellens (Ed.), *Miracles: God, science, and psychology in the paranormal: Vol. 3. Parapsychological perspectives* (pp. 16–37). Westport, CT: Praeger.

Hood, R. W., Jr. (2008b). Spirituality and religion. In P. B. Clarke & P. Beyer (Eds.), *The world's religions* (pp. 675–689). New York, NY: Routledge.

Hood, R. W., Jr. (2008c). Theoretical fruits from the empirical study of mysticism: A Jamesian perspective. *Journal für Psychologie, 16*, Jfp-3.

Hood, R. W., Jr. (2010). Towards cultural psychology of religion: Principles, approaches, and applications: An appreciative response to Belzen's invitation. *Mental Health, Religion and Culture, 13*, 397–408.

Hood, R. W., Jr. (2011). The psychology of evil. In J. H. Ellens (Ed.), *Explaining evil* (Vol. 1, pp. 13–32). Santa Barbara, CA: Praeger.

Hood, R. W., Jr. (2012a). History and current status of research in the psychology of religion. In L. Miller (Ed.), *The Oxford handbook of psychology and spirituality* (pp. 7–20). New York, NY: Oxford University Press.

Hood, R. W., Jr. (2012b). Methodological agnosticism for the social sciences?: Lessons from Sorokin's and James's allusions to psychoanalysis, mysticism, and Godly love. In M. T. Lee & A. Yong (Eds.), *The science and theology of Godly love* (pp. 121–140). DeKalb: Northern Illinois University Press.

Hood, R. W., Jr. (2013). Methodological diversity in the psychology of religion. In K. I. Pargament, J. J. Exline, & J. W. Jones (Eds.), *APA handbook of the psychology of religion and spirituality* (Vol. 1, pp. 79–102). Washington, DC: American Psychological Association.

Hood, R. W., Jr. (2014a). Chemically assisted mysticism and the question of veridicality. In J. H. Ellens (Ed.), *Seeking the sacred with psychoactive substances: Chemical paths to spirituality and God* (Vol. 1, pp. 395–410). Santa Barbara, CA: Praeger.

Hood, R. W., Jr. (2014b). Methodological issues in the use of psychedelics in religious rituals. In J. H. Ellens (Ed.), *Seeking the sacred with psychoactive substances: Chemical paths to spirituality and God* (Vol. II, pp. 179–199). Santa Barbara, CA: Praeger.

Hood, R. W., Jr., & Belzen, J. A. (2005). Research methods in the psychology of religion. In R. F. Paloutzian & C. L. Park (Eds.), *Handbook of the psychology of religion and spirituality* (pp. 62–79). New York, NY: Guilford Press.

Hood, R. W., Jr., & Byrom, G. (2010). Mysticism, madness, and mental health. In J. H. Ellens (Ed.), *The healing power of spirituality: How faith helps humans thrive: Vol. 3. Psychodynamics* (pp. 171–191). Westport, CT: Praeger.

Hood, R. W., Jr., Ghorbani, N., Watson, P. J., Ghramaleki, A. F., Bing, M. B., Davison, H. R., et al. (2001). Dimensions of the Mysticism Scale: Confirming the three factor structure in the United States and Iran. *Journal for the Scientific Study of Religion, 40*, 691–705.

Hood, R. W., Jr., & Hall, J. R. (1980). Gender differences in the description of erotic and mystical experience. *Review of Religious Research, 21*, 195–207.

Hood, R. W., Jr., Hill, P. C., & Williamson, W. P. (2005). *The psychology of religious fundamentalism.* New York, NY: Guilford Press.

Hood, R. W., Jr., & Kimbrough, D. (1995). Serpent-handling Holiness sects: Theoretical considerations. *Journal for the Scientific Study of Religion, 34*, 311–322.

Hood, R. W., Jr., & Morris, R. J. (1981a). Knowledge and experience criteria in the report of mystical experience. *Review of Religious Research, 23*, 76–84.

Hood, R. W., Jr., & Morris, R. J. (1981b). Sensory isolation and the differential elicitation of imagery in intrinsic and extrinsic persons. *Journal for the Scientific Study of Religion, 20*, 261–273.

Hood, R. W., Jr., & Morris, R. J. (1983). Toward a theory of death transcendence. *Journal for the Scientific Study of Religion, 22*, 353–365.

Hood, R. W., Jr., Morris, R. J., & Harvey, D. K. (1993, October). *Religiosity, prayer and their relationship to mystical experience.* Paper presented at the annual meeting of the Religious Research Association, Raleigh, NC.

Hood, R. W., Jr., Morris, R. J., Hickman, S. E., & Watson, P. J. (1995). Martin and Malcolm as cultural icons: An empirical study comparing lower class African American and white males. *Review of Religious Research, 36*, 382–388.

Hood, R. W., Jr., Morris, R. J., & Watson, P. J. (1985). Boundary maintenance, socio-political views, and presidential preference. *Review of Religious Research, 27*, 134–145.

Hood, R. W., Jr., Morris, R. J., & Watson, P. J. (1986). Maintenance of religious fundamentalism. *Psychological Reports, 9*, 547–559.

Hood, R. W., Jr., Morris, R. J., & Watson, P. J. (1989). Prayer experience and religious orientation. *Review of Religious Research, 31*, 39–45.

Hood, R. W., Jr., Morris, R. J., & Watson, P. J. (1990). Quasi-experimental elicitation of the differential report of religious experience among intrinsic and indiscriminately pro-religious types. *Journal for the Scientific Study of Religion, 29*, 164–172.

Hood, R. W., Jr., Morris, R. J., & Watson, P. J. (1991). Male commitment to the cult of the Virgin Mary and the passion of Christ as a function of early maternal bonding. *International Journal for the Psychology of Religion, 1*, 221–231.

Hood, R. W., Jr., Morris, R. J., & Watson, P. J. (1993). Further factor analysis of Hood's Mysticism Scale. *Psychological Reports, 3*, 1176–1178.

Hood, R. W., Jr., Spilka, B., Hunsberger, B., & Gorsuch, R. L. (1996). *The psychology of religion: An empirical approach* (2nd ed.). New York, NY: Guilford Press.

Hood, R. W., Jr., & Williamson, W. P. (2000). An empirical test of the unity thesis: The structure of mystical descriptors in various faith samples. *Journal of Christianity and Psychology, 19*, 222–244.

Hood, R. W., Jr., & Williamson, W. P. (2008a). Contemporary Christian serpent handlers and the new paradigm for the psychology of religion. *Research in the Social Scientific Study of Religion, 19*, 59–89.

Hood, R. W., Jr., & Williamson, W. P. (2008b). *Them that believe: The power and meaning of the Christian serpent-handling tradition*. Berkeley: University of California Press.

Hood, R. W., Jr., & Williamson, W. P. (2014). Case study of the intratextual model of fundamentalism: Serpent handlers and Mark 16:17–18. *Journal of Psychology and Christianity, 33*, 58–69.

Hood, R. W., Jr., Williamson, W. P., & Morris, R. J. (1999). Evaluation of the legitimacy of conversion experience as a function of the five signs of Mark 16. *Review of Religious Research, 41*, 96–109.

Hood, R. W., Jr., Williamson, W. P., & Morris, R. J. (2000). Changing views of serpent handling: A quasi-experimental study. *Journal for the Scientific Study of Religion, 39*, 287–296.

Hooper, T., & Spilka, B. (1970). Some meanings and correlates of future time and death perspectives among college students. *Omega, 1*, 49–56.

Hopkins, E. W. (1923). *Origin and evolution of religion*. New Haven, CT: Yale University Press.

Hopkins, W. L., & Sundararajan, L. (2015). Müntzer and mysticism: A contested connection. *The Humanistic Psychologist, 43*, 103–108.

Horgan, J. (1999). *The undiscovered mind*. New York, NY: Free Press.

Horgan, J. (2006, November 20). The God experiments. *Discover Magazine*. Retrieved from *http://discovermagazine.com/2006/dec/god-experiments*.

Hornbeck, R. G., & Barrett, J. L. (2013). Refining and testing "counterintuitiveness" in virtual reality: Cross-cultural evidence for recall of counterintuitive representations. *International Journal for the Psychology of Religion, 23*, 15–28.

Horner, J., & Dobb, E. (1997). *Dinosaur lives*. New York, NY: HarperCollins.

Horowitz, I. L. (1983a). Symposium on scholarship and sponsorship: Universal standards, not universal beliefs: Further reflections on scientific method and religious sponsors. *Sociological Analysis, 44*, 179–182.

Horowitz, I. L. (1983b). A reply to critics and crusaders. *Sociological Analysis, 44*, 221–225.

Hostetler, J. A. (1974). *Hutterite society*. Baltimore: Johns Hopkins University Press.

Hostetler, J. A. (1980). *Amish society* (3rd ed.). Baltimore: Johns Hopkins University Press.

Hoult, T. F. (1958). *The sociology of religion*. New York, NY: Dryden.

House, J. A. (2008). *Americans' changing lives: Waves I, II, III, and IV codebook*. Ann Arbor: Inter-University Consortium for Political and Social Research, University of Michigan.

Houtman, D., & Aupers, S. (2007). The spiritual turn and decline of tradition: The spread of post-Christian spirituality in 14 Western countries, 1981–2000. *Journal for the Scientific Study of Religion, 46*, 305–320.

Hovi, T. (2004). Religious conviction shaped and maintained by narration. *Archiv für Religionspsychologie, 26*, 35–50.

Howkins, K. G. (1966). *Religious thinking and religious education*. London, UK: Tyndale Press.

Hoyert, D. L., Kochanek, K. D., & Murphy, S. L. (1999). Deaths: Final data for 1997 (DHHS Publication No. 99-1120). *National Vital Statistics Report 47*(19).

Huber, S., Reich, K. H., & Schenker, D. (2000, July). *Studying empirically religious development: Interview, repertory grid, and specific questionnaire techniques*. Paper presented at the Symposium for Psychologists of Religion, Sigtuna, Sweden.

Hudson, W. H. (1939). *Far away and long ago*. London, UK: Dent.

Huelsman, M. A., Piroch, J., & Wasieleski, D. (2006). Relation of religiosity with academic dishonesty in a sample of college students. *Psychological Reports, 99*, 739–742.

Huffman, J. C., Beale, E. E., Celano, C. M., Beach, S. R., Belcher, A. M., Moore, S. V., et al. (2016). Effects of optimism and gratitude on physical activity, biomarkers, and readmissions after an acute coronary syndrome. *Circulation: Cardiovascular Quality and Outcomes, 9*, 55–63.

Hufford, D. J. (1982). *The terror that comes in the night: An experience-centered study of supernatural assault traditions*. Philadelphia, PA: University of Pennsylvania Press.

Hughes, D. E., & Peake, T. H. (2002). Investigating the value of spiritual well-being and psychosocial development in mitigating senior adulthood depression. *Activities, Adaptation, and Aging, 26*(3), 15–35.

Hughes, P. (1954). *A popular history of the Catholic church*. Garden City, NY: Doubleday.

Hundleby, J. D. (1987). Adolescent drug use in a behavioral matrix: A confirmation and comparison of the sexes. *Addictive Behaviors, 12*, 103–112.

Hunsberger, B. (1976). Background religious denomination, parental emphasis, and the religious orientation of university students. *Journal for the Scientific Study of Religion, 15*, 251–255.

Hunsberger, B. (1977). A reconsideration of parochial schools: The case of Mennonites and Roman Catholics. *Mennonite Quarterly Review, 51*, 140–151.

Hunsberger, B. (1978). The religiosity of college students: Stability and change over years at university. *Journal for the Scientific Study of Religion, 17*, 159–164.

Hunsberger, B. (1980). A reexamination of the antecedents of apostasy. *Review of Religious Research, 21*, 158–170.

Hunsberger, B. (1983a). Apostasy: A social learning perspective. *Review of Religious Research, 25*, 21–38.

Hunsberger, B. (1983b). *Current religious position and self-reports of religious socialization influences.* Paper presented at the annual convention of the Society for the Scientific Study of Religion, Knoxville, TN.

Hunsberger, B. (1985a). Parent–university student agreement on religious and nonreligious issues. *Journal for the Scientific Study of Religion, 24*, 314–320.

Hunsberger, B. (1985b). Religion, age, life satisfaction, and perceived sources of religiousness: A study of older persons. *Journal of Gerontology, 40*, 615–620.

Hunsberger, B. (1989). A short version of the Christian orthodoxy scale. *Journal for the Scientific Study of Religion, 28*, 360–365.

Hunsberger, B. (1996). Religious fundamentalism, right-wing authoritarianism, and hostility toward homosexuals in nonChristian religious groups. *International Journal for the Psychology of Religion, 6*, 39–49.

Hunsberger, B. (2000). Swimming against the current: Exceptional cases of apostates and converts. In L. J. Francis & Y. J. Katz (Eds.), *Joining and leaving religion: Research perspectives* (pp. 233–248). Leominster, UK: Gracewing.

Hunsberger, B., Alisat, S., Pancer, S. M., & Pratt, M. (1996). Religious fundamentalism and religious doubts: Content, connections, and complexity of thinking. *International Journal for the Psychology of Religion, 6*, 201–220.

Hunsberger, B. E., & Altemeyer, B. (2006). *Atheists: A groundbreaking study of America's nonbelievers.* Amherst, NY: Prometheus Books.

Hunsberger, B., & Brown, L. B. (1984). Religious socialization, apostasy, and the impact of family background. *Journal for the Scientific Study of Religion, 23*, 239–251.

Hunsberger, B., & Jackson, L. (2005). Religion, meaning, and prejudice. *Journal of Social Issues, 61*, 807–826.

Hunsberger, B., Lea, J., Pancer, S. M., Pratt, M., & McKenzie, B. (1992). Making life complicated: Prompting the use of integratively complex thinking. *Journal of Personality, 60*, 95–114.

Hunsberger, B., McKenzie, B., Pratt, M., & Pancer, S. M. (1993). Religious doubt: A social psychological analysis. *Research in the Social Scientific Study of Religion, 5*, 27–51.

Hunsberger, B., Owusu, V., & Duck, R. (1999). Religion and prejudice in Ghana and Canada: Religious fundamentalism, right-wing authoritarianism and attitudes toward homosexuals and women. *International Journal for the Psychology of Religion, 9*, 181–194.

Hunsberger, B., & Platonow, E. (1986). Religion and helping charitable causes. *Journal of Psychology, 120*, 517–528.

Hunsberger, B., Pratt, M., & Pancer, S. M. (1994). Religious fundamentalism and integrative complexity of thought: A relationship for existential content only? *Journal for the Scientific Study of Religion, 33*, 335–346.

Hunsberger, B., Pratt, M., & Pancer, S. M. (2001a). Adolescent identity formation: Religious exploration and commitment. *Identity: An International Journal of Theory and Research, 1*, 365–387.

Hunsberger, B., Pratt, M., & Pancer, S. M. (2001b). Religious versus nonreligious socialization: Does religious background have implications for adjustment? *International Journal for the Psychology of Religion, 11*, 105–128.

Hunsberger, B., Pratt, M., & Pancer, S. M. (2002). A longitudinal study of religious doubts in high school and beyond: Relationships, stability, and searching for answers. *Journal for the Scientific Study of Religion, 41*, 255–266.

Hunsberger, B., & Watson, B. (1986, November). *The Devil made me do it: Attributions of responsibility to God and Satan.* Paper presented at the annual convention of the Society for the Scientific Study of Religion, Washington, DC.

Hunt, M. (1959). *The natural history of love.* New York, NY: Knopf.

Hunt, R. A. (1972). Mythological–symbolic religious commitment: The LAM scales. *Journal for the Scientific Study of Religion, 11*, 42–52.

Hunt, R. A., & King, M. B. (1978). Religiosity and marriage. *Journal for the Scientific Study of Religion, 17*, 399–406.

Hunter, E. (1951). *Brainwashing in red China*. New York, NY: Vanguard.

Hunter, J. D. (1991). *Culture wars: The struggle to control the family, art, education, law, and politics in America*. New York, NY: Basic Books.

Hunter, W. F. (Ed.). (1989). The case for theological literacy in the psychology of religion [Special issue]. *Journal of Psychology and Theology, 17*.

Hutch, R. A. (1980). The personal ritual of glossolalia. *Journal for the Scientific Study of Religion, 19*, 255–256.

Hutsebaut, D., & Verhoeven, D. (1995). Studying dimensions of God representation: Choosing closed or open-ended research questions. *International Journal for the Psychology of Religion, 5*, 49–60.

Huxley, A. (1962). *Island*. New York, NY: Harper Perennial.

Huxley, J. (1966). A discussion on ritualization of behavior in animals and man: Introduction. *Philosophical Transactions of the Royal Society of London, Series B, Biological Sciences, 251*, 249–272.

Huxley, J. (1968). Ritual in human society. In D. R. Cutler (Ed.), *The religious situation: 1968* (pp. 696–711). Boston, MA: Beacon Press.

Hyde, K. E. (1990). *Religion in childhood and adolescence: A comprehensive review of the research*. Birmingham, AL: Religious Education Press.

Hynson, L. M., Jr. (1975). Religion, attendance, and belief in an afterlife. *Journal for the Scientific Study of Religion, 14*, 285–287.

Iannaccone, L. (1994). Why strict churches are strong. *American Journal of Sociology, 99*, 1180–1211.

Iannaccone, L. (1996). Reassessing church growth: Statistical pitfalls and their consequences. *Journal for the Scientific Study of Religion, 36*, 141–157.

Ibrahim, N., & Abdalla, M. (2010). A critical examination of Qur'an 4:34 and its relevance to intimate partner violence in Muslim families. *Journal of Muslim Mental Health, 5*, 327–349.

Ibrahim, S. E. (1980). Anatomy of Egypt's militant groups. *International Journal of Middle East Studies, 12*, 423–453.

Ibrahim, S. E. (1982). Islamic militancy as a social movement. In A. E. M. Dessouki (Ed.), *Islamic resurgence in the Arab world* (pp. 117–137). New York, NY: Praeger.

Idler, E. L., & Kasl, S. V. (1992). Religion, disability, depression and the timing of death. *American Journal of Sociology, 97*, 1052–1079.

Illich, I. (1976). *Medical nemesis: The expropriation of health*. New York, NY: Pantheon Books.

Inge, D. (1899). *Christian mysticism*. London, UK: Methuen.

Inglehart, R., & Baker, W. E. (2000). Modernization, cultural change, and the persistence of traditional values. *American Sociological Review, 65*, 19–51.

Intermountain Jewish News. (2006, February 24). DNA lab at CU screens for 10 Ashkenazi disorders. p. 12.

Ironson, G., Stuetzle, R., & Fletcher, M. A. (2006). An increase in religiousness/spirituality occurs after HIV diagnosis and predicts slower disease progression over 4 years in people with HIV. *Journal of General Internal Medicine, 21*(Suppl. 5), S62–S68.

Isley, P. J. (1997). Child sexual abuse and the Catholic church: An historical and contemporary review. *Pastoral Psychology, 45*, 277–289.

Ismail, H., Wright, J., Rhodes, P., & Small, N. (2005). Religious beliefs about causes and treatment of epilepsy. *British Journal of General Practice, 55*, 26–31.

Isralowitz, R. E., & Ong, T. (1990). Religious values and beliefs and place of residence as predictors of alcohol use among Chinese college students in Singapore. *International Journal of the Addictions, 25*, 515–529.

Jackson, C. W., Jr., & Kelly, E. L. (1962). Influence of suggestion and subject's prior knowledge in research on sensory deprivation. *Science, 132*, 211–212.

Jackson, G. (1908). *The fact of conversion: The Cole Lectures for 1908*. New York, NY: Revell.

Jackson, L. M. (2001, May). Problems and promise in religious intergroup relations. In V. Saroglou (Chair), *Pluralism and identity*. Symposium conducted at the University Catholique de Louvain, Louvain, Belgium.

Jackson, L. M., & Esses, V. M. (1997). Of scripture and ascription: The relation between religious fundamentalism and intergroup helping. *Personality and Social Psychology Bulletin, 23*, 893–906.

Jackson, L. M., & Hunsberger, B. (1999). An intergroup perspective on religion and prejudice. *Journal for the Scientific Study of Religion, 38*, 509–523.

Jackson, N. J., & Spilka, B. (1980, April 10). *Correlates of religious mystical experience: A selective study*. Paper presented at the annual convention of the Rocky Mountain Psychological Association, Tucson, AZ.

Jacobs, D. M. (1992). *Secret life: First-hand accounts of UFO abductions*. New York, NY: Simon & Schuster.

Jacobs, J. L. (1984). The economy of love in religious commitment: The deconversion of women from nontraditional religious movements. *Journal for the Scientific Study of Religion, 23*, 155–171.

Jacobs, J. L. (1987). Deconversion from religious movements: An analysis of charismatic bonding and spiritual commitment. *Journal for the Scientific Study of Religion, 26*, 294–308.

Jacobs, J. L. (1989). *Divine disenchantment.* Bloomington, IN: Indiana University Press.

Jacobs, J. L. (1996). Women, ritual, and secrecy: The creation of crypto-Jewish culture. *Journal for the Scientific Study of Religion, 35,* 97–108.

Jacobs, J. L. (2002). *The hidden heritage: The legacy of the Crypto-Jews.* Berkeley: University of California Press.

Jacobs, T. (2015, May 5). Why atheists terrify believers. *Pacific Standard.* Retrieved from *www.psmag. com/health-and-behavior/why-atheists-terrify-believers.*

Jacobson, C. J., Jr., Luckhaupt, S. E., Delaney, S., & Tsevat, J. (2006). Religio-biography, coping, and meaning-making among persons with HIV/AIDS. *Journal for the Scientific Study of Religion, 45,* 39–56.

Jacobson, E., & Bruno, J. (1994). Narrative variants and major psychiatric illnesses in close encounter and abduction narrators. In A. Pritchard, D. E. Prichard, J. E. Mack, P. Kasey, & C. Yapp (Eds.), *Alien discussions: Proceedings of the Abduction Study Conference, MIT* (pp. 304–309). Cambridge, MA: North Cambridge Press.

James, W. (1950). *The principles of psychology* (2 vols.). New York, NY: Dover. (Original work published 1890)

James, W. (1985). *The varieties of religious experience.* Cambridge, MA: Harvard University Press. (Original work published 1902)

Jang, S. J., & Franzen, A. B. (2013). Is being "spiritual" enough without being religious?: A study of violent and property crimes among emerging adults. *Criminology, 51,* 595–627.

Jankowski, P. J., Hardy, S. A., Zamboanga, B. L., Ham, L. S., Schwartz, S. J., Kim, S. Y., et al. (2015). Religiousness and level of hazardous alcohol use: A latent profile analysis. *Journal of Youth and Adolescence, 44,* 1968–1983.

Jankowski, P. J., Sandage, S. J., & Hill, P. C. (2013). Differentiation-based models of forgiveness, mental health, and social justice commitment: Mediator effects for differentiation of self and humility. *Journal of Positive Psychology, 8,* 412–424.

Janssen, J., de Hart, J., & den Draak, C. (1990). A content analysis of the praying practices of Dutch youth. *Journal for the Scientific Study of Religion, 29,* 99–107.

Janssen, J., de Hart, J., & Gerardts, M. (1994). Images of God in adolescence. *International Journal for the Psychology of Religion, 4,* 105–121.

Jantzen, G. M. (1995). *Power, gender, and Christian mysticism.* Cambridge, UK: Cambridge University Press.

Janus, S. S., & Janus, C. L. (1993). *The Janus report on sexual behavior.* New York, NY: Wiley.

Jarusiewicz, B. (2000). Spirituality and addiction: Relationship to recovery and relapse. *Alcoholism Treatment Quarterly, 18,* 99–109.

Jaynes, J. (1976). *The origin of consciousness in the breakdown of the bicameral mind.* Boston, MA: Houghton Mifflin.

Jenkins, R. A., & Pargament, K. I. (1988). The relationship between cognitive appraisals and psychological adjustment in cancer patients. *Social Science and Medicine, 26,* 625–633.

Jewish Telegraphic Agency. (2015, June 28). US Jews among biggest supporters of same-sex marriage, data shows. Retrieved from *www.JTA. org/2015/06/38/nred-opinion/united-states/data.*

Jim, H. S. L., Pustejovsky, J. E., Park, C. L., Danhauer, S. C., Sherman, A. C., Fitchett, G., et al. (2015). Religion, spirituality, and physical health in cancer patients: A meta-analysis. *Cancer, 121*(21) 3760–3768.

Jindra, I. W. (2008). Religious stage development among converts to different religious groups. *International Journal for the Psychology of Religion, 18,* 195–215.

John Jay College of Criminal Justice. (2004). *The nature and scope of the problem of sexual abuse of minors by Catholic priests and deacons in the United States.* New York, NY: Author.

Johnson, B. (1961). Do Holiness sects socialize in dominant values? *Social Forces, 39,* 309–317.

Johnson, B. (1963). On church and sect. *American Sociological Review, 28,* 539–549.

Johnson, B. (1971). Church and sect revisited. *Journal for the Scientific Study of Religion, 10,* 124–137.

Johnson, B. (2001). Spiritual marketplace: Baby boomers and the remaking of American religion [Book review]. *Sociology of Religion, 62,* 140–142.

Johnson, B. L., Eberly, S., Duke, J. T., & Sartain, D. H. (1988). Wives' employment status and marital happiness of religious couples. *Review of Religious Research, 29,* 259–270.

Johnson, B. R., Jang, S. J., Larson, D. B., & Li, S. D. (2001). Does adolescent religious commitment matter?: A reexamination of the effects of religiosity on delinquency. *Journal of Research in Crime and Delinquency, 38,* 22–44.

Johnson, D. M., Williams, J. S., & Bromley, D. G. (1986). Religion, health and healing: Findings from a Southern city. *Sociological Analysis, 47,* 66–73.

Johnson, D. P. (1979). Dilemmas of charismatic leadership: The case of the People's Temple. *Sociological Analysis, 40,* 315–323.

Johnson, D. P., & Mullins, L. C. (1989). Subjective and social dimensions of religiosity and loneliness among the well elderly. *Review of Religious Research, 31,* 3–15.

Johnson, E. L., & Watson, P. J. (2012). Worldview

communities and the science of psychology. *Research in the Social Scientific Study of Religion, 23,* 269–283.

Johnson, K. A., Cohen, A. B., & Okun, M. A. (2016). God is watching you . . . but also watching over you: The influence of benevolent God representations on secular volunteerism among Christians. *Psychology of Religion and Spirituality, 7,* 363–374.

Johnson, K. A., Li, Y. J., Cohen, A. B., & Okun, M. A. (2013). Friends in high places: The influence of authoritarian and benevolent God concepts on social attitudes and behaviors. *Psychology of Religion and Spirituality, 5,* 15–22.

Johnson, K. A., Memon, R., Alladin, A., Cohen, A. B., & Okun, M. A. (2015). Who helps the Samaritan?: The influence of religious vs. secular primes on spontaneous helping of members of religious outgroups. *Journal of Cognition and Culture, 15,* 217–231.

Johnson, K. A., Okun, M. A., & Cohen, A. B. (2015). The mind of the Lord: Measuring authoritarian and benevolent God representations. *Psychology of Religion and Spirituality, 7,* 227–238.

Johnson, M. A. (1973). Family life and religious commitment. *Review of Religious Research, 14,* 144–150.

Johnson, M. K., Rowatt, W. C., & LaBouff, J. P. (2012). Religiosity and prejudice revisited: In-group favoritism, out-group derogation, or both? *Psychology of Religion and Spirituality, 4,* 154–168.

Johnson, M. K., Rowatt, W. C., & LaBouff, J. P., Patock-Peckham, J., & Carlisle, R. D. (2012). Facets of right-wing authoritarianism mediate the relationship between religious fundamentalism and attitudes toward Arabs and African-Americans. *Journal for the Scientific Study of Religion, 51,* 128–142.

Johnson, P. E. (1959). *Psychology of religion* (rev. ed.). New York, NY: Abingdon Press.

Johnson, S., & Spilka, B. (1988, October 30). *Coping with breast cancer: The role of religion.* Paper presented at the annual convention of the Society for the Scientific Study of Religion, Chicago, IL.

Johnson, S., & Spilka, B. (1991). Religion and the breast cancer patient: The roles of clergy and faith. *Journal of Religion and Health, 30,* 21–33.

Johnson, T. J., Sheets, V. L., & Kristeller, J. L. (2008). Identifying mediators of the relationship between religious/spirituality and alcohol use. *Journal of Studies on Alcohol and Drugs, 69,* 160–170.

Johnson, W. (1974). *The search for transcendence.* New York, NY: Harper & Row.

Johnston, J. C., de Groot, H., & Spanos, N. P. (1995). The structure of paranormal belief: A factor-analytic investigation. *Imagination, Cognition and Personality, 14,* 165–174.

Johnstone, R. L. (1966). *The effectiveness of Lutheran elementary and secondary schools as agencies of Christian education.* St. Louis, MO: Concordia Seminary Research Center.

Jones, J. W. (2008). *Blood that cries out from the earth: The psychology of religious terrorism.* New York, NY: Oxford University Press.

Jones, R. H. (1986). *Science and mysticism.* London, UK: Associated Universities Press.

Jones, R. H. (2016). *Philosophy of mysticism: Raids on the ineffable.* Albany, NY: State University of New York Press.

Jones, S. L. (1994). A constructive relationship for religion with the science and profession of psychology: Perhaps the boldest model yet. *American Psychologist, 49,* 184–199.

Jones, W. H. S. (Trans.). (1923). *Hippocrates* (Vol. 2). Cambridge, MA: Harvard University Press.

Jong, J. (2014, November 11). How not to criticize the (evolutionary) cognitive science of religion. *Los Angeles Review of Books.* Retrieved from *http://marginalia.lareviewofbooks.org/criticize-evolutionary-cognitive-science-religion.*

Jong, J., Halberstadt, J., & Bluemke, M. (2012). Foxhole atheism, revisited: The effects of mortality salience on explicit and implicit religious belief. *Journal of Experimental Social Psychology, 48,* 983–989.

Jong, J., Zahl, B. P., & Sharp, C. A. (2017). Indirect and implicit measures of religiosity. In R. Finke & C. D. Bader (Eds.), *Faithful measures: New methods in the measurement of religion* (pp. 78–107). New York, NY: New York University Press.

Jowett, B. (1907). *The dialogues of Plato* (Vol. 1). New York, NY: Scribner.

Joyce, C. R. B., & Weldon, R. M. C. (1965). The objective efficacy of prayer: A double-blind clinical trial. *Journal of Chronic Diseases, 18,* 367–377.

Judah, J. S. (1974). *Hare Krishna and the counterculture.* New York, NY: Wiley.

Juergensmeyer, M. (2000). *Terror in the mind of God: The global rise of religious violence.* Berkeley: University of California Press.

Jull-Johnson, D. S. (1995). The use of social bereavement rituals by gay men confronting HIV-related loss. *Dissertation Abstracts International, 56*(6), 3449B.

Jung, C. G. (1933). *Modern man in search of a soul* (W. S. Dell & C. F. Baynes, Trans.). New York, NY: Harcourt, Brace.

Jung, C. G. (1964). Flying saucers: A modern myth of things seen in the skies. In H. Read, M. Fordham, & G. Adler (Eds.) & R. F. C. Hull (Trans.), *The collected works of C. G. Jung* (Vol. 10, pp. 309–433). Princeton, NJ: Princeton University Press. (Original work published 1958)

Jung, C. G. (1969). A psychological approach to the dogma of the Trinity. In H. Read, M. Fordham, & G. Adler (Eds.) & R. F. C. Hull (Trans.), *The collected works of C. G. Jung* (2nd ed., Vol. 11, pp. 107–200). Princeton, NJ: Princeton University Press. (Original work published 1948)

Jung, J. H. (2015). Sense of divine involvement and sense of meaning in life: Religious tradition as a contingency. *Journal for the Scientific Study of Religion, 54*, 119–133.

Kagan, J. (1998). *Three seductive ideas*. Cambridge, MA: Harvard University Press.

Kahneman, D. (2003). A perspective on judgment and choice. *American Psychologist, 58*, 697–720.

Kaldor, P., Francis, L. J., & Fisher, J. W. (2002). Personality and spirituality: Christian prayer and Eastern meditation are not the same. *Pastoral Psychology, 50*, 167–172.

Kalish, R. A. (1981). *Death, grief, and caring relationships*. New York: Brooks/Cole.

Kalton, M. C. (2000). Green spirituality: Horizontal transcendence. In P. Young-Eisendrath & M. E. Miller (Eds.), *The psychology of nature spirituality: Integrity, wisdom, and transcendence* (pp. 187–200). London, UK: Routledge.

Kamble, S. V., Watson, P. J., Marigoudar, S., & Chen, Z. (2014). Varieties of openness and religious commitment in India: Relationships of attitudes toward Hinduism, Hindu religious reflection, and religious schema. *Archive for the Psychology of Religion, 36*, 172–198.

Kandel, D. B., & Sudit, M. (1982). Drinking practices among urban adults in Israel: A cross-cultural comparison. *Journal of Studies on Alcohol, 43*, 1–16.

Kane, D., Cheston, S. E., & Greer, J. (1993). Perceptions of God by survivors of childhood sexual abuse: An exploratory study in an underresearched area. *Journal of Psychology and Theology, 21*, 228–237.

Kanekar, S., & Merchant, S. M. (2001). Helping norms in relation to religious affiliation. *Journal of Social Psychology, 141*, 617–626.

Kanpol, B., & Poplin, M. (Eds.). (2017). *Christianity and the secular border patrol: The loss of Judeo-Christian knowledge* (Critical Education & Ethics, Vol. 9). New York, NY: Peter Lang.

Kapogiannis, D., Barbey, A. K., Su, M., Krueger, F., & Grafman, J. (2009). Neuroanatomical variability of religiosity. *PLOS One, 4*(9), e7180.

Kapogiannis, D., Dehpande, G., Krueger, F., Thornburg, M. P., & Grafman, J. H. (2014). Brain networks shaping religious belief. *Brain Connectivity, 4*, 70–79.

Karasu, T. B. (1999). Spiritual psychotherapy. *American Journal of Psychotherapy, 53*, 143–162.

Karlsen, C. F. (1989). *The devil in the shape of a woman*. New York, NY: Random House.

Karsh, E. (2002, December). Intifada II: The long trail of Arab anti-Semitism. *Commentary*, pp. 49–53.

Kass, J. D., Friedman, R., Leserman, J., Zuttermeister, P. C., & Benson, H. (1991). Health outcomes and a new index of spiritual experience. *Journal for the Scientific Study of Religion, 30*, 203–211.

Kastenbaum, R. J. (1981). *Death, society, and human experience*. St. Louis, MO: Mosby.

Katchadourian, H. A. (1989). *Fundamentals of human sexuality*. New York, NY: Holt, Rinehart & Winston.

Katz, S. T. (1977). *Mysticism and philosophical analysis*. New York, NY: Oxford University Press.

Katz, S. T. (1983). *Mysticism and religious traditions*. New York, NY: Oxford University Press.

Katz, S. T. (1992). *Mysticism and language*. New York, NY: Oxford University Press.

Katz, Y. J., & Schmida, M. (1992). Validation of the Student Religiosity Questionnaire. *Educational and Psychological Measurement, 52*, 353–356.

Kay, A. C., Gaucher, D., McGregor, I., & Nash, K. (2010). Religious belief as compensatory control. *Personality and Social Psychology Review, 14*, 37–48.

Kay, W. K. (1996). Bringing child psychology to religious curricula: The cautionary tale of Goldman and Piaget. *Educational Review, 48*, 205–215.

Kay, W. K., & Francis, L. J. (1999). The young British atheist: A social-psychological profile. *Journal of Empirical Theology, 8*, 5–26.

Kazantzakis, N. (1961). *Report to Greco*. New York, NY: Simon & Schuster.

Kearl, M. (1989). *Endings: A sociology of death and dying*. New York, NY: Oxford University Press.

Kearl, M. (2002). Euthanasia and the right to die. Retrieved February 21, 2002, from *www.trinity.edu/~mkearl/dtheuth.html*.

Kedem, P., & Cohen, D. W. (1987). The effects of religious education on moral judgment. *Journal of Psychology and Judaism, 11*, 4–14.

Kegeles, S. M., Coates, C. J., Christopher, T. A., & Lazarus, J. L., (1989). Perceptions of AIDS: The continuing saga of AIDS-related stigma. *AIDS, 3*(Suppl.), S253–S258.

Kelemen, D. (1999). Why are rocks pointy?: Children's preferences for teleological explanations of the natural world. *Developmental Psychology, 35*, 1440–1452.

Kelemen, D. (2004). Are children "intuitive theists"?: Reasoning about purpose and design in nature. *Psychological Science, 15*, 295–301.

Kelemen, D., & Rosset, E. (2009). The human function compunction: Teleological explanation in adults. *Cognition, 111*, 138–143.

Kelley, D. M. (1972). *Why conservative churches are growing*. New York, NY: Harper & Row.

Kelley, H. H. (1967). Attribution theory in social psychology. In D. Levine (Ed.), *Nebraska Symposium on Motivation* (Vol. 15, pp. 192–238). Lincoln: University of Nebraska Press.

Kelley, M. L., Power, T. G., & Wimbush, D. D. (1992). Determinants of disciplinary practices in low-income black mothers. *Child Development, 63,* 573–582.

Kelly, E. F., Kelly, E. W., Crabtree, A., Gauld, A., Grosso, M., & Greyson, B. (Eds.). (2007). *Irreducible mind: Toward a psychology for the 21st century.* Lanham, MD: Rowan & Littlefield.

Kelsey, M. T. (1964). *Tongue speaking: An experiment in spiritual experience.* Garden City, NY: Doubleday.

Kemper, T. D. (1978). *A social interaction theory of emotions.* New York, NY: Wiley.

Keniston, K. (1968). *Young radicals.* New York, NY: Harcourt, Brace & World.

Keniston, K. (1971). *Youth and dissent.* New York, NY: Harcourt Brace Jovanovich.

Kennedy, J. E., Rosati, K. G., Spann, L. H., Neelon, F. A., & Rosati, R. A. (n.d.). *Changing for the better: Spirituality supports healthy lifestyle choices.* Unpublished manuscript, Rice Diet Program and Department of Medicine, Duke University Medical Center, Durham, NC.

Kent, S. A. (2001). *From slogans to mantras: Social protest and religious conversion in the late Vietnam war era.* Syracuse, NY: Syracuse University Press.

Kerr, C. W., Donnelly, J. P., Wright, S. T., Kuszczak, S. M., Banas, A., Grant, P. C., & Luczkiewicz, D. L. (2014). End-of-life dreams and visions: A longitudinal study of hospice patients' experiences. *Journal of Palliative Medicine, 17,* 296.

Keysar, A. (2007). Who are America's atheists and agnostics? In B. A. Kosmin & A. Keysar (Eds.), *Secularism and secularity: Contemporary international perspectives* (pp. 33–39). Hartford, CT: Institute for the Study of Secularism in Society and Culture.

Keysar, A., & Kosmin, B. A. (1995). The impact of religious identification on differences in educational attainment among American women in 1990. *Journal for the Scientific Study of Religion, 34,* 49–62.

Keysar, A., & Kosmin, B. A. (2007). The free thinkers and a free market of religion. In B. A. Kosmin & A. Keysar (Eds.), *Secularism and secularity: Contemporary international perspectives* (pp. 17–39). Hartford, CT: Institute for the Study of Secularism in Society and Culture.

Keysar, A., & Kosmin, B. A. (2008). *International survey: Worldviews and opinions of scientists, India 2007–08 summary report.* Hartford, CT: Institute for the Study of Secularism in Society and Culture.

Khan, Z. H., Sultana, S., & Watson, P. J. (2009). Pakistani Muslims dealing with cancer: Relationships with religious coping, religious orientation, and psychological distress. *Research in the Social Scientific Study of Religion, 20,* 217–237.

Khan, Z. H., & Watson, P. J. (2006). Construction of the Pakistani Religious Coping Practices Scale: Correlations with religious coping, religious orientation, and reactions to stress among Muslim university students. *International Journal for the Psychology of Religion, 16,* 101–112.

Khan, Z. H., Watson, P. J., & Chen, Z. (2016). Muslim spirituality, religious coping, and reactions to terrorism among Pakistani university students. *Journal of Religion and Health, 55*(6), 2086–2098.

Khwaja, G. A., Singh, G., & Chaudry, N. (2007). Epilepsy and religion. *Annals of Indian Academy of Neurology, 10,* 165–168.

Kidorf, I. W. (1966). The shiva: A form of group psychotherapy. *Journal of Religion and Health, 5,* 43–46.

Kieren, D. K., & Munro, B. (1987). Following the leaders: Parents' influence on adolescent religious activity. *Journal for the Scientific Study of Religion, 26,* 249–255.

Kiev, A. (1966). Prescientific psychiatry. In S. Arieti (Ed.), *American handbook of psychiatry* (Vol. 3, pp. 166–179). New York, NY: Basic Books.

Kilbourne, B. K. (1983). The Conway and Siegelman claim against religious cults: An assessment of their data. *Journal for the Scientific Study of Religion, 22,* 380–385.

Kilbourne, B. K., & Richardson, J. T. (1984). Psychotherapy and new religions in a pluralistic society. *American Psychologist, 39,* 237–251.

Kilbourne, B. K., & Richardson, J. T. (1986). Cultphobia. *Thought, 61,* 258–266.

Kilbourne, B. K., & Richardson, J. T. (1989). Paradigm conflict, types of conversion, and conversion theories. *Sociological Analysis, 50,* 1–21.

Kildahl, J. P. (1972). *The psychology of speaking in tongues.* New York, NY: Harper & Row.

Kim, B. (1979). Religious deprogramming and subjective reality. *Sociological Analysis, 40,* 197–207.

Kimball, C. N., Cook, K. V., Boyatzis, C. J., & Leonard, K. C. (2016). Exploring emerging adults' relational spirituality: A longitudinal, mixed-methods analysis. *Psychology of Religion and Spirituality, 8,* 110–118.

Kimble, M. A. (1995). Pastoral care. In M. A. Kimble, S. H. McFadden, J. W. Ellor, & J. J. Seeber (Eds.), *Aging, spirituality and religion* (pp. 131–147). Minneapolis, MN: Fortress Press.

Kimbrough, D. L. (1995). *Taking up serpents: Snake handling in eastern Kentucky.* Chapel Hill: University of North Carolina Press.

Kim-Spoon, J., Farley, J. P., Holmes, C., Longo, G. S., & McCullough, M. E. (2014). Processes linking parents' and adolescents' religiousness and adolescent substance use: Monitoring and self-control. *Journal of Youth and Adolescence, 43*, 745–756.

Kim-Spoon, J., McCullough, M. E., Bickel, W. K., Farley, J. P., & Longo, G. S. (2015). Longitudinal associations among religiousness, delay discounting, and substance use initiation in early adolescence. *Journal of Research on Adolescence. 25*, 36–43.

King, D. G. (1990). Religion and health relationships: A review. *Journal of Religion and Health, 29*, 101–112.

King, M., Jones, L., Barnes, K., Low, J., Walker, C., Wilkinson, S., et al. (2006). Measuring spiritual belief: Development and standardization of a Beliefs and Values Scale. *Psychological Medicine, 36*, 417–425.

King, P. E. (2003). The influence of religion on fathers' relationships with their children. *Journal of Marriage and the Family, 65*, 382–395.

King, P. E., Furrow, J. L., & Roth, N. (2002). The influence of families and peers on adolescent religiousness. *Journal of Psychology and Christianity, 21*, 109–120.

King, V., Elder, G. H., Jr., & Whitbeck, L. B. (1997). Religious involvement among rural youth: An ecological and life-course perspective. *Journal of Research on Adolescence, 7*, 431–456.

Kirk, S. A., & Kutchins, H. (1992). *The selling of DSM: The rhetoric of science in psychiatry.* New York, NY: Aldine de Gruyter.

Kirkpatrick, L. A. (1988). The Conway–Siegelman data on religious cults: Kilbourne's analysis reassessed (again). *Journal for the Scientific Study of Religion, 27*, 117–121.

Kirkpatrick, L. A. (1992). An attachment-theory approach to the psychology of religion. *International Journal for the Psychology of Religion, 2*, 3–28.

Kirkpatrick, L. A. (1993). Fundamentalism, Christian orthodoxy, and intrinsic religious orientation as predictors of discriminatory attitudes. *Journal for the Scientific Study of Religion, 32*, 256–268.

Kirkpatrick, L. A. (1994). The role of attachment in religious belief and behavior. *Advances in Personal Relationships, 5*, 239–265.

Kirkpatrick, L. A. (1995). Attachment theory and religious experience. In R. W. Hood, Jr. (Ed.), *Handbook of religious experience* (pp. 446–475). Birmingham, AL: Religious Education Press.

Kirkpatrick, L. A. (1997). A longitudinal study of changes in religious belief and behavior as a function of individual differences in attachment style. *Journal for the Scientific Study of Religion, 36*, 207–217.

Kirkpatrick, L. A. (1998). God as a substitute attachment figure: A longitudinal study of adult attachment style and religious change in college students. *Personality and Social Psychology Bulletin, 24*, 961–973.

Kirkpatrick, L. A. (1999). Attachment and religious representations and behavior. In J. Cassidy & P. R. Shaver (Eds.), *Handbook of attachment: Theory, research, and clinical applications* (pp. 803–822). New York, NY: Guilford Press.

Kirkpatrick, L. A. (2005). *Attachment, evolution, and the psychology of religion.* New York, NY: Guilford Press.

Kirkpatrick, L. A. (2006a). Rejoinder: Response to Beit-Hallahmi and Watts. *Archive for the Psychology of Religion, 28*, 71–79.

Kirkpatrick, L. A. (2006b). Religion is not an adaptation. In P. McNamara (Ed.), *Where God and science meet* (Vol. 1, pp. 159–179). Westport, CT: Praeger.

Kirkpatrick, L. A., & Hood, R. W., Jr. (1990). Intrinsic–extrinsic religious orientation: The boon or bane of contemporary psychology of religion? *Journal for the Scientific Study of Religion, 29*, 442–462.

Kirkpatrick, L. A., Hood, R. W., Jr., & Hartz, G. W. (1991). Fundamentalist religion conceptualized in terms of Rokeach's theory of the open and closed mind: New perspectives on some old ideas. In M. L. Lynn & D. O. Moberg (Eds.), *Research in the social scientific study of religion* (Vol. 3, pp. 157–179). Greenwich, CT: JAI Press.

Kirkpatrick, L. A., & Shaver, P. R. (1990). Attachment theory and religion: Childhood attachments, religious beliefs, and conversion. *Journal for the Scientific Study of Religion, 29*, 315–334.

Kirkpatrick, L. A., & Shaver, P. R. (1992). An attachment-theoretical approach to romantic love and religious belief. *Personality and Social Psychology Bulletin, 18*, 266–275.

Kittrie, N. (1971). *The right to be different.* Baltimore: John Hopkins University Press.

Klaczynski, P. A., & Gordon, D. H. (1996). Self-serving influences on adolescents' evaluations of belief-relevant evidence. *Journal of Experimental Child Psychology, 62*, 317–339.

Klass, M. (1995). *Ordered universes: Approaches to the anthropology of religion.* Boulder, CO: Westview Press.

Klassen, D. W., & McDonald, M. J. (2002). Quest and identity development: Re-examining pathways for existential research. *International Journal for the Psychology of Religion, 12*, 189–200.

Klausner, S. Z. (1964). *Psychiatry and religion.* New York, NY: Free Press.

Kliewer, W., & Murrelle, L. (2007). Risk and protective factors for adolescent substance use: Findings from a study in selected Central American countries. *Journal of Adolescent Health, 40,* 448–455.

Klingberg, G. (1959). A study of religious experience in children from nine to thirteen years of age. *Religious Education, 54,* 211–216.

Klinger, E. (1971). *Structure and functions of fantasy.* New York, NY: Wiley.

Klopfer, F. J., & Price, W. F. (1979). Euthanasia acceptance as related to afterlife belief and other attitudes. *Omega, 9,* 245–253.

Kluegel, J. R. (1980). Denominational mobility: Current patterns and recent trends. *Journal for the Scientific Study of Religion, 19,* 26–39.

Kobau, R., Sniezek, J., Zack, M. M., Lucas, R. E., & Burns, A. (2010). Well-being assessment: An evaluation of well-being scales for public health and population estimates of well-being among US adults. *Applied Psychology: Health and Well-Being, 2,* 272–297.

Koch, P. (1994). *Solitude: A philosophical encounter.* Chicago, IL: Open Court.

Koenig, H., Patterson, G. R., & Meador, K. G. (1997). Religion index for psychiatric research: A 5-item measure for use in health outcome studies. *American Journal of Psychiatry, 154,* 885.

Koenig, H. G. (1994a). *Aging and God: Spiritual pathways to mental health in midlife and later years.* New York, NY: Haworth Press.

Koenig, H. G. (1994b). *Self-destructive behaviors related to death in physically ill elderly men: Pilot data.* Unpublished manuscript, Duke University Medical Center, Durham, NC.

Koenig, H. G. (1995). Use of acute hospital services and mortality among religious and non-religious copers with medical illness. *Journal of Religious Gerontology, 9*(3), 1–22.

Koenig, H. G. (1997). *Is religion good for your health?* New York, NY: Haworth Press.

Koenig, H. G. (Ed.). (1998). *Handbook of religion and mental health.* San Diego, CA: Academic Press.

Koenig, H. G. (2000). Religion, well-being, and health in the elderly: The scientific evidence for an association. In J. A. Thorson (Ed.), *Perspectives on spiritual well-being and aging* (pp. 84–97). Springfield, IL: Charles C Thomas.

Koenig, H. G. (2012). Religion, spirituality, and health: The research and clinical implications. *International Scholarly Research Network, 2012,* 1–33.

Koenig, H. G., George, L. K., & Siegler, I. C. (1988). The use of religion and other emotion-regulating coping strategies among older adults. *The Gerontologist, 28,* 303–310.

Koenig, H. G., King, D. E., & Carson, V. B. (2012). *Handbook of religion and health* (2nd ed.). New York, NY: Oxford University Press.

Koenig, H. G., Kvale, J. N., & Ferrel, C. (1988). Religion and well-being in later life. *The Gerontologist, 28,* 18–28.

Koenig, H. G., & Larson, D. B. (2001). Religion and mental health: Evidence for an association. *International Review of Psychiatry, 13,* 67–78.

Koenig, H. G., Larson, D. B., Hays, J. C., McCullough, M. E., George, L. K., Branch, P. S., et al. (1998). Religion and the survival of 1010 hospitalized veterans. *Journal of Religion and Health, 37,* 15–30.

Koenig, H. G., McCullough, M. E., & Larson, D. B. (2001). *Handbook of religion and health.* New York, NY: Oxford University Press.

Koenig, H. G., Smiley, M., & Gonzales, J. A. P. (1988). *Religion, health, and aging.* New York, NY: Greenwood Press.

Kohlberg, L. (1964). Development of moral character and moral ideology. In M. L. Hoffman & L. W. Hoffman (Eds.), *Review of child development research* (pp. 383–431). New York, NY: Russell Sage Foundation.

Kohlberg, L. (1969). Stage and sequence: The cognitive-developmental approach to socialization. In D. A. Goslin (Ed.), *Handbook of socialization theory and research* (pp. 347–480). Chicago, IL: Rand McNally.

Kohlberg, L. (1980). Stages of moral development as a basis for moral education. In B. Munsey (Ed.), *Moral development, moral education, and Kohlberg* (pp. 15–98). Birmingham, AL: Religious Education Press.

Kohlberg, L. (1981). *Essays on moral development: Vol. 1. The philosophy of moral development: Moral stages and the idea of justice.* San Francisco, CA: Harper & Row.

Kohlberg, L. (1984). *Essays on moral development: Vol. 2. The psychology of moral development: The nature and validity of moral stages.* San Francisco, CA: Harper & Row.

Kohls, N., Hack, A., & Walach, H. (2008). Measuring the unmeasurable by ticking boxes and actually opening Pandora's box: Mixed methods research as a useful tool for investigating exceptional spiritual experiences. *Archive for the Psychology of Religion, 30,* 155–187.

Kohls, N., & Walach, H. (2006). Exceptional experiences and spiritual practice: A new measurement approach. *Spirituality and Health International, 7,* 125–150.

Kohls, N., & Walach, H. (2007). Psychological distress, experiences of ego loss and spirituality: Exploring the effects of spiritual practice. *Social Behavior and Personality, 35,* 1301–1316.

Kohls, N., Walach, H., & Wirtz, M. (2009). The relationship between spiritual experiences, transpersonal trust, social support, and sense of coherence and mental distress: A comparison of spiritually practising and non-practising samples. *Mental Health, Religion and Culture, 12*(1), 1–23.

Kolakowski, L. (1985). *Bergson.* New York, NY: Oxford University Press.

Koltko, M. E. (1993, August 21). *Religion and vocational development: The neglected relationship.* Paper presented at the annual convention of the American Psychological Association, Toronto, Ontario, Canada.

Konig, R., Eisinga, R., & Scheepers, P. (2000). Explaining the relationship between Christian religion and anti-Semitism in the Netherlands. *Review of Religious Research, 41,* 373–393.

Kooistra, W. P., & Pargament, K. I. (1999). Religious doubting in parochial school adolescents. *Journal of Psychology and Theology, 27,* 33–42.

Koole, S. L., McCullough, M. E., Kuhl, J., & Roelofsma, P. H. M. P. (2010). Why religion's burdens are light: From religiosity to implicit self-regulation. *Personality and Social Psychology Review, 14,* 95–107.

Kopplin, D. (1976). *Religious orientations of college students and related personality characteristics.* Paper presented at the annual convention of the American Psychological Association, Washington, DC.

Körver, J. W. (2015). [Review of the book *APA handbook of psychology, religion and spirituality* (Vols. 1–2) by K. I. Pargament]. *International Journal for the Psychology of Religion, 25,* 250–254.

Köse, A., & Loewenthal, K. M. (2000). Conversion motifs among British converts to Islam. *International Journal for the Psychology of Religion, 10*(2), 101–110.

Kosmin, B. A., & Keysar, A. (Eds.). (2007). *Secularism and secularity: Contemporary international perspectives.* Hartford, CT: Institute for the Study of Secularism in Society and Culture.

Kosmin, B. A., & Lachman, S. P. (1993). *One nation under God.* New York, NY: Harmony Books.

Kosmin, B. A., Mayer, E., & Keysar, A. (2001, December 19). *American Religious Identification Survey 2001.* New York, NY: Graduate Center of the City University of New York.

Koster, J. P. (1989). *The atheist syndrome.* Brentwood, TN: Wolgemuth & Hyatt.

Kotre, J. N. (1971). *The view from the border.* Chicago, IL: Aldine/Atherton.

Kramer, D. A. (2000). Wisdom as a classical source of human strength: Conceptualization and empirical inquiry. *Journal of Social and Clinical Psychology, 19,* 83–101.

Kramrisch, S., Otto, J., Ruck, C., & Wasson, R. (1986). *Persephone's quest: Etheogens and the origin of religion.* New Haven, CT: Yale University Press.

Krause, N. (1999). Religious support. In *Multidimensional measurement of religiousness/spirituality for use in health research: A report of the Fetzer Institute/National Institute on Aging Working Group* (pp. 57–64). Kalamazoo, MI: Fetzer Institute.

Krause, N. (2002). Common facets of religion, unique facets of religion, and life satisfaction among older African Americans. *Journal of Gerontology, 57B,* S332–S347.

Krause, N. (2003). Religious meaning and subjective well-being in late life. *Journals of Gerontology, 58B,* S160–S170.

Krause, N. (2004a). Assessing the relationships among prayer expectancies, race, and self-esteem in late life. *Journal for the Scientific Study of Religion, 43,* 395–408.

Krause, N. (2004b). Common facets of religion, unique facets of religion, and life satisfaction among older African Americans. *Journals of Gerontology, 59B,* 109–117.

Krause, N. (2007a). Evaluating the stress-buffering function of meaning in life among older people. *Journal of Aging and Health, 19,* 792–812.

Krause, N. (2007b). Longitudinal study of social support and meaning in life. *Psychology and Aging, 22,* 456–469.

Krause, N. (2009). Meaning in life and mortality. *Journal of Gerontology: Social Sciences, 64B,* 517–527.

Krause, N. (2011a). Assessing the prayer lives of older whites, older blacks, and older Mexican Americans: A descriptive analysis. *International Journal for the Psychology of Religion, 22*(1), 60–78.

Krause, N. (2011b). Reported contact with the dead, religious involvement, and death anxiety in late life. *Review of Religious Research, 52,* 347–364.

Krause, N. (2012). Meaning in life and healthy aging. In P. T. P. Wong (Ed.), *The human quest for meaning: Theories, research, and applications* (2nd ed., pp. 409–432). New York, NY: Routledge/Taylor & Francis.

Krause, N. (2013). Religious involvement in the later years of life. In K. Pargament, J. J. Exline, & J. W. Jones (Eds.), *APA handbook of psychology, religion, and spirituality* (Vol. 1, pp. 529–545). Washington, DC: American Psychological Association.

Krause, N., & Bastida, E. (2011). Church-based social relationships, belonging, and health among older Mexican Americans. *Journal for the Scientific Study of Religion, 50,* 397–409.

Krause, N., & Ellison, C. G. (2003). Forgiveness by God, forgiveness of others, and psychological well-being in late life. *Journal for the Scientific Study of Religion, 42,* 77–93.

Krause, N., & Ellison, C. G. (2009). The social environment of the church and feelings of gratitude toward God. *Psychology of Religion and Spirituality, 3,* 191–205.

Krause, N., Ellison, C. G., & Wulff, K. M. (1998). Church-based support, negative interaction, and well-being. *Journal for the Scientific Study of Religion, 37,* 725–741.

Krause, N., Emmons, R. A., & Ironson, G. (2015). Benevolent images of God, gratitude, and physical health status. *Journal of Religion and Health, 54,* 1503–1519.

Krause, N., & Hayward, R. D. (2014). Religious involvement, practical wisdom, and self-rated health. *Journal of Aging and Health, 26,* 540–558.

Krause, N., & Hayward, R. D. (2015). Assessing whether practical wisdom and awe of God are associated with life satisfaction. *Psychology of Religion and Spirituality, 7,* 51–59.

Krause, N., Hayward, R. D., Bruce, D., & Woolever, C. (2014). Gratitude to God, self-rated health, and depressive symptoms. *Journal for the Scientific Study of Religion, 53,* 341–355.

Krause, N., Ingersoll-Dayton, B., Ellison, C. G., & Wulff, K. M. (1999). Aging, religious doubt, and psychological well-being. *The Gerontologist, 39,* 525–533.

Krause, N., Ironson, G., & Hill, P. C. (2018). Religious involvement and happiness: Assessing the mediating role of compassion and helping others. *Journal of Social Psychology, 158,* 256–270.

Krause, N., & Van Tranh, T. (1989). Stress and religious involvement among older blacks. *Journal of Gerontology: Social Sciences, 44,* S4–S13.

Kraya, N. A., & Patrick, C. (1997). Folie a deux in forensic setting. *Australian and New Zealand Journal of Psychiatry, 31,* 883–888.

Kraybill, D. B. (1977). *Ethnic education: The impact of Mennonite schooling.* San Francisco, CA: R & E Research Associates.

Kraybill, D. B. (1994). Plotting social change across four affiliations. In D. B. Kraybill & M. A. Olshan (Eds.), *The Amish struggle with modernity* (pp. 53–74). Hanover, NH: University Press of New England.

Krejci, M. J. (1998). Gender comparison of God schemas: A multidimensional scaling analysis. *International Journal for the Psychology of Religion, 8,* 57–66.

Kressel, N. J. (2007). *Bad faith: The danger of religious extremism.* Amherst, NY: Prometheus Books.

Kripal, J. J. (2001). *Roads of excess, palaces of wisdom and the reflexivity in the study of mysticism.* Chicago, IL: University of Chicago Press.

Krishnan, V. (1993). Gender of children and contraceptive use. *Journal of Biosocial Science, 25,* 213–221.

Kristeller, J., & Rapgay, L. (2013). Buddhism: A blend of religion, spirituality, and psychology. In K. I.

Pargament, J. J. Exline, & J. W. Jones (Eds.), *APA handbook of psychology, religion, and spirituality* (Vol. 1, pp. 635–652). Washington, DC: American Psychological Association.

Kristensen, K. B., Pedersen, D. M., & Williams, R. N. (2001). Profiling religious maturity: The relationships of religious attitude components to religious orientations. *Journal for the Scientific Study of Religion, 40,* 75–86.

Kristof, N. (2010, January 10). Religion and women. *The New York Times,* p. WK11.

Kroeger, C. C., & Beck, J. R. (Eds.). (1996). *Women, abuse, and the Bible: How scripture can be used to hurt or to heal.* Grand Rapids, MI: Baker Books.

Kroll, J., & Bachrach, B. (1982). Visions and psychopathology in the Middle Ages. *Journal of Nervous and Mental Disease, 170,* 41–49.

Kroll, M. D. (1994). A commentary on optimism, fundamentalism, and egoism. *Psychological Science, 5,* 56.

Kroll-Smith, J. S. (1980). The testimony as performance: The relationship of an expressive event to the belief system of a Holiness sect. *Journal for the Scientific Study of Religion, 19,* 16–25.

Kruglanski, A. W., Hasmel, I. Z., Maides, S. A., & Schwartz, J. M. (1978). Attribution theory as a special case of lay epistemology. In J. H. Harvey, W. Ickes, & R. F. Kidd (Eds.), *New directions in attribution research* (Vol. 2, pp. 299–333). Hillsdale, NJ: Erlbaum.

Krumrei, E. J., Mahoney, A., & Pargament, K. I. (2011). Demonization as a spiritual struggle with divorce: Prevalence rates and links to post-divorce adjustment. *Family Relations, 60,* 90–103.

Kuhn, T. (1962). *The structure of scientific revolutions.* Chicago, IL: University of Chicago Press.

Kundera, M. (1983). *The unbearable lightness of being.* London, UK: Faber & Faber.

Kunkel, L. E., & Temple, L. L. (1992). Attitudes towards AIDS and homosexuals: Gender, marital status, and religion. *Journal of Applied Social Psychology, 22,* 1030–1040.

Kunkel, M. A., Cook, S., Meshel, D. S., Daughtry, D., & Hauenstein, A. (1999). God images: A concept map. *Journal for the Scientific Study of Religion, 38,* 193–202.

Kunst, J. L., Bjorck, J. P., & Tan, S.-Y. (2000). Causal attributions for uncontrollable negative events. *Journal of Psychology and Christianity, 19,* 47–60.

Kunz, J. (2009). Is there a particular role for ideational aspects of religions in human behavioral ecology? In E. Voland & W. Schiefenhovel (Eds.), *The biological evolution of religious mind and behavior* (pp. 89–104). New York, NY: Springer.

Kupky, O. (1928). *The religious development of adolescents.* New York, NY: Macmillan.

Kupor, M., Laurin, K., & Levav, J. (2015). Anticipating

divine protection?: Reminders of God can increase nonmoral risk taking. *Psychological Science, 26,* 374–384.

Kushner, H. (1981). *When bad things happen to good people.* New York, NY: Schocken Books.

Kutter, C. J., & McDermott, D. S. (1997). The role of the church in adolescent drug education. *Journal of Drug Education, 27,* 293–305.

Kwilecki, S. (1999). *Becoming religious: Understanding devotion to the unseen.* Lewisburg, PA: Bucknell University Press.

LaBarre, W. (1969). *The peyote cult* (enlarged ed.). New York, NY: Schocken Books.

LaBarre, W. (1972a). Hallucinations and the shamanantic origins of religion. In P. T. Furst (Ed.), *The flesh of the gods* (pp. 261–278). New York, NY: Praeger.

LaBarre, W. (1972b). *The ghost dance: The origins of religion* (rev. ed.). New York, NY: Delta.

LaBouff, J. P., Rowatt, W. C., Johnson, M. K., & Finkle, C. (2012). Differences in attitudes toward outgroups in religious and nonreligious contexts in a multinational sample: A situational context priming study. *International Journal for the Psychology of Religion, 22,* 1–9.

LaBouff, J. P., Rowatt, W. C., Johnson, M. K., Thedford, M., & Tsang, J. (2010). Development and initial validation of an implicit measure of religiousness–spirituality. *Journal for the Scientific Study of Religion, 49,* 439–455.

LaBouff, J. P., Rowatt, W. C., Johnson, M. K., Tsang, J.-A., & McCullough, G. (2012). Humble people are more helpful than less humble persons: Evidence from three studies. *Journal of Positive Psychology, 7,* 16–29.

Ladd, K. L., McIntosh, D. N., & Spilka, B. (1998). Children's God concepts: Influences of denomination, age, and gender. *International Journal for the Psychology of Religion, 8,* 49–56.

Ladd, K. L., Milmoe, S., & Spilka, B. (1994, April). *Religious schemata: Coping with breast cancer.* Paper presented at the annual convention of the Rocky Mountain Psychological Association, Las Vegas, NV.

Ladd, K. L., & Spilka, B. (2002). Inward, outward, and upward: Cognitive aspects of prayer. *Journal for the Scientific Study of Religion, 41,* 475–484.

Ladd, K. L., & Spilka, B. (2006). Inward, outward, upward prayer: Scale reliability and validation. *Journal for the Scientific Study of Religion, 45,* 233–251.

Lafal, J., Monahan, J., & Richman, P. (1974). Communication of meaning in glossolalia. *Journal of Social Psychology, 92,* 277–291.

Lafferty, J. (1990). Religion and racism in South Africa: Conflict between faith and culture. *Social Thought, 16,* 36–49.

Lam, P.-Y. (2002). As the flocks gather: How religion affects voluntary association participation. *Journal for the Scientific Study of Religion, 41,* 405–422.

Lambert, N. M., Fincham, F. D., Braithwaite, S. R., Graham, S. M., & Beach, S. R. H. (2009). Can prayer increase gratitude? *Psychology of Religion and Spirituality, 1,* 139–149.

Lambert, N. M., Fincham, F. D., LaVallee, D. C., & Brantley, C. W. (2012). Praying together and staying together: Couple prayer and trust. *Psychology of Religion and Spirituality, 4,* 1–9.

Lambert, N. M., Fincham, F. D., Stillman, T. F., Graham, S. M., & Beach, S. R. M. (2010). Motivating change in relationships: Can prayer increase forgiveness? *Psychological Science, 21,* 126–132.

Lambert, N. M., Stillman, T. F., Baumeister, R. F., Fincham, F. D., Hicks, J. A., & Graham, S. M. (2010). Family as a salient source of meaning in young adulthood. *Journal of Positive Psychology, 5,* 367–376.

Lamm, M. (1969). *The Jewish way in death and mourning.* New York, NY: Jonathan David.

Lammers, C., Ireland, M., Resnick, M., & Blum, R. (2000). Influences on adolescents' decision to postpone onset of sexual intercourse: A survival analysis of virginity among youths aged 13 to 18 years. *Journal of Adolescent Health, 26,* 42–48.

Landor, A. M., & Simons, L. G. (2014). Why virginity pledges succeed or fail: The moderating effect of religious commitment versus religious participation. *Journal of Child and Family Studies, 23,* 1102–1113.

Lange, R., & Thalbourne, M. A. (2007). The Rasch scaling of mystical experiences: Construct validity and correlates of the Mystical Experience Scale. *International Journal for the Psychology of Religion, 17,* 121–140.

Langer, E. J. (1983). *The psychology of control.* Beverly Hills, CA: SAGE.

Langford, B. J., & Langford, C. C. (1974). Review of the polls. *Journal for the Scientific Study of Religion, 13,* 221–222.

Langone, J. (2004, November 2). In search of the "God gene." *The New York Times,* Health and Fitness section, p. 6.

LaPierre, L. L. (1994). A model for describing spirituality. *Journal of Religion and Health, 33,* 153–161.

Larsen, K. S., & Long, E. (1988). Attitudes toward sex-roles: Traditional or egalitarian? *Sex Roles, 19,* 1–12.

Larsen, S. (1976). *The shaman's doorway.* New York, NY: Harper & Row.

Larson, D. B., Koenig, H. G., Kaplan, B. H., Greenberg, R. S., Logue, E., & Tyroler, H. A. (1989). The impact of religion on men's blood pressure. *Journal of Religion and Health, 28,* 265–277.

Larson, E. J., & Witham, L. (1998, July 23). Correspondence: Leading scientists still reject God. *Nature, 394,* 313.

Laski, M. (1961). *Ecstasy: A study of some secular and religious experiences.* Bloomington: Indiana University Press.

Latkin, C. A. (1995). New directions in applying psychological theory to the study of new religions. *International Journal for the Psychology of Religion, 5,* 177–180.

Laubach, M. (2004). The social effects of psychism: Spiritual experience and the construction of privatized religion. *Sociology of Religion, 65,* 239–263.

Laumann, E. O., Gagnon, J. H., Michael, R. T., & Michaels, S. (1994). *The social organization of sexuality: Sexual practices in the United States.* Chicago, IL: University of Chicago Press.

Laurencelle, R. M., Abell, S. C., & Schwartz, D. J. (2002). The relation between intrinsic faith and psychological well-being. *International Journal for the Psychology of Religion, 12,* 109–123.

Laurin, K., Kay, A. C., & Fitzsimmons, G. M. (2012). Divergent effects of activating thoughts of God on self-regulation. *Journal of Personality and Social Psychology, 102,* 4–21.

Lavery, J. V., Dickens, B. M., Boyle, J. M., & Singer, P. A. (1997). Bioethics for clinicians: II. Euthanasia and assisted suicide. *Canadian Medical Association Journal, 156,* 1405–1408.

Lawson, E. T., & McCauley, R. N. (1990). *Rethinking religion: Connecting cognition and culture.* Cambridge, UK: Cambridge University Press.

Lawson, R., Drebing, C., Berg, G., Vincellette, A., & Penk, W. (1998). The long term impact of child abuse on religious behavior and spirituality in men. *Child Abuse and Neglect, 22,* 369–380.

Lawton, L. E., & Bures, R. (2001). Parental divorce and the "switching" of religious identity. *Journal for the Scientific Study of Religion, 40,* 99–111.

Laythe, B., Finkel, D., & Kirkpatrick, L. A. (2001). Predicting prejudice from religious fundamentalism and right-wing authoritarianism: A multiple-regression approach. *Journal for the Scientific Study of Religion, 40,* 1–10.

Lazar, A. (2006). Fear of personal death as a predictor of motivation for religious behavior. *Review of Religious Research, 48,* 179–189.

Lazar, A., & Kravetz, S. (2005). Response to the mysticism scale by religious Jewish persons: A comparison of structural models of mystical experience. *International Journal for the Psychology of Religion, 2,* 155–168.

Lazarus, R. S. (1990). Constructs of the mind in adaptation. In N. L. Stein, B. Leventhal, & T. Trabasso (Eds.), *Psychological and biological approaches to emotion* (pp. 3–20). Hillsdale, NJ: Erlbaum.

Lazarus, R. S., & Folkman, S. (1984). *Stress, appraisal, and coping.* New York, NY: Springer.

Leach, M. M., & Soto, T. (2013). A content analysis of the *Psychology of Religion and Spirituality* journal: The initial four years. *Psychology of Religion and Spirituality, 5,* 61–68.

Leak, G. K., & Fish, S. (1989). Religious orientation, impression management, and self-deception: Toward a clarification of the link between religiosity and social desirability. *Journal for the Scientific Study of Religion, 28,* 355–359.

Leak, G. K., & Fish, S. B. (1999). Development and initial validation of a measure of religious maturity. *International Journal for the Psychology of Religion, 9,* 83–103.

Leak, G. K., Loucks, A. A., & Bowlin, P. (1999). Development and initial validation of an objective measure of faith development. *International Journal for the Psychology of Religion, 9,* 105–124.

Leak, G. K., & Randall, B. A. (1995). Clarification of the link between right-wing authoritarianism and religiousness: The role of religious maturity. *Journal for the Scientific Study of Religion, 34,* 245–252.

Leane, W., & Shute, R. (1998). Youth suicide: The knowledge and attitudes of Australian teachers and clergy. *Suicide and Life-Threatening Behavior, 28,* 165–169.

Leary, T. (1964). Religious experience: Its production and interpretation. *Psychedelic Review, 1,* 324–346.

Lebacqz, K., & Barton, R. G. (1991). *Sex in the parish.* Louisville, KY: Westminster John Knox Press.

Lebra, T. S. (1970). Religious conversion as a breakthrough for transculturation: A Japanese sect in Hawaii. *Journal for the Scientific Study of Religion, 9,* 181–186.

Lee, J. W., Rice, G. T., & Gillespie, V. B. (1997). Family worship patterns and their correlation with adolescent behavior and beliefs. *Journal for the Scientific Study of Religion, 36,* 372–381.

Leech, K. (1985). *Experiencing God: Theology as spirituality.* New York, NY: Harper & Row.

Lefcourt, H. M. (1973). The function of the illusions of control and freedom. *American Psychologist, 28,* 417–425.

Legare, C. H., Evans, E. M., Rosengren, K. S., & Harris, P. L. (2012). The coexistence of natural and supernatural explanations across cultures and development. *Child Development, 83,* 779–793.

Legare, C. H., & Gelman, S. A. (2008). Bewitchment, biology, or both: The co-existence of natural and supernatural explanatory frameworks across development. *Cognitive Science, 32,* 607–642.

Lehrer, E. L. (2004). Religion as a determinant of economic and demographic behavior in the United

States. *Population and Development Review, 30,* 707–726.

Lehrer, E. L., & Chiswick, C. U. (1993). Religion as a determinant of marital stability. *Demography, 30,* 385–403.

Lemoult, J. (1978). Deprogramming members of religious sects. *Fordham Law Review, 46,* 599–640.

Lenski, G. E. (1961). *The religious factor: A sociological study of religious impact on politics, economics and family life.* Garden City, NY: Doubleday.

Lenz, F. (1995). *Surfing the Himalayas: A spiritual adventure.* New York, NY: St. Martin's Press.

Lepp, I. (1963) *Atheism in our time* (B. Murchland, Trans.). New York, NY: Macmillan.

Lerner, R. M., & Spanier, G. B. (1980). *Adolescent development: A life-span perspective.* New York, NY: McGraw-Hill.

Lester, D. (1967). Experimental and correlational studies of the fear of death. *Psychological Bulletin, 67,* 27–36.

Lester, D. (1972). Religious behaviors and attitudes toward death. In A. Godin (Ed.), *Death and presence* (pp. 107–124). Brussels, Belgium: Lumen Vitae Press.

Leuba, J. H. (1896). A study in the psychology of religious phenomena. *American Journal of Psychology, 7,* 309–385.

Leuba, J. H. (1916). *Belief in God and immortality: An anthropological and statistical study.* Boston, MA: Sherman & French.

Leuba, J. H. (1925). *The psychology of religious mysticism.* New York, NY: Harcourt, Brace.

Leuba, J. H. (1934). Religious beliefs of American scientists. *Harper's Magazine, 169,* 291–300.

Levenson, H. (1973). Multidimensional locus of control in psychiatric patients. *Journal of Consulting and Clinical Psychology, 41,* 397–404.

Levenson, H. (1974). Activism and powerful others: Distinctions within the concept of internal–external control. *Journal of Personality Assessment, 38,* 377–383.

Levenson, M. R., Aldwin, C. M., & D'Mello, M. (2005). Religious development from adolescence to middle adulthood. In R. F. Paloutzian & C. L. Park (Eds.), *Handbook of the psychology of religion and spirituality* (pp. 144–161). New York, NY: Guilford Press.

Levin, J. S. (2015). Religious differences in self-rated health among US Jews: Findings from five urban population surveys. *Journal of Religion and Health, 54,* 765–782.

Levin, J. S., & Markides, K. S. (1986). Religious attendance and subjective health. *Journal for the Scientific Study of Religion, 25,* 31–49.

Levin, J. S., & Schiller, P. L. (1987). Is there a religious factor in health? *Journal of Religion and Health, 26,* 9–36.

Levin, T. M., & Zegans, L. S. (1974). Adolescent identity and religious conversion: Implications for psychotherapy. *British Journal of Medical Psychology, 47,* 73–82.

Levinger, G. (1979). A social psychological perspective on marital dissolution. In G. Levinger & O. C. Moles (Eds.), *Divorce and separation: Contexts, causes, and consequences* (pp. 37–60). New York, NY: Basic Books.

Levy, B. R., Slade, M. D., & Ranasinghe, P. (2009). Causal thinking after a tsunami wave: Karma beliefs, pessimistic explanatory style and health among Sri Lankan survivors. *Journal of Religion and Health, 48,* 38–45.

Levy, D. L., & Reeves, P. (2011). Resolving identity conflict: Gay, lesbian, and queer individuals with a Christian upbringing. *Journal of Gay and Lesbian Social Services, 23,* 53–68.

Levy, L. H., Martinkowski, K. S., & Derby, J. F. (1994). Differences in patterns of adaptation in conjugal bereavement: Their sources and potential significance. *Omega, 29,* 71–87.

Lewellen, T. C. (1979). Deviant religion and cultural evolution: The Aymara case. *Journal for the Scientific Study of Religion, 81,* 243–251.

Lewis, C. A., & Joseph, S. (1994). Religiosity: Psychoticism and obsessionality in Northern Irish university students. *Personality and Individual Differences, 17,* 685–687.

Lewis, C. A., & Maltby, J. (1995). Religiosity and personality among U.S. adults. *Personality and Individual Differences, 18,* 293–295.

Lewis, C. S. (1956). *Surprised by joy: The shape of my early life.* New York, NY: Harcourt, Brace.

Lewis, C. S. (2000). The Screwtape letters. In *The complete C. S. Lewis signature classics* (pp. 121–204). San Francisco, CA: Harper San Francisco. (Original work published 1942)

Lewis, I. M. (1971). *Ecstatic religion: An anthropological study of spirit possession and shamanism.* Baltimore: Penguin.

Lewis, J. R. (1989). Apostates and the legitimation of repression: Some historical and empirical perspectives on the cult controversy. *Sociological Analysis, 49,* 386–396.

Lewis, J. R., & Bromley, D. G. (1987). The cult withdrawal syndrome: A case of misattribution of cause. *Journal for the Scientific Study of Religion, 26,* 508–522.

Lewis, M., Kaita, H., Giblett, E. R., Anderson, J., Philipps, S., Steinberg, A. G., et al. (2005). Multiplicity of genetic polymorphisms of blood in the Schmiedeleut Hutterites. *American Journal of Medical Genetics, 22,* 477–485.

Leyn, R. M. (1976). Terminally ill children and their families: A study of the variety of responses to fatal illness. *Maternal–Child Nursing Journal, 5,* 179–188.

Lifton, R. J. (1961). *Thought reform and the psychology of totalism.* New York, NY: Norton.

Lifton, R. J. (1973). The sense of immortality: On death and the continuity of life. *American Journal of Psychoanalysis, 33,* 3–15.

Lifton, R. J. (1985). Cult processes, religious liberty and religious totalism. In T. Robbins, W. Shepherd, & J. McBride (Eds.), *Cults, culture, and law* (pp. 59–70). Chico, CA: Scholars Press.

Lilly, J. C. (1956). Mental effects on reduction of ordinary levels of physical stimuli on intact healthy persons. *Psychiatric Research Reports, 5,* 1–19.

Lilly, J. C. (1977). *The deep self.* New York, NY: Warner Books.

Lilly, J. C., & Lilly, A. (1976). *The dyadic cyclone.* New York, NY: Simon & Schuster.

Lind, E. A., Kanfer, R., & Earley, P. C. (1990). Voice, control, and procedural justice: Instrumental and noninstrumental concerns in fairness judgments. *Journal of Personality and Social Psychology, 59,* 952–959.

Linder Gunnoe, M., Hetherington, E. M., & Reiss, D. (1999). Parental religiosity, parenting style, and adolescent social responsibility. *Journal of Early Adolescence, 19,* 199–225.

Lindgren, J. (2014, August 1). Atheists or Christians—Which group is more common among those with fairly high IQ scores? *The Washington Post.* Retrieved from *www.washingtonpost.com/news/volokh-conspiracy/wp/2014/08/01/atheists-or-christians-which-are-more-common-among-those-with-fairly-high-iq-scores/?utm_term=.0ff12bb576d2.*

Lindquist, M. A., & Gelman, A. (2009). Correlations and multiple comparisons in functional imaging. *Perspectives on Psychological Science, 4,* 310–313.

Lipka, M. (2015, May 13). A closer look at America's rapidly growing religious "nones." *Pew Research Center.* Retrieved from *www.pewresearch.org/fact-tank/2015/05/13/a-closer-look-at-americas-rapidly-growing-religious-nones.*

Lippman, L. H., & Keith, J. D. (2006). The demographics of spirituality among youth: International perspectives. In E. C. Roehlkepartain, P. E. King, L. Wagener, & P. L. Benson (Eds.), *The handbook of spiritual development in childhood and adolescence* (pp. 109–123). Thousand Oaks, CA: SAGE.

Lippy, C. H. (1994). *Being religious, American style.* Westport, CT: Praeger.

Litchfield, A. W., Thomas, D. L., & Li, B. D. (1997). Dimensions of religiosity as mediators of the relations between parenting and adolescent deviant behavior. *Journal of Adolescent Research, 12,* 199–226.

Litke, J. (1983, August 5). Ideas about afterlife a heavenly mix, survey indicates. *The Denver Post,* p. 15D.

Loehr, F. (1959). *The power of prayer on plants.* Garden City, NY: Doubleday.

Loewenthal, K. M. (2013). Religion, spirituality, and culture: Clarifying the direction of effects. In K. I. Pargament, A. Mahoney, & E. P. Shafranske (Eds.), *APA handbook of psychology, religion, and spirituality* (Vol. 2, pp. 239–255). Washington, DC: American Psychological Association.

Loewenthal, K. M., & Cornwall, N. (1993). Religiosity and perceived control of life events. *International Journal for the Psychology of Religion, 3,* 39–45.

Lofland, J. (1977). *Doomsday cult* (rev. ed.). New York, NY: Irvington Press.

Lofland, J., & Skonovd, N. (1981). Conversion motifs. *Journal for the Scientific Study of Religion, 20,* 373–385.

Lofland, J., & Stark, R. (1965). Becoming a world saver: A theory of conversion to a deviant perspective. *American Sociological Review, 30,* 862–874.

Loftus, E. F., & Guyer, M. J. (2002). Who abused Jane Doe?: The hazards of the single case history. Part 1. *Skeptical Inquirer, 26*(3), 24–32.

London, P. (1964). *The modes and morals of psychotherapy.* New York, NY: Holt, Rinehart & Winston.

Long, D., Elkind, D., & Spilka, B. (1967). The child's conception of prayer. *Journal for the Scientific Study of Religion, 6,* 101–109.

Long, T. E., & Hadden, J. K. (Eds.). (1983). *Religion and religiosity in America.* New York, NY: Crossroad.

Lorenz, K. S. (1966). Evolution of ritualization in the biological and cultural spheres. *Philosophical Transactions of the Royal Society of London, Series B, Biological Sciences, 251,* 273–284.

Lottes, I., Weinberg, M., & Weller, I. (1993). Reactions to pornography on a college campus: For or against? *Sex Roles, 29,* 69–89.

Lovekin, A., & Malony, H. N. (1977). Religious glossolalia: A longitudinal study of personality changes. *Journal for the Scientific Study of Religion, 16,* 383–393.

Loveland, G. G. (1968). The effects of bereavement on certain religious attitudes. *Sociological Symposium, 1,* 17–27.

Lowe, C. M. (1955). Religious beliefs and religious delusions. *American Journal of Psychotherapy, 9,* 54–61.

Lowe, C. M., & Braaten, R. O. (1966). Differences in religious attitudes in mental illness. *Journal for the Scientific Study of Religion, 5,* 435–445.

Lown, E. A., & Vega, W. A. (2001). Prevalence and

predictors of physical partner abuse among Mexican American women. *American Journal of Public Health, 91,* 441–445.

Ludwig, D. J., Weber, T., & Iben, D. (1974). Letters to God: A study of children's religious concepts. *Journal of Psychology and Theology, 2,* 31–35.

Luft, G. A., & Sorell, G. T. (1987). Parenting style and parent–adolescent religious value consensus. *Journal of Adolescent Research, 2,* 53–68.

Luhrmann, T. M. (2012). *When God talks back: Understanding the American evangelical relationship with God.* New York, NY: Knopf.

Lukoff, D., & Lu, F. G. (1988). Transpersonal psychology research review topic: Mystical experience. *Journal of Transpersonal Psychology, 20,* 161–184.

Lukoff, D., Zanger, R., & Lu, F. (1990). Transpersonal psychology research review: Psychoactive substances and transpersonal states. *Journal of Transpersonal Psychology, 22,* 107–148.

Lumsden, C. J., & Wilson, E. O. (1983). *Promethean fire: Reflections on the origin of mind.* Cambridge, MA: Harvard University Press.

Lundmark, M. (2010). When Mrs. B met Jesus during radiotherapy: A single case study of a Christic vision—psychological prerequisites and functions and considerations on narrative methodology. *Archive for the Psychology of Religion, 32*(1), 27–68.

Lupfer, M. B., Brock, K. F., & DePaola, S. J. (1992). The use of secular and religious attributions to explain everyday behavior. *Journal for the Scientific Study of Religion, 31,* 486–503.

Lupfer, M. B., DePaola, S., Brock, K. F., & Clement, L. (1994). Making secular and religious attributions: The availability hypothesis revisited. *Journal for the Scientific Study of Religion, 33,* 162–171.

Lupfer, M. B., Tolliver, D., & Jackson, M. (1996). Explaining life-altering occurrences: A test of the "God-of-the-gaps" hypothesis. *Journal for the Scientific Study of Religion, 35,* 379–391.

Luquis, R. R., Brelsford, G. M., & Rojas-Guyler, L. (2012). Religiosity, spirituality, sexual attitudes, and sex behaviors among college students. *Journal of Religion and Health, 51,* 601–614.

Luyten, P., & Corveleyn, J. (2007). Attachment and religion: The need to leave our secure base: A comment on the discussion between Granqvist, Rizzuto and Wulff. *International Journal for the Psychology of Religion, 17,* 81–97.

Lynch, B. (1996). Religious and spirituality conflicts. In D. Davies & C. Neal (Eds.), *Pink therapy: A guide for counselors and therapists working with lesbian, gay and bisexual clients* (pp. 199–207). Bristol, PA: Open University.

Lynn, C. D. (2013). "The wrong Holy Ghost": Discerning the apostolic gift of discernment using a signaling and systems theoretical approach. *Ethos, 41,* 223–247.

Lynn, R., & Longley, D. (2006). On the high intelligence and cognitive achievements of Jews in Britain. *Intelligence, 34*(6), 541–547.

Lynxwiler, J., & Gay, D. (2000). Moral boundaries and deviant music: Public attitudes toward heavy metal and rap. *Deviant Behavior, 21,* 63–85.

Lyons, L. (2005, January 11). *Religiosity measure shows stalled recovery.* Washington, DC: Gallup Poll News Service.

MacDonald, C. B., & Luckett, J. B. (1983). Religious affiliation and psychiatric diagnoses. *Journal for the Scientific Study of Religion, 22,* 15–37.

MacDonald, D. A. (2000). Spirituality: Description, measurement, and relation to the five-factor model of personality. *Journal of Personality, 68,* 153–197.

MacDonald, D. A., & Holland, D. (2002). Spirituality and boredom proneness. *Personality and Individual Differences, 32,* 1113–1119.

MacDonald, D. A., LeClair, L., Holland, C. J., Alter, A., & Friedman, H. L. (1995). A survey of measures of transpersonal constructs. *Journal of Transpersonal Psychology, 27,* 171–235.

MacIntyre, A. (1988). *Whose justice?: Which rationality?* Notre Dame, IN: University of Notre Dame Press.

MacLean, K. A., Leoutsakos, J. M. S., Johnson, M. V., & Griffiths, R. R. (2012). Factor analysis of the Mystical Experience Questionnaire: A study of experiences occasioned by the hallucinogen psilocybin. *Journal for the Scientific Study of Religion, 51,* 721–737.

Macmillan Science Library: Genetics. (2004). Tay–Sachs disease. Retrieved December 2, 2008, from *www.bookrags.com/research/tay-sachs-disease-gen-04.*

Madge, V. (1965). *Children in search of meaning.* New York, NY: Morehouse-Barlow.

Madsen, G. E., & Vernon, G. M. (1983). Maintaining the faith during college: A study of campus religious group participation. *Review of Religious Research, 25,* 127–141.

Mafra, C. (2000). Shared accounts: Experiences of conversion to Pentecostalism among Brazilians and Portuguese. *Mana, 6,* 57–86.

Magnusson, D. (Ed.). (1981). *Toward a psychology of situations.* Hillsdale, NJ: Erlbaum.

Mahoney, A. (2010). Religion in families, 1999–2009: A relational spirituality framework. *Journal of Marriage and Family, 72,* 805–827.

Mahoney, A., Pargament, K. I., Murray-Swank, A., & Murray-Swank, N. (2003). Religion and the sanctification of family relationships. *Review of Religious Research, 44* 220–236.

Mahoney, A., Pargament, K. I., Tarakeshwar, N., & Swank, A. B. (2001). Religion in the home in the 1980s and 1990s: A meta-analytic review and conceptual analysis of links between religion, marriage, and parenting. *Journal of Family Psychology, 15*, 559–596.

Mahoney, A., & Tarakeshwar, N. (2005). Religion's role in marriage and parenting in daily life and during family crises. In R. F. Paloutzian & C. L. Park (Eds.), *Handbook of the psychology of religion and spirituality* (pp. 177–195). New York, NY: Guilford Press.

Mak, H. K., & Tsang, J. (2008). Separating the "sinner" from the "sin": Religious orientation and prejudiced behavior toward sexual orientation and promiscuous sex. *Journal for the Scientific Study of Religion, 47*, 379–392.

Makarec, K., & Persinger, M. A. (1985). Temporal lobe signs: Electroencephalographic validity and enhanced scores in special populations. *Perceptual and Motor Skills, 60*, 831–842.

Makepeace, J. M. (1987). Social and victim–offender differences in courtship violence. *Family Relations Journal of Applied Family and Child Studies, 36*, 87–91.

Malinowski, B. (1965). The role of magic and religion. In W. A. Lessa & E. Z. Vogt (Eds.), *A reader in contemporary religion* (pp. 63–72). New York, NY: Harper & Row.

Malony, H. N., & Lovekin, A. A. (1985). *Glossolalia: Behavioral science perspectives on speaking in tongues.* New York, NY: Oxford University Press.

Maltby, L. E., & Hill, P. C. (2008). "So firm a foundation": What the comparative study of religion offers positive psychology. *Research in the Social Scientific Study of Religion, 19*, 117–142.

Manfredi, C., & Pickett, M. (1987). Perceived stressful situations and coping strategies utilized by the elderly. *Journal of Community Mental Health Nursing, 4*, 99–110.

Mann, M. (2015). Triangle atheists: Stigma, identity and community among atheists in North Carolina's triangle region. *Secularism and Nonreligion, 4*, 1–12.

Manning, C. (1999). *God gave us the right: Conservative Catholic, evangelical Protestant, and Orthodox Jewish women grapple with feminism.* New Brunswick, NJ: Rutgers University Press.

Marcellino, E. M. (1996). Internalized homonegativity, self concept and images of God in gay and lesbian individuals. *Dissertation Abstracts International, 57*(1), 273A.

Marcia, J. (1966). Development and validation of ego-identity status. *Journal of Personality and Social Psychology, 3*, 551–558.

Marcia, J., Waterman, A., Matteson, D., Archer, S., & Orlofsky, J. (Eds.). (1993). *Ego identity: A handbook for psychosocial research.* New York, NY: Springer-Verlag.

Marcum, J. P. (1999). Measuring church attendance: A further look. *Review of Religious Research, 41*, 121–129.

Marcuse, H. (1955). *Eros and civilization: A philosophical inquiry into Freud.* Boston, MA: Beacon Press.

Margolis, R. D., & Elifson, K. W. (1979). Typology of religious experience. *Journal for the Scientific Study of Religion, 18*, 61–67.

Marin, G. (1976). Social-psychological correlates of drug use among Colombian university students. *International Journal of the Addictions, 11*, 199–207.

Markstrom, C. A. (1999). Religious involvement and adolescent psychosocial development. *Journal of Adolescence, 22*, 205–221.

Markstrom-Adams, C., Hofstra, G., & Dougher, K. (1994). The ego-virtue of fidelity: A case for the study of religion and identity formation in adolescence. *Journal of Youth and Adolescence, 23*, 453–469.

Markstrom-Adams, C., & Smith, M. (1996). Identity formation and religious orientation among high school students from the United States and Canada. *Journal of Adolescence, 19*, 247–261.

Marlasch, C. (1979). The emotional consequences of arousal without reason. In C. E. Izard (Ed.), *Emotions in personality and psychophysiology* (pp. 565–590). New York, NY: Plenum Press.

Marler, P. L., & Hadaway, C. K. (2002). "Being religious" or "being spiritual" in America: A zero-sum proposition? *Journal for the Scientific Study of Religion, 41*, 289–300.

Marques, S. C., Lopez, S. J., & Mitchell, J. (2013). The role of hope, spirituality and religious practice in adolescents' life satisfaction: Longitudinal findings. *Journal of Happiness Studies, 14*, 251–261.

Marshall, J. L. (1996). Sexual identity and pastoral concerns: Caring with women who are developing lesbian identities. In J. S. Moessner (Ed.), *Through the eyes of women* (pp. 143–166). Minneapolis, MN: Fortress.

Marshall, P. (2005). *Mystical encounters with the natural world: Experiences and explanations.* New York, NY: Oxford University Press.

Marshall, P. (2015). Mystical experiences as windows on reality. In E. F. Kelly, A. Crabtree, & P. Marshall (Eds.), *Beyond physicalism: Toward reconciliation of science and spirituality* (pp. 39–76). Lanham, MD: Rowan & Littlefield.

Marshall, S. K., & Markstrom-Adams, C. (1995). Attitudes on interfaith dating among Jewish adolescents: Contextual and developmental considerations. *Journal of Family Issues, 16,* 787–811.

Marsiglia, F. F., Kulis, S., Nieri, T., & Parsai, M. (2005). God forbid!: Substance use among religious and nonreligious youth. *American Journal of Orthopsychiatry, 75,* 585–598.

Marsiglio, W. (1993). Attitudes toward homosexual activity and gays as friends: A national survey of heterosexual 15- to 19-year-old males. *Journal of Sex Research, 30,* 12–17.

Martin, D., & Wrightsman, L. S., Jr. (1964). Religion and fears about death: A critical review. *Religious Education, 59,* 174–176.

Martin, M. (2002). *Atheism, morality and meaning.* Amherst, NY: Prometheus Books.

Martin, M. (2007). Atheism and religion. In M. Martin (Ed.), *The Cambridge companion to atheism* (pp. 217–232). New York, NY: Cambridge University Press.

Martin, R. A., Ellingsen, V. J., Tzilos, G. K., & Rohsenow, D. J. (2015). General and religious coping predict drinking outcomes for alcohol dependent adults in treatment. *American Journal on Addictions, 24,* 240–245.

Martin, W. T. (1984). Religiosity and United States suicide rates, 1972–1978. *Journal of Clinical Psychology, 40,* 1166–1169.

Marty, M. E. (1975). *The pro and con book of religious America: A bicentennial argument.* Waco, TX: Word.

Marty, M. E., & Appleby, R. S. (Eds.). (1991). *Fundamentalisms observed.* Chicago, IL: University of Chicago Press.

Marty, M. E., & Appleby, R. S. (Eds.). (1994). *Accounting for fundamentalisms.* Chicago, IL: University of Chicago Press.

Masci, D. (2013, November 21). To end our days. *Pew Research Center.* Retrieved from *www.pewforum. org/2013/11/21/to-end-our-days.*

Masci, D. (2014, September 25). National Congregations Study finds more church acceptance of gays and lesbians. *Pew Research Center.* Retrieved from *www.pewresearch.org/fact-tank/2014/09/25/new-study-finds-a-greater-church-acceptance-of-gays-and-lesbians-2.*

Maslow, A. H. (1964). *Religions, values, and peak experiences.* Columbus: Ohio State University Press.

Mason, M. J., Schmidt, C., & Mennis, J. (2012). Dimensions of religiosity and access to religious social capital: Correlates with substance use among urban adolescents. *Journal of Primary Prevention, 33,* 229–237.

Mason, M., Singleton, A., & Webber, R. (2007). *The spirit of Generation Y: Young people's spirituality in a changing Australia.* Mulgrave, Victoria, Australia: John Garratt.

Mason, W. A., & Windle, M. (2002). A longitudinal study of the effects of religiosity on adolescent alcohol use and alcohol-related problems. *Journal of Adolescent Research, 17,* 346–363.

Masterman, M. (1970). The nature of paradigm. In I. Lakotos & A. Musgraves (Eds.), *Criticism and the growth of knowledge* (pp. 59–89). Cambridge, UK: Cambridge University Press.

Masters, K. S. (2005). Research on the healing power of distant intercessory prayer: Disconnect between science and faith. *Journal of Psychology and Theology, 33,* 268–277.

Masters, K. S., & Bergin, A. E. (1992). Religious orientation and mental health. In J. F. Schumaker (Ed.), *Religion and mental health* (pp. 221–232). New York, NY: Oxford University Press.

Masters, K. S., & Hooker, S. A. (2013). Religion, spirituality, and health. In R. F. Paloutzian & C. L. Park (Eds.), *Handbook of the psychology of religion and spirituality* (2nd ed., pp. 519–539). New York, NY: Guilford Press.

Masters, K. S., Spielmans, G. I., & Goodson, J. T. (2006). Are there demonstrable effects of intercessory prayer?: A meta-analytic review. *Annals of Behavioral Medicine, 32,* 21–26.

Masters, R. E. L., & Houston, J. (1966). *The varieties of psychedelic experience.* New York, NY: Delta.

Masters, R. E. L., & Houston, J. (1973). Subjective realities. In B. Schwartz (Ed.), *Human connection and the new media* (pp. 88–106). Englewood Cliffs, NJ: Prentice-Hall.

Masters, W. H., & Johnson, V. E. (1970). *Human sexual inadequacy.* Boston, MA: Little, Brown.

Mathes, E. W. (1982). Mystical experience, romantic love, and hypnotic susceptibility. *Psychological Reports, 50,* 701–702.

Mathews, A. P. (1994). *The sexuality of submissive wives.* Paper presented at the annual convention of the Society for the Scientific Study of Religion, Albuquerque, NM.

Mathews, S., & Smith, G. B. (Eds.). (1923). *A dictionary of religion and ethics.* New York, NY: Macmillan.

Maton, K. I. (1989). The stress-buffering role of spiritual support: Cross-sectional and prospective investigations. *Journal for the Scientific Study of Religion, 28,* 310–323.

Maton, K. I., & Wells, E. A. (1995). Religion as a community resource for well-being: Prevention, healing and empowerment. *Journal of Social Issues, 51,* 177–193.

Mattis, J. S. (2002). Religion and spirituality in the meaning-making and coping experiences of African-American women: A qualitative analysis. *Psychology of Women Quarterly, 26,* 309–321.

Mattis, J. S., Ahluwalia, M. K., Cowie, S.-A. E., &

Kirkland-Harris, A. M. (2006). Ethnicity, culture, and spiritual development. In E. C. Roehlkepartain, P. E. King, L. Wagner, & P. L. Benson (Eds.), *The handbook of spiritual development in childhood and adolescence* (pp. 283–296). Thousand Oaks, CA: SAGE.

Maugans, T. A. (1996). The SPIRITual History. *Archives of Family Medicine, 5,* 11–16.

Mavor, K. I., & Gallois, C. (2008). Social group and moral orientation factors as mediators of religiosity and multiple attitude targets. *Journal for the Scientific Study of Religion, 47,* 361–377.

Maxwell, M., & Tschudin, V. (Eds.). (1990). *Seeing the invisible: Modern religious and other transcendent experiences.* London, UK: Penguin.

May, C. L. (1956). A survey of glossolalia and related phenomena in non-Christian religions. *American Anthropologist, 58,* 75–96.

Mayer, A., & Sharp, H. (1962). Religious preference and worldly success. *American Sociological Review, 27,* 218–227.

Mayer, E. (1985). Children of intermarriage. In E. Mayer (Ed.), *Love tradition: Marriage between Jews and Christians* (pp. 245–277). New York, NY: Plenum Press.

Maynard, E. A., Gorsuch, R. L., & Bjorck, J. P. (2001). Religious coping style, concept of God, and personal religious variables in threat, loss, and challenge situations. *Journal for the Scientific Study of Religion, 40,* 65–74.

McAdams, D. P., Booth, L., & Selvik, R. (1981). Religious identity among students at a private college: Social motives, ego stage, and development. *Merrill–Palmer Quarterly, 27,* 219–239.

McAlexander, J. H., Dufault, B. L., Martin, D. M., & Schouten, J. W. (2014, October). The marketization of religion: Field, capital, and consumer identity. *Journal of Consumer Research, 41,* 858–875.

McCallister, B. J. (1995). Cognitive theory and religious experience. In R. W. Hood, Jr. (Ed.), *Handbook of religious experience* (pp. 312–352). Birmingham, AL: Religious Education Press.

McCauley, R. N. (2011). *Why religion is natural and science is not.* New York, NY: Oxford University Press.

McCauley, R. N., & Lawson, E. T. (2002). *Bringing ritual to mind.* Cambridge, UK: Cambridge University Press.

McCleary, D. F., Quillivan, C. C., Foster L. N., & Williams, R. l. (2011). Meta-analysis of correlational relationships between perspectives of truth in religion and major psychological constructs. *Psychology of Religion and Spirituality, 3,* 163–180.

McClelland, D. C. (1961). *The achieving society.* Princeton, NJ: Van Nostrand.

McClenon, J. (1984). *Deviant science.* Philadelphia, PA: University of Pennsylvania Press.

McClenon, J. (1990). Chinese and American anomalous experiences. *Sociological Analysis, 51,* 53–67.

McClenon, J., & Nooney, J. (1999). Biological evolution and prevalent theories regarding the origin of religion: A review and critique. *Journal of the International Society of Life Information Science, 17,* 12–19.

McClosky, H., & Brill, A. (1983). *Dimensions of tolerance: What Americans believe about civil liberties.* New York, NY: Russell Sage Foundation.

McConahay, J. B., & Hough, J. C., Jr. (1973). Love and guilt-oriented dimensions of Christian belief. *Journal for the Scientific Study of Religion, 12,* 53–64.

McCosh, J. (1890). *The religious aspect of evolution.* New York, NY: Scribner.

McCrae, R. R. (Ed.). (1992). The five-factor model: Issues and applications [Special issue]. *Journal of Personality, 60.*

McCullough, M. E. (2001). Religious involvement and mortality. In T. G. Plante & A. C. Sherman (Eds.), *Faith and health: Psychological perspectives* (pp. 53–74). New York, NY: Guilford Press.

McCullough, M. E., Bono, G., & Root, L. M. (2005). Religion and forgiveness. In R. F. Paloutzian & C. L. Park (Eds.), *Handbook of the psychology of religion and spirituality* (pp. 394–411). New York, NY: Guilford Press.

McCullough, M. E., & Carter, E. C. (2013). Religion, self-control, and self-regulation: How and why are they related? In K. I. Pargament, J. J. Exline, & J. W. Jones (Eds.), *APA handbook of psychology, religion, and spirituality* (Vol. 1, pp. 123–138). Washington, DC: American Psychological Association.

McCullough, M. E., Emmons, R. A., & Tsang, J. (2002). The grateful disposition: A conceptual and empirical topography. *Journal of Personality and Social Psychology, 82,* 112–127.

McCullough, M. E., Friedman, H. S., Enders, C. K., & Martin, L. R. (2009). Does devoutness delay death?: Psychological investment in religion and its association with longevity in the Terman sample. *Journal of Personality and Social Psychology, 97,* 866–882.

McCullough, M. E., Hoyt, W. T., Larson, D. B., Koenig, H. G., & Thoresen, C. (2000). Religious involvement and mortality: A meta-analytic view. *Health Psychology, 19,* 211–222.

McCullough, M. E., Kimeldorf, M. B., & Cohen, A. D. (2008). An adaptation for altruism?: The social causes, social effects, and social evolution of gratitude. *Current Directions in Psychological Science, 17,* 281–285.

McCullough, M. E., & Larson, D. B. (1999). Prayer. In W. R. Miller (Ed.), *Integrating spirituality into treatment* (pp. 85–110). Washington, DC: American Psychological Association.

McCullough, M. E., & Snyder, C. R. (2000). Classical sources of human strength: Revisiting an old home and building a new one. *Journal of Social and Clinical Psychology, 19,* 1–10.

McCullough, M. E., & Willoughby, B. L. B. (2009). Religion, self-regulation, and self-control: Associations, explanations, and implications. *Psychological Bulletin, 135,* 69–93.

McCutcheon, A. L. (1988). Denominations and religious intermarriage: Trends among white Americans in the twentieth century. *Review of Religious Research, 29,* 213–227.

McDargh, J. (1983). *Psychoanalytic object relations theory and the study of religion.* Lanham, MD: University Press of America.

McDargh, J. (2001). Faith development theory and the postmodern problem of foundations. *International Journal for the Psychology of Religion, 11,* 185–199.

McDonald, W. L. (1992). Idionecrophanies: The social construction of perceived contact with the dead. *Journal for the Scientific Study of Religion, 31,* 215–223.

McFarland, M. J., Uecker, J. E., & Regnerus, M. D. (2011). The role of religion in shaping sexual frequency and satisfaction: Evidence from married and unmarried older adults. *Journal of Sex Research, 48,* 297–308.

McFarland, S. G. (1989). Religious orientations and the targets of discrimination. *Journal for the Scientific Study of Religion, 28,* 324–336.

McFarland, S. G. (1990). *Religiously oriented prejudice in communism and Christianity: The role of Quest.* Paper presented at the annual convention of the Southeastern Psychological Association, Atlanta, GA.

McFarland, S. G., & Warren, J. C., Jr. (1992). Religious orientations and selective exposure among fundamentalist Christians. *Journal for the Scientific Study of Religion, 31,* 163–174.

McGowan, J. C., Midlarksy, E., Morin, R. T., & Graber, L. S. (2016). Religiousness and psychological distress in Jewish and Christian older adults. *Clinical Gerontologist, 39*(5), 489–507.

McGinn, B. (1989). Preface. In M. Idel & B. McGinn (Eds.), *Mystical union and monotheistic faith: An ecumenical dialogue* (pp. vii–ix). New York, NY: Macmillan.

McGinn, B. (1991). Appendix: Theoretical foundations: The modern study of mysticism. In B. McGinn (Ed.), *The foundations of mysticism* (pp. 265–343). New York, NY: Crossroad.

McGuire, M. B. (1990). Religion and the body: Rematerializing the human body in the social sciences of religion. *Journal for the Scientific Study of Religion, 29,* 283–296.

McGuire, M. B. (1992). *Religion: The social context* (3rd ed.). Belmont, CA: Wadsworth.

McIntosh, D. N. (1995). Religion-as-schema, with implications for the relation between religion and coping. *International Journal for the Psychology of Religion, 5,* 1–16.

McIntosh, D. N., Kojetin, B. A., & Spilka, B. (1985). *Form of personal faith and general and specific locus of control.* Paper presented at the annual convention of the Rocky Mountain Psychological Association, Tucson, AZ.

McIntosh, D. N., Silver, R. C., & Wortman, C. B. (1993). Religion's role in adjustment to a negative life event: Coping with the loss of a child. *Journal of Personality and Social Psychology, 65,* 812–821.

McIntosh, D. N., & Spilka, B. (1990). Religion and physical health: The role of personal faith and control beliefs. In M. L. Lynn & D. O. Moberg (Eds.), *Research in the social scientific study of religion* (Vol. 2, pp. 167–194). Greenwich, CT: JAI Press.

McKay, M. J. (2005, June 8). Genetic disorders hit Amish hard. *CBS News 60.* Retrieved from *www.cbsnews.com/news/genetic-disorders-hit-amish-hard.*

McKeon, R. (Ed.). (1941). *The basic works of Aristotle.* New York, NY: Random House.

McKinney, J. P., & McKinney, K. G. (1999). Prayer in the lives of late adolescents. *Journal of Adolescence, 22,* 279–290.

McKusick, V. A. (Ed.). (1978). *Medical genetic studies of the Amish.* Baltimore: Johns Hopkins University Press.

McLaughlin, S. A., & Malony, H. N. (1984). Near-death experiences and religion: A further investigation. *Journal of Religion and Health, 23,* 149–159.

McLoughlin, W. F. (1978). *Revivals, awakenings, and reform.* Chicago, IL: University of Chicago Press.

McNamara, P., Durso, R., Brown, A., & Harris, E. (2006). The chemistry of religiosity: Evidence from patients with Parkinson's disease. In P. McNamara (Ed.), *Where God and science meet* (Vol. 2, pp. 1–14). Westport, CT: Praeger.

McNeill, J. T. (1951). *A history of the cure of souls.* New York, NY: Harper.

Mead, F. S. (Ed.). (1965). *The encyclopedia of quotations.* Westwood, NJ: Revell.

Meadow, M. J., & Kahoe, R. D. (1984). *Psychology of religion: Religion in individual lives.* New York, NY: Harper & Row.

Meadow, M. J., & Rayburn, C. A. (Eds.). (1985). *A time to weep, a time to sing.* Minneapolis, MN: Winston.

Meehl, P. E. (1954). *Clinical vs. statistical prediction.* Minneapolis, MN: University of Minnesota Press.

Meier, P. D. (1977). *Christian child-rearing and*

personality development. Grand Rapids, MI: Baker House.

Meisenhelder, J. B., & Marcum, J. P. (2004). Responses of clergy to 9/11: Posttraumatic stress, coping, and religious outcomes. *Journal for the Scientific Study of Religion, 43*, 547–554.

Melton, J. G. (1985). Spiritualization and reaffirmation: What really happens when prophecy fails. *American Studies, 26*, 17–29.

Mercer, C., & Durham, T. W. (1999). Religious mysticism and gender orientation. *Journal for the Scientific Study of Religion, 38*, 175–182.

Merkur, D. (2000). *The mystery of manna: The psychedelic sacrament of the Bible*. Rochester, VT: Park Street Press.

Merrill, R. M., Salazar, R. D., & Gardner, N. W. (2001). Relationship between family religiosity and drug use behavior among youth. *Social Behavior and Personality, 29*, 347–358.

Metzenberg, H. (2005, June 7). An unnatural history of Jewish population genetics. Retrieved September 17, 2007, from *home.comcast.net/~neoeugenics/IQgenes.htm*.

Meusner, T. M., Davies, R. M., & Marwit, S. J. (1994–1995). Personality and conjugal bereavement in older widow(er)s. *Omega, 30*, 223–235.

Michael, R. T., Gagnon, J. H., & Laumann, E. O. (1994). *Sex in America: A definitive survey*. Boston, MA: Little, Brown.

Michalak, L., Trocki, K., & Bond, J. (2007). Religion and alcohol in the U.S. National Alcohol Survey: How important is religion for abstention and drinking? *Drug and Alcohol Dependence, 87*, 268–280.

Miles, G. (2007). *Science and religious experiences: Are they similar forms of knowledge?* Brighton, UK: Sussex Academic Press.

Miles, J. (2004). The disbarment of God. In J. H. Ellens (Ed.), *The destructive power of religion: Violence in Judaism, Christianity, and Islam* (Vol. 1, pp. 123–167). Westport, CT: Praeger.

Millenson, M. L. (2015, October 18). We need a new Jewish ritual for the terminally ill. Retrieved from *https://forward.com/opinion/322676/we-need-a-new-jewish-ritual-for-the-terminally-ill*.

Miller, A. S., & Hoffman, J. P. (1995). Risk and religion: An explanation of gender differences in religiosity. *Journal for the Scientific Study of Religion, 34*, 63–75.

Miller, B. C., Norton, M. C., Curtis, T., Hill, E. J., Schvaneveldt, P., & Young, M. H. (1997). The timing of sexual intercourse among adolescents: Family, peer, and other antecedents. *Youth and Society, 29*, 54–83.

Miller, D. E., & Miller, A. M. (2000). Introduction: Understanding Generation X: Values, politics, and religious commitments. In R. W. Flory & D. E. Miller (Eds.), *Gen X religion* (pp. 1–12). New York, NY: Routledge.

Miller, G. (2003). *Incorporating spirituality in counseling and psychotherapy*. Hoboken, NJ: Wiley.

Miller, K. R. (1999). *Finding Darwin's God*. New York, NY: HarperCollins.

Miller, L. J. (2012a). (Ed.). *The Oxford handbook of psychology and spirituality*. New York, NY: Oxford University Press.

Miller, L. J. (2012b). Introduction. In L. J. Miller (Ed.), *The Oxford handbook of psychology and spirituality* (pp. 1–4). New York, NY: Oxford University Press.

Miller, L. (2015). *The spiritual child: The new science on parenting for health and lifelong thriving*. New York, NY: Picador.

Miller, L., & Kelley, B. S. (2005). Relationships of religiosity and spirituality with mental health and psychopathology. In R. F. Paloutzian & C. L. Park (Eds.), *Handbook of the psychology of religion and spirituality* (pp. 460–478). New York, NY: Guilford Press.

Miller, L., Weissman, M., Gur, M., & Adams, P. (2001). Religiousness and substance use in children of opiate addicts. *Journal of Substance Abuse, 13*, 232–236.

Miller, W. R. (Ed.). (1999). *Integrating spirituality into treatment*. Washington, DC: American Psychological Association.

Miller, W. R., & C'deBaca, J. (1994). Quantum change: Toward a psychology of transformation. In T. F. Heatherton & J. L. Weinberger (Eds.), *Can personality change?* (pp. 253–280). Washington, DC: American Psychological Association.

Miller, W. R., & Thoresen, C. E. (2003). Spirituality, religion, and health: An emerging research field. *American Psychologist, 58*, 24–35.

Millikan, R. A. (1935). *Evolution in science and religion*. London, UK: Humphrey Milford, Oxford University Press.

Miner, M. H., & McKnight, J. (1999). Religious attributions: Situational factors and effects on coping. *Journal for the Scientific Study of Religion, 38*, 274–286.

Mitchell, C. E. (1988). Paralleling cognitive and moral development with spiritual development and denominational choice. *Psychology: A Quarterly Journal of Human Behavior, 25*, 1–9.

Mitchell, K. (2015, January 15). Values clash at lesbian's funeral. *The Denver Post*, pp. 1A, 9A.

Mitroff, L., & Denton, E. (1999). *A spiritual audit of corporate America: A hard look at spirituality, religion, and values in the workplace*. San Francisco, CA: Jossey-Bass.

Moadel, A., Morgan, C., Fatone, A., Grennan, J., Carter, J., Laruffa, G., et al. (1999). Seeking meaning and hope: Self-reported spiritual and existential needs among an ethnically diverse cancer patient population. *Psycho-oncology, 8,* 378–385.

Moberg, D. O. (1962). *The church as a social institution.* Englewood Cliffs, NJ: Prentice-Hall.

Moberg, D. O. (1965). The integration of older members in the church congregation. In A. M. Rose & W. A. Peterson (Eds.), *Older people and their social worlds* (pp. 125–140). Philadelphia, PA: Davis.

Moberg, D. O. (1971). Religious practices. In M. P. Strommen (Ed.), *Research on religious development: A comprehensive handbook* (pp. 551–598). New York, NY: Hawthorn Books.

Moberg, D. O. (2001). Research on spirituality. In D. O. Moberg (Ed.), *Aging and spirituality* (pp. 55–69). New York, NY: Haworth Press.

Moberg, D. O., & Hoge, D. R. (1986). Catholic college students' religious and moral attitudes, 1961 to 1982: Effects of the sixties and seventies. *Review of Religious Research, 28,* 104–117.

Moghaddam, F. M. (2005). The staircase to terrorism: A psychological exploration. *American Psychologist, 60*(2), 161–169.

Moghaddam, F. M. (2006). *From the terrorists' point of view: What they experience and why they come to destroy.* Westport, CT: Praeger.

Moghaddam, F. M., Warren, Z., & Love, K. (2013). Religion and the staircase to terrorism. In R. F. Paloutzian & C. L. Parks (Eds.), *Handbook of the psychology of religion and spirituality* (2nd ed., pp. 632–648). New York, NY: Guilford Press.

Mohler, A. (2004). "The God gene": Bad science meets bad theology. Retrieved June 9, 2007, from *www-beliefnet.com/story/154/story_15458_1.html.*

Mohr, S. (2013). Religion, spirituality, and severe mental disorder: From research to clinical practice. In K. I. Pargament, A. Mahoney, & E. P. Shafranske (Eds.), *APA handbook of psychology, religion, and spirituality* (Vol. 2, pp. 257–274). Washington, DC: American Psychological Association.

Monitor on Psychology. (2015, June). APA applauds President Obama's call to end use of therapies intended to change sexual orientation. p. 10.

Montgomery, R. L. (1991). The spread of religions and macrosocial relations. *Sociological Analysis, 52,* 14–22.

Moody, R. (1976). *Life after life.* New York, NY: Bantam.

Moore, K. A., & Glei, D. (1995). Taking the plunge: An examination of positive youth development. *Journal of Adolescent Research, 10,* 15–40.

Mora, G. (1969). The scrupulosity syndrome. In E. M. Pattison (Ed.), *Clinical psychiatry and religion* (pp. 163–174). Boston, MA: Little, Brown.

Moreland, J. P. (2018). What is euthanasia? *Christian Research Journal.*

Morin, R. (2000, April 2). Unconventional wisdom: New facts and hot stats from the social sciences. *The Washington Post,* p. B5.

Morin, S. M., & Welsh, L. A. (1996). Adolescents' perceptions and experiences of death and grieving. *Adolescence, 31,* 585–595.

Morinis, A. (1985). The religious experience: Pain and the transformation of consciousness in ordeals of initiation. *Ethos, 13,* 150–174.

Morreim, D. C. (1991). *Changed lives: The story of Alcoholics Anonymous.* Minneapolis, MN: Augsburg.

Morris, C. G., & Maisto, A. A. (1998). *Psychology: An introduction* (10th ed.). Upper Saddle River, NJ: Prentice-Hall.

Morris, P. (1996). Community beyond tradition. In P. Heelas, S. Lash, & P. Morris (Eds.), *Detraditionalization: Critical reflections on authority and identity* (pp. 222–249). Cambridge, MA: Blackwell.

Morris, R. J., Hood, R. W., & Watson, P. J. (1989). A second look at religious orientation, social desirability and prejudice. *Bulletin of the Psychonomic Society, 27,* 81–84.

Moulton, B. E., & Sherkat, D. E. (2012). Specifying the effects of religious participation and educational attainment on mortality risk for U.S. adults. *Sociological Spectrum, 32,* 1–19.

Mowrer, O. H. (1958). Discussion: Symposium on relationships between religion and mental health. *American Psychologist, 13,* 576–579.

Moyer, C. A., Donnelly, M. P. W., Anderson, J. C., Valek, K. C., Huckaby, S. J., Wiederholt, D. A., et al. (2011). Frontal electroencephalographic asymmetry associated with positive emotion is produced by very brief meditation training. *Biological Science, 22,* 1277–1279.

Mudd, T., Naijle, M., Ng, B., & Gervais, W. (2015). The roots of right and wrong: Do concepts of innate morality reduce intuitive associations of mortality with atheism? *Secularism and Nonreligion, 4,* 1–6.

Mueller, D. J. (1967). Effects and effectiveness of parochial elementary schools: An empirical study. *Review of Religious Research, 9,* 48–51.

Mueller, G. H. (1978). The Protestant and the Catholic ethic. *Annual Review of the Social Sciences of Religion, 2,* 143–166.

Mullen, K., & Francis, L. J. (1995). Religiosity and attitudes towards drug use among Dutch school children. *Journal of Alcohol and Drug Education, 41,* 16–25.

Muller, F. M. (1879). *Lectures on the origin and growth of religion as illustrated by the religions of India.* New York, NY: Scribner.

Muller, F. M. (1889). *Natural religion.* London, UK: Longmans, Green.

Murphy, C. (2015, June 2). Interfaith marriage is

common in U.S., particularly among the recently wed. Retrieved from *www.pewresearch.org/fact-tank/2015/06/02/interfaith-marriage*.

Murphy, P. E., Ciarrocchi, J. W., Piedmont, R. L., Cheston, S., Peyrot, M., & Fitchett, G. (2000). The relation of religious beliefs and practices, depression, and hopelessness in persons with clinical depression. *Journal of Consulting and Clinical Psychology, 68,* 1102–1106.

Murphy-Berman, V., Berman, J. J., Pachauri, A., & Kumar, P. (1985). Religious attitudes and perceptions of justice. *Psychologia: An International Journal of Psychology in the Orient, 18,* 29–34.

Murray, K. M., Ciarrocchi, J. W., & Murray-Swank, N. A. (2007). Spirituality, religiosity, shame and guilt as predictors of sexual attitudes and experience. *Journal of Psychology and Theology, 35,* 222–234.

Musick, M., & Wilson, J. (1995). Religious switching for marital reasons. *Sociology of Religion, 56,* 257–270.

Myers, D. G. (1992). *The pursuit of happiness.* New York, NY: Morrow.

Myers, D. G. (1998). *Psychology* (5th ed.). New York, NY: Worth.

Myers, D. G., & Diener, E. (1995). Who is happy? *Psychological Science, 6,* 10–19.

Myers, D. G., & Spencer, S. J. (2001). *Social psychology* (Canadian ed.). Toronto, Ontario, Canada: McGraw-Hill.

Myers, F. W. H. (1961). *Human personality and its survival of bodily death.* New Hyde Park, NY: University Books. (Original work published 1903)

Myers, S. M. (1996). An interactive model of religiosity inheritance: The importance of family context. *American Sociological Review, 61,* 858–866.

Nagi, M. H., Pugh, M. D., & Lazerine, N. G. (1977–1978). Attitudes of Catholic and Protestant clergy toward euthanasia. *Omega, 8,* 153–164.

Najman, J. M., Williams, G. M., Keeping, J. D., Morrison, J., & Anderson, M. L. (1988). Religious values, practices and pregnancy outcomes: A comparison of the impact of sect and mainstream Christian affiliation. *Social Science and Medicine, 26,* 401–407.

Naranjo, C., & Ornstein, R. E. (1971). *On the psychology of meditation.* New York, NY: Viking.

Nasim, A., Utsey, S. O., Corona, R., & Belgrave, F. Z. (2006). Religiosity, refusal efficacy, and substance use among African American adolescents and young adults. *Journal of Ethnicity in Substance Abuse, 5*(3), 29–49.

Nason-Clark, N. (1997). *The battered wife: How Christians confront family violence.* Louisville, KY: Westminster John Knox Press.

Natera, G., Renconco, M., Alemendares, R., Rosowsky, H., & Alemendares, J. (1983). Patterns of alcohol consumption in two semirural areas between Honduras and Mexico. *Acta Psiquiatrica y Psicologica de America Latina, 29,* 116–127.

National Center for Injury Prevention and Control, Division of Violence Prevention. (2015). Suicide facts at a glance. Retrieved from *www.cdc.gov/violenceprevention*.

Needleman, J., & Baker, G. (Eds.). (1978). *Understanding the new religions.* New York, NY: Seabury.

Nelsen, H. M. (1980). Religious transmission versus religious formation: Preadolescent–parent interaction. *Sociological Quarterly, 21,* 207–218.

Nelsen, H. M. (1981a). Life without afterlife: Toward congruency of belief across generations. *Journal for the Scientific Study of Religion, 20,* 109–118.

Nelsen, H. M. (1981b). Religious conformity in an age of disbelief: Contextual effects of time, denomination, and family processes upon church decline and apostasy. *American Sociological Review, 46,* 632–640.

Nelsen, H. M. (1982). The influence of social and theological factors upon the goals of religious education. *Review of Religious Research, 23,* 255–263.

Nelsen, H. M. (1990). The religious identification of children of interfaith marriages. *Review of Religious Research, 32,* 122–134.

Nelsen, H. M., Cheek, N. H., & Au, P. (1985). Gender differences in images of God. *Journal for the Scientific Study of Religion, 24,* 396–402.

Nelsen, H. M., & Kroliczak, A. (1984). Parental use of the threat "God will punish": Replication and extension. *Journal for the Scientific Study of Religion, 23,* 267–277.

Nelsen, H. M., & Potvin, R. H. (1981). Gender and regional differences in the religiosity of Protestant adolescents. *Review of Religious Research, 22,* 268–285.

Nelsen, H. M., Potvin, R. H., & Shields, J. (1976). *The religion of children.* Unpublished manuscript, Catholic University of America.

Nelson, B. (2002, March 12). 6 days of creation: The search of evidence. *Newsday.*

Nelson, L. D. (1988). Disaffiliation, desacralization, and political values. In D. G. Bromley (Ed.), *Falling from the faith: Causes and consequences of religious apostasy* (pp. 122–139). Newbury Park, CA: SAGE.

Nelson, L. D., & Dynes, R. R. (1976). The impact of devotionalism and attendance on ordinary and emergency helping behavior. *Journal for the Scientific Study of Religion, 15,* 47–59.

Nelson, M. O. (1971). The concept of God and feelings toward parents. *Journal of Individual Psychology, 27,* 46–49.

Neubauer, R. L. (2014). Prayer as an interpersonal

relationship: A neuroimaging study. *Brain and Behavior, 4*, 92–103.

Neville, R. C. (Ed.). (2001). *Ultimate realities The comparative religious ideas project* (Vol. 2). Albany, NY: State University of New York Press.

Newberg, A. (2006a). Religious and spiritual practices: A neurochemical perspective. In P. McNamara (Ed.), *Where God and science meet* (Vol. 2, pp. 15–31). Westport, CT: Praeger.

Newberg, A. (2006b). The neurobiology of spiritual transformation. In J. D. Koss-Chioino & P. Hefner (Eds.), *Spiritual transformation and healing* (pp. 189–205). Lanham, MD: AltaMira Press.

Newberg, A., Alavi, A., Baime, M., Pourdehnad, M. J., Santanna, J., & d'Aquili, E. (2001). The measurement of regional cerebral blood flow during the complex cognitive task of meditation: A preliminary SPECT study. *Psychiatry Research, 106*, 113–122.

Newberg, A., d'Aquili, E., & Rause, V. (2001). *Why God won't go away: Brain science and the biology of belief.* New York, NY: Ballantine.

Newberg, A., & Newberg, S. (2010). Psychology and neurobiology in a postmaterialist world. *Journal of Religion and Spirituality, 2*, 119–121.

Newberg, A., Pourdehnad, M., Alavi, A., & d'Aquili, E. (2003). Cerebral blood flow during meditative prayer: Preliminary findings and methodological issues. *Perceptual and Motor Skills, 97*, 625–630.

Newport, F. (2006a, June 23). *Who believes in God and who doesn't?* Washington, DC: Gallup Poll News Service.

Newport, F. (2006c, November 29). *Religion most important to blacks, women, and older Americans.* Washington, DC: Gallup Poll News Service.

Newport, F. (2007b, December 24). *Questions and answers about Americans' religion.* Retrieved from *www.gallup.com/poll/103459/questions-answers-about-americans-religion.aspx.*

The New York Times. (2002, August 26). Confession had his signature; DNA did not. Retrieved from *www.nytimes.com/2002/08/26/us/confession-had-his-signature-dna-did-not.html.*

Nichols, D. E., & Chemel, B. R. (2006). The neuropharmacology of religious experience: Hallucinogens and the experience of the divine. In P. McNamara (Ed.), *Where God and science meet* (Vol. 3, pp. 1–34). Westport, CT: Praeger.

Niebuhr, H. R. (1929). *The social sources of denominationalism.* New York, NY: Holt, Rinehart & Winston.

Nielsen, M. E. (1998). An assessment of religious conflicts and their resolution. *Journal for the Scientific Study of Religion, 37*, 181–190.

Nielsen, M. E. (2001, September 14). Religion's role in the terroristic attack of September 11, 2001.

Retrieved December 1, 2001, from *www.psywww.com/psyrelig/fundamental/html.*

Nietzsche, F. (1967). On the genealogy of morals. In W. Kaufmann (Ed.), *On the genealogy of morals and ecce homo* (pp. 13–163). New York, NY: Random House. (Original work published 1887)

Nipkow, K. E., & Schweitzer, F. (1991). Adolescents' justifications for faith or doubt in God: A study of fulfilled and unfulfilled expectations. In F. K. Oser & W. G. Scarlett (Eds.), *Religious development in childhood and adolescence* (New Directions for Child Development, No. 52, pp. 91–100). San Francisco, CA: Jossey-Bass.

Nolan, W. M. (1990). Scrupulosity. In R. J. Hunter, H. N. Malony, L. O. Mills, & J. Patton (Eds.), *Dictionary of pastoral care and counseling* (p. 1120). Nashville, TN: Abingdon Press.

Nonnemaker, J., McNeely, C. A., & Blum, R. W. (2006). Public and private domains of religiosity and adolescent smoking transitions. *Social Science and Medicine, 62*, 3084–3095.

Nordquist, T. A. (1978). *Ananda cooperative village: A study in the beliefs, values and attitudes of a New Age religious community.* Uppsala, Sweden: Borgstroms Tryckeri.

Norenzayan, A. (2014). Does religion make people moral? *Behaviour, 151*, 365–384.

Norenzayan, A., Gervais, W. M., & Trzesniewski, K. H. (2012). Mentalizing deficits constrain belief in a personal god. *PLOS One, 7*, e36880.

Norlander, T., GÅrd, L., Lindholm, L., & Archer, T. (2003). New age: Exploration of outlook-on-life frameworks from a phenomenological perspective. *Mental Health, Religion, and Culture, 6*, 1–20.

Novotney, A. (2014, September). Reproducing results. *Monitor on Psychology*, pp. 32–35.

Novotni, M., & Petersen, R. (2001). *Angry with God.* Colorado Springs, CO: Piñon Press.

Nucci, L., & Turiel, E. (1993). God's word, religious rules, and their relation to Christian and Jewish children's concepts of morality. *Child Development, 64*, 1475–1491.

Nuenke, M. (2005, June 18). Closing in on the intelligence genes—at least some Jewish ones. Retrieved September 9, 2007, from *majorityrights.com/index.php/weblog/comments/closing_in_on_intelligence_genes.*

Nunn, C. Z. (1964). Child-control through a "coalition with God." *Child Development, 35*, 417–432.

Nye, R. M. (1999). Relational consciousness and the spiritual lives of children: Convergence with children's theory of mind. In K. H. Reich, F. K. Oser, & W. G. Scarlett (Eds.), *Psychological studies on spiritual development: Vol. 2. Being human: The case of religion* (pp. 57–82). Lengerich, Germany: Pabst Sciences.

Nye, W. C., & Carlson, J. S. (1984). The development of the concept of God in children. *Journal of Genetic Psychology, 145,* 137–142.

Oakes, K. E., Allen, J. P., & Ciarrocchi, J. W. (2000). Spirituality, religious problem-solving, and sobriety in Alcoholics Anonymous. *Alcoholism Treatment Quarterly, 18,* 37–50.

Obisesan, T., Livingston, I., Trulear, H. D., & Gillum, F. (2006). Frequency of attendance at religious services, cardiovascular disease, metabolic risk factors, and dietary intake in Americans: An age-stratified exploratory analysis. *International Journal of Psychiatry in Medicine, 36,* 435–448.

O'Brien, E. (Ed.). (1965). *The varieties of mystical experience.* Garden City, NY: Doubleday/Anchor.

Ochsmann, R. (1984). Belief in an afterlife as a moderator of fear of death? *European Journal of Social Psychology, 14,* 53–67.

O'Donnell, J. P. (1993). Predicting tolerance for new religious movements: A multivariate analysis. *Journal for the Scientific Study of Religion, 32,* 356–365.

O'Faolain, J., & Martines, L. (Eds.). (1973). *Not in God's image.* New York, NY: Harper & Row.

Ogata, A., & Miyakawa, T. (1998). Religious experiences in epileptic patients with a focus on ictus-related episodes. *Psychiatry and Clinical Neurosciences, 52,* 321–325.

O'Hara, J. P. (1980). A research note on the sources of adult church commitment among those who were regular attenders during childhood. *Review of Religious Research, 21,* 462–467.

Oishi, S., & Diener, E. (2014). Residents of poor nations have a greater sense of meaning in life than residents of wealthy nations. *Psychological Science, 25,* 422–430.

Ojha, H., & Pramanick, M. (1992). Religio-cultural variation in childrearing practices. *Psychological Studies, 37,* 65–72.

Okagaki, L., & Bevis, C. (1999). Transmission of religious values: Relations between parents' and daughters' beliefs. *Journal of Genetic Psychology, 160,* 303–318.

Oksanen, A. (1994). *Religious conversion: A meta-analytical study.* Lund, Sweden: Lund University Press.

Oldmixon, E. A., & Calfano, B. R. (2007). The religious dynamics of decision making on gay rights issues in the U.S. House of Representatives, 1993–2002. *Journal for the Scientific Study of Religion, 46,* 55–70.

Oliner, S. P., & Oliner, P. M. (1988). *The altruistic personality: Rescuers of Jews in Nazi Europe.* New York, NY: Free Press.

Olshan, M. A. (1994). Conclusion: What good are the Amish? In D. B. Kraybill & M. A. Olshan (Eds.), *The Amish struggle with modernity* (pp. 231–242). Hanover, NH: University Press of New England.

Olson, D. V. A. (1989). Church friendships: Boon or barrier to church growth? *Journal for the Scientific Study of Religion, 28,* 432–447.

Olson, D. V. A., & Perl, P. (2001). Variations in strictness and religious commitment among five denominations. *Journal for the Scientific Study of Religion, 40,* 757–764.

Olson, L. R., Cadge, W., & Harrison, J. T. (2006). Religion and public opinion about same sex marriage. *Social Science Quarterly, 87,* 340–360.

Olson, P. J. (2006). The public perception of "cults" and new religious movements. *Journal for the Scientific Study of Religion, 45,* 97–106.

Olson, T., & Christiansen, G. (1966). *Thirty-one hours: The Grindstone experiment.* Toronto, Ontario, Canada: American Friends Service Committee.

Oman, D., & Reed, D. (1998). Religion and mortality among the community dwelling elderly. *American Journal of Public Health, 88,* 1469–1475.

Oman, D., & Thoresen, C. E. (2003). Spiritual modeling: A key to spiritual and religious growth? *International Journal for the Psychology of Religion, 13,* 149–165.

Oman, D., & Thoresen, C. E. (2005). Do religion and spirituality influence health? In R. F. Paloutzian & C. L. Park (Eds.), *Handbook of the psychology of religion and spirituality* (pp. 435–459). New York, NY: Guilford Press.

Oman, D., & Thoresen, C. E. (2006). Religion, spirituality, and children's physical health. In E. C. Roehlkepartain, P. E. King, L. Wagener, & P. L. Benson (Eds.), *The handbook of spiritual development in childhood and adolescence* (pp. 399–415). Thousand Oaks, CA: SAGE.

Oman, D., & Thoresen, C. E. (2007). How does one learn to be spiritual?: The neglected role of spiritual modeling in health. In T. G. Plante & C. E. Thoresen (Eds.), *Spirit, science, and health: How the spiritual mind fuels physical wellness* (pp. 39–54). Westport, CT: Praeger.

O'Neil, T. (2014, January 27). Christians are following secular trends in premarital sex, cohabitation outside of marriage, says dating site survey. Retrieved from *www.christianpost.com/news/christians-are-following-secular-trends-in-premarital-sex-cohabitation-outside-of-marriage-says-dating-site-survey-113373.*

Onions, C. T. (Ed.). (1955). *The Oxford universal dictionary on historical principles* (3rd ed.). London, UK: Oxford University Press.

Oppenheimer, M. (2014, July 19). Examining the growth of the "spiritual but not religious." *The New York Times,* p. A14.

Oppenheimer, M. (2015, January 3). Gay marriage

prompts call for clergy to shun civil ceremonies. *The New York Times*. Retrieved from *www.nytimes.com/2015/01/03/us/gay-marriage-prompts-a-call-for-clergy-to-shun-civil-ceremonies.html*.

Orenstein, A. (2002). Religion and paranormal belief. *Journal for the Scientific Study of Religion, 41*, 301–311.

Ortberg, J. C., Jr., Gorsuch, R. L., & Kim, G. J. (2001). Changing attitude and moral obligation: Their independent effects on behavior. *Journal for the Scientific Study of Religion, 40*, 489–496.

Osarchuk, M., & Tatz, S. J. (1973). Effect of induced fear of death on belief in an afterlife. *Journal of Personality and Social Psychology, 27*, 256–260.

Osborne, H. (2013, March 13). Amish community have a mutated gene that causes developmental delay. *International Business Times*. Retrieved from *www.ibtimes.co.uk/Amish-gene-mutation-mental-retardation-developmental-delay-445578*.

Oser, F. K. (1991). The development of religious judgment. In F. K. Oser & W. G. Scarlett (Eds.), *Religious development in childhood and adolescence* (New Directions for Child Development, No. 52, pp. 5–25). San Francisco, CA: Jossey-Bass.

Oser, F. K. (1994). The development of religious judgment. In B. Puka (Ed.), *Moral development: A compendium. Vol. 2. Fundamental research in moral development* (pp. 375–395). New York, NY: Garland Press.

Oser, F. K., & Gmunder, P. (1991). *Religious judgment: A developmental approach* (H. F. Hahn, Trans.). Birmingham, AL: Religious Education Press.

Oser, F. K., & Reich, K. H. (1990). Moral judgment, religious judgment, worldview, and logical thought: A review of their relationship. *British Journal of Religious Education, 12*, 94–101.

Oser, F. K., & Reich, K. H. (1996). Psychological perspectives on religious development. *World Psychology, 2*, 365–396.

Oser, F. K., Reich, K. H., & Bucher, A. A. (1994). Development of belief and unbelief in childhood and adolescence. In J. Corveleyn & D. Hutsebaut (Eds.), *Belief and unbelief: Psychological perspectives* (Vol. 3, pp. 39–62). Atlanta, GA: Rodopi.

Oser, F. K., Scarlett, W. G., & Bucher, A. (2006). Religious and spiritual development throughout the life span. In W. Damon & R. M. Lerner (Series Eds.) & R. M. Lerner (Vol. Ed.), *Handbook of child psychology: Vol. 1. Theoretical models of human development* (6th ed., pp. 942–998). Hoboken, NJ: Wiley.

Oshodin, O. G. (1983). Alcohol abuse: A case study of secondary school students in a rural area of Benin District, Nigeria. *Journal of Alcohol and Drug Education, 29*, 40–47.

Osis, K., & Haraldson, E. (1977). *At the hour of death*. New York, NY: Avon.

Ostow, M. (1990). The fundamentalist phenomenon: A psychological perspective. In N. J. Cohen (Ed.), *The fundamentalist phenomenon* (pp. 99–125). Grand Rapids, MI: Eerdmans.

Ostrer, H. (2000). Genetic analysis of Jewish origins. *Avotaynu, 16*(1), 15–16.

Othman, N. (2011). Exploring the ummatic personality dimensions from the psycho-spiritual paradigm. *International Journal of Psychological Studies, 3*(2), 37–47.

Ott, U., Hölzel, B. K., & Vaitl, D. (2011). Brain structure and meditation: How spiritual practice shapes the brain. In H. Walach, S. Schmidt, & W. B. Jonas (Eds.), *Neuroscience, consciousness and spirituality: Proceedings of the Expert Meeting in Freiburg/Breisgau, 2008* (pp. 119–128). Berlin, Germany: Springer.

Otto, R. (1923). *The idea of the Holy* (J. W. Harvey, Trans.). London, UK: Oxford University Press. (Original work published 1917)

Owens, C. M. (1972). The mystical experience: Facts and values. In J. White (Ed.), *The highest state of consciousness* (pp. 135–152). Garden City, NY: Doubleday/Anchor.

Oxman, T. E., Freeman, D. H., & Manheimer, E. D. (1995). Lack of social participation or religious strength and comfort as risk factors for death after cardiac surgery in the elderly. *Psychosomatic Medicine, 57*, 5–15.

Oxman, T. E., Rosenberg, S. D., Schnurr, P. P., Tucker, G. J., & Gala, G. G. (1988). The language of altered states. *Journal of Nervous and Mental Disease, 176*, 401–408.

Ozorak, E. W. (1989). Social and cognitive influences on the development of religious beliefs and commitment in adolescence. *Journal for the Scientific Study of Religion, 28*, 448–463.

Ozorak, E. W. (1996). The power, but not the glory: How women empower themselves through religion. *Journal for the Scientific Study of Religion, 35*, 17–29.

Packard, E. (2007, October). Stress may set off tumor development. *APA Monitor*, p. 42.

Paffard, M. (1973). *Inglorious Wordsworths: A study of some transcendental experiences itn childhood and adolescence*. London, UK: Hodder & Stoughton.

Pagelow, M. D., & Johnson, P. (1988). Abuse in the American family: The role of religion. In A. L. Horton & J. A. Williamson (Eds.), *Abuse and religion: When praying isn't enough* (pp. 1–12). Lexington, MA: Lexington Books.

Pahnke, W. N. (1966). Drugs and mysticism. *International Journal of Parapsychology, 8*, 295–320.

Pahnke, W. N. (1969). The psychedelic mystical experience in the human encounter with death. *Harvard Theological Review, 62*, 1–32.

Palkovitz, R., & Palm, G. (1998). Fatherhood and faith in formation: The developmental effects of fathering on religiosity, morals, and values. *Journal of Men's Studies, 7,* 33–51.

Palmer, C. E., & Noble, D. N. (1986). Premature death: Dilemmas of infant mortality. *Social Casework, 67,* 332–339.

Paloutzian, R. F. (1981). Purpose-in-life and value changes following religious conversion. *Journal of Personality and Social Psychology, 41,* 1153–1168.

Paloutzian, R. F. (1996). *Invitation to the psychology of religion* (2nd ed.). Needham Heights, MA: Allyn & Bacon.

Paloutzian, R. F. (2005). Religious conversion and spiritual transformation: A meaning-system analysis. In R. F. Paloutzian & C. L. Park (Eds.), *Handbook of the psychology of religion and spirituality* (pp. 331–347). New York, NY: Guilford Press.

Paloutzian, R. F. (2014). Psychology of religious conversion and spiritual transformation. In L. R. Rambo & C. E. Farhadian (Eds.), *The Oxford handbook of religious conversion* (pp. 209–239). New York, NY: Oxford University Press.

Paloutzian, R. F., & Ellison, C. W. (1982). Loneliness, spiritual well-being, and quality of life. In L. A. Peplau & D. Perlman (Eds.), *Loneliness: A sourcebook of current theory, research and therapy.* New York, NY: Wiley-Interscience.

Paloutzian, R. F., Jackson, S. L., & Crandell, J. E. (1978). Conversion experience, belief system, and personal and ethical attitudes. *Journal of Psychology and Theology, 6,* 266–275.

Paloutzian, R. F., & Park, C. L. (Eds.). (2005). *Handbook of the psychology of religion and spirituality.* New York, NY: Guilford Press.

Paloutzian, R. F., & Park, C. L. (Eds.). (2013a). *Handbook of the psychology of religion and spirituality* (2nd ed.). New York, NY: Guilford Press.

Paloutzian, R. F., & Park, C. L. (2013b). Recent progress and core issues in the science of the psychology of religion and spirituality. In R. F. Paloutzian & C. L. Park (Eds.), *Handbook of the psychology of religion and spirituality* (2nd ed., pp. 3–22). New York, NY: Guilford Press.

Paloutzian, R. F., Richardson, J. T., & Rambo, L. R. (1999). Religious conversion and personality change. *Journal of Personality, 67,* 1047–1079.

Paloutzian, R. F., Swenson, E. L., & McNamara, P. (2006). Religious conversion, spiritual transformation, and the neurocognition of meaning making. In P. McNamara (Ed.), *The neurology of religious experience* (pp. 151–169). Westport, CT: Praeger.

Pancer, S. M., Jackson, L. M., Hunsberger, B., Pratt, M., & Lea, J. (1995). Religious orthodoxy and the complexity of thought about religious and non-religious issues. *Journal of Personality, 63,* 213–232.

Pancer, S. M., & Pratt, M. (1999). Social and family determinants of community service involvement in Canadians. In M. Yates & J. Youniss (Eds.), *Roots of civic identity: Intervention perspectives on community service and activism in youth* (pp. 32–55). New York, NY: Cambridge University Press.

Pape, R. (2005). *Dying to win*: New York, NY: Random House.

Pargament, K. I. (1988). Religion and the problem-solving process: Three styles of coping. *Journal for the Scientific Study of Religion, 27,* 90–104.

Pargament, K. I. (1997). *The psychology of religion and coping.* New York, NY: Guilford Press.

Pargament, K. I. (1999). The psychology of religion and spirituality?: Yes and no. *International Journal for the Psychology of Religion, 9,* 3–16.

Pargament, K. I. (2007). *Spiritually integrated psychotherapy.* New York, NY: Guilford Press.

Pargament, K. I. (2011). Religion and coping: The current state of knowledge. In S. Folkman (Ed.), *The Oxford handbook of stress, health, and coping* (pp. 269–288). New York, NY: Oxford University Press.

Pargament, K. I., & Abu-Raiya, H. (2007). A decade of research of religion and coping: Things we assumed and lessons we learned. *Psyke and Logos, 28,* 742–766.

Pargament, K. I., Ensing, D. S., Falgout, K., Olsen, H., Reilly, B., Van Haitsma, K., & Warren, R. (1990). God help me: I. Coping efforts as predictors of the outcomes to significant negative life events. *American Journal of Community Psychology, 18,* 793–824.

Pargament, K. I., Exline, J. I., & Jones, J. W. (Eds.). (2013). *APA handbook of psychology, religion, and spirituality* (Vol. 1). Washington, DC: American Psychological Association.

Pargament, K. I., Falb, M. D., Ano, G. G., & Wachholtz, A. B. (2013). The religious dimension of coping: Advances in theory, research, and practice. In R. F. Paloutzian & C. L. Park (Eds.), *Handbook of the psychology of religion and spirituality* (2nd ed., pp. 560–579). New York, NY: Guilford Press.

Pargament, K. I., Kennell, J., Hathaway, W., Grevengoed, N., Newman, J., & Jones, W. (1988). Religion and the problem-solving process: Three styles of coping. *Journal for the Scientific Study of Religion, 27,* 90–104.

Pargament, K. I., Koenig, H. G., & Perez, L. M. (2000). The many methods of religious coping: Development and initial validation of the RCOPE. *Journal of Clinical Psychology, 56,* 519–543.

Pargament, K. I., & Mahoney, A. (2002). Spirituality: Discovering and conserving the sacred. In C. R.

Snyder & S. J. Lopez (Eds.), *Handbook of positive psychology* (pp. 646–659). New York, NY: Oxford University Press.

Pargament, K. I., Mahoney, A., & Shafranske, E. P. (Eds.). (2013). *APA handbook of psychology, religion, and spirituality* (Vol. 2). Washington, DC: American Psychological Association.

Pargament, K. I., Poloma, M. M., & Tarakeshwar, N. (2001). Methods of coping from the religions of the world: The bar mitzvah, karma, and spiritual healing. In C. R. Snyder (Ed.), *Coping with stress: Effective people and processes* (pp. 259–284). New York, NY: Oxford University Press.

Pargament, K. I., Silverman, W., Johnson, S., Echemendia, R., & Snyder, S. (1983). The psychosocial climate of religious congregations. *American Journal of Community Psychology, 11*, 351–381.

Park, C. L. (2005). Religion and meaning. In R. F. Paloutzian & C. L. Park (Eds.), *Handbook of the psychology of religion and spirituality* (pp. 295–314). New York, NY: Guilford Press.

Park, C. L. (2010). Making sense of the meaning literature: An integrative review of meaning making and its effects on adjustment to stressful life events. *Psychological Bulletin, 136*, 255–301.

Park, C. L., & Cohen, L. H. (1993). Religious and nonreligious coping with the death of a friend. *Cognitive Therapy and Research, 17*, 561–577.

Park, C. L., Edmondson, D., & Hale-Smith, A. (2013). Why religion?: Meaning as motivation. In K. Pargament, J. J. Exline, & J. W. Jones (Eds.), *APA handbook of psychology, religion, and spirituality* (Vol. 1, pp. 157–171). Washington, DC: American Psychological Association.

Park, C. L., & Slattery, J. M. (2013). Religion, spirituality, and mental health. In R. F. Paloutzian & C. L. Park (Eds.), *Handbook of the psychology of religion and spirituality* (2nd ed., pp. 540–559). New York, NY: Guilford Press.

Park, H.-S., Bauer, S., & Oescher, J. (2001). Religiousness as a predictor of alcohol use in high school students. *Journal of Drug Education, 31*, 289–303.

Parker, C. A. (1971). Changes in religious beliefs of college students. In M. P. Strommen (Ed.), *Research on religious development: A comprehensive handbook* (pp. 724–776). New York, NY: Hawthorn Books.

Parker, G. (1983). *Parental overprotection.* New York, NY: Grune & Stratton.

Parker, G., Tupling, H., & Brown, L. B. (1979). A parental bonding instrument. *British Journal of Medical Psychology, 52*, 1–10.

Parker, M., & Gaier, E. L. (1980). Religion, religious beliefs, and religious practices among Conservative Jewish adolescents. *Adolescence, 15*, 361–374.

Parkes, C. M. (1972). *Bereavement: Studies of grief in later life.* New York, NY: International Universities Press.

Parnell, J. O., & Sprinkle, R. L. (1990). Personality characteristics of persons who claim UFO experiences. *Journal of UFO Studies, 2*, 105–137.

Parnia, S., & Fenwick, P. (2002). Near death experiences in cardiac arrest visions of a dying brain or visions of a new science of consciousness. *Resuscitation, 52*, 5–11.

Parrinder, G. (1980). *Sex in the world's religions.* New York, NY: Oxford University Press.

Parsons, W. B. (1999). *The enigma of the oceanic feeling: Revisioning the psychoanalytic theory of mysticism.* New York, NY: Oxford University Press.

Pasquale, F. (2007). The "nonreligious" in the American Northwest. In B. A. Kosmin & A. Keysar (Eds.), *Secularism and secularity: Contemporary international perspectives* (pp. 41–58). Hartford, CT: Institute for the Study of Secularism in Society and Culture.

Pastorino, E., Dunham, R. M., Kidwell, J., Bacho, R., & Lamborn, S. D. (1997). Domain-specific gender comparisons in identity development among college youth: Ideology and relationships. *Adolescence, 32*, 559–577.

Patrick, T., & Dulack, T. (1977). *Let our children go!* New York, NY: Ballantine Books.

Paul, C., Fitzjohn, J., Eberhart-Phillips, J., Herbison, P., & Dickson, N. (2000). Sexual abstinence at age 21 in New Zealand: The importance of religion. *Social Science and Medicine, 51*, 1–10.

Paul, J. (2015, January 14). Pastor halts lesbian's funeral. *The Denver Post*, pp. 1A, 9A.

Paw Prints. (n.d.). Dear God: Children's letters to God. Retrieved December 3, 2008, from *pawprints.kashalinka.com/quotes/quotes_dear_god.shtml*.

Payne, M., Rupar, C. A., Siu, G. M., & Siu, V. M. (2011). Amish, Mennonite, and Hutterite genetic disorder database. *Pediatric Child Health, 16*, e23–e24.

Pearce, L. P., & Axinn, W. G. (1998). The impact of family religious life on the quality of mother–child relations. *American Sociological Review, 63*, 810–828.

Peatling, J. H. (1974). Cognitive development in pupils in grades four through twelve: The incidence of concrete and religious thinking. *Character Potential: A Record of Research, 7*, 52–61.

Peatling, J. H. (1977). Cognitive development: Religious thinking in children, youth and adults. *Character Potential: A Record of Research, 8*, 100–115.

Peatling, J. H., & Laabs, C. W. (1975). Cognitive development in pupils in grades four through twelve: The incidence of concrete and abstract religious thinking. *Character Potential: A Record of Research, 7*, 107–115.

Peatling, J. H., Laabs, C. W., & Newton, T. B. (1975). Cognitive development: A three-sample comparison of means on the Peatling Scale of Religious Thinking. *Character Potential: A Record of Research, 7,* 159–162.

Peek, C. W., Curry, E. W., & Chalfant, H. P. (1985). Religiosity and delinquency over time: Deviance, deterrence and deviance amplification. *Social Science Quarterly, 66,* 120–131.

Peel, R. (1987). *Spiritual healing in a scientific age.* San Francisco, CA: Harper & Row.

Pekala, R. J., Steinberg, J., & Kumar, V. K. (1986). Measurement of phenomenological experience: Phenomenology of Consciousness Inventory. *Perceptual and Motor Skills, 63,* 983–989.

Pelletier, K. R., & Garfield, C. (1976). *Consciousness: East and West.* New York, NY: Harper & Row.

Pelton, R. W., & Carden, K. W. (1974). *Snake handlers: God-fearers or fanatics?* Nashville, TN: Nelson.

Pennachio, J. (1986). Near-death experience as mystical experience. *Journal of Religion and Health, 25,* 64–72.

Pennycook, G., Cheyne, J. A., Seli, P., Koehler, D. J., & Fugelsang, J. A. (2012). Analytic cognitive style predicts religious and paranormal belief. *Cognition, 123,* 335–346.

Perez, R. L. (2000). Fiesta as tradition, fiesta as change: Ritual, alcohol and violence in a Mexican community. *Addiction, 95,* 365–373.

Perkins, H. W. (1991). Religious commitment, yuppie values, and well-being in post-collegiate life. *Review of Religious Research, 32,* 244–251.

Perrin, R. D. (2000). Religiosity and honesty: Continuing the search for the consequential dimension. *Review of Religious Research, 41,* 534–544.

Perry, E. L., Davis, J. H., Doyle, R. T., & Dyble, J. E. (1980). Toward a typology of unchurched Protestants. *Review of Religious Research, 21,* 388–404.

Perry, E. L., & Hoge, D. R. (1981). Faith priorities of pastor and laity as a factor in the growth and decline of Presbyterian congregations. *Review of Religious Research, 22,* 221–241.

Perry, N., & Echeverría, L. (1988). *Under the heel of Mary.* London, UK: Routledge & Kegan Paul.

Perry, R. B. (1935). *The thought and character of William James* (2 vols.). Boston, MA: Little, Brown.

Persinger, M. A. (1987). *Neurophysiological basis of God beliefs.* New York, NY: Praeger.

Persinger, M. A. (1993). Vectorial cerebral hemisphericity as differential sources for the sensed presence, mystical experiences, and religious conversions. *Perceptual and Motor Skills, 76,* 915–930.

Persinger, M. A. (2002). The temporal lobe: The biological basis of the God experience. In R. Joseph (Ed.), *Neurotheology* (pp. 273–278). San José, CA: University Press.

Persinger, M. A., Bureau, Y. R. J., Peredery, O. P., & Richards, P. M. (1994). The sensed presence as right hemispheric intrusions into the left hemispheric awareness of self: An illustrative case study. *Perceptual and Motor Skills, 78,* 999–1009.

Persinger, M. A., & Makarec, K. (1987). Temporal lobe epileptic signs and correlative behaviors displayed by normal populations. *Journal of General Psychology, 114,* 179–195.

Peter, L. J. (Ed.). (1977). *Peter's quotations.* New York, NY: Bantam.

Peterman, A. H., Fitchett, G., Brady, M. J., Hernandez, L., & Cella, D. (2002). Measuring spiritual well-being in people with cancer: The Functional Assessment of Chronic Illness-Spiritual Well-Being Scale (FACIT-Sp). *Annals of Behavioral Medicine, 24,* 49–58.

Petersen, A. C. (1988). Adolescent development. *Annual Review of Psychology, 39,* 583–607.

Petersen, L. R., & Donnenwerth, G. V. (1997). Secularization and the influence of religion on beliefs about premarital sex. *Social Forces, 75,* 1071–1088.

Peterson, B. E., & Lane, M. D. (2001). Implications of authoritarianism for young adulthood: Longitudinal analysis of college experiences and future goals. *Personality and Social Psychology Bulletin, 27,* 678–690.

Peterson, C., & Seligman, M. E. P. (2004). *Character strength and virtues: A handbook and classification.* New York, NY: Oxford University Press.

Peterson, C., Seligman, M. E. P., & Vaillant, G. E. (1988). Pessimistic explanatory style is a risk factor for physical illness: A thirty-five year longitudinal study. *Journal of Personality and Social Psychology, 55,* 23–27.

Peterson, J. B. (1999). *Maps of meaning: The architecture of belief.* New York, NY: Routledge.

Peterson, L. (1975). *Hearts made glad: The changes of intemperance against Joseph Smith the Mormon Prophet.* Salt Lake City, UT: Author.

Petraitis, J., Flay, B. R., & Miller, T. Q. (1995). Reviewing theories of adolescent substance use: Organizing pieces in the puzzle. *Psychological Bulletin, 117,* 67–86.

Petsonk, J., & Remsen, J. (1988). *The intermarriage handbook: A guide for Jews and Christians.* New York, NY: Morrow/Quill.

Pettersson, T. (1991). Religion and criminality: Structural relationships between church involvement and crime rates in contemporary Sweden. *Journal for the Scientific Study of Religion, 30,* 279–291.

Petts, R. J. (2009). Family and religious characteristics' influence on delinquency trajectories from adolescence to young adulthood. *American Sociological Review, 74*, 465–483.

Petts, R. J. (2014). Families, religious attendance, and trajectories of psychological well-being among youth. *Journal of Family Psychology, 26*, 759–768.

Petts, R. J., & Knoester, C. (2007). Parents' religious heterogamy and children's well-being. *Journal for the Scientific Study of Religion, 46*, 373–389.

Pevey, C. (1994, November 4). *Submission and power among Southern Baptist ladies.* Paper presented at the annual convention of the Society for the Scientific Study of Religion, Albuquerque, NM.

Pew Research Center, Forum on Religion and Public Life. (2008, June). U.S. religious landscape study. Retrieved August 12, 2008, from *religions.pewforum.org/reports.*

Pew Research Center, Forum on Religion and Public Life. (2009, April 27). Faith in flux. Retrieved from *www.pewforum.org/2009/04/27/faith-in-flux.*

Pew Research Center, Forum on Religion and Public Life. (2010, September 28). U.S. religious knowledge survey: Who knows what about religion. Retrieved from *www.pewforum.org/2010/09/28/us-religious-knowledge-survey-who-knows-what-about-religion.*

Pew Research Center, Forum on Religion and Public Life. (2013a, May 17). The religious affiliation of U.S. immigrants: Majority Christian, rising share of other faiths. Retrieved from *www.pewforum.org/geography/the-religious-affiliation-of-US-immigrants.aspx.*

Pew Research Center, Forum on Religion and Public Life. (2013b, July 2). Growth of the nonreligious. Retrieved from *www.pewforum.org/2013/07/02/growth-of-the-nonreligious-many-say-trend-is-bad-for-american-society.*

Pew Research Center, Forum on Religion and Public Life. (2013c, October 1). A portrait of Jewish Americans. Retrieved from *www.pewforum.org/2013/10/01/jewish-american-beliefs-attitudes-culture-survey.*

Pew Research Center, Forum on Religion and Public Life. (2013d, December 30). Public's views on human evolution. Retrieved from *www.pewforum.org/2013/12/30/publics-views-on-human-evolution.*

Pew Research Center, Forum on Religion and Public Life. (2015a, April 2). The future of world religions: Population growth projections, 2010–2050. Retrieved from *www.pewforum.org/2015/04/02/religious-projections-2010-2050.*

Pew Research Center, Forum on Religion and Public Life. (2015b, May 12). America's changing religious landscape. Retrieved from *www.pewforum.org/2015/05/12/americas-changing-religious-landscape.*

Pfeifer, J. E. (1992). The psychological framing of cults: Schematic representations and cult evaluations. *Journal of Applied Social Psychology, 22*, 531–544.

Pfeifer, S., & Waelty, U. (1995). Psychopathology and religious commitment: A controlled study. *Psychopathology, 28*, 70–77.

Pfeiffer, J. E. (1982). *The creative explosion.* New York, NY: Harper & Row.

Phares, E. J. (1976). *Locus of control in personality.* Morristown, NJ: General Learning Press.

Philibert, P. J., & Hoge, D. R. (1982). Teachers, pedagogy and the process of religious education. *Review of Religious Research, 23*, 264–285.

Philipchalk, R., & Mueller, D. (2000). Glossolalia and temperature change in the right and left cerebral hemispheres. *International Journal for the Psychology of Religion, 10*, 181–185.

Phillips, R. E., III, Cheng, C. M., Oemig, C., Hietbrink, L., & Vonnegut, E. (2012). Validation of a Buddhist coping measure among primarily non-Asian Buddhists in the United States. *Journal for the Scientific Study of Religion, 51*, 156–172.

Phillips, R. E., III, Cheng, C. M., Pargament, K. I., Oemig, C., Colvin, S. D., Abarr, A. N., et al. (2009). Spiritual coping in American Buddhists: An exploratory study. *International Journal for the Psychology of Religion, 19*, 231–243.

Piaget, J. (1948). *The moral judgment of the child* (M. Gabain, Trans.). Glencoe, IL: Free Press. (Original work published 1932)

Piaget, J. (1952). *The origins of intelligence in children* (M. Cook, Trans.). New York, NY: International Universities Press. (Original work published 1936)

Piaget, J. (1954). *The construction of reality in the child* (M. Cook, Trans.). New York, NY: Basic Books. (Original work published 1937)

Pichon, I., Boccato, G., & Saroglou, V. (2007). Nonconscious influences of religion on prosociality: A priming study. *European Journal of Social Psychology, 37*, 1032–1045.

Pichon, I., & Saroglou, V. (2009). Religion and helping: Impact of target thinking styles and just-world beliefs. *Archiv für Religionspsychologie/Archive for the Psychology of Religion, 31*, 215–236.

Pickren, W. E. (2009). Indigenization and the history of psychology. *Psychological Studies, 54*, 87–95.

Piedmont, R. L. (1999). Does spirituality represent the sixth factor of personality?: Spiritual transcendence and the five-factor model. *Journal of Personality, 67*, 985–1013.

Piedmont, R. L., & Wilkins, T. A. (2013). Spirituality, religiousness, and personality: Theoretical foundations and empirical applications. In K. I. Pargament, J. J. Exline, & J. W. Jones (Eds.), *APA handbook of psychology, religion, and spirituality*

(Vol. 1, pp. 173–186). Washington, DC: American Psychological Association.

Pierce, B. J., & Cox, W. F. (1995). Development of faith and religious understanding in children. *Psychological Reports, 76,* 957–958.

Pigliucci, M. (2006, April 28). Neurotheology: A rather skeptical perspective. Retrieved from *http://web. archive.org/web/20060428215415/http://life.bio. sunysb.edu/~massimo/essays/neurotheology.html.*

Pilarzyk, K. T. (1978). The origin, development and decline of a youth culture movement: An application of sectarianization theory. *Review of Religious Research, 20,* 23–43.

Pilkington, G. W., Poppleton, P. K., Gould, J. B., & McCourt, M. M. (1976). Changes in religious beliefs, practices and attitudes among university students over an eleven-year period in relation to sex differences, denominational differences and differences between faculties and years of study. *British Journal of Social and Clinical Psychology, 15,* 1–9.

Pirutinsky, S. (2014). Does religiousness increase self-control and reduce criminal behavior?: A longitudinal analysis of adolescent offenders. *Criminal Justice and Behavior, 41,* 1290–1307.

Pirutinsky, S., Rosmarin, D., Pargament, K. I., & Midlarsky, E. (2011). Does negative religious coping accompany, precede, or follow depression among Orthodox Jews? *Journal of Affective Disorders, 132,* 401–405.

Plante, T. G. (1999). Introduction: What do we know about Roman Catholic priests who sexually abuse minors? In T. G. Plante (Ed.), *Bless me father for I have sinned: Perspectives on sexual abuse committed by Roman Catholic priests* (pp. 1–6). Westport, CT: Praeger.

Plante, T. G., & Aldridge, A. (2004). Psychological patterns among Roman Catholic clergy accused of sexual misconduct. *Pastoral Psychology, 54,* 73–80.

Plante, T. G., & Sharma, N. K. (2001). Religious faith and mental health outcomes. In T. G. Plante & A. C. Sherman (Eds.), *Faith and health: Psychological perspectives* (pp. 240–261). New York, NY: Guilford Press.

Plante, T. G., Vallaeys, C. L., Sherman, A. C., & Wallston, K. A. (2002). The development of a brief version of the Santa Clara Strength of Religious Faith Questionnaire. *Pastoral Psychology, 50,* 359–368.

Plaskow, J., & Romero, J. A. (Eds.). (1974). *Women and religion* (rev. ed.). Missoula, MT: Scholars Press.

Plutchik, R., & Ax, F. A. (1967). A critique of "Determinants of emotional state" by Schachter and Singer. *Psychophysiology, 4,* 79–82.

Polanyi, M. (1958). *The study of man.* Chicago, IL: University of Chicago Press.

Pollio, H. R., Henley, T. B., & Thompson, C. J. (1997). *The phenomenology of everyday life.* New York, NY: Cambridge University Press.

Pollner, M. (1987). *Mundane reason: Reality in everyday and sociological discourse.* Cambridge, UK: Cambridge University Press.

Pollner, M. (1989). Divine relations, social relations, and well-being. *Journal of Health and Social Behavior, 30,* 92–104.

Poloma, M. M. (1991). A comparison of Christian Science and mainline Christian healing ideologies and practices. *Review of Religious Research, 32,* 337–350.

Poloma, M. M. (1995). The sociological context of religious experience. In R. W. Hood, Jr. (Ed.), *Handbook of religious experience* (pp. 161–182). Birmingham, AL: Religious Education Press.

Poloma, M. M. (2003). *Main Street mystics: The Toronto Blessing and reviving Pentecostalism.* Walnut Creek, CA: AltaMira Press.

Poloma, M. M., & Gallup, G. H., Jr. (1991). *Varieties of prayer: A survey report.* Philadelphia, PA: Trinity Press International.

Poloma, M. M., & Hood, R. W., Jr. (2008). *Blood and fire: Godly love in a Pentecostal emerging church.* New York, NY: New York University Press.

Poloma, M. M., & Pendleton, B. F. (1989). Exploring types of prayer and quality of life research: A research note. *Review of Religious Research, 31,* 46–53.

Poloma, M. M., & Pendleton, B. F. (1991). *Exploring neglected dimensions of quality of life research.* Lewiston, NY: Edwin Mellen Press.

Ponton, M. O., & Gorsuch, R. L. (1988). Prejudice and religion revisited: A cross-cultural investigation with a Venezuelan sample. *Journal for the Scientific Study of Religion, 27,* 260–271.

Porpora, D. V. (2006). Methodological atheism, methodological agnosticism and religious experience. *Journal for the Theory of Social Behavior, 36,* 57–75.

Porter, N. (1883). *Elements of intellectual science.* New York, NY: Scribner.

Porterfield, A. (2001). *The transformation of American religion.* New York, NY: Oxford University Press.

Post, R. H. (1973). Jews, genetics, and disease. In A. Shiloh & I. C. Selavan (Eds.), *Ethnic groups of America: Their morbidity, mortality, and behavior disorders: Vol. 1. The Jews* (pp. 67–71). Springfield, IL: Charles C Thomas.

Poston, L. (1992). *Islamic da'wah in the West.* Oxford, UK: Oxford University Press.

Potvin, R. H. (1977). Adolescent God images. *Review of Religious Research, 19,* 43–53.

Potvin, R. H., & Sloane, D. M. (1985). Parental

control, age, and religious practice. *Review of Religious Research, 27,* 3–14.

Powell, L. H., Shahabi, L., & Thoresen, C. E. (2003). Religion and spirituality: Linkages to physical health. *American Psychologist, 58,* 36–52.

Powers, C., Nam, R. K., Rowatt, W. C., & Hill, P. C. (2007). Associations between humility, spiritual transcendence, and forgiveness. *Research in the Social Scientific Study of Religion, 18,* 75–94.

Pratt, J. B. (1920). *The religious consciousness: A psychological study.* New York, NY: Macmillan.

Pratt, M. W., Hunsberger, B., Pancer, S. M., & Roth, D. (1992). Reflections on religion: Aging, belief orthodoxy, and interpersonal conflict in adult thinking about religious issues. *Journal for the Scientific Study of Religion, 31,* 514–522.

Prentice, N. M., Manosevitz, M., & Hubbs, L. (1978). Imaginary figures of early childhood: Santa Claus, Easter Bunny, and the Tooth Fairy. *American Journal of Orthopsychiatry, 48,* 618–628.

Pressman, P., Lyons, J. S., Larson, D. B., & Gartner, J. (1992). Religion, anxiety, and fear of death. In J. F. Schumaker (Ed.), *Religion and mental health* (pp. 98–109). New York, NY: Oxford University Press.

Pressman, P., Lyons, J. S., Larson, D. B., & Strain, J. J. (1990). Religious belief, depression, and ambulation status in elderly women with broken hips. *American Journal of Psychiatry, 147,* 758–760.

Preston, D. L. (1981). Becoming a Zen practitioner. *Sociological Analysis, 42,* 47–55.

Preston, D. L. (1982). Meditative–ritual practice and spiritual conversion–commitment: Theoretical implications based upon the case of Zen. *Sociological Analysis, 43,* 257–270.

Preston, D. L. (1988). *The social organization of Zen practice.* Cambridge, UK: Cambridge University Press.

Preston, J. L., & Ritter, R. S. (2013). Different effects of religion and God on prosociality with the ingroup and the outgroup. *Personality and Social Psychology Bulletin, 39,* 1471–1483.

Preus, J. S. (1987). *Explaining religion.* New Haven, CT: Yale University Press.

Prince, R. H. (1992). Religious experience and psychopathology. In J. F. Schumaker (Ed.), *Religion and mental health* (pp. 281–290). New York, NY: Oxford University Press.

Pritt, A. F. (1998). Spiritual correlates of reported sexual abuse among Mormon women. *Journal for the Scientific Study of Religion, 37,* 273–285.

Proudfoot, W. (1985). *Religious experience.* Berkeley, CA: University of California Press.

Proudfoot, W., & Shaver, P. (1975). Attribution theory and the psychology of religion. *Journal for the Scientific Study of Religion, 14,* 317–330.

Pruyser, P. W. (1968). *A dynamic psychology of religion.* New York, NY: Harper & Row.

Pruyser, P. W. (1977). The seamy side of current religious beliefs. *Bulletin of the Menninger Clinic, 41,* 329–348.

Puhakka, K. (1995). Hinduism and religious experience. In R. W. Hood, Jr. (Ed.), *Handbook of religious experience* (pp. 122–143). Birmingham, AL: Religious Education Press.

Purves, W. K., Orians, G. H., & Heller, H. C. (1995). *Life: The science of biology.* Sunderland, MA: Sinauer.

Putnam, R. D. (2000). *Bowling alone: The collapse and revival of American community.* New York, NY: Simon & Schuster.

Putney, S., & Middleton, R. (1961). Dimensions and correlates of religious ideologies. *Social Forces, 39,* 285–290.

Pylyshyn, Z. W. (1973). What a mind's eye tells the mind's brain. *Psychological Bulletin, 80,* 1–24.

Qin, J., Goodman, G. S., Bottoms, B. L., & Shaver, P. R. (1998). Repressed memories of ritualistic and religion-related abuse. In S. J. Lynn & K. M. McConkey (Eds.), *Truth in memory* (pp. 260–283). New York, NY: Guilford Press.

Quinn, D. M. (1993). Plural marriage and Mormon fundamentalism. In M. E. Marty & R. S. Appleby (Eds.), *Fundamentalism and society* (pp. 240–293). Chicago, IL: University of Chicago Press.

Qureshi, N. A., & Al-Habeeb, T. A. (2000). Sociodemographic parameters and clinical pattern of drug abuse in Al-Qassim region—Saudi Arabia. *Arab Journal of Psychiatry, 11,* 10–21.

Ragan, C., Malony, H. N., & Beit-Hallahmi, B. (1980). Psychologists and religion: Professional factors and personal belief. *Review of Religious Research, 21,* 208–217.

Rahman, F. (1988). Islamization of knowledge: A response. *American Journal of Islamic Social Science, 5,* 3–11.

Ramachandran, V. S., & Blakeslee, S. (1998). *Phantoms in the brain.* New York, NY: Morrow.

Rambo, L. R. (1982). Current research on religious conversion. *Religious Studies Review, 8,* 146–159.

Rambo, L. R. (1993). *Understanding religious conversion.* New Haven, CT: Yale University Press.

Rambo, L. R., & Farhadian, C. E. (2014a). Introduction. In L. R. Rambo & C. E. Farhadian (Eds.), *The Oxford handbook of religious conversion* (pp. 1–24). New York, NY: Oxford University Press.

Rambo, L. R., & Farhadian, C. E. (Eds.). (2014b). *The Oxford handbook of religious conversion.* New York, NY: Oxford University Press.

Randall, T. M., & Desrosiers, M. (1980). Measurement of supernatural belief: Sex differences and locus of control. *Journal of Personality Assessment, 44*, 493–498.

Randolph-Seng, B., & Nielsen, M. E. (2007). Honesty: One effect of primed religious representations. *International Journal for the Psychology of Religion, 17*, 303–315.

Rasmussen, C. H., & Johnson, M. E. (1994). Spirituality and religiosity: Relative relationships to death anxiety. *Omega, 29*, 313–318.

Ratcliffe, M. (2006). *Feelings of being: Phenomenology, psychiatry, and the sense of reality.* Oxford, UK: Oxford University Press.

Rätsch, C. (Ed.). (1990). *Gateway to inner space: Sacred plants, mysticism and psychotherapy.* Bridport, UK: Prism Press.

Ray, S. D., Lockman, J. D., Jones, E. J., & Kelly, M. H. (2015). Attributions to God and Satan about life-altering events. *Psychology of Religion and Spirituality, 7*, 60–69.

Razib. (2005, June 15). Bad science. Retrieved July 30, 2007, from *www.gnxp.com/MT2/archives/004077.html.*

Razmyar, S., & Reeve, C. L. (2013). Individual differences in religiosity as a function of cognitive ability and cognitive style. *Intelligence, 41*, 667–673.

Rea, M. P., Greenspoon, S., & Spilka, B. (1975). Physicians and the terminal patient: Some selected attitudes and behavior. *Omega, 6*, 291–302.

Redekop, C. A. (1974). A new look at sect development. *Journal for the Scientific Study of Religion, 13*, 345–352.

Reed, G. (1974). *The psychology of anomalous experience.* Boston, MA: Houghton Mifflin.

Reeves, N. C., & Boersma, F. J. (1989–1990). The therapeutic use of ritual in maladaptive grieving. *Omega, 20*, 281–291.

Regnerus, M. D., Smith, C., & Sikkink, D. (1998). Who gives to the poor?: The influence of religious tradition and political location on the personal generosity of Americans toward the poor. *Journal for the Scientific Study of Religion, 37*, 481–493.

Regnerus, M. D., Smith, C., & Smith, B. (2004). Social context in the development of adolescent religiosity. *Applied Developmental Science, 8*, 27–38.

Reich, K. H. (1989). Between religion and science: Complementarity in the religious thinking of young people. *British Journal of Religious Education, 11*, 62–69.

Reich, K. H. (1991). The role of complementarity reasoning in religious development. In F. K. Oser & W. G. Scarlett (Eds.), *Religious development in childhood and adolescence* (New Directions for Child Development, No. 52, pp. 77–89). San Francisco, CA: Jossey-Bass.

Reich, K. H. (1992). Religious development across the lifespan: Conventional and cognitive developmental approaches. In D. L. Featherman, R. M. Lerner, & M. Perlmutter (Eds.), *Life-span development and behavior* (Vol. 11, pp. 145–188). Hillsdale, NJ: Erlbaum.

Reich, K. H. (1993a). Cognitive-developmental approaches to religiousness: Which version for which purpose? *International Journal for the Psychology of Religion, 3*, 145–171.

Reich, K. H. (1993b). Integrating differing theories: The case of religious development. *Journal of Empirical Theology, 6*, 39–49.

Reich, K. H. (1994). Can one rationally understand Christian doctrines?: An empirical study. *British Journal of Religious Education, 16*, 114–126.

Reich, K. H. (1997). Do we need a theory for the religious development of women? *International Journal for the Psychology of Religion, 7*, 67–86.

Reich, K. H. (2000). Scientist vs. believer: On navigating between the Scilla of scientific norms and the Charybdis of personal experience. *Journal of Psychology and Theology, 28*, 190–200.

Reich, S. H., & Hill, P. C. (Eds.). (2008). Perspectives for the future of the psychology of religion [Special section]. *Archive for the Psychology of Religion, 30*, 5–134.

Reid, T. (1969). *The active powers of the human mind.* Cambridge, MA: MIT Press.

Reifsnyder, W. E., & Campbell, E. I. (1960). Religious attitudes of male neuropsychiatric patients: I. Most frequently expressed attitudes. *Journal of Pastoral Care, 14*, 92–97.

Reimer, K. S., & Furrow, J. L. (2001). A qualitative exploration of relational consciousness in Christian children. *International Journal of Children's Spirituality, 6*, 7–23.

Reimer, S. (2010). Higher education and theological liberalism: Revisiting the old issue. *Sociology of Religion, 71*, 393–408.

Reinert, D. F., & Smith, C. E. (1997). Childhood sexual abuse and female spiritual development. *Counseling and Values, 41*, 235–245.

Reinert, D. F., & Stifler, K. R. (1993). Hood's Mysticism Scale revisited: A factor-analytic replication. *Journal for the Scientific Study of Religion, 32*, 383–388.

Reiss, I. L. (1976). *The family system in America* (2nd ed.). New York, NY: Holt, Rinehart & Winston.

Reiss, S. (2000). Why people turn to religion: A motivational analysis. *Journal for the Scientific Study of Religion, 39*, 47–52.

Reiss, S. (2004). The 16 strivings for God. *Zygon, 39*, 303–320.

Reiss, S. (2013). *The Reiss Motivational Profile: What motivates you?* Columbus, OH: IDS.

Reiss, S. (2015). *The 16 strivings for God.* Macon, GA: Mercer University Press.

Reiss, S., & Havercamp, S. M. (2005). Motivation in

developmental context: A new method for studying self-actualization. *Journal of Humanistic Psychology, 45,* 41–53.

Rest, J. R. (1979). *Development in judging moral issues.* Minneapolis, MN: University of Minnesota Press.

Rest, J. R. (1983). Morality. In P. H. Mussen (Series Ed.) & J. H. Flavell & E. M. Markham (Vol. Eds.), *Handbook of child psychology: Vol. 3. Cognitive development* (4th ed., pp. 556–629). New York, NY: Wiley.

Rest, J. R., Cooper, D., Coder, R., Masanz, J., & Anderson, D. (1974). Judging the important issues in moral dilemmas: An objective measure of development. *Developmental Psychology, 10,* 491–501.

Rest, J. R., Narvaez, D., Thoma, S. J., & Bebeau, M. J. (1999). DIT2: Devising and testing a revised instrument of moral judgment. *Journal of Educational Psychology, 91,* 644–659.

Reynolds, D. I. (1994). Religious influence and premarital sexual experience: Critical observations on the validity of a relationship. *Journal for the Scientific Study of Religion, 33,* 382–387.

Reynolds, D. K., & Nelson, F. L. (1981). Personality, life situation, and life expectancy. *Suicide and Life-Threatening Behavior, 11,* 99–110.

Reynolds, F. E., & Waugh, E. H. (1977). *Religious encounters with death.* University Park, PA: Pennsylvania State University Press.

Riccio, J. A. (1979). Religious affiliation and socioeconomic achievement. In R. Wuthnow (Ed.), *The religious dimension: New directions in quantitative research* (pp. 199–228). New York, NY: Academic Press.

Rice, S. A. (2007). *Encyclopedia of evolution.* New York, NY: Facts on File.

Richards, P. S. (1991). The relation between conservative religious ideology and principled moral reasoning: A review. *Review of Religious Research, 32,* 359–368.

Richards, P. S., & Bergin, A. E. (1997). *A spiritual strategy for counseling and psychotherapy.* Washington, DC: American Psychological Association.

Richards, P. S., & Bergin, A. E. (Eds.). (2000). *Handbook of psychotherapy and religious diversity.* Washington, DC: American Psychological Association.

Richards, P. S., & Davison, M. L. (1992). Religious bias in moral development research: A psychometric investigation. *Journal for the Scientific Study of Religion, 31,* 467–485.

Richards, T. A., Wrubel, J., & Folkman, S. (1999–2000). Death rites in the San Francisco gay community: Cultural developments of the AIDS epidemic. *Omega, 40,* 335–350.

Richards, W. A. (2008). The phenomenology and potential religious import of states of consciousness facilitated by psilocybin. *Archive for the Psychology of Religion, 30,* 189–199.

Richards, W. A. (2016). *Sacred knowledge: Psychedelics and religious experiences.* New York, NY: Columbia University Press.

Richardson, A. H. (1973). Social and medical correlates of survival among octogenarians: United Automobile Worker retirees and Spanish American War veterans. *Journal of Gerontology, 28,* 207–215.

Richardson, H. (Ed.). (1980). *New religions and mental health.* New York, NY: Edwin Mellen Press.

Richardson, J. T. (1973). Psychological interpretation of glossolalia: A reexamination of research. *Journal for the Scientific Study of Religion, 12,* 199–207.

Richardson, J. T. (1978a). An oppositional and general conceptualization of cult. *Social Research, 41,* 299–327.

Richardson, J. T. (Ed.). (1978b). *Conversion careers: In and out of the new religions.* Beverly Hills, CA: SAGE.

Richardson, J. T. (1979). From cult to sect: Creative eclecticism in new religious movements. *Pacific Sociological Review, 22,* 139–166.

Richardson, J. T. (1985a, October). *Legal and practical reasons for claiming to be a religion.* Paper presented at the annual meeting of the Society for the Scientific Study of Religion, Savannah, GA.

Richardson, J. T. (1985b). The active vs. passive convert: Paradigm conflict in conversion/recruitment research. *Journal for the Scientific Study of Religion, 24,* 163–179.

Richardson, J. T. (1993). Definitions of cult: From sociological–technical to popular–negative. *Review of Religious Research, 34,* 348–356.

Richardson, J. T. (1995). Clinical and personality assessment of participants in new religions. *International Journal for the Psychology of Religion, 5,* 145–170.

Richardson, J. T. (1999). Social control of new religions: From "brainwashing" claims to sexual abuse accusations. In S. Palmer & C. Hardman (Eds.), *Children in new religions* (pp. 172–186). New Brunswick, NJ: Rutgers University Press.

Richardson, J. T., Best, J., & Bromley, D. G. (Eds.). (1991). *The Satanism scare.* Hawthorne, NY: Aldine/de Gruyter.

Richardson, J. T., & Introvigne, M. (2001). "Brainwashing" theories in European parliamentary and administrative reports on "cults" and "sects." *Journal for the Scientific Study of Religion, 40,* 143–168.

Richardson, J. T., Stewart, T. M., & Simmonds, R. (1979). *Organized miracles: A study of a communal youth fundamentalist group.* New Brunswick, NJ: Transaction Books.

Richardson, J. T., & van Driel, B. (1984). Public

support for anti-cult legislation. *Journal for the Scientific Study of Religion, 23,* 412–418.

Richardson, K. (2000). *The making of intelligence.* New York, NY: Columbia University Press.

Richert, R. A., & Granqvist, P. (2013). Religious and spiritual development in childhood. In R. F. Paloutzian & C. L. Park (Eds.), *Handbook of the psychology of religion and spirituality* (2nd ed., pp. 145–182). New York, NY: Guilford Press.

Richert, R. A., & Smith, E. I. (2009). Cognitive foundations in the development of a religious mind. In E. Voland & W. Schiefenhovel (Eds.), *The biological evolution of religious mind and behavior* (pp. 181–192). Berlin, Germany: Springer.

Riedl, M. (2015, June 14). Kansas, Nebraska United Methodists support change to homosexual doctrines. *The Wichita Eagle,* p. A10.

Riley, N. S. (2013a, April 6). Interfaith unions: A mixed blessing. *The New York Times,* p. A17.

Riley, N. S. (2013b). *'Til faith do us part: How interfaith marriage is transforming America.* New York, NY: Oxford University Press.

Ring, K. (1984). *Heading toward omega: In search of the meaning of the near death experience.* New York, NY: Morrow.

Ritzema, R. J. (1979). Religiosity and altruism: Faith without works? *Journal of Psychology and Theology, 7,* 105–113.

Ritzema, R. J., & Young, C. (1983). Causal schemata and the attribution of supernatural causality. *Journal of Psychology and Theology, 11,* 36–43.

Rizzuto, A.-M. (1979). *The birth of the living God: A psychoanalytic study.* Chicago, IL: University of Chicago Press.

Rizzuto, A.-M. (1982). The father and the child's representation of God: A developmental approach. In S. H. Cath, A. R. Gurwitt, & J. M. Ross (Eds.), *Father and child: Development and clinical perspectives* (pp. 357–382). Boston, MA: Little, Brown.

Rizzuto, A.-M. (2001). Religious development beyond the modern paradigm discussion: The psychoanalytic point of view. *International Journal for the Psychology of Religion, 11,* 201–214.

Rizzuto, A.-M. (2006). Discussion on Granqvist's article "On the relation between secular and divine relationships: An emerging attachment perspective and a critique of the 'depth' approaches." *International Journal for the Psychology of Religion, 16,* 19–28.

Robbins, T. (1977, February 26). Even a Moonie has civil rights. *The Nation,* pp. 233–242.

Robbins, T. (1983). The beach is washing away: Controversial religion and the sociology of religion. *Sociological Analysis, 7,* 197–206.

Robbins, T. (1985). New religious movements, brainwashing and deprogramming: The view from the law journals. *Religious Studies Review, 11,* 361–370.

Robbins, T. (2001). Combating "cults" and "brainwashing" in the United States and Western Europe: A comment on Richardson and Introvigne's report. *Journal for the Scientific Study of Religion, 40,* 169–175.

Robbins, T., & Anthony, D. (1979). Cults, brainwashing, and countersubversion. *Annals of the American Academy of Political and Social Science, 446,* 78–90.

Robbins, T., & Anthony, D. (1980). The limits of "coercive persuasion" as an explanation for conversion to authoritarian sects. *Political Psychology, 3,* 22–37.

Robbins, T., & Anthony, D. (1982). Deprogramming, brainwashing and the medicalization of deviant religious groups. *Social Problems, 29,* 284–296.

Roberts, A. E., Koch, J. R., & Johnson, D. P. (2001). Religious reference groups and the persistence of normative behavior: An empirical test. *Sociological Spectrum, 21,* 81–98.

Roberts, C. W. (1989). Imagining God: Who is created in whose image? *Review of Religious Research, 30,* 375–386.

Roberts, K. A. (1984). *Religion in sociological perspective.* Homewood, IL: Dorsey Press.

Roberts, M. K., & Davidson, J. D. (1984). The nature and sources of religious involvement. *Review of Religious Research, 25,* 334–350.

Roberts, T. B., & Hruby, P. J. (1995). *Religion and psychoactive sacraments: A bibliographic guide.* San Francisco, CA: Council on Spiritual Practices.

Robertson, R. (1975). On the analysis of mysticism: Pre-Weberian, Weberian, and post-Weberian perspectives. *Sociological Analysis, 36,* 241–266.

Robinson, D. N. (1981). *An intellectual history of psychology.* New York, NY: Macmillan.

Robinson, D. N. (2002). *A student's guide to psychology.* Wilmington, Delaware: ISI Books.

Robinson, E. A. R., Cranford, J. A., & Webb, J. R. (2007). Six-month changes in spirituality, religiousness, and heavy drinking in a treatment-seeking sample. *Journal of Studies on Alcohol and Drugs, 68,* 282–290.

Rochford, E. B., Jr., Purvis, S., & NeMar, E. (1989). New religions, mental health, and social control. *Research in the Social Scientific Study of Religion, 1,* 57–82.

Roco, M., & Ticu, B. (1996). Preliminary research on the phases of religious judgment. *Revue Roumaine de Psychologie, 40,* 141–161.

Roehlkepartain, E. C., Benson, P. L., King, P. E., & Wagener, L. (2006). Spiritual development in childhood and adolescence: Moving to the scientific mainstream. In E. C. Roehlkepartain, P. E. King, L. Wagener, & P. L. Benson (Eds.), *The handbook of spiritual development in childhood and adolescence* (pp. 1–15). Thousand Oaks, CA: SAGE.

Rogers, M. (Ed.). (1983). *Contradictory quotations.* Harlow, UK: Longman.

Rohner, R. P. (1994). Patterns of parenting: The warmth dimension in worldwide perspective. In W. J. Lonner & R. Malpass (Eds.), *Psychology and culture* (pp. 113–120). Boston, MA: Allyn & Bacon.

Rohrbaugh, J., & Jessor, R. (1975). Religiosity in youth: A personal control against deviant behavior. *Journal of Personality, 43,* 136–155.

Rokeach, M. (1968). *Beliefs, attitudes, and values.* San Francisco, CA: Jossey-Bass.

Rokeach, M. (1969). Value systems and religion. *Review of Religious Research, 11,* 24–38.

Romme, M., & Escher, A. (1989). Hearing voices. *Schizophrenia Bulletin, 15,* 209–216.

Romme, M., & Escher, A. (1996). Empowering people who hear voices. In G. Haddock & P. D. Slade (Eds.), *Cognitive and behavioral interventions with psychotic disorders* (pp. 137–150). London, UK: Routledge.

Roof, W. C. (1990). Return of the baby boomers to organized religion. In C. J. Jacquet (Ed.), *Yearbook of American and Canadian churches* (pp. 284–289). Nashville, TN: Abingdon Press.

Roof, W. C. (1993). *A generation of seekers: The spiritual journeys of the boom generation.* San Francisco, CA: Harper San Francisco.

Roof, W. C. (1999). *Spiritual marketplace.* Princeton, NJ: Princeton University Press.

Roof, W. C., & McKinney, W. (1987). *American mainline religion: Its changing shape and future.* New Brunswick, NJ: Rutgers University Press.

Roozen, D. A. (1980). Church dropouts: Changing patterns of disengagement and re-entry. *Review of Religious Research, 21,* 427–450.

Rosegrant, J. (1976). The impact of set and setting on religious experience in nature. *Journal for the Scientific Study of Religion, 15,* 301–310.

Rosen, B. C. (1950). Race, ethnicity, and the achievement syndrome. *American Sociological Review, 24,* 47–60.

Rosenau, P. M. (1992). *Postmodernism and the social sciences: Insights, inroads, and intrusions.* Princeton, NJ: University of Princeton Press.

Rosenberg, M. (1962). The dissonant religious context and emotional disturbance. *American Journal of Sociology, 68,* 1–10.

Roshdieh, S., Templer, D. I., Cannon, W. G., & Canfield, M. (1998–1999). The relationships of death anxiety and death depression to religion and civilian war-related experiences in Iranians. *Omega, 38,* 201–210.

Rosik, C. H. (2007a). Ideological concern in the operationalization of homophobia: Part I. An analysis of Hererk's ATLG-R scale. *Journal of Psychology and Theology, 35,* 132–144.

Rosik, C. H. (2007b). Ideological concern in the operationalization of homophobia: Part II. The need for interpretive sensitivity with conservatively religious persons. *Journal of Psychology and Theology, 35,* 145–152.

Rosik, C. H., Griffith, B. A., & Cruz, Z. (2007). Homophobia and conservative religion: Toward a more nuanced understanding. *American Journal of Orthopsychiatry, 77,* 10–19.

Rosmarin, D. H., Krumrei, E. J., & Andersson, G. (2009). Religion as a predictor of psychological distress in two religious communities. *Cognitive Behaviour Therapy, 38,* 54–64.

Rosmarin, D. H., Pargament, K. I., & Flannelly, K. J. (2009). Do spiritual struggles predict poorer physical/mental health among Jews? *International Journal for the Psychology of Religion, 19,* 244–258.

Rosmarin, D. H., Pargament, K. I., Krumrei, E. J., & Flannelly, K. J. (2010). Religious coping among Jews: Development and initial validation of the JCOPE. *Journal of Clinical Psychology, 65,* 670–683.

Rosmarin, D. H., Pirutinsky, S., Cohen, A. B., Galler, Y., & Krumrei, E. J. (2011). Grateful to God or just plain grateful?: A comparison of religious and general gratitude. *Journal of Positive Psychology, 6,* 389–396.

Ross, C. E. (1990). Religion and psychological distress. *Journal for the Scientific Study of Religion, 29,* 236–245.

Ross, C. F. J., Weiss, D., & Jackson, L. M. (1996). The relation of Jungian psychological type to religious attitudes and practices. *International Journal for the Psychology of Religion, 6,* 263–279.

Ross, L., Greene, D., & House, P. (1977). The "false-consensus effect": An egocentric bias in social perception and attribution process. *Journal of Experimental Social Psychology, 13,* 279–301.

Ross, L., & Nisbett, R. E. (1991). *The person and the situation: Perspectives of social psychology.* New York, NY: McGraw-Hill.

Ross, M. W. (1983). Clinical profiles of Hare Krishna devotees. *American Journal of Psychiatry, 140,* 416–420.

Rossetti, S. J. (1995). The impact of child sexual abuse on attitudes toward God and the Catholic Church. *Child Abuse and Neglect, 19,* 1469–1481.

Rossi, A. M., Sturrock, J. B., & Solomon, P. (1963). Suggestion effects on reported imagery in sensory deprivation. *Perceptual and Motor Skills, 16,* 39–45.

Rosten, L. (1972). *Rosten's treasury of Jewish quotations.* New York, NY: McGraw-Hill.

Roszak, T. (1968). *The making of a counterculture.* Garden City, NY: Doubleday.

Roszak, T. (1975). *The unfinished animal.* New York, NY: Harper & Row.

Rotenberg, M. (1978). *Damnation and deviance: The Protestant ethic and the spirit of failure.* New York, NY: Free Press.

Roth, H. D. (1995). Some issues in the study of early Chinese mysticism: A review essay. *Chinese Review International, 2,* 154–173.

Roth, H. D. (1999). *Original Tao: Inward training (Nei-yeh) and the foundations of Taoist mysticism.* New York, NY: Columbia University Press.

Roth, P. A. (1987). *Meaning and method in the social sciences: The case for methodological pluralism.* Ithaca, NY: Cornell University Press.

Rothbaum, F., Weisz, J., Pott, M., Miyake, K., & Morelli, G. (2000). Attachment and culture: Security in the United States and Japan. *American Psychologist, 55,* 1093–1104.

Rothbaum, F., Weisz, J. R., & Snyder, S. S. (1982). Changing the world and changing the self: A two process model of perceived control. *Journal of Personality and Social Psychology. 42,* 5–37.

Rotter, J. B. (1966). Generalized expectancies for internal versus external control of reinforcement. *Psychological Monographs, 80*(1, Whole No. 609).

Rotter, J. B. (1990). Internal versus external control of reinforcement: A case history of a variable. *American Psychologist, 45,* 489–493.

Rounding, K., Lee, A., Jacobson, J. A., & Ji, L. J. (2012). Religion replenishes self-control. *Psychological Science, 23,* 635–642.

Rowatt, W. C., & Franklin, L. (2004). Christian orthodoxy, religious fundamentalism, and right-wing authoritarianism as predictors of implicit racial prejudice. *International Journal for the Psychology of Religion, 14,* 125–138.

Rowatt, W. C., Franklin, L., & Cotton, M. (2005). Patterns and personality correlates of implicit and explicit attitudes toward Christians and Muslims. *Journal for the Scientific Study of Religion, 44,* 29–43.

Rowatt, W. C., Kang, L. L., Haggard, M. C., & LaBouff, J. P. (2014). A social-personality perspective on humility, religiousness, and spirituality. *Journal of Psychology and Theology, 42,* 31–40.

Rowatt, W. C., & Kirkpatrick, L. A. (2002). Two dimensions of attachment to God and their relation to affect, religiosity, and personality constructs. *Journal for the Scientific Study of Religion, 41,* 637–651.

Rowatt, W. C., LaBouff, J. P., Johnson, M., Froese, P., & Tsang, J. (2009). Associations among religiousness, social attitudes, and prejudice in a national sample of American adults. *Psychology of Religion and Spirituality, 1,* 14–24.

Rowatt, W. C., Ottenbreit, A., Nesselroade, K. P., & Cunningham, P. A. (2002). On being holier-than-thou or humbler-than-thee: A social-psychological perspective on religiousness and humility. *Journal for the Scientific Study of Religion, 41,* 227–237.

Rowatt, W. C., Powers, C., Targhetta, V., Comer, J., Kennedy, S., & LaBouff, J. (2006). Development and initial validation of an implicit measure of humility relative to arrogance. *Journal of Positive Psychology, 1,* 198–211.

Rowatt, W. C., Shen, M. J., LaBouff, J. P., & Gonzalez, A. (2013). Religious fundamentalism, right-wing authoritarianism, and prejudice. In R. F. Paloutzian & C. L. Park (Eds.), *Handbook of the psychology of religion and spirituality* (2nd ed., pp. 457–475). New York, NY: Guilford Press.

Rowatt, W. C., Tsang, J., Kelly, J., LaMartina, B., McCullers, M., & McKinley, A. (2006). Associations between religious personality dimensions and implicit homosexual prejudice. *Journal for the Scientific Study of Religion, 45,* 397–406.

Rubin, Z. (1970). Measurement of romantic love. *Journal of Personality and Social Psychology, 16,* 265–273.

Ruether, R. R. (1972, September). *St. Augustine's penis: Sources of misogynism in Christian theology and prospects for liberation today.* Paper presented at the International Congress of Learned Societies in the Field of Religion, Los Angeles, CA.

Ruether, R. R. (Ed.). (1974). *Religion and sexism: Images of women in the Jewish and Christian traditions.* New York, NY: Simon & Schuster.

Ruether, R. R. (1975). *New woman, new earth: Sexist ideologies and human liberation.* Minneapolis, MN: Winston.

Ruether, R. R., & McLaughlin, E. (Eds.). (1979). *Women of spirit.* New York, NY: Simon & Schuster.

Ruffing, J. K. (Ed.). (2001). *Mysticism and social transformation.* Syracuse, NY: Syracuse University Press.

Ruffle, B. J., & Sosis, R. (2006). Cooperation and the in-group–out-group bias: A field test on Israeli kibbutz members and city residents. *Journal of Economic Behavior and Organization, 60,* 147–163.

Ruffle, B. J., & Sosis, R. (2007). Does it pay to pray?: Costly ritual and cooperation. *B.E. Journal of Economic Analysis and Policy, 7,* 1–35.

Ruse, M. (2006). *Darwinism and its discontents.* New York, NY: Cambridge University Press.

Ruse, M. (2013). Naturalism and the scientific method. In S. Bullivant & M. Ruse (Eds.), *The Oxford handbook of atheism* (pp. 383–397). Oxford, UK: Oxford University Press.

Russell, B. (1935). *Religion and science.* London, UK: Oxford University Press.

Ruthven, M. (1984). *Islam in the world.* New York, NY: Oxford University Press.

Ryan, R. M., Rigby, S., & King, K. (1993). Two types of religious internalization and their relations to religious orientations and mental health. *Journal of Personality and Social Psychology, 65,* 586–596.

Ryff, C. D., & Singer, B. H. (1996). Psychological

well-being: Meaning, measurement, and implications for psychotherapy research, *Psychotherapy and Psychosomatics, 65,* 14–23.

Ryle, G. (1954). The world of science and the everyday world. In G. Ryle (Ed.), *Dilemmas* (pp. 68–81). Cambridge, UK: Cambridge University Press.

Saad, L. (2013, May 29). U.S. support for euthanasia hinges on how it's described. *The Gallup Poll.* Retrieved from *http://news.gallup.com/poll/162815/support-euthanasia-hinges-described.aspx.*

Sachs, S. (2002a, April 27). Anti-Semitism is deepening among Muslims. *The New York Times,* p. B9.

Sachs, S. (2002b, June 15). Baptist pastor attacks Islam, inciting cries of intolerance. *The New York Times,* p. A10.

Salas-Wright, C. P., Vaughn, M. G., Hodge, D. R., & Perron, B. E. (2012). Religiosity profiles of American youth in relation to substance use, violence, and delinquency. *Journal of Youth and Adolescence, 41,* 1560–1575.

Salas-Wright, C. P., Vaughn, M. G., & Maynard, B. R. (2014). Religiosity and violence among adolescents in the United States: Findings from the National Survey on Drug Use and Health 2006–2010. *Journal of Interpersonal Violence, 29,* 1178–1200.

Salsman, J. M., Putejovsky, J. E., Jim, H. S., Munoz, A. R., Merluzzi, T. V., George, L., et al. (2015). A meta-analytic approach to examining the correlation between religion/spirituality and mental health in cancer. *Cancer, 121,* 3769–3778.

Samarin, W. J. (1959). Glossolalia as learned behavior. *Canadian Journal of Theology, 19,* 60–64.

Samarin, W. J. (1972). *Tongues of men and angels.* New York, NY: Macmillan.

Sandage, S. J., & Morgan, J. (2014). Hope and positive religious coping as predictors of social justice commitment. *Mental Health, Religion and Culture, 17,* 557–567.

Sanders, C. M. (1979–1980). A comparison of adult bereavement in the death of a spouse, child, and parent. *Omega, 10,* 303–322.

Sands, R. G., Marcus, S. C., & Danzig, R. A. (2008). Spirituality and religiousness among American Jews. *International Journal for the Psychology of Religion, 18,* 238–255.

Sapp, G. L. (1986). Moral judgment and religious orientation. In G. L. Sapp (Ed.), *Handbook of moral development* (pp. 271–286). Birmingham, AL: Religious Education Press.

Sarafino, E. P. (1990). *Health psychology.* New York, NY: Wiley.

Sargent, W. (1957). *Battle for the mind.* London, UK: Heinemann.

Saroglou, V. (2002a). Beyond dogmatism: The need for closure related to religion. *Mental Health, Religion and Culture, 5,* 183–194.

Saroglou, V. (2002b). Religion and the five factors of personality: A meta-analytic review. *Personality and Individual Differences, 32,* 15–25.

Saroglou, V. (2010). Religiousness as a cultural adaptation of basic traits: A five-factor model perspective. *Personality and Social Psychology Review, 14,* 108–125.

Saroglou, V. (2012). Comment: Is religion not prosocial at all? Comment on Galen (2012). *Psychological Bulletin, 138,* 907–912.

Saroglou, V. (2013). Religion, spirituality, and altruism. In K. I. Pargament, J. J. Exline, & J. W. Jones (Eds.), *APA handbook of psychology, religion, and spirituality* (Vol. 1, pp. 439–457). Washington, DC: American Psychological Association.

Saroglou, V. (2014a). Conclusion: Understanding religion and irreligion. In V. Saroglou (Ed.), *Religion, personality, and social behavior* (pp. 361–391). New York, NY: Psychology Press.

Saroglou, V. (Ed.). (2014b). *Religion, personality, and social behavior.* New York, NY: Psychology Press.

Saroglou, V., Corneille, O., & Van Cappellen, P. (2009). "Speak, Lord, your servant is listening": Religious priming activates submissive thoughts and behaviors. *International Journal for the Psychology of Religion, 19,* 143–154.

Saroglou, V., Delpierre, V., & Dernelle, R. (2004). Values and religiosity: A meta-analysis of studies using Schwartz's model. *Personality and Individual Differences, 37,* 721–734.

Saroglou, V., & Muñoz-García, A. (2008). Individual differences in religion and spirituality: An issue of personality traits and/or values. *Journal for the Scientific Study of Religion, 47,* 83–101.

Saroglou, V., Pichon, I., Trompette, L., Verschueren, M., & Dernelle, R. (2005). Prosocial behavior and religion: New evidence based on projective measures and peer-ratings. *Journal for the Scientific Study of Religion, 44,* 323–348.

Saroyan, W. (1937). *My name is Aram.* New York, NY: Harcourt, Brace.

Sasaki, M. A. (1979). Status inconsistency and religious commitment. In R. Wuthnow (Ed.), *The religious dimension: New directions in quantitative research* (pp. 135–156). New York, NY: Academic Press.

Saucier, G., & Skrzypińska, K. (2006). Spiritual but not religious?: Evidence for two independent dispositions. *Journal of Personality, 74*(5), 1257–1292.

Saunders, J. (2001, July 6). Furor erupts as police seize spanked children. *The Globe and Mail* [Toronto], p. A1.

Savage, D. A., & Torgler, B. (2013). The emergence of emotions and religious sentiments during the September 11 disaster. *Motivation and Emotion, 37,* 586–599.

Savage, S., Collins-Mayo, S., Mayo, B., & Cray, G.

(2006). *Making sense of Generation Y: The world view of 15–25 year-olds*. London, UK: Church House.

Scarboro, A., Campbell, N., & Stave, S. (1994). *Living witchcraft: An American coven*. Westport, CT: Praeger.

Scarlett, W. G. (1994). Cognitive-developmental and psychoanalytic comments on Tamminen's essay. *International Journal for the Psychology of Religion, 4*, 87–90.

Scarlett, W. G., & Perriello, L. (1991). The development of prayer in adolescence. In F. K. Oser & W. G. Scarlett (Eds.), *Religious development in childhood and adolescence* (New Directions for Child Development, No. 52, pp. 63–76). San Francisco, CA: Jossey-Bass.

Schachter, S. (1964). The interaction of cognitive and physiological determinants of emotional states. In L. Berkowitz (Ed.), *Advances in experimental social psychology* (Vol. 1, pp. 49–80). New York, NY: Academic Press.

Schachter, S. (1971). *Emotion, obesity, and crime*. New York, NY: Academic Press.

Schachter, S. C. (2006). Religion and the brain: Evidence from temporal lobe epilepsy, In P. McNamara (Ed.), *Where God and science meet* (Vol. 2, pp. 171–188). Westport, CT: Praeger.

Schachter, S., & Singer, J. E. (1962). Cognitive, social, and physiological determinants of emotional states. *Psychological Review, 69*, 379–399.

Schaefer, C. A., & Gorsuch, R. L. (1991). Psychological adjustment and religiousness: The multivariate belief–motivation theory of religiousness. *Journal for the Scientific Study of Religion, 30*, 448–461.

Schaefer, C. A., & Gorsuch, R. L. (1992). Dimensionality of religion: Belief and motivation as predictors of behavior. *Journal of Psychology and Christianity, 11*, 244–254.

Schaffer, M. D. (1990, August 15). Sex a special challenge for many clergy members. *The Denver Post*, p. 6B.

Schaler, J. A. (1996). Spiritual thinking in addiction-treatment providers: The spiritual belief scale. *Alcoholism Treatment Quarterly, 14*(3), 7–33.

Scharfstein, B.-A. (1973). *Mystical experience*. Indianapolis, IN: Bobbs-Merrill.

Scharfstein, B.-A. (1993). *Ineffability*. Albany, NY: State University of New York Press.

Scheflin, A., & Opton, E. (1978). *The mind manipulators*. New York, NY: Paddington.

Schein, E., Schneier, I., & Barker, C. H. (1971). *Coercive persuasion*. New York, NY: Norton.

Schellenberg, J. A. (1990). William James and symbolic interactionism. *Personality and Social Psychology Bulletin, 16*, 769–773.

Schieman, S., Bierman, A., & Ellison, E. G. (2010). Religious involvement, beliefs about God, and the sense of mattering among older adults. *Journal for the Scientific Study of Religion, 49*, 517–535.

Schimmel, S. (1997). *The seven deadly sins: Jewish, Christian, and classical reflections on human nature*. New York, NY: Free Press.

Schjoedt, U., Stetkilde-Jorgensen, H., Geertz, A. W., & Roepstorff, A. (2009). Highly religious participants recruit areas of social cognition in personal prayer. *Social Cognitive and Affective Neuroscience, 4*, 199–207.

Schlenhofer, M. M., Omotto, A. M., & Adelman, J. R. (2008). How do "religion" and "spirituality" differ?: Lay definitions among older adults. *Journal for the Scientific Study of Religion, 47*, 411–425.

Schoenrade, P., Ludwig, C., Atkinson, T., & Shane, R. (1990, November). *Whose loss?: Intrinsic religion and the consideration of one's own or another's death*. Paper presented at the annual convention of the Society for the Scientific Study of Religion, Virginia Beach, VA.

Scholem, G. G. (1969). *On the Kabbalah and its symbolism* (R. Manheim, Trans.). New York, NY: Schocken Books.

Schulz, R., & Heckhausen, J. (1996). A life span model of successful aging. *American Psychologist, 51*, 702–714.

Schumaker, J. F. (1995). *The corruption of reality*. Amherst, NY: Prometheus Books.

Schuon, F. (1975). *The transcendent unity of religion* (rev. ed., P. Townsend, Trans.). New York, NY: Harper & Row.

Schur, E. (1976). *The awareness trap: Self absorption instead of social change*. Chicago, IL: Quadrangle.

Schurig, V., Van Orman, A., Bowen, P., & Opitz, J. M. (2005). Nonprogressive cerebellar disorder with mental retardation and autosomal recessive inheritance in Hutterites. *American Journal of Medical Genetics, 9*, 43–53.

Schwartz, L. L., & Kaslow, F. W. (1979). Religious cults, the individual and the family. *Journal of Marital and Family Therapy, 5*, 15–26.

Schwartz, S. H. (1992). Universals in the content and structure of values: Theoretical advances and empirical tests in 20 countries. In M. Zanna (Ed.), *Advances in experimental social psychology* (Vol. 25, pp. 1–65). San Diego, CA: Academic Press.

Schweitzer, F. (1997). Why we might still need a theory for the religious development of women. *International Journal for the Psychology of Religion, 7*, 87–91.

Schweitzer, F. (2000). Religious affiliation and disaffiliation in late adolescence and early adulthood: The impact of a neglected period of life. In L. J. Francis & Y. J. Katz (Eds.), *Joining and leaving religion: Research perspectives* (pp. 87–101). Leominster, UK: Gracewing.

Science Daily. (2014, August 24). Neuroscience

and big data: How to find simplicity in the brain. Retrieved from *www.sciencedaily.com/releases/2014/08/140824152349.htm*.

Scobie, G. E. W. (1973). Types of religious conversion. *Journal of Behavioral Science, 1,* 265–271.

Scobie, G. E. W. (1975). *Psychology of religion.* New York, NY: Wiley.

Scott, E. (1999). The science and religion movement. *The Skeptical Inquirer,* 29–31.

Scott, J. (1989). Conflicting beliefs about abortion: Legal approval and moral doubts. *Social Psychology Quarterly, 52,* 319–326.

Seals, B. F., Ekwo, E. E., Williamson, R. A., & Hanson, J. W. (1985). Moral and religious influences on the amniocentesis decision. *Social Biology, 32,* 13–30.

Sears, C. E. (1924). *Days of delusion: A strange bit of history.* Boston, MA: Houghton Mifflin.

Sears, R. E. (2015). The construction, preliminary validation, and correlates of a dream-specific scale for mystical experience. *Journal for the Scientific Study of Religion, 54,* 134–155.

Sears, R. E., & Hood, R. W., Jr. (2016). Dreaming mystical experience amongst Christians and Hindus: The impact of culture, language, and religious participation on responses to the Dreaming Mysticism Scale. *Mental Health, Religion and Culture, 19*(8), 833–845.

Seeman, T. E., Dubin, L. F., & Seeman, M. (2003). Religion/spirituality and health: A critical review of the evidence for biological pathways. *American Psychologist, 58,* 53–63.

Segal, R. A. (1985). Have the social sciences been converted? *Journal for the Scientific Study of Religion, 24,* 321–324.

Seggar, J., & Kunz, P. (1972). Conversion: Analysis of a step-like process for problem solving. *Review of Religious Research, 13,* 178–184.

Seigfried, C. H. (1990). *William James's radical reconstruction of philosophy.* Albany, NY: State University of New York Press.

Selig, S., & Teller, G. (1975). The moral development of children in three different school settings. *Religious Education, 70,* 406–415.

Seligman, M. E. P. (1975). *Helplessness: On depression, development, and death.* San Francisco, CA: Freeman.

Seligman, M. E. P. (1999). The president's address. *American Psychologist, 54,* 559–562.

Seligman, M. E. P., & Csikszentmihalyi, M. (2000). Positive psychology: An introduction. *American Psychologist, 55,* 5–14.

Sensky, T. (1983). Religiosity, mystical experience and epilepsy. In F. C. Rose (Ed.), *Research in epilepsy* (pp. 214–220). New York, NY: Pitman.

Sensky, T., Wilson, A., Petty, R., Fenwick, P. B. C., & Rose, F. C. (1984). The interictal personality traits of temporal lobe epileptics: Religious belief and its association with reported mystical experiences. In R. J. Porter et al. (Eds.), *Advances in epileptology: XVth Epilepsy International Symposium* (pp. 545–549). New York, NY: Raven Press.

Sethi, S., & Seligman, M. E. P. (1993). Optimism and fundamentalism. *Psychological Science, 4,* 256–259.

Sethi, S., & Seligman, M. E. P. (1994). The hope of fundamentalists. *Psychological Science, 5,* 58.

Sevinc, K., Hood, R. W., Jr., & Coleman, T. J., III. (2017). Secularism in Turkey. In P. Zuckerman & J. R. Shook (Eds.), *The Oxford handbook of secularism* (pp. 155–171). New York, NY: Oxford University Press.

Seybold, K. S. (2016). *Questions in the psychology of religion.* Eugene, OR: Cascade Books.

Seybold, K. S., & Hill, P. C. (2001). The role of religion and spirituality in mental and physical health. *Current Directions in Psychological Science, 10,* 21–24.

Shafranske, E. P. (1992). Religion and mental health in early life. In J. F. Schumaker (Ed.), *Religion and mental health* (pp. 163–176). New York, NY: Oxford University Press.

Shafranske, E. P. (1995). Freudian theory and religious experience. In R. W. Hood, Jr. (Ed.), *Handbook of religious experience* (pp. 200–232). Birmingham, AL: Religious Education Press.

Shafranske, E. P. (1996a). Religious beliefs, practices and affiliations of clinical psychologists. In E. P. Shanfranske (Ed.), *Religion and the clinical practice of psychology* (pp. 149–164). Washington, DC: American Psychological Association.

Shafranske, E. P. (2013). Addressing religiousness and spirituality in psychotherapy: Advancing evidence-based practice. In R. F. Paloutzian & C. L. Park (Eds.), *Handbook of the psychology of religion and spirituality* (2nd ed., pp. 595–616). New York, NY: Guilford Press.

Shafranske, E. P., & Malony, H. N. (1985, February). *Religion, spirituality, and psychotherapy: A study of California psychologists.* Paper presented at the meeting of the California State Psychological Association, San Francisco, CA.

Shahabi, L., Powell, L., Musick, M. A., Pargament, K. I., Thoresen, C. E., Williams, D., et al. (2002). Correlates of self-perceptions of spirituality among American adults. *Annals of Behavioral Medicine, 24,* 59–68.

Shakespeare, W. (1964). *Measure for measure.* New York, NY: New American Library. (Original work produced 1604)

Shand, J. D. (1990). A forty-year followup of the religious beliefs and attitudes of a sample of Amherst College grads. In M. L. Lynn & D. O. Moberg (Eds.), *Research in the social scientific study of religion* (Vol. 2, pp. 117–136) Greenwich, CT: JAI Press.

Shanon, B. (2008). Biblical entheogens: A speculative hypothesis. *Time and Mind: The Journal of Archaeology, Consciousness and Culture, 1*, 51–74.

Shapiro, E. (1977). Destructive cultism. *American Family Physician, 15*, 80–83.

Sharf, R. H. (2000). The rhetoric of religion in the study of religious experience. In J. Andresen & R. K. Forman (Eds.), *Cognitive models and spiritual maps: Interdisciplinary explorations of religious experience* (pp. 267–287). Bowling Green, OH: Imprint Academic.

Shariff, A. F., & Norenzayan, A. (2007). God is watching you: Priming God concepts increases social behavior in an anonymous economic game. *Psychological Science, 18*, 803–809.

Shariff, A. F., & Norenzayan, A. (2011). Mean gods make good people: Different views of God predict cheating behavior. *International Journal for the Psychology of Religion, 21*, 85–96.

Shaw, G. B. (1931). Briefer views. In A. M. Drummond & R. H. Wagner (Eds.), *Problems and opinions* (p. 378). New York, NY: Century.

Sheldon, K. M., & King, L. (2001). Why positive psychology is necessary. *American Psychologist, 56*, 216–217.

Sheldrake, R. (2012). *Science set free*. New York, NY: Random House.

Shenhav, A., Rand, D. G., & Greene, J. D. (2012). Divine intuition: Cognitive style influences belief in God. *Journal of Experimental Psychology: General, 141*, 423–428.

Shephard, R. N. (1978). The mental image. *American Psychologist, 33*, 125–137.

Sheridan, T. B. (2014). *What is God?: Can religion be modeled?* Washington, DC: New Academia.

Sherif, M. (1953). *Groups in harmony and tension*. New York, NY: Harper & Row.

Sherif, M. (1966). *In common predicament: Social psychology of intergoup conflict and cooperation*. Boston, MA: Houghton Mifflin.

Sherkat, D. E. (2000). "That they be keepers of the home": The effect of conservative religion on early and late transitions into housewifery. *Review of Religious Research, 41*, 344–358.

Sherkat, D. E., & Darnell, A. (1999). The effect of parents' fundamentalism on children's educational attainment: Examining differences by gender and children's fundamentalism. *Journal for the Scientific Study of Religion, 38*, 23–35.

Sherman, A. C., Merluzzi, T. V., Pustejovsky, J. E., Park, C. L., George, L., Fitchett, G., et al. (2015). A meta-analytic review of religious or spiritual involvement and social health among cancer patients. *Cancer, 121*, 3779–3788.

Shermer, M. (2000). *How we believe: The search for God in an age of science*. New York, NY: Freeman.

Shermer, M. (2009, June 1). Why people believe invisible agents control the world. *Scientific American*. Retrieved from *www.scientificamerican.com/article/skeptic-agenticity*.

Shermer, M. (2010, April 1). The sensed-presence effect. *Scientific American*. Retrieved from *www.scientificamerican.com/article/the-sensed-presence-effect*.

Sheskin, A., & Wallace, S. E. (1980). Differing bereavements: Suicide, natural, and accidental death. In R. A. Kalish (Ed.), *Death, dying, transcending* (pp. 74–87). Farmingdale, NY: Baywood.

Shidlo, A., & Schroeder, M. (2002). Changing sexual orientation: A consumer's report. *Professional Psychology: Research and Practice, 33*, 249–259.

Shields, J. J., Broome, K. M., Delany, P. J., Fletcher, B. W., & Flynn, P. M. (2007). Religion and substance abuse treatment: Individual and program effects. *Journal for the Scientific Study of Religion, 46*, 355–371.

Shokeir, M. H. K., Rozdilsky, B., Opitz, J. M., & Reynolds, J. F. (2005). Muscular dystrophy in Saskatchewan Hutterites. *American Journal of Medical Genetics, 22*, 487–493.

Shor, E., & Roelfs, D. J. (2013). The longevity effects of religious and nonreligious participation: A meta-analysis and meta-regression. *Journal for the Scientific Study of Religion, 52*, 120–145.

Shor, R. E., & Orne, E. C. (1962). *Harvard Group Scale of Hypnotic Susceptibility*. Palo Alto, CA: Consulting Psychologists Press.

Shortz, J. L., & Worthington, E. L. (1994). Young adults' recall of religiosity, attributions, and coping in a parental divorce. *Journal for the Scientific Study of Religion, 33*, 173–179.

Šhram, Z. (2017). Psychopathy and depression as predictors of the satanic syndrome. *Open Theology, 3*, 90–126.

Shrauger, J. S., & Silverman, R. E. (1971). The relationship of religious background and participation to locus of control. *Journal for the Scientific Study of Religion, 10*, 11–16.

Shrell-Fox, P. (2015). When rabbis lose faith: Twelve rabbis tell about loss of belief in God. *Science, Religion and Culture, 2*, 131–146.

Shuman, C. R., Fournet, G. P., Zelhart, P. F., Roland, B. C., & Estes, R. E. (1992). Attitudes of registered nurses toward euthanasia. *Death Studies, 16*, 1–15.

Shupe, A. D., Jr., & Bromley, D. (1985). Social response to cults. In P. Hammond (Ed.), *The sacred in a secular age* (pp. 58–69). Berkeley, CA: University of California Press.

Shupe, A. D., Jr., Bromley, D. G., & Oliver, D. L. (1984). *The anti-cult movement in America*. New York, NY: Garland Press.

Shupe, A. D., Jr., Spielman, R., & Stigall, S. (1977). Deprogramming. *American Behavioral Scientist, 20,* 941–956.

Shweder, R. A., Goodnow, J., Hatano, G., Levine, R., Markus, H., & Miller, P. (2006). The cultural psychology of development: One mind, many mentalities. In W. Damon & R. M. Lerner (Series Eds.) & R. M. Lerner (Vol. Ed.), *Handbook of child psychology: Vol. 1. Theoretical models of human development* (6th ed., pp. 716–792). Hoboken, NJ: Wiley.

Sidgewick, H. A. (1894). Report of the census on hallucinations. *Proceedings of the Society for Psychical Research, 26,* 259–394.

Sieben, I. (2001). Schooling or social origin?: The impact of educational attainment on religious, political, and social orientations after controlling for family background. *Mens en Maatschappij, 76,* 22–43.

Siegel, R. K. (1977). Religious behavior in animals and man: Drug-induced effects. *Journal of Drug Issues, 7,* 219–236.

Silberman, C. E. (1985). *A certain people: American Jews and their lives today.* New York, NY: Summit Books.

Silberman, I. (2003). Spiritual role modeling: The teaching of meaning systems. *International Journal for the Psychology of Religion, 13,* 175–195.

Silberman, I. (2005a). Religion as a meaning system: Implications for a new millennium. *Journal of Social Issues, 61,* 641–663.

Silberman, I. (2005b). Religious violence, terrorism, and peace: A meaning-system analysis. In R. F. Paloutzian & C. L. Park (Eds.), *Handbook of the psychology of religion and spirituality* (pp. 529–549). New York, NY: Guilford Press.

Silton, N. R., Flannelly, K. J., Ellison, C. G., Galek, K., Jacobs, M. R., Marcum, J. P., & Simon, F. J. (2011). The association between religious beliefs and practices and end-of-life fears among members of the Presbyterian Church (U.S.A.). *Review of Religious Research, 53,* 357–370.

Silver, C. F., Coleman, T. J., Hood, R. W., Jr., & Holcombe, J. M. (2014). The six types of non-belief: A quantitative and qualitative study of type and narrative. *Mental Health, Religion and Culture, 17,* 990–1001.

Silver, C. F., Olson, M. A., Larsen, J. T., & Hood, R. W., Jr. (2017). *Jesus in context: Are mental images of Jesus malleable?* Poster session presented at the annual convention of the Society for Personality and Social Psychology, San Antonio, TX.

Silverman, M. K., & Pargament, K. I. (1990). *God help me: III. Longitudinal and prospective studies on effects of religious coping efforts on the outcomes of significant negative life events.* Paper presented at the annual convention of the American Psychological Association, San Francisco, CA.

Silverman, W. H., Pargament, K. I., Johnson, S. M., Echemendia, R. J., & Snyder, S. (1983). Measuring member satisfaction with the church. *Journal of Applied Psychology, 68,* 664–677.

Silvestri, P. J. (1979). Locus of control and God dependence. *Psychological Reports, 45,* 89–90.

Simmonds, R. B. (1977a). Conversion or addiction? *American Behavioral Scientist, 20,* 909–924.

Simmonds, R. B. (1977b). *The people of the Jesus movement: A personality assessment of members of a fundamentalist religious community.* Unpublished doctoral dissertation, University of Nevada at Reno, Reno, NV.

Simon, B. (1978). *Mind and madness in ancient Greece.* Ithaca, NY: Cornell University Press.

Simpkinson, A. A. (1996, November–December). Soul betrayal. *Common Boundary,* pp. 24–37.

Simpson, J. B. (Ed.). (1964). *Contemporary quotations.* New York, NY: Galahad Books.

Singer, J. L. (1966). *Daydreaming: An introduction to the experimental study of inner experience.* New York, NY: Random House.

Singer, M. T. (1978a, January). Coming out of the cults. *Psychology Today,* pp. 72–82.

Singer, M. T. (1978b). Therapy with ex-cult members. *Journal of the National Association of Private Psychiatric Hospitals, 9,* 14–18.

Singer, M. T., & Ofshe, R. (1990). Thought reform programs and the production of psychiatric casualties. *Psychiatric Annals, 20,* 188–193.

Singer, M. T., & West, L. J. (1980). Cults, quacks, and non-professional therapies. In H. I. Kaplan & J. B. Sadock (Eds.), *Comprehensive textbook of psychiatry* (3rd ed., Vol. 3, pp. 3245–3258). Baltimore: Williams & Wilkins.

Sipe, A. W. R. (1990). *A secret world: Sexuality and the search for celibacy.* New York, NY: Brunner/Mazel.

Sipe, A. W. R. (1995). *Sex, priests, and power: Anatomy of a crisis.* New York, NY: Brunner/Mazel.

Sisemore, T. A. (2016). *The psychology of religion and spirituality: From the inside out.* Hoboken, NJ: Wiley.

Skal, D. J. (1998). *Screams of reason.* New York, NY: Norton.

Skinner, B. F. (1948). "Superstition" in the pigeon. *Journal of Experimental Psychology, 38,* 168–172.

Skinner, B. F. (1969). *Contingencies of reinforcement.* New York, NY: Appleton-Century-Crofts.

Skinner, E. (1996). A guide to constructs of control. *Journal of Personality and Social Psychology, 71,* 549–570.

Skonovd, N. (1983). Leaving the cultic religious milieu. In D. Bromley & J. Richardson (Eds.),

The brainwashing/deprogramming controversy: Sociological, psychological, legal and historical perspectives (pp. 91–105). Lewiston, NY: Edwin Mellen Press.

Skorikov, V., & Vondracek, F. W. (1998). Vocational identity development: Its relationship to other identity domains and to overall identity development. *Journal of Career Assessment, 6*, 13–35.

Sloan, R. P., & Bagiella, E. (2002). Claims about religious involvement and health outcomes. *Annals of Behavioral Medicine, 24*, 14–21.

Sloan, R. P., Bagiella, E., & Powell, T. (1999). Religion, spirituality, and medicine. *Lancet, 353*, 664–667.

Smith, C., & Denton, M. L. (2005). *Soul searching: The religious and spiritual lives of American teenagers.* New York, NY: Oxford University Press.

Smith, C., Lundquist Denton, M. L., Faris, R., & Regnerus, M. (2002). Mapping American adolescent religious participation. *Journal for the Scientific Study of Religion, 41*, 597–612.

Smith, E. R., & Mackie, D. M. (1995). *Social psychology.* New York, NY: Worth.

Smith, H. (2000). *Cleansing the doors of perception: The religious significance of entheogenic plants and chemicals.* New York, NY: Tarcher/Putnam.

Smith, J. H., & Handelman, S. A. (1990). *Psychoanalysis and religion.* Baltimore: Johns Hopkins University Press.

Smith, J. Z. (1996). The bare facts of ritual. In R. L. Grimes (Ed.), *Readings in ritual studies* (pp. 473–483). Upper Saddle River, NJ: Prentice-Hall. (Original work published 1982)

Smith, M. (1977). *An introduction to mysticism.* New York, NY: Oxford University Press.

Smith, P. C., Range, L. M., & Ulmer, A. (1991–1992). Belief in afterlife as a buffer in suicidal and other bereavement. *Omega, 24*, 217–225.

Smith, R. E., Wheeler, G., & Diener, E. (1975). Faith without works: Jesus people, resistance to temptation, and altruism. *Journal of Applied Social Psychology, 5*, 320–330.

Smith, T. W. (2006). The National Spiritual Transformation Study. *Journal for the Scientific Study of Religion, 45*, 283–296.

Smith, T. W. (2012). *Beliefs about God across time and countries.* Chicago, IL: NORC/University of Chicago.

Snarey, J. R. (1985). Cross-cultural universality of social–moral development: A critical review of Kohlbergian research. *Psychological Bulletin, 97*, 202–233.

Snook, J. B. (1974). An alternative to church–sect. *Journal for the Scientific Study of Religion, 13*, 191–204.

Snook, S. C., & Gorsuch, R. L. (1985). *Religion and racial prejudice in South Africa.* Paper presented

at the annual convention of the American Psychological Association, Los Angeles, CA.

Snow, D. A., & Machalek, R. (1983). The convert as a social type. In R. Collins (Ed.), *Sociological theory* (pp. 259–289). San Francisco, CA: Jossey-Bass.

Snow, D. A., & Machalek, R. (1984). The sociology of conversion. *Annual Review of Sociology, 10*, 167–190.

Snow, D. A., Zurcher, L. A., Jr., & Ekland-Olson, S. (1980). Social networks and social movements: A microstructural approach to differential recruitment. *American Sociological Review, 45*, 797–801.

Snow, D. A., Zurcher, L. A., Jr., & Ekland-Olson, S. (1983). Further thoughts on social networks and movement recruitment. *Sociology, 17*, 112–120.

Snyder, C. R. (1994). *The psychology of hope: You can get there from here.* New York, NY: Free Press.

Snyder, C. R. (2001). *Coping with stress: Effective people and processes.* New York: Oxford University Press.

Snyder, C. R., Sigmon, D., & Feldman, D. B. (2002). Hope for the sacred and vice-versa: Positive goal-directed thinking and religion. *Psychological Inquiry, 13*, 234–238.

Sober, E. (1984). *The nature of selection: Evolutionary theory in philosophical focus.* Cambridge, MA: MIT Press.

Socha, P. (1999). The existential human situation: Spirituality as a way of coping. In K. H. Reich, F. Oser, & W. G. Scarlett (Eds.), *Psychological studies on spiritual and religious development: Vol. 2. Being human: The case of religion* (pp. 50–56). Berlin, Germany: Pabst Science.

Söderblom, N. (1963). *Uppenbarelsereligion.* Stockholm, Sweden: Prisma.

Somit, A. (1968). Brainwashing. In D. Solls (Ed.), *International encyclopaedia of the social sciences* (Vol. 2, pp. 138–143). New York, NY: Macmillan.

Soper, J. C. (2001). Tribal instinct and religious persecution: Why do western European states behave so badly? *Journal for the Scientific Study of Religion, 40*, 177–180.

Sorokin, P. A. (2002). *The ways and power of love: Types, factors, and techniques of moral transformation.* Philadelphia, PA: Templeton Foundation Press. (Original work published 1954)

Sparks, G. G. (2001, September–October). The relationship between paranormal beliefs and religious beliefs. *Skeptical Inquirer*, pp. 50–56.

Sparrow, G. S. (1995). *I am with you always: True stories of encounters with Jesus.* New York, NY: Bantam.

Spellman, C. M., Baskett, G. D., & Byrne, D. (1971). Manifest anxiety as a contributing factor in religious conversion. *Journal of Consulting and Clinical Psychology, 36*, 245–247.

Spencer, C., & Agahi, C. (1982). Social background, personal relationships, and self-descriptions as predictors of drug-user status: A study of adolescents in post-revolutionary Iran. *Drug and Alcohol Dependence, 10,* 77–84.

Spilka, B. (1970). Images of man and dimensions of personal religion: Values for an empirical psychology of religion. *Review of Religious Research, 11,* 171–182.

Spilka, B. (1976). "The compleat person": Some theoretical views and research findings for a theological-psychology of religion. *Journal of Psychology and Theology, 4,* 15–24.

Spilka, B. (1977). Utilitarianism and personal faith. *Journal of Psychology and Theology, 5,* 226–233.

Spilka, B. (1993, August). *Spirituality: Problems and directions in operationalizing a fuzzy concept.* Paper presented at the annual meeting of the American Psychological Association, Toronto, Ontario, Canada.

Spilka, B. (2007). *Reanalysis of General Social Survey data on contact with the dead.* Unpublished manuscript.

Spilka, B., Addison, J., & Rosensohn, M. (1975). Parents, self, and God: A test of competing theories of individual–religion relationships. *Review of Religious Research, 16,* 154–165.

Spilka, B., Armatas, P., & Nussbaum, J. (1964). The concept of God: A factor analytic approach. *Review of Religious Research, 6,* 28–36.

Spilka, B., Brown, G. A., & Cassidy, S. E. (1993). The structure of mystical experience in relation to pre- and post-experience lifestyle correlates. *International Journal for the Psychology of Religion, 2,* 241–257.

Spilka, B., Hood, R. W., Jr., & Gorsuch, R. L. (1985). *The psychology of religion: An empirical approach.* Englewood Cliffs, NJ: Prentice-Hall.

Spilka, B., Kojetin, B., & McIntosh, D. (1985). Forms and measures of personal faith: Questions, correlates and distinctions. *Journal for the Scientific Study of Religion, 24,* 437–442.

Spilka, B., & Ladd, K. L. (2013). *The psychology of prayer: A scientific approach.* New York, NY: Guilford Press.

Spilka, B., Ladd, K. L., McIntosh, D. N., Milmoe, S., & Bickel, C. O. (1996). The content of religious experience: The roles of expectancy and desirability. *International Journal for the Psychology of Religion, 6,* 95–105.

Spilka, B., & Loffredo, L. (1982). *Classroom cheating among religious students: Some factors affecting perspectives, actions and justifications.* Paper presented at the annual convention of the Rocky Mountain Psychological Association, Albuquerque, NM.

Spilka, B., & McIntosh, D. N. (1995). Attribution theory and religious experience. In R. W. Hood, Jr. (Ed.), *Handbook of religious experience* (pp. 421–445). Birmingham, AL: Religious Education Press.

Spilka, B., & Schmidt, G. (1983a). General attribution theory for the psychology of religion: The influence of event-character on attributions to God. *Journal for the Scientific Study of Religion, 22,* 326–339.

Spilka, B., & Schmidt, G. (1983b). *Stylistic factors in attributions: The role of religion and locus of control.* Paper presented at the annual convention of the Rocky Mountain Psychological Association, Snowbird, UT.

Spilka, B., Shaver, P., & Kirkpatrick, L. A. (1985). A general attribution theory for the psychology of religion. *Journal for the Scientific Study of Religion, 24,* 1–20.

Spilka, B., Spangler, J. D., & Nelson, C. B. (1983). Spiritual support in life-threatening illness. *Journal of Religion and Health, 22,* 98–104.

Spilka, B., Spangler, J. D., & Rea, M. P. (1981). The role of theology in pastoral care for the dying. *Theology Today, 38,* 16–29.

Spilka, B., Spangler, J. D., Rea, M. P., & Nelson, C. B. (1981). Religion and death: The clerical perspective. *Journal of Religion and Health, 20,* 299–306.

Spilka, B., & Werme, P. (1971). Religion and mental disorder: A critical review and theoretical perspective. In M. Strommen (Ed.), *Research on religious development: A comprehensive handbook* (pp. 461–484). New York, NY: Hawthorn Books.

Spilka, B., Zwartjes, W. J., & Zwartjes, G. M. (1991). The role of religion in coping with childhood cancer. *Pastoral Psychology, 39,* 285–304.

Spinella, M., & Wain, O. (2006). The neural substrates of moral, religious, and paranormal beliefs. *Skeptical Inquirer, 30*(5), 35–38.

Spinetta, J. J. (1977). Adjustment in children with cancer. *Journal of Pediatric Psychology, 2*(2), 49–51.

Sprinthall, N. A., & Collins, W. A. (1995). *Adolescent psychology: A developmental view* (3rd ed.). New York, NY: McGraw-Hill.

Stace, W. T. (1960). *Mysticism and philosophy.* Philadelphia, PA: Lippincott.

Stack, S., & Wasserman, I. (1992). The effect of religion on suicide ideology: An analysis of the networks perspective. *Journal for the Scientific Study of Religion, 31,* 457–466.

Stambrook, M., & Parker, K. C. H. (1987). The development of the concept of death in childhood: A review of the literature. *Merrill–Palmer Quarterly, 33,* 133–157.

Stander, F. (1987). Some rigors of our time: The First Amendment and real life and death. *Cultic Studies Journal, 4,* 1–17.

Starbuck, E. D. (1897). A study of conversion. *American Journal of Psychology, 8,* 268–308.

Starbuck, E. D. (1899). *The psychology of religion.* New York, NY: Scribner.

Starbuck, E. D. (1904). The varieties of religious experience. *The Biblical World, 24*(N.S.), 100–111.

Stark, R. (1963). On the incompatibility of religion and science: A survey of American graduate students. *Journal for the Scientific Study of Religion, 3,* 3–20.

Stark, R. (1965). A taxonomy of religious experience. *Journal for the Scientific Study of Religion, 5,* 97–116.

Stark, R. (1971). Psychopathology and religious commitment. *Review of Religious Research, 12,* 165–176.

Stark, R. (1985). Church and sect. In P. E. Hammond (Ed.), *The sacred in a secular age* (pp. 139–149). Berkeley, CA: University of California Press.

Stark, R. (1996). Why religious movements succeed or fail: A revised general model. *Journal of Contemporary Religion, 11,* 133–146.

Stark, R. (1998). *Sociology* (7th ed.). Belmont, CA: Wadsworth.

Stark, R. (1999). A theory of revelations. *Journal for the Scientific Study of Religion, 38,* 287–308.

Stark, R., & Bainbridge, W. S. (1979). Of churches, sects and cults: Preliminary concepts for a theory of religious movements. *Journal for the Scientific Study of Religion, 18,* 117–133.

Stark, R., & Bainbridge, W. S. (1980a). Networks of faith: Interpersonal bonds and recruitment to cults and sects. *American Journal of Sociology, 85,* 1376–1395.

Stark, R., & Bainbridge, W. S. (1980b). Towards a theory of religion. *Journal for the Scientific Study of Religion, 19,* 114–128.

Stark, R., & Bainbridge, W. S. (1985). *The future of religion.* Berkeley, CA: University of California Press.

Stark, R., & Bainbridge, W. S. (1987). *A theory of religion.* New York, NY: Peter Lang.

Stark, R., Doyle, D. P., & Rushing, J. L. (1983). Beyond Durkheim: Religion and suicide. *Journal for the Scientific Study of Religion, 22,* 120–131.

Stark, R., & Glock, C. Y. (1968). *American piety: The nature of religious commitment.* Berkeley, CA: University of California Press.

Staudinger, U. M., & Baltes, P. B. (1996). Interactive minds: A facilitative setting for wisdom-related performance? *Journal of Personality and Social Psychology, 71,* 746–762.

Staudinger, U. M., & Leipold, B. (2003). The assessment of wisdom-related performance. In S. J. Lopex & C. R. Snyder (Eds.), *Positive psychological assessment: A handbook of models and measures* (pp. 171–184). Washington, DC: American Psychological Association.

Steeman, T. M. (1975). Church, sect, mysticism, denomination: Periodological aspects of Troeltsch's types. *Sociological Analysis, 26,* 181–204.

Steger, M. F., Dik, B. J., & Duffy, R. D. (2012). Measuring meaningful work: The Work and Meaning Inventory (WAMI). *Journal of Career Assessment, 20,* 322–337.

Steger, M. F., Fitch-Martin, A. R., Donnelly, J., & Rickard, K. M. (2015). Meaning in life and health: Proactive health orientation links meaning in life to health variables among American undergraduates. *Journal of Happiness Studies, 16,* 583–597.

Steinberg, L. (1983). *The sexuality of Christ in Renaissance art and in modern oblivion.* New York, NY: Pantheon.

Steinberg, L., Lamborn, S. D., Dornbusch, S. M., & Darling, N. (1992). Impact of parenting practices on adolescent achievement: Authoritative parenting, school involvement, and encouragement to succeed. *Child Development, 63,* 1266–1281.

Stengel, E. (1964). *Suicide and attempted suicide.* Baltimore: Penguin.

Stephan, C. W., & Stephan, W. G. (1985). *Two social psychologies.* Homewood, IL: Dorsey Press.

Sterling, R. C., Weinstein, S., Hill, P. C., & Gottheil, E., Gordon, S. M., & Shorie, K. (2006). Levels of spirituality and treatment outcome: A preliminary investigation. *Journal of Studies on Alcohol, 67,* 600–606.

Sterling, R. C., Weinstein, S., Losardo, D., Raively, K., Hill, P. C., Petrone, A., & Gottheil, E. (2007). A retrospective case control study of alcohol relapse and spiritual growth. *American Journal on Addictions, 16,* 56–61.

Sternberg, R. J. (2007). A systems model of leadership: WICS. *American Psychologist, 62,* 34–42.

Stevens, J. (1987). *Storming heaven: LSD and the American dream.* New York, NY: Harper & Row.

Stewart, C. (2001). The influence of spirituality on substance use of college students. *Journal of Drug Education, 31,* 343–351.

Stifler, K., Greer, J., Sneck, W., & Dovenmuehle, R. (1993). An empirical investigation of the discriminability of reported mystical experiences among religious contemplatives, psychotic inpatients, and normal adults. *Journal for the Scientific Study of Religion, 32,* 366–372.

Stifoss-Hanssen, H. (1994). Rigid religiosity and mental health: An empirical study. In L. B. Brown (Ed.), *Religion, personality, and mental health* (pp. 138–143). New York, NY: Springer-Verlag.

Stinespring, J., & Cragun, R. T. (2015). Simple Markov model for estimating the growth of nonreligion in the United States. *Science, Religion, and Culture, 2,* 96–103.

Stobart, St. C. (1971). *Torchbearers of spiritualism.* New York, NY: Kennikat.

Stone, J. R. (2000). *Expecting Armageddon: Essential readings in failed prophecy.* New York, NY: Routledge.

Stone, P. J., Dunphy, D. C., Smith, M. S., & Ogilvie, D. M. (1966). *The general inquirer: A computer approach to content analysis.* Cambridge, MA: MIT Press.

Stoppler, M. C. (n.d.). Cortisol: The "stress" hormone. Retrieved April 29, 2002, from *www.stress.about.com/library/weeklyaa012901a.htm.*

Storch, E. A., & Storch, J. B. (2001). Organizational, nonorganizational, and intrinsic religiosity and academic dishonesty. *Psychological Reports, 88,* 548–552.

Storr, A. (1988). *Solitude: A return to the self.* New York, NY: Ballantine Books.

Stouffer, S. (1955). *Communism, conformity, and civil liberty.* Garden City, NY: Doubleday.

Stout-Miller, R., Miller, L. S., & Langenbrunner, M. R. (1997). Religiosity and child sexual abuse: A risk factor assessment. *Journal of Child Sexual Abuse, 6,* 15–34.

Strang, S., & Strang, P. (2001). Spiritual thoughts, coping and 'sense of coherence' in brain tumor patients and their spouses. *Palliative Medicine, 15,* 127–134.

Strassman, R. (2001). *DMT: The spirit molecule.* Rochester, VT: Park Street Press.

Straus, R. A. (1976). Changing oneself: Seekers and the creative transformation of experience. In J. Lofland (Ed.), *Doing social life* (pp. 252–272). New York, NY: Wiley.

Straus, R. A. (1979). Religious conversion as a personal and collective accomplishment. *Sociological Analysis, 40,* 158–165.

Strawbridge, W. J., Cohen, R. D., Shema, S. J., & Kaplan, G. A. (1997). Frequent attendance at religious services and mortality over 28 years. *American Journal of Public Health, 87,* 957–961.

Strawbridge, W. J., Shema, S. J., Cohen, R. D., & Kaplan, G. A. (2001). Religious attendance increases survival by improving and maintaining good health behaviors, mental health, and social relationships. *Annals of Behavioral Medicine, 23,* 68–74.

Strawson, P. F. (1959). *Individuals: An essay in descriptive metaphysics.* London, UK: Methuen.

Streib, H. (2001a). Faith development theory revisited: The religious styles perspective. *International Journal for the Psychology of Religion, 11,* 143–158.

Streib, H. (2001b). Fundamentalism as a challenge to religious education. *Religious Education, 96,* 227–244.

Streib, H. (2007). Religious praxis—de-institutionalized: Theoretical and empirical considerations. In H. Streib (Ed.), *Religion inside and outside traditional institutions* (pp. 147–174). Leiden, The Netherlands: Brill.

Streib, H. (2008). More spiritual than religious: Changes in the religious field require new approaches. In H. Streib, A. Dinter, & K. Söderblom (Eds.), *Lived religion: Conceptual, empirical, and practical-theological approaches: Essays in honor of Hans-Günter Heimbroell* (pp. 53–67). Leiden, The Netherlands: Brill.

Streib, H. (2014). Deconversion. In L. R. Rambo & C. E. Farhadian (Eds.), *The Oxford handbook of conversion* (pp. 271–296). New York, NY: Oxford University Press.

Streib, H., & Hood, R. W., Jr. (2011). "Spirituality" as privatized experience-oriented religion: Empirical and conceptual perspectives. *Journal of Implicit Religion, 14,* 433–453.

Streib, H., & Hood, R. W., Jr. (Eds.). (2016). *Semantics and psychology of spirituality: A cross-cultural analysis comparing Germany and America.* New York, NY: Springer.

Streib, H., Hood, R. W., Jr., & Keller, B. (2016). Deconversion and "spirituality"—migrations in the religious field. In H. Streib & R. W. Hood, Jr. (Eds.), *Semantics and psychology of spirituality: A cross-cultural analysis* (pp. 19–26). New York, NY: Springer.

Streib, H., Hood, R. W., Jr., Keller, B., Csöff, R.-M., & Silver, C. (2009). *Deconversion: Qualitative and quantitative results from cross-cultural research in Germany and the United States* (Research in Contemporary Religion, Vol. 4). Göttingen, Germany: Vandenhoeck & Ruprecht.

Streib, H., Hood, R. W., Jr., & Klein, C. (2010). The Religious Schema Scale: Construction and initial validation of a quantitative measure for religious styles. *International Journal for the Psychology of Religion, 20,* 151–172.

Streib, H., & Klein, C. (2013). Atheists, agnostics, and apostates. In K. I. Pargament, J. J. Exline, & J. W. Jones (Eds.), *APA handbook of psychology, religion, and spirituality* (Vol. 1, pp. 713–728). Washington, DC: American Psychological Association.

Strength, J. M. (1999). Grieving the loss of a child. *Journal of Psychology and Christianity, 18,* 338–353.

Strickland, M. P. (1924). *Psychology of religious experience.* New York, NY: Abingdon Press.

Strickler, J., & Danigelis, N. L. (2002). Changing frameworks in attitudes toward abortion. *Sociological Forum, 17,* 187–201.

Strommen, M. P., Brekke, M. L., Underwager, R. C., & Johnson, A. L. (1972). *A study of generations.* Minneapolis, MN: Augsburg.

Stroope, S., Draper, S., & Whitehead, A. L. (2013). Images of a loving God and sense of meaning in life. *Social Indicators Research, 111,* 25–44.

Struch, N., & Schwartz, S. H. (1989). Intergroup aggression: Its predictors and distinctness from ingroup bias. *Journal of Personality and Social Psychology, 56,* 364–373.

Suedfeld, P. (1975). The benefits of boredom: Sensory deprivation reconsidered. *American Scientist, 63,* 60–69.

Suedfeld, P., & Vernon, J. (1964). Visual hallucination in sensory deprivation: A problem of criteria. *Science, 145,* 412–413.

Sullivan, J. L., Pierson, J. E., & Marcus, G. E. (1982). *Political tolerance in American democracy.* Chicago, IL: University of Chicago Press.

Sundararajan, L., & Kim, C. (2014). Spiritual suffering from medieval German mysticism to Mother Teresa: A psycholinguistic analysis. *The Humanistic Psychologist, 42,* 172–198.

Surwillo, W. W., & Hobson, D. P. (1978). Brain electrical activity during prayer. *Psychological Reports, 43,* 135–143.

Sutherland, I., & Shepherd, J. P. (2001). Social dimensions of adolescent substance use. *Addiction, 96,* 445–458.

Sutherland, P. (1988). A longitudinal study of religious and moral values in late adolescence. *British Educational Research Journal, 14,* 73–78.

Suttie, I. D. (1952). *The origins of love and hate.* New York, NY: Julian Press.

Suzuki, D. T. (1957). *Mysticism: Christian and Buddhist.* New York, NY: Harper. (Original work published 1927)

Swatos, W. H. (1981). Church, sect and cult: Bringing mysticism back in. *Sociological Analysis, 42,* 17–26.

Swatos, W. H., Jr. (1992). Adolescent Satanism: A research note on exploratory survey data. *Review of Religious Research, 34,* 161–169.

Swatos, W. H., Jr. (1998). *Encyclopedia of religion and society.* Walnut Creek, CA: Altamira Press.

Swinburne, R. (1981). The evidential value of religious experience. In A. R. Peacoke (Ed.), *The sciences and theology in the twentieth century* (pp. 182–196). Notre Dame, IN: University of Notre Dame Press.

Symonds, P. M. (1946). *Dynamics of human adjustment.* New York, NY: Appleton-Century.

Szasz, T. (1970). *Ideology and insanity: Essays on the psychiatric dehumanization of man.* Garden City, NY: Doubleday.

Szasz, T. (1983). *The manufacture of madness.* New York, NY: Harper & Row.

Szasz, T. (1984). *The therapeutic states: Psychiatry in the mirror of current events.* Buffalo, NY: Prometheus Books.

Tajfel, H., & Turner, J. C. (1986). The social identity theory of intergroup behavior. In S. Worchel & W. G. Austin (Eds.), *Psychology of intergroup relations* (pp. 7–24). Chicago, IL: Nelson-Hall.

Tamminen, K. (1976). Research concerning the development of religious thinking in Finnish students: A report of results. *Character Potential: A Record of Research, 7,* 206–219.

Tamminen, K. (1991). *Religious development in childhood and youth: An empirical study.* Helsinki, Finland: Suomalainen Tiedeakatemia.

Tamminen, K. (1994). Religious experiences in childhood and adolescence: A viewpoint of religious development between the ages of 7 and 20. *International Journal for the Psychology of Religion, 4,* 61–85.

Tamminen, K., & Nurmi, K. E. (1995). Developmental theories and religious experience. In R. W. Hood, Jr. (Ed.), *Handbook of religious experience* (pp. 169–311). Birmingham, AL: Religious Education Press.

Tamminen, K., Vianello, R., Jaspard, J.-M., & Ratcliff, D. (1988). The religious concepts of preschoolers. In D. Ratcliff (Ed.), *Handbook of preschool religious education* (pp. 97–108). Birmingham, AL: Religious Education Press.

Tamney, J. (2002). *The resilience of conservative religion: The case of popular, conservative Protestant congregations.* Cambridge, UK: Cambridge University Press.

Tangney, J. P. (2009). Humility. In C. R. Snyder & S. J. Lopez (Eds.), *Handbook of positive psychology* (2nd ed., pp. 483–490). New York, NY: Oxford University Press.

Tarakeshwar, N. (2013). What does it mean to be a Hindu?: A review of common Hindu beliefs and practices and their implications for health. In K. I. Pargament, J. J. Exline, & J. W. Jones (Eds.), *APA handbook of psychology, religion, and spirituality* (Vol. 1, pp. 653–664). Washington, DC: American Psychological Association.

Tarakeshwar, N., Pargament, K. I., & Mahoney, A. (2003). Initial development of a measure of religious coping among Hindus. *Journal of Community Psychology, 31,* 607–628.

Targ, E., Schlitz, M., & Irwin, H. J. (2000). Psi-related experiences. In E. Cardeña, S. J. Lynn, & S. Krippner (Eds.), *Varieties of anomalous experience* (pp. 219–252). Washington, DC: American Psychological Association.

Tart, C. (1975). Science, state of consciousness, and spiritual experiences: The need for state-specific sciences. In C. Tart (Ed.), *Transpersonal psychologies* (pp. 9–58). New York, NY: Harper & Row.

Taslimi, C. R., Hood, R. W., Jr., & Watson, P. J. (1991). Assessment of former members of Shiloh: The Adjective Check List 17 years later. *Journal for the Scientific Study of Religion, 30,* 306–311.

Tate, D. G., & Forchheimer, M. (2002). Quality of life, life satisfaction, and spirituality: Comparing outcomes between rehabilitation and cancer patients. *American Journal of Physical and Medical Rehabilitation, 8,* 400–410.

Tate, E. D., & Miller, G. R. (1971). Differences in value systems of persons with varying religious orientations. *Journal for the Scientific Study of Religion, 10,* 357–365.

Taves, A. (1999). *Fits, trances, and visions: Experiencing religion and explaining experience from Wesley to James.* Princeton, NJ: Princeton University Press.

Taves, A. (2009). *Religious experience reconsidered: A building block approach to the study of religion and other special things.* Princeton, NJ: Princeton University Press.

Tavris, C., & Sadd, S. (1977). *The Redbook report on female sexuality.* New York, NY: Dell.

Tawney, R. H. (1926). *Religion and the rise of capitalism.* New York, NY: Harcourt, Brace.

Taylor, C. (2002). *Varieties of religion today: William James revisited.* Cambridge, MA: Harvard University Press.

Taylor, C. (2007). *A secular age.* Cambridge, MA: Harvard University Press/Belknap Press.

Taylor, H. (1998, August 12). Large majority of people believe they will go to heaven; only one in fifty thinks they will go to hell (Harris Poll No. 41). Retrieved December 21, 2001, from *www.harrisinteractive.com/harris poll/index.asp?PID=167.*

Taylor, S. M. (2007). *Green sisters: A spiritual ecology.* Cambridge, MA: Harvard University Press.

Teachman, J. (2003). Premarital sex, premarital cohabitation, and the risk of subsequent marital dissolution among women. *Journal of Marriage and Family, 65,* 444–445.

Tekke, M., Watson, P. J., İsmail, N. A., & Chen, Z. J. (2015). Muslim religious openness and *ilm*: Relationships with Islamic religious reflection, religious schema, and religious commitments in Malaysia. *Archive for the Psychology of Religion, 37,* 295–320.

Telegraph Media Group Limited. (2010, April 6). Jesus appeared in my chewing gum. *The Telegraph.*

Tellegen, A., & Atkinson, G. (1974). Openness to absorbing and self-altering experiences ("absorption"), a trait related to hypnotic susceptibility. *Journal of Abnormal Psychology, 83,* 268–277.

Templeton, J. (2000). *Possibilities for over one hundredfold more spiritual information: The human approach in theology and science.* Philadelphia, PA: Templeton Foundation Press.

Templin, D. P., & Martin, M. J. (1999). The relationship between religious orientation, gender, and drinking patterns among Catholic college students. *College Student Journal, 33,* 488–495.

Tennant, F. (1968). *The sources of the doctrine of the fall and original sin.* New York, NY: Schocken Books. (Original work published 1903)

ter Voert, M., Felling, A., & Peters, J. (1994). The effect of religion on self-interest morality. *Review of Religious Research, 35,* 302–323.

Terry, K. J., & Freilich, J. D. (2012). Understanding child sexual abuse by Catholic priests from a situational perspective. *Journal of Child Sexual Abuse, 21,* 437–455.

Thalbourne, M. A. (1998). Transliminality: Further correlates and a short scale. *Journal of the American Society for Psychical Research, 92,* 402–419.

Thalbourne, M. A., Bartemucci, L., Delin, P. S., Fox, B., & Nofi, O. (1997). Transliminality: Its nature and correlates. *Journal of the American Society for Psychical Research, 91,* 305–331.

Thalbourne, M. A., & Delin, P. S. (1994). A common thread underlying belief in the paranormal, creative personality, mystical experience, and psychopathology. *Journal of Parapsychology, 58,* 3–38.

Thalbourne, M. A., & Delin, P. S. (1999). Transliminality: Its relation to dream life, religiosity, and mystical experience. *International Journal for the Psychology of Religion, 9,* 35–43.

Thearle, M. J., Vance, J. C., Najman, J. M., Embelton, G., & Foster, W. J. (1995). Church attendance, religious affiliation and parental responses to sudden infant death, neonatal death and stillbirth. *Omega, 31,* 51–58.

Thibaut, J., & Walker, L. (1975). *Procedural justice: A psychological analysis.* Hillsdale, NJ: Erlbaum.

Thoits, P. A. (2010). Stress and health: Major findings and policy implications. *Journal of Health and Social Behavior, 51*(1, Suppl.), S41–S53.

Thomas, L. E. (1974). Generational discontinuity in beliefs: An exploration of the generation gap. *Journal of Social Issues, 30,* 1–22.

Thomas, L. E., & Cooper, P. E. (1978). Measurement and incidence of mystical experiences: An exploratory study. *Journal for the Scientific Study of Religion, 17,* 433–437.

Thomas, L. E., & Cooper, P. E. (1980). Incidence and psychological correlates of intense spiritual experiences. *Journal of Transpersonal Psychology, 12,* 75–85.

Thoresen, C. E. (2007). Spirituality, religion, and health: What's the deal? In T. G. Plante & C. E. Thoresen (Eds.), *Spirit, science, and health: How the spiritual mind fuels physical wellness* (pp. 3–10). Westport, CT: Praeger.

Thorner, I. (1966). Prophetic and mystic experiences: Comparisons and consequences. *Journal for the Scientific Study of Religion, 5,* 2–96.

Thornton, E. E. (1970). *Professional education for the ministry: A history of clinical pastoral education.* Nashville, TN: Abingdon Press.

Thorson, J. A. (1991). Afterlife constructs, death anxiety, and life reviewing: The importance of religion as a moderating variable. *Journal of Psychology and Theology, 19*, 278–284.

Thurstone, L. L., & Chave, E. J. (1929). *The measurement of attitude: A psychophysical method and some experiments with a scale for measuring attitude toward the church.* Chicago, IL: University of Chicago Press.

Tien, A. Y. (1991). Distribution of hallucinations in the population. *Social Psychiatry and Psychiatric Epidemiology, 26*, 287–292.

Tillich, P. (1952). *The courage to be.* New Haven, CT: Yale University Press.

Tillich, P. (1957). *Dynamics of faith.* New York, NY: Harper & Row.

Tippett, A. R. (1977). Conversion as a dynamic process in Christian mission. *Missiology, 2*, 203–221.

Tipton, R. M., Harrison, B. M., & Mahoney, J. (1980). Faith and locus of control. *Psychological Reports, 46*, 1151–1154.

Tipton, S. M. (1982). *Getting saved from the sixties: Moral meaning in conversion and cultural change.* Berkeley, CA: University of California Press.

Tobias, K. P. (2015). Does religious belief infect philosophical analysis? *Religion, Brain, and Behavior, 16*, 56–66.

Toburen, T., & Meier, B. P. (2010). Priming God-related concepts increases anxiety and task persistence. *Journal of Social and Clinical Psychology, 29*, 127–143.

Todd, N. R., McConnell, E. A., & Suffrin, R. L. (2014). The role of attitudes toward white privilege and religious beliefs in predicting social justice interest and commitment. *American Journal of Community Psychology, 53*, 109–121.

Tonigan, J. S., Miller, W. R., & Schermer, C. (2002) Atheists, agnostics and alcoholics anonymous. *Journal of Studies on Alcohol, 63*, 534–541.

Toussaint, L. T., Williams, D. R., Musick, M. A., & Everson, S. A. (2001). Forgiveness and health: Age differences in a U.S. probability sample. *Journal of Adult Development, 8*, 249–257.

Travisano, R. (1970). Alternation and conversion as qualitatively different transformations. In G. P. Stone & H. A. Faberman (Eds.), *Social psychology through symbolic interaction* (pp. 594–606). Waltham, MA: Ginn-Blaisdell.

Trier, K. K., & Shupe, A. (1991). Prayer, religiosity and healing in the heartland, USA: A research note. *Review of Religious Research, 32*, 351–358.

Troeltsch, E. (1931). *The social teachings of the Christian churches* (2 vols., O. Wyon, Trans.). New York, NY: Macmillan.

Tsang, J., & McCullough, M. E. (2003). Measuring religious constructs: A hierarchical approach to construct organization and scale selection. In S. J. Lopez & C. R. Snyder (Eds.), *Positive psychological assessment: A handbook of models and measures* (pp. 345–360). Washington, DC: American Psychological Association.

Tsang, J., & Rowatt, W. C. (2007). The relationship between religious orientation, right-wing authoritarianism, and implicit sexual prejudice. *International Journal for the Psychology of Religion, 17*, 99–120.

Tsuang, M. T., Williams, W. M., Simpson, J. C., & Lyons, M. J. (2002). Pilot study of spirituality and mental health in twins. *American Journal of Psychiatry, 159*, 486–488.

Tucker, D. M., Novelly, R. A., & Walker, P. J. (1987). Hyperreligiosity in temporal lobe epilepsy: Redefining the relationship. *Journal of Nervous and Mental Disease, 175*(3), 181–184.

Tumminia, D. (1998). How prophecy never fails: Interpretive reason in a flying saucer group. *Sociology of Religion, 59*, 157–170.

Turiel, E., & Neff, K. (2000). Religion, culture, and beliefs about reality in moral reasoning. In K. S. Rosengren, C. N. Johnson, & P. L. Harris (Eds.), *Imagining the impossible: Magical, scientific, and religious thinking in children* (pp. 269–304). Cambridge, UK: Cambridge University Press.

Turner, P. R. (1979). Religious conversion and community development. *Journal for the Scientific Study of Religion, 18*, 252–269.

Twenge, J. M., Exline, J. J., Grubbs, J. B., Sastry, R., & Campbell, W. K. (2015). Generational and time period differences in American adolescents?: Religious orientation, 1966–2014. *PLOS One, 10*(5), e0121454.

Tylor, E. B. (1873). *Primitive culture* (Vol. 2). London, UK: Murray.

Tylor, E. B. (1896). *Anthropology.* New York, NY: Appleton.

Tyrrell, B. J. (1985). Christotherapy: An approach to facilitating psychospiritual healing and growth. In R. J. Wicks, R. D. Parsons, & D. Capps (Eds.), *Clinical handbook of pastoral counseling* (pp. 58–75). New York, NY: Paulist Press.

Tzuriel, D. (1984). Sex role typing and ego identity in Israeli, Oriental, and Western adolescents. *Journal of Personality and Social Psychology, 46*, 440–457.

U.S. Bureau of the Census. (2007). *Statistical abstract of the United States: 2007.* Washington, DC: U.S. Government Printing Office.

U.S. Bureau of the Census. (2008). *Statistical abstract of the United States: 2008.* Washington, DC: U.S. Government Printing Office.

Udry, J. R. (1971). *The social context of marriage* (2nd ed.). Philadelphia, PA: Lippincott.

Uecker, J. E. (2008a). Religion, pledging, and the

premarital sexual behavior of married young adults. *Journal of Marriage and Family, 70,* 728–744.

Uecker, J. E. (2008b). Religious and spiritual responses to 9/11: Evidence from the Add Health study. *Sociological Spectrum, 28,* 477–509.

Ullman, C. (1982). Cognitive and emotional antecedents of religious conversion. *Journal of Personality and Social Psychology, 43,* 183–192.

Unamuno, M. de. (1954). *The tragic sense of life* (J. E. Crawford Fitch, Trans.). New York, NY: Dover. (Original work published 1921)

Underhill, E. (1933). *The golden sequence: A fourfold study of the spiritual life* (3rd ed.). London, UK: Methuen.

Underhill, R. M. (1936). *The autobiography of a Papago woman* (Memoirs of the American Anthropological Association, No. 46). Menasha, WI: American Anthropological Association.

Underwood, A. (2001, May 7). Religion and the brain. *Newsweek,* pp. 50–57.

Underwood, L. G. (1999). Daily spiritual experiences. In *Multidimensional measurement of religiousness/spirituality for use in health research: A report of the Fetzer Institute/National Institute of Aging Working Group* (pp. 11–17). Kalamazoo, MI: Fetzer Institute.

Ungerleider, J. T., & Welish, D. K. (1979). Coercive persuasion (brainwashing), religious cults, and deprogramming. *American Journal of Psychiatry, 136,* 279–282.

Uslaner, E. M. (2002). Religion and civic engagement in Canada and the United States. *Journal for the Scientific Study of Religion, 41,* 239–254.

Vaas, R. (2009). Gods, gains, and genes. In E. Voland & W. Schiefenhovel (Eds.), *The biological evolution of religious mind and behavior* (pp. 25–50). New York, NY: Springer.

Vail, K. E., III, Rothschild, Z. K., Weise, D. R., Solomon, S., Pyszczynski, T., & Greenberg, J. (2010). A terror management analysis of the psychological functions of religion. *Personality and Social Psychology Review, 14,* 84–94.

Valdesolo, P., & Graham, J. (2013). Awe, uncertainty, and agency detection. *Psychological Science, 25,* 170–178.

Van Cappellen, P., & Saroglou, V. (2012). Awe activates religious and spiritual feelings and behavioral intentions. *Psychology of Religion and Spirituality, 4,* 223–236.

van der Lans, J. (1985). Frame of reference as a prerequisite for the induction of religious experience through meditation: An experimental study. In L. B. Brown (Ed.), *Advances in the psychology of religion* (pp. 127–134). Oxford, UK: Pergamon Press.

van der Lans, J. (1987). The value of Sunden's role-theory demonstrated and tested with respect to religious experiences in meditation. *Journal for the Scientific Study of Religion, 26,* 401–412.

van Driel, B., & Richardson, J. T. (1988). Categorization of new religions in American print media. *Sociological Analysis, 49,* 171–183.

Van Fossen, A. B. (1988). How do movements survive failures of prophecy? *Research in Social Movements, Conflicts and Change, 10,* 193–202.

Van Owen, R. (Ed.). (1973). *Chinese mystics.* New York, NY: Harper & Row.

Van Tongeren, D., Hill, P. C., Krause, N., Ironson, G., & Pargament, K. I. (2017). The mediating role of meaning in the association between stress and health. *Annals of Behavioral Medicine, 51*(5), 775–781.

Vande Kemp, H. (1976). Teaching psychology/religion in the seventies: Monopoly or cooperation? *Teaching of Psychology, 3,* 15–18.

VandeCreek, L., Pargament, K., Belavich, T., Cowell, B., & Friedel, L. (1999). The unique benefits of religious support during cardiac bypass surgery. *Journal of Pastoral Care, 53,* 19–29.

VanderStoep, S. W., & Green, C. W. (1988). Religiosity and homonegativism: A path-analytic study. *Basic and Applied Social Psychology, 9,* 135–147.

Vaos, D., & McAndrew, S. (2012). Three puzzles of non-religion in Britain. *Journal of Contemporary Religion, 27,* 29–48.

Vasilenko, S. A., & Lefkowitz, E. S. (2014). Changes in religiosity after first intercourse in the transition to adulthood. *Psychology of Religion and Spirituality, 6,* 310–315.

Vaux, K. (1990). Theology as the queen (bee) of the disciplines. *Zygon, 25,* 317–322.

Verdier, P. (1977). *Brainwashing and the cults.* Redondo Beach, CA: Institute of Behavioral Conditioning.

Vergote, A. (1997). *Religion, belief, and unbelief: A psychological study.* Amsterdam, The Netherlands: Rodopi.

Vergote, A., & Tamayo, A. (Eds.). (1981). *The parental figures and the representation of God: A psychological and cross-cultural study.* The Hague, The Netherlands: Mouton.

Vernon, G. M. (1968). The religious "nones": A neglected category. *Journal for the Scientific Study of Religion, 7,* 219–229.

Vitell, S. J., Bing, M. N., Davison, H. K., Ammeter, A. P., Garner, B. L., & Novicevic, M. M. (2009). Religiosity and moral identity: The mediating role of self-control. *Journal of Business Ethics, 88,* 601–613.

Vitz, P. C. (1977). *Psychology as religion.* Grand Rapids, MI: Eerdmans.

Vitz, P. C. (2000). *Faith of the fatherless: The psychology of atheism.* Dallas, TX: Spence.

Vohs, K. D., & Baumeister, R. F. (Eds.). (2011). *Handbook of self-regulation: Research, theory, and applications.* New York, NY: Guilford Press.

Volcano Press. (1995). *Family violence and religion.* Volcano, CA: Author.

Volinn, E. (1985). Eastern meditative groups: Why join? *Sociological Analysis, 46,* 147–156.

Volken, L. (1961). *Vision, revelations, and the church.* New York, NY: J. P. Kennedy.

Von Eckardt, B. (1995). *What is cognitive science?* Cambridge, MA: MIT Press.

Vul, E., Harris, C., Winkielman, P., & Pashler, H. (2009). Puzzlingly high correlations in fMRI studies of emotion, personality, and social cognition. *Perspectives on Psychological Science, 4,* 274–290.

Vyse, S. A. (1997). *Believing in magic: The psychology of superstition.* New York, NY: Oxford University Press.

Wachholtz, A., & Sambamoorthi, U. (2011). National trends in prayer use as a coping mechanism for health concerns: Changes from 2002 to 2007. *Psychology of Religion and Spirituality, 3,* 67–77.

Wade, N. (2005, June 3). Researchers say intelligence and diseases may be linked in Ashkenazic genes. *The New York Times,* p. A21.

Wade, N. (2009). *The faith instinct: How religion evolved and why it endures.* New York, NY: Penguin.

Wagner, G. J., Serafini, J., Rabkin, J., Remien, R., & Williams, J. (1994). Integration of one's religion and homosexuality: A weapon against internalized homophobia? *Journal of Homosexuality, 26,* 91–110.

Walach, H., Kohls, N., von Stillfried, N., Hinterberger, T., & Schmidt, S. (2009). Spirituality: The legacy of parapsychology. *Archive for the Psychology of Religion, 31,* 277–308.

Walker, C., Ainette, M. G., Wills, T. A., & Mendoza, D. (2007). Religiosity and substance use: Test of an indirect-effect model in early and middle adolescence. *Psychology of Addictive Behaviors, 21,* 84–96.

Walker, S. R., Tonigan, J. S., Miller, W. R., Comer, S., & Kahlich, L. (1997). Intercessory prayer in the treatment of alcohol abuse and dependence: A pilot investigation. *Alternative Therapies, 3,* 79–86.

Wallace, A. F. C. (1956). Revitalization movements. *American Anthropologist, 58,* 264–281.

Wallace, C. W. (1966). *Religion: An anthropological view.* New York, NY: Random House.

Wallace, J. M., Jr., Brown, T. N., Bachman, J. G., & Laviest, T. A. (2003). The influence of race and religion on abstinence from alcohol, cigarettes, and marijuana among adolescents. *Journal of Studies on Alcohol, 64,* 843–848.

Wallace, J. M., Jr., & Forman, T. A. (1998). Religion's role in promoting health and reducing risk among American youth. *Health Education and Behavior, 25,* 721–741.

Wallace, J. M., Jr., & Williams, D. R. (1997). Religion and adolescent health-compromising behavior. In J. Schulenberg, J. Maggs, & K. Hurrelmann (Eds.), *Health risks and developmental transitions during adolescence* (pp. 444–468). Cambridge, UK: Cambridge University Press.

Waller, N. G., Kojetin, B. A., Bouchard, T. J., Jr., Lykken, D. T., & Tellegen, A. (1990). Genetic and environmental influences on religious interests, attitudes, and values: A study of twins reared apart and together. *Psychological Science, 1,* 138–142.

Wallis, R. (1974). Ideology, authority, and the development of cultic movements. *Social Research, 41,* 299–327.

Wallis, R. (1976). *The road to total freedom: A sociological analysis of Scientology.* New York, NY: Columbia University Press.

Wallis, R. (1986). Figuring out cult receptivity. *Journal for the Scientific Study of Religion, 25,* 494–503.

Wallston, K. A., Malcarne, V. L., Flores, L., Hansdottir, I., Smith, C. A., Stein, M. J., et al. (1999). Does God determine your health?: The God Locus of Health Control Scale. *Cognitive Therapy and Research, 23,* 131–142.

Walsh, A. (2002). Returning to normalcy. *Religion in the News, 5,* 26–28.

Walsh, F. (2013). Religion and spirituality: A family systems perspective in clinical practice. In K. I. Pargament, A. Mahoney, & E. P. Shafranske (Eds.), *APA handbook of psychology, religion, and spirituality* (Vol. 2, pp. 189–205). Washington, DC: American Psychological Association.

Walsh, R. (1982). Psychedelics and psychological well-being. *Journal of Humanistic Psychology, 22,* 22–32.

Walsh, W. J. (1906). *The apparitions of the shrines of heaven's bright queen* (4 vols.). New York, NY: Cary-Stafford.

Wang, M., Horne, S. G., Levitt, H. M., & Klesges, L. M. (2009). Christian women in IPV relationships: An exploratory study of religious factors. *Journal of Psychology and Christianity, 28,* 224–235.

Wangerin, R. (1993). *The children of God.* Westport, CT: Bergin & Garvey.

Ware, A. P. (Ed.). (1985). *Midwives of the future.* Kansas City, MO: Leaven Press.

Warner, M. (1976). *Alone of all her sex: The myth and the cult of the Virgin Mary.* New York, NY: Knopf.

Warren, R. (2002). *The purpose-driven life.* Grand Rapids, MI: Zondervan.

Wasserman, I., & Stack, S. (1993). The effect of religion on suicide: An analysis of cultural context. *Omega, 27,* 295–305.

Wasson, R. G. (1969). *Soma: Divine mushroom of*

immortality. New York, NY: Harcourt Brace Jovanovich.

Wasson, R. G., Hofmann, A., & Ruck, C. (1978). *The road to Eleusis: Unveiling the secret of mysteries*. New York, NY: Harcourt Brace Jovanovich.

Waterman, A. (1985). *Identity in adolescence: Processes and contents*. San Francisco, CA: Jossey-Bass.

Watkins, M. M. (1976). *Waking dreams*. New York, NY: Harper & Row.

Watkins, P. C. (2004). Gratitude and subjective well-being. In R. A. Emmons & M. E. McCullough (Eds.), *The psychology of gratitude* (pp. 167–192). New York, NY: Oxford University Press.

Watkins, P. C. (2014). *Gratitude and the good life: Toward a psychology of appreciation*. New York, NY: Springer.

Watkins, P. C., & McCurrach, D. (2016). Exploring how gratitude trains cognitive processes important to well-being. In D. Carr (Ed.), *Perspectives on gratitude: An interdisciplinary approach* (pp. 27–40). New York, NY: Routledge.

Watkins, P. C., Woodward, K., Stone, T., & Kolts, R. L. (2003). Gratitude and happiness: Development of a measure of gratitude and relationships with subjective well-being. *Social Behavior and Personality*, *31*, 431–452.

Watson, P. J. (1993). Apologetics and ethnocentricism: Psychology and religion within an ideological surround. *International Journal for the Psychology of Religion*, *3*, 1–20.

Watson, P. J. (2011). Whose psychology? Which rationality?: Christian psychology within an ideological surround after postmodernism. *Journal of Psychology and Christianity*, *30*, 307–316.

Watson, P. J., Chen, Z., Ghorbani, N., & Vartanian, M. (2015). Religious openness hypothesis: I. Religious reflection, schemas, and orientations within religious fundamentalist and biblical foundationalist ideological surrounds. *Journal of Psychology and Christianity*, *34*, 99–113.

Watson, P. J., Chen, Z., & Hood, R. W., Jr. (2011). Biblical foundationalism and religious reflection: Polarization of faith and intellect oriented epistemologies within a Christian ideological surround. *Journal of Psychology and Theology*, *39*, 111–121.

Watson, P. J., Chen, Z., & Morris, R. J. (2014). Varieties of quest and the religious openness hypothesis within religious fundamentalist and biblical foundationalist ideological surrounds. *Religions*, *5*, 1–20.

Watson, P. J., Chen, Z., Morris, R. J., & Stephenson, E. (2015). Religious openness hypothesis: III. Defense against secularism within fundamentalist and biblical foundationalist ideological surrounds. *Journal of Psychology and Christianity*, *34*, 125–140.

Watson, P. J., Ghorbani, N., Vartanian, M., & Chen, Z. (2015). Religious openness hypothesis: II. Religious reflection and orientations, mystical experience, and psychological openness of Christians in Iran. *Journal of Psychology and Christianity*, *34*, 114–124.

Watson, P. J., Hood, R. W., Jr., & Morris, R. J. (1985). Dimensions of religiosity and empathy. *Journal of Psychology and Christianity*, *4*, 73–85.

Watson, P. J., Hood, R. W., Jr., Morris, R. J., & Hall, J. R. (1984). Empathy, religious orientation, and social desirability. *Journal of Psychology*, *117*, 211–216.

Watson, P. J., Howard, R., Hood, R. W., Jr., & Morris, R. J. (1988). Age and religious orientation. *Review of Religious Research*, *29*, 271–280.

Watson, P. J., Morris, R. J., Foster, J. E., & Hood, R. W., Jr. (1986). Religiosity and social desirability. *Journal for the Scientific Study of Religion*, *25*, 215–232.

Watson, P. J., Morris, R. J., & Hood, R. W., Jr. (1993). Mental health, religion and the ideology of irrationality. In M. L. Lynn & D. O. Moberg (Eds.), *Research in the social scientific study of religion* (Vol. 5, pp. 53–88). Greenwich, CT: JAI Press.

Watson, P. J., Sawyers, P., Morris, R. J., Carpenter, M. J., Jimenez, R. S., Jonas, K. A., & Robinson, D. L. (2003). Reanalysis within a Christian ideological surround: Relationships of intrinsic religious orientation with fundamentalism and right-wing authoritarianism. *Journal of Psychology and Theology*, *31*, 315–328.

Watt, C., & Nagtegaal, M. (2004). Reporting of blind methods: An interdisciplinary survey. *Journal of the Society for Psychical Research*, *68*, 105–114.

Watterson, K., & Geisler, R. B. (2012). Religiosity and self-control: When the going gets tough, the religious get self-regulating. *Psychology of Religion and Spirituality*, *4*, 193–205.

Watts, F. (2002). *Theology and psychology*. Aldershot, UK: Ashgate.

Watts, F. (2006). Attachment, evolution, and the psychology of religion: A response to Lee Kirkpatrick. *Archive for the Psychology of Religion*, *28*, 63–69.

Watts, F. (2014). Religion and the emergence of differential cognition. In F. Watts & L. Turner (Eds.), *Evolution, religion, and cognitive science: Critical and constructive essays* (pp. 109–131). Oxford, UK: Oxford University Press.

Watts, I. (1707). *When I survey the wondrous cross* [Hymn].

Wax, M. L. (1984). Religion as universal: Tribulations of an anthropological enterprise. *Zygon*, *19*, 5–20.

Waxman, C. I. (1994). Religious and ethnic patterns of Jewish baby boomers. *Journal for the Scientific Study of Religion*, *33*, 74–80.

Weaver, A. J., Berry, J. W., & Pittel, S. M. (1994).

Ego development in fundamentalist and non-fundamentalist Protestants. *Journal of Psychology and Theology, 22,* 215–225.

Weaver, A. J., Samford, J. A., Morgan, V. J., Larson, D. B., Koenig, H. G., & Flannelly, K. J. (2002). A systematic review of research on religion in six primary marriage and family journals: 1995–1999. *American Journal of Family Therapy, 30,* 293–309.

Webb, M., & Otto Whitmer, K. J. (2001). Abuse history, world assumptions, and religious problem solving. *Journal for the Scientific Study of Religion, 40,* 445–453.

Weber, C. (n.d.). *The purpose of cortisol and corticosterone.* Retrieved July 12, 2002, from *www.member.tripod.com/~Charles_W/cortisol.html.*

Weber, M. (1930). *The Protestant ethic and the spirit of capitalism* (T. Parsons, Trans.). New York, NY: Scribner. (Original work published 1904)

Webster, D. (2015). The effects of spirituality on drug use. *Journal of Human Behavior in the Social Environment, 25,* 322–332.

Webster, H., Freedman, M., & Heist, P. (1962). Personality changes in college students. In N. Sanford (Ed.), *The American college: A psychological and social interpretation of the higher learning* (pp. 811–846). New York, NY: Wiley.

Weigert, A. J., D'Antonio, W. V., & Rubel, A. J. (1971). Protestantism and assimilation among Mexican Americans: An exploratory study of ministers' reports. *Journal for the Scientific Study of Religion, 10,* 219–232.

Weigert, A. J., & Thomas, D. L. (1969). Religiosity in 5-D: A critical note. *Social Forces, 48,* 260–263.

Weil, A. (1986). *The natural mind* (rev. ed.). Boston, MA: Houghton Mifflin.

Weiser, N. (1974). The effects of prophetic disconfirmation of the committed. *Review of Religious Research, 16,* 19–30.

Welch, M. R. (1977). Empirical examination of Wilson's sect typology. *Journal for the Scientific Study of Religion, 16,* 125–139.

Wells, M. G. (1999). Religion. In W. K. Silverman & T. H. Ollendick (Eds.), *Developmental issues in the clinical treatment of children* (pp. 199–212). Boston, MA: Allyn & Bacon.

Wells, T., & Triplett, W. (1992). *Drug wars: An oral history from the trenches.* New York, NY: Morrow.

Welton, G. L., Adkins, A. G., Ingle, S. L., & Dixon, W. A. (1996). God control: The fourth dimension. *Journal of Psychology and Theology, 24,* 13–25.

Wenger, J. L. (2004). The automatic activation of religious concepts: Implications for religious orientations. *International Journal for the Psychology of Religion, 14,* 109–123.

Wernik, U. (1975). Frustrated beliefs and early Christianity: A psychological enquiry into the gospels of the New Testament. *Numen, 22,* 96–130.

Westermeyer, J., & Walzer, V. (1975). Drug usage: An alternative to religion? *Diseases of the Nervous System, 36,* 492–495.

Whalen, J., & Flacks, R. (1989). *Beyond the barricades: The sixties generation grows up.* Philadelphia, PA: Temple University Press.

Whitcomb, D., Battaly, H., Baehr, J., & Howard-Snyder, D. (2017). Intellectual humility: Owning our limitations. *Philosophy and Phenomenological Research, 94*(3), 509–539.

White, C. (1991). *Clergy attitudes about death and response to those who are dying or bereaved.* Unpublished doctoral dissertation, University of Cincinnati, Cincinnati, OH.

Whitehead, A. N. (1926). *Religion in the making.* New York, NY: Macmillan.

Whiteley, J., & Loxley, J. (1980). A curriculum for the development of character and community in college students. In L. Erickson & J. Whiteley (Eds.), *Developmental counseling and teaching* (pp. 262–297). Monterey, CA: Brooks/Cole.

Whitley, B. E., Jr. (2009). Religiosity and attitudes toward lesbians and gay men: A meta-analysis. *International Journal for the Psychology of Religion, 19,* 21–38.

Whitman, W. (1942). Starting from Paumanok. In *Leaves of grass.* Garden City, NY: Doubleday, Doran. (Original work published 1855)

Whitney, G. (1976). Genetic substrates for the initial evolution of human sociality: I. Sex chromosome mechanisms. *American Naturalist, 110,* 867–875.

Whooley, M. A., Boyd, A. L., Gardin, J. M., & Williams, D. R. (2002). Religious involvement and cigarette smoking in young adults: The CARDIA study. *Archives of Internal Medicine, 162,* 1604–1610.

Wicks, R. J., Parsons, R. D., & Capps, D. (Eds.). (1985). *Clinical handbook of pastoral counseling.* New York, NY: Paulist Press.

Wiebe, P. H. (1997). *Visions of Jesus: Direct encounters from the New Testament to today.* New York, NY: Oxford University Press.

Wiebe, P. H. (2000). Critical reflections on Christic visions. In J. Andresen & R. K. Forman (Eds.), *Cognitive models and spiritual maps: Interdisciplinary explorations of religious experience* (pp. 119–141). Bowling Green, OH: Imprint Academic.

Wiebe, P. H. (2015). *Intuitive knowing as spiritual experience.* New York, NY: Palgrave Macmillan.

Wiehe, V. R. (1990). Religious influence on parental attitudes toward the use of corporal punishment. *Journal of Family Violence, 5,* 173–186.

Wikstrom, O. (1987). Attribution, roles and religion: A theoretical analysis of Sunden's role theory of religion and the attributional approach to religious experience. *Journal for the Scientific Study of Religion, 26,* 390–400.

Wilcox, C., Ferrara, J., O'Donnell, J., Bendyna, M., Gehan, S., & Taylor, R. (1992). Public attitudes toward church–state issues: Elite–masses differences. *Journal of Church and State, 34,* 259–277.

Wilcox, C., & Jelen, T. G. (1991). The effects of employment and religion on women's feminist attitudes. *International Journal for the Psychology of Religion, 1,* 161–171.

Wilcox, W. B. (1998). Conservative Protestant childrearing: Authoritarian or authoritative? *American Sociological Review, 63,* 796–809.

Wildman, W. J. (2011). *Religious and spiritual experiences.* New York, NY: Cambridge University Press.

Wildman, W. J., & McNamara, P. (2010). Evaluating reliance on narratives in the psychological study of religious experiences. *International Journal for the Psychology of Religion, 20,* 223–254.

Wilkinson, W. W. (2004). Religiosity, authoritarianism, and homophobia: A multidimensional approach. *International Journal for the Psychology of Religion, 14,* 55–67.

Williams, G. C. (1966). *Adaptation and natural selection.* Princeton, NJ: Princeton University Press.

Williams, R. (1971). A theory of God-concept readiness: From the Piagetian theories of child artificialism and the origin of religious feeling in children. *Religious Education, 66,* 62–66.

Williams, R. N., & Faulconer, J. E. (1994). Religion and mental health: A hermeneutic reconsideration. *Review of Religious Research, 35,* 335–349.

Williamson, W. P. (1995). *An attributional basis of the Church of God's rejection of serpent handling.* Paper presented at the annual convention of the Southeastern Psychological Association, Savannah, GA.

Williamson, W. P. (2000). The experience of religious serpent handling: A phenomenological study. *Dissertation Abstracts International, 62,* 1136B.

Williamson, W. P., & Assadi, A. (2005). Religious orientation, incentive, self-esteem, and gender as predictors of academic dishonesty: An experimental approach. *Archive for the Psychology of Religion, 28,* 137–159.

Williamson, W. P., & Hood, R. W., Jr. (2004). Differential maintenance and growth of religious organizations based on high cost behaviors. *Review of Religious Research, 45,* 50–168.

Williamson, W. P., Hood, R. W., Jr., Ahmad, A., Sadiq, M., & Hill, P. C. (2010). The Intratextual Fundamentalism Scale: Cross-cultural application, validity evidence, and relationship with religious orientation and the Big Five Factor markers. *Mental Health, Religion and Culture, 13,* 721–747.

Williamson, W. P., & Pollio, H. R. (1999). The phenomenology of religious serpent handling: A rationale and thematic study of extemporaneous sermons. *Journal for the Scientific Study of Religion, 38,* 203–218.

Williamson, W. P., Pollio, H. R., & Hood, R. W., Jr. (2000). A phenomenological analysis of anointing among serpent handlers. *Journal for the Scientific Study of Religion, 10,* 221–240.

Wilson, B. R. (1970). *Religious sects.* New York, NY: McGraw-Hill.

Wilson, B. R. (1983). Sympathetic detachment and disinterested involvement: A note on academic integrity. *Sociological Analysis, 44,* 183–188.

Wilson, E. O. (1978). *On human nature.* Cambridge, MA: Harvard University Press.

Wilson, J., & Sherkat, D. E. (1994). Returning to the fold. *Journal for the Scientific Study of Religion, 33,* 148–161.

Wilson, S. R. (1982). In pursuit of spiritual energy: Spiritual growth in a yoga ashram. *Journal of Humanistic Psychology, 22,* 43–55.

Wimberley, R. C., & Christenson, J. A. (1981). Civil religion and other religious identities. *Sociological Analysis, 42,* 91–100.

Winfield, L. (2002, January 23). Reparative therapy doesn't work. *The Denver Post,* p. 11B.

Wink, P., Ciciolla, L., Dillon, M., & Tracy, A. (2007). Religiousness, spiritual seeking, and personality: Findings from a longitudinal study. *Journal of Personality, 75,* 1051–1070.

Wink, P., Dillon, M., & Fay, K. (2005). Spiritual seeking, narcissism, and psychotherapy: How are they related? *Journal for the Scientific Study of Religion, 44,* 143–158.

Wink, P., Dillon, M., & Prettyman, A. (2007). Religiousness, spiritual seeking, and authoritarianism: Findings from a longitudinal study. *Journal for the Scientific Study of Religion, 46,* 321–335.

Wink, P., & Helson, R. (1997). Practical and transcendent wisdom: Their nature and some longitudinal findings. *Journal of Adult Development, 4,* 1–15.

Wink, P., & Scott, J. (2005). Does religiousness buffer against the fear of death and dying in late adulthood?: Findings from a longitudinal study. *Journal of Gerontology, 60B,* 207–214.

Winokuer, H. R. (2000). The impact of expected versus unexpected death on the surviving spouse. *Dissertation Abstracts International, 61,* 553B.

Winseman, A. L. (2005, December 6). *Religion in America: Who has none?* Washington, DC: Gallup Poll News Service.

Winter, T., Karvonen, S., & Rose, R. J. (2002). Does religiousness explain regional differences in alcohol use in Finland? *Alcohol and Alcoholism, 37,* 330–339.

Wirth, L. (1928). *The ghetto.* Chicago, IL: University of Chicago Press.

Wittberg, P. (1996). *Pathways to re-creating religious communities.* Mahwah, NJ: Paulist Press.

Witter, R. A., Stock, W. A., Okun, M. A., & Haring, M. J. (1985). Religion and subjective well-being in adulthood: A quantitative analysis. *Review of Religious Research, 26*, 332–342.

Wittgenstein, L. (1953). *Philosophical investigations* (G. E. M. Anscombe, Trans.). New York, NY: Routledge & Kegan Paul. (Original work published 1945–1949)

Witzig, T. F., Jr., & Pollard, C. A. (2013). Obsessional beliefs, religious beliefs, and scrupulosity among fundamentalist Protestant Christians. *Journal of Obsessive–Compulsive and Related Disorders, 2*, 331–337.

Wolcott, H. F. (1994). *Transforming qualitative data: Description, analysis, and interpretation.* Thousand Oaks, CA: SAGE.

Wolpert, L. (2006). *Six impossible things before breakfast: The evolutionary origins of belief.* New York, NY: Norton.

Wong, L. P., Fung, H. H., & Jiang, D. (2013). Associations between religiosity and death attitudes: Different between Christians and Buddhists? *Psychology of Religion and Spirituality, 7*, 70–79.

Wong, P. T. P. (1979). Frustration, exploration, and learning. *Canadian Psychological Review, 20*, 133–144.

Wong, P. T. P. (1998). Spirituality, meaning, and successful aging. In P. T. P. Wong & P. S. Fry (Eds.), *The human quest for meaning: A handbook of psychological research and clinical applications* (pp. 359–394). Mahwah, NJ: Erlbaum.

Wong, P. T. P., & Weiner, B. (1981). When people ask 'why' questions, and the heuristics of attributional search. *Journal of Personality and Social Psychology, 40*, 650–663.

Wong-McDonald, A., & Gorsuch, R. (1997). *Surrender to God: An additional coping style?* Paper presented at the annual convention of the Society for the Scientific Study of Religion, San Diego, CA.

Wong-McDonald, A., & Gorsuch, R. L. (2000). Surrender to God: An additional coping style? *Journal of Psychology and Theology, 28*, 149–161.

Wong-McDonald, A., & Gorsuch, R. L. (2004). A multivariate theory of God concept, religious motivation, locus of control, coping, and spiritual well-being. *Journal of Psychology and Theology, 32*, 318–334.

Wood, A. M., Froh, J., & Geraghty, A. W. (2010). Gratitude and well-being: A review and theoretical integration. *Clinical Psychology Review, 30*, 890–905.

Wood, W. W. (1965). *Culture and personality aspects of the pentecostal holiness religion.* The Hague, The Netherlands: Mouton.

Woodberry, J. D. (1992). Conversion in Islam. In H. N. Malony & S. Southard (Eds.), *Handbook of religious conversion* (pp. 22–40). Birmingham, AL: Religious Education Press.

Woodroof, J. T. (1985). Premarital sexual behavior and religious adolescents. *Journal for the Scientific Study of Religion, 24*, 343–366.

Woodruff, M. L. (1993). Report: Electroencephalograph taken from Pastor Liston Pack, 4:00 p.m., 7 Nov. 1985. In T. Burton, *Serpent-handling believers* (pp. 142–144). Knoxville, TN: University of Tennessee Press.

Woodward, K. L. (1970, April 6). How America lives with death. *Time*, pp. 81–88.

Woody, W. D. (2009). Use of cult in the teaching of psychology of religion and spirituality. *Psychology of Religion and Spirituality, 1*, 218–232.

Woolley, J. D. (2000). The development of beliefs about direct mental–physical causality in imagination, magic, and religion. In K. S. Rosengren, C. N. Johnson, & P. L. Harris (Eds.), *Imagining the impossible: Magical, scientific, and religious thinking in children* (pp. 99–129). Cambridge, UK: Cambridge University Press.

Woolley, J. D., & Phelps, K. E. (2001). The development of children's beliefs about prayer. *Journal of Cognition and Culture, 1*, 139–167.

Worten, S. A., & Dollinger, S. J. (1986). Mothers' intrinsic religious motivation, disciplinary preferences, and children's conceptions of prayer. *Psychological Reports, 58*, 218.

Worthington, B. (2018). Elder suicide: A needless tragedy. *Today's Geriatric Medicine.*

Worthington, E. L., Jr. (Ed.). (2005). *Handbook of forgiveness.* New York, NY: Routledge.

Worthington, E. L., Jr. (2006). *Forgiveness and reconciliation: Theory and application.* New York, NY: Routledge.

Worthington, E. L., Jr., Wade, N. G., Hight, T. L., Ripley, J. S., McCullough, M. E., Berry, J. W., et al. (2003). The Religious Commitment Inventory–10: Development, refinement, and validation of a brief scale for research and counseling. *Journal of Counseling Psychology, 50*, 84–96.

Wortman, C. B. (1976). Causal attributions and personal control. In J. H. Harvey, W. J. Ickes, & R. F. Kidd (Eds.), *New directions in attribution research* (Vol. 1, pp. 23–52). Hillsdale, NJ: Erlbaum.

Wotherspoon, C. M. (2000). The relationship between spiritual well-being and health in later life. In J. A. Thorson (Ed.), *Perspectives on spiritual well-being and aging* (pp. 69–83). Springfield, IL: Charles C Thomas.

Wright, L. S., Frost, C. J., & Wisecarver, S. J. (1993). Church attendance, meaningfulness of religion, and depressive symptomatology among adolescents. *Journal of Youth and Adolescence, 22*, 559–568.

Wright, S. A. (1986). Dyadic intimacy and social control in three cult movements. *Sociological Analysis, 47*, 137–150.

Wright, S. A. (1987). *Leaving cults: The dynamics of defection* (Monograph No. 7). Washington, DC: Society for the Scientific Study of Religion.

Wu, Z., Detels, R., Zhang, J., & Duan, S. (1996). Risk factors for intravenous drug use and sharing equipment among young male drug users in Lonchuan County, southwest China. *AIDS, 10,* 1017–1024.

Wu, A., Wang, J. Y., & Jia, C. X. (2015). Religion and completed suicide: A meta-analysis. *PLOS One, 10*(6).

Wulf, J., Prentice, D., Hansum, D., Ferrar, A., & Spilka, B. (1984). Religiosity, and sexual attitudes and behavior among evangelical Christian singles. *Review of Religious Research, 26,* 119–131.

Wulff, D. M. (1993). On the origins and goals of religious development. *International Journal for the Psychology of Religion, 3,* 181–186.

Wulff, D. M. (1995). Phenomenological psychology. In R. W. Hood, Jr. (Ed.), *Handbook of religious experience* (pp. 183–199). Birmingham, AL: Religious Education Press.

Wulff, D. M. (1997). *Psychology of religion: Classic and contemporary views* (2nd ed.). New York, NY: Wiley.

Wulff, D. M. (2000). Mystical experience. In E. Cardeña, S. J. Lynn, & S. S. Krippner (Eds.), *Varieties of anomalous experience* (pp. 397–440). Washington, DC: American Psychological Association.

Wulff, D. M. (2003). A field in crisis: Is it time to start over? In H. M. Poelofsma, J. M. Corveleyn, & J. W. van Sane (Eds.), *One hundred years of the psychology of religion* (pp. 11–32). Amsterdam, The Netherlands: VU University Press.

Wulff, D. M. (2006). How attached should we be to attachment theory? *International Journal for the Psychology of Religion, 16,* 29–36.

Wulff, K. (2011). Are pastors the cause of the loss of church membership? *Review of Religious Research, 53,* 1–7.

Wundt, W. (1901). *Lectures on human and animal psychology* (J. E. Creighton & E. B. Titchener, Trans.). New York, NY: Macmillan.

Wundt, W. (1916). *Elements of folk psychology.* London, UK: Allen & Unwin.

Wuthnow, R. (1978). *Experimentation in American religion.* Berkeley, CA: University of California Press.

Wuthnow, R. (1993). *Christianity in the twenty-first century.* New York, NY: Oxford University Press.

Wuthnow, R. (1994). *God and mammon in America.* New York, NY: Free Press.

Wuthnow, R. (1998). *After heaven: Spirituality in America since the 1950s.* Berkeley, CA: University of California Press.

Wuthnow, R., & Glock, C. Y. (1973). Religious loyalty, defection, and experimentation among college youth. *Journal for the Scientific Study of Religion, 12,* 157–180.

Wuthnow, R., & Mellinger, G. (1978). Religious loyalty, defection, and experimentation: A longitudinal analysis of university men. *Review of Religious Research, 19,* 231–245.

Wylie, R. C. (1979). *The self concept* (2 vols., 2nd ed.). Lincoln, NE: University of Nebraska Press.

Xygalatas, D. (2016). Cognitive science of religion. In D. A. Leeming (Ed.), *Encyclopedia of psychology and religion* (pp. 343–347). Boston, MA: Springer.

Yamane, D. (2000). Narrative and religious experience. *Sociology of Religion, 61,* 171–189.

Yamane, D. (2007). Introduction: *Habits of the Heart* at 20. *Sociology of Religion, 69,* 179–187.

Yamane, D., & Polzer, M. (1994). Ways of seeing ecstasy in modern society: Experimental–expressive and cultural–linguistic views. *Sociology of Religion, 55,* 1–25.

Yensen, R. (1990). LSD and psychotherapy. *Journal of Psychoactive Drugs, 17,* 267–277.

Yeung, J. W. K., Chan, Y., & Lee, B. L. (2009). Youth religiosity and substance use: A meta-analysis from 1995–2007. *Psychological Reports, 105,* 255–266.

Yinger, J. M. (1967). Pluralism, religion, and secularism. *Journal for the Scientific Study of Religion, 6,* 17–28.

Young, D. (1991). *Origins of the sacred.* New York, NY: St. Martin's Press.

Youniss, J., McLellan, J. A., Su, Y., & Yates, M. (1999). The role of community service in identity development: Normative, unconventional, and deviant orientations. *Journal of Adolescent Research, 14,* 248–261.

Youniss, J., McLellan, J. A., & Yates, M. (1999). Religion, community service, and identity in American youth. *Journal of Adolescence, 22,* 243–253.

Zablocki, B., & Robbins, T. (2001). *Misunderstanding cults: Searching for objectivity in a controversial field.* Toronto, Ontario, Canada: University of Toronto Press.

Zachry, W. H. (1990). Correlation of abstract religious thought and formal operations in high school and college students. *Review of Religious Research, 31,* 405–412.

Zaehner, R. C. (1957). *Mysticism, sacred and profane: An inquiry into some varieties of praeternatural experience.* London, UK: Oxford University Press.

Zaehner, R. C. (1972). *Zen, drugs and mysticism.* New York, NY: Pantheon.

Zaehner, R. C. (1974). *Our savage God.* New York, NY: Sheed & Ward.

Zaleski, C. (1987). *Otherworld journeys: Accounts*

of near-death experience in medieval and modern times. New York, NY: Oxford University Press.

Zaleski, E. H., & Schiaffino, K. M. (2000). Religiosity and sexual risk-taking behavior during the transition to college. *Journal of Adolescence, 23,* 223–227.

Zarrelli, N. (2016, October 18). Dial-a-Ghost on Thomas Edison's least successful inventions: The Spirit Phone. Available at *www.atlasobscura.com/ articles/dial-a-ghost-on-thomas-edisons-least-successful-invention-the-spirit-phone.*

Zemore, S. E., & Kaskutas, L. A. (2004). Helping, spirituality and Alcoholics Anonymous in recovery. *Journal of Studies on Alcohol, 65,* 383–391.

Zenk, T. (2013). New atheism. In S. Bullivant & M. Ruse (Eds.), *The Oxford handbook of atheism* (pp. 243–260). Oxford, UK: Oxford University Press.

Zern, D. S. (1984). Religiousness related to cultural complexity and pressures to obey cultural norms. *Genetic Psychology Monographs, 110,* 207–227.

Zern, D. S. (1987). Positive links among obedience pressure, religiosity, and measures of cognitive accomplishment: Evidence for the secular value of being religious. *Journal of Psychology and Theology, 15,* 31–39.

Zhai, J. E., Ellison, C. G., Stokes, C. E., & Glenn, N. D. (2008). "Spiritual, but not religious": The impact of parental divorce on the religious and spiritual identities of young adults in the United States. *Review of Religious Research, 49,* 379–394.

Zilboorg, G., & Henry, G. W. (1941). *A history of medical psychology.* New York, NY: Norton.

Zimbardo, P. G., & Hartley, C. F. (1985). Cults go to high school: A theoretical and empirical analysis of the initial stage in the recruitment process. *Cultic Studies Journal, 2,* 91–147.

Zimmer, C. (2004). A search for the genetic basis of spirituality. *Scientific American, 291*(4), 110–111.

Zinberg, N. (Ed.). (1977). *Alternate states of consciousness.* New York, NY: Free Press.

Zinnbauer, B. J., & Pargament, K. I. (1998). Spiritual conversion: A study of religious change among college students. *Journal for the Scientific Study of Religion, 37,* 161–180.

Zinnbauer, B. J., & Pargament, K. I. (2005). Religiousness and spirituality. In R. F. Paloutzian & C. L. Park (Eds.), *Handbook of the psychology of religion*

and spirituality (pp. 21–42). New York, NY: Guilford Press.

Zinnbauer, B. J., Pargament, K. I., Cole, B., Rye, M. S., Butter, E. M., Belavich, T. G., et al. (1997). Religion and spirituality: Unfuzzying the fuzzy. *Journal for the Scientific Study of Religion, 36,* 549–564.

Zinnbauer, B. J., Pargament, K. I., & Scott, A. B. (1999). The emerging meanings of religiousness and spirituality: Problems and prospects. *Journal of Personality, 67,* 889–919.

Zollschan, G. K., Schumaker, J. F., & Walsh, G. F. (Eds.). (1995). *Exploring the paranormal.* Bridport, UK: Prism Press.

Zondag, H. J., & Belzen, J. A. (1999). Between reduction of uncertainty and reflection: The range and dynamics of religious judgment. *International Journal for the Psychology of Religion, 9,* 63–81.

Zubeck, J. P. (Ed.). (1969). *Sensory deprivation: Fifty years of research.* New York, NY: Appleton-Century-Crofts.

Zuckerman, D. M., Kasl, S. V., & Ostfeld, A. M. (1984). Psychosocial predictors of mortality among the elderly poor. *American Journal of Epidemiology, 119,* 410–423.

Zuckerman, P. (2007). Atheism: Contemporary numbers and patterns. In M. Martin (Ed.), *The Cambridge companion to atheism* (pp. 47–65). Cambridge, UK: Cambridge University Press.

Zuckerman, P. (2014). *Living the secular life:* New York, NY: Penguin Press.

Zugger, C. L. (2001). *The forgotten: Catholics of the Soviet empire from Lenin through Stalin.* Syracuse, NY: Syracuse University Press.

Zukerman, M., Silberman, J., & Hall, J. A. (2013). The relationship between intelligence and religiosity: A meta-analysis and some proposed explanations. *Personality and Social Psychology Review, 17,* 325–354.

Zusne, L., & Jones, W. H. (1989). *Anomalistic thinking: A study of magical thinking* (2nd ed.). Hillsdale, NJ: Erlbaum.

Zwartjes, W. J., Spilka, B., Zwartjes, G. M., Heideman, D. R., & Cilli, K. A. (1979). *School problems of children with malignant neoplasms* (Final Report, Project No. 212-46-1061). Washington, DC: National Cancer Institute.

Zygmunt, J. F. (1972). When prophecy fails: A theoretical perspective on the comparative evidence. *American Behavioral Scientist, 16,* 245–268.

Author Index

Author Index

Subject Index

Note. *f* or *t* following a page number indicates a figure or a table.